STRESS, HEALTH & WELL-BEING

THRIVING IN THE 21ST CENTURY

RICK HARRINGTON

University of Houston, Victoria

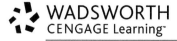

WADSWORTH
CENGAGE Learning™

Australia • Brazil • Japan • Korea • Mexico • Singapore • Spain • United Kingdom • United States

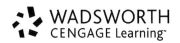

Stress, Health & Well-Being: Thriving in the 21st Century
Rick Harrington

Publisher: Jon-David Hague

Developmental Editor: Ken King

Assistant Editor: Kelly Miller

Editorial Assistant: Sheli DeNola

Media Editor: Lauren Keyes

Marketing Manager: Sean Foy

Marketing Coordinator: Janay Pryor

Marketing Communications Manager:
   Laura Localio

Content Project Manager:
   Charlene M. Carpentier

Design Director: Rob Hugel

Art Director: Vernon Boes

Manufacturing Planner: Karen Hunt

Rights Acquisitions Specialist:
   Thomas McDonough

Production Service: MPS Limited,
   a Macmillan Company

Text Designer: Lisa Henry

Photo Researcher: Bill Smith Group

Text Researcher: Sue C. Howard

Copy Editor: Araceli S. Popen

Illustrator: MPS Limited,
   a Macmillan Company

Cover Designer: Lisa Henry

Cover Image: Daryl Benson/Masterfile

Compositor: MPS Limited,
   a Macmillan Company

For product information and technology assistance, contact us at
Cengage Learning Customer & Sales Support, 1-800-354-9706.

For permission to use material from this text or product, submit all requests online at **www.cengage.com/permissions.**
Further permissions questions can be e-mailed to
permissionrequest@cengage.com.

Library of Congress Control Number: 2011928038
Student Edition:
ISBN-13: 978-1-111-83161-5
ISBN-10: 1-111-83161-0

Wadsworth
20 Davis Drive
Belmont, CA 94002-3098
USA

Cengage Learning is a leading provider of customized learning solutions with office locations around the globe, including Singapore, the United Kingdom, Australia, Mexico, Brazil, and Japan. Locate your local office at **www.cengage.com/global.**

Cengage Learning products are represented in Canada by Nelson Education, Ltd.

To learn more about Wadsworth, visit **www.cengage.com/ Wadsworth.**

Purchase any of our products at your local college store or at our preferred online store **www.CengageBrain.com.**

Printed in the United States of America
5 6 7 8 9 10 11 21 20 19 18 17

To Cindy,

Thank you for all of your love and support. You are the best!

—RICK

BRIEF CONTENTS

CONTENTS

Part 2   The Biology of Stress and Illness   67

Part 7 Guidelines for Stress Management and Well-Being Enhancement 453

Welcome to *Stress, Health & Well-Being: Thriving in the 21st Century*. It is my hope that this book will provide readers an understanding of and appreciation for the interconnection of stress, health, and well-being and how the strategies employed regarding stress can optimize health and well-being.

Since my graduate student days conducting a dissertation on the effects of heart rate biofeedback on the experience of anxiety, I have been fascinated by the mind-body connection, especially as it relates to managing stress. Upon receiving my doctorate, as part of my licensure in psychology training and beyond, I was able to help others apply this information through their participation in the numerous stress management groups I conducted. Later, as a psychology professor, it has been my good fortune to teach an exciting course called Stress and Health where I can share my knowledge, experience, and enthusiasm for this subject with students.

Another exciting course I teach, called the Psychology of Happiness, is a class that inspires intense interest in the "good life." The more general related field of study, a burgeoning new area called positive psychology, has a lot to say about how to enhance well-being. I have discovered, as have others, that positive psychology is a natural partner to the stress and health field. It begins to fill the gaps, to provide understanding for how a person can move beyond managing distress toward a greater sense of well-being, and ultimately toward the goal of flourishing and thriving, a goal we can all relate to.

This text is designed with that integrative perspective in mind. It surveys the topics of stress and health while adding positive psychology theory and research to fill the gaps and enrich our understanding. It is tailor-made for an upper-level undergraduate class in stress and health or stress management, and it also is suitable for a course in health psychology that has a particular emphasis on stress in all its dimensions.

While giving full coverage to the negative side of stress, this book also adds balance by introducing more information on the positive side of issues related to stress and health. It addresses questions like "What is the adaptive value of stress?" "What kind of benefits, if any, can come from a traumatic encounter?" "How can stress and challenge lead to greater well-being?" "How can a person go beyond managing stress toward the goal of thriving?"

Further, the book focuses not only on health risk and vulnerability factors, but also on health-protective factors within the context of stress and lifestyle. Living a healthy lifestyle is a fundamental foundation for all the factors discussed, and this book lays out many of the strategies for accomplishing this goal, including how to stack the deck in favor of living a long, quality life.

This text has many applied features and therefore provides information on how to enhance well-being along with providing a comprehensive coverage of stress management. However, it also includes more in-depth discussion of areas like stress and the nervous system, the biology of the immune system, psychoneuroimmunology, the impact of stress on health conditions, job stress, and personality and stress that expand its depth and scope beyond that found in typical stress management books.

Other areas covered in this book that expand the scope or fill gaps include the following topics and themes: anxiety, anger, and depression reactions to stress and how these are similar or different to related symptoms of particular clinical disorders; gender, cultural, racial, or ethnic differences in the experience of stress along with any related health issues; preventive and coping strategies for dealing with stress-related health conditions; functional foods, antioxidants, and healthy eating plans; and the role of meaning and purpose in coping with stress and positive growth to name a few. In keeping with its emphasis on the importance of living a healthy lifestyle as a foundation for good stress management, this book devotes a full chapter to exercise and another to nutrition.

In addition, this text is empirically grounded. The book presents consolidated quantitative information from meta-analytic reviews of multiple studies when feasible. Although the text gives due consideration to seminal studies, it also strives to stay on top of the most current findings in each area. When appropriate, methodological considerations are discussed and students are encouraged to use their critical thinking skills when examining these and other issues.

The book is organized into seven parts including the topic areas of (1) Stress, Health, and Positive Psychology, (2) The Biology of Stress and Illness, (3) Stress, Personality, and Emotions, (4) Interpersonal and Job Stress, (5) Emotional and Behavioral Self-Regulation, (6) Mind-Body Strategies, and (7) Guidelines for Stress Management and Well-Being Enhancement. The organization of each chapter is designed to maximize learning by including the following features:

- **Vignettes**—Each chapter starts with a vignette to involve the reader in a relevant scenario before discussing the theory and research in that area.
- **Highlighted key terms and concepts**—Key terms and concepts are set in bold type so that the reader can immediately recognize their importance. They also are listed at the end of the chapter.
- **A running glossary**—Many key terms and concepts are placed in the margins along with their definitions to serve as a running glossary.
- **A full glossary**—A full glossary of key terms is included in the back of the book.

- **Insight exercises**—Many chapters have insight exercises that are designed to raise the reader's awareness at the personal level of the concepts discussed.

- **Stress management exercises**—A number of chapters include stress management exercises that engage the reader and facilitate experiential learning and application of the concepts discussed.

- **A chapter summary and concept review**—Concluding each chapter is a chapter summary and concept review that includes bullet points of important information.

- **Critical thinking questions**—A series of critical thinking questions is included at the end of each chapter to facilitate deeper understanding of the concepts and stimulate thinking about how to implement useful lifestyle and stress management ideas.

In addition to the in-book features, the text is supported by a suite of digital resources. PowerPoint Presentations and a Test Bank accompany the text for professors. Students have the option to purchase an additional online resource: Psychology CourseMate.

Psychology CourseMate with Engagement Tracker, a first-of-its-kind tool that monitors student engagement in the course, includes:

- an interactive eBook
- interactive teaching and learning tools including:
  - Quizzes
  - Flashcards
  - Videos
  - and more

POWERPOINT PRESENTATIONS

Ready-to-use Microsoft® PowerPoint® slides allow instructors to assemble, edit, publish, and present custom lectures for this course. They may be used as a teaching aid for classroom presentation, a chapter review for students, or a reference to be printed for classroom distribution. The slides include lecture outlines covering material from major sections of the text as well as selected figures. Instructors should feel free to add their own slides for additional topics that they would like to introduce to the class.

TEST BANKS

The Test Banks contain 50 questions per chapter, including 20 multiple choice questions, 20 short answer questions, and 10 essay questions. An additional set of Test Banks with 20 multiple choice questions per chapter is provided for web quizzing. Both sets are available in Microsoft Word®. The questions cover the learning objectives in each chapter, address various levels of thinking, and contain references to the primary level headings in the chapter from which the question material is taken.

ACKNOWLEDGMENTS

Any book author needs supportive individuals who believe in the author's vision for the author's imagined book to come to realization. I have been fortunate to have benefitted from such supportive people. To each person who made this book possible, I want to express my sincere gratitude.

My heartfelt thanks go to my editor, Jon-David Hague, who from the beginning understood and appreciated the tone, feel, and vision of the book and whose generous spirit and guiding hand brought it to life beyond my expectations. I also cannot say enough about Ken King, my development editor and mentor through this process, who offered me frank, insightful suggestions for each chapter that were immeasurably helpful. In addition I want to thank Cengage Project Manager Charlene Carpentier and MPS Content Services Project Manager Liah Rose for overseeing the production, Art Director Vernon Boes for the art design, Editorial Assistant Sheli DeNola for her support and guidance, and Assistant Editor Kelly Miller for developing supplemental materials.

I am grateful to the following reviewers for their helpful comments and suggestions: **Amy Bohmann**, Texas A&M San Antonio; **Kurt Organista**, UC Berkeley; **Todd Kashdan**, George Mason University; **Elvrid Lawrence**, DePaul University School for New Learning; **Kenneth Hart**, University of Windsor; **Todd Wilkinson**, University of Wisconsin–River Falls; **James Byron-Daniel**, University of the West of England–Bristol; **Jamie Dusold**, Roosevelt University; **William J. Papin**, Western Carolina University; **Mary Fox**, University of Maryland, Baltimore County; **Micah Sadigh**, Cedar Crest College; **Rachelle Duncan**, Oklahoma State University–Institute of Technology; and **Robin Powers**, Gannon University.

I'd also like to thank the following instructors who agreed to review the manuscript in prepublication: **Karen Cardillo**, Monroe Community College; **Paul Gluch**, California State University, Fullerton; **Gretchen Reevy**, CSU East Bay; **Lisa Cheung**, Open Polytechnic University, New Zealand; **Kathy Pignatelli**, Bergen Community College; **Steve Hoover**, Saint Cloud State University; **Barry Zwibelman**, University of Miami; **Jon Peters**, Indiana University, Bloomington; **Ron Olson**, Kingsborough Community College; **Julie Gast**, Utah State University; **Barbara Konopka**, Oakland Community College Auburn Hills; **Loeen Irons**, Baylor University; **Shirley Wood**, Centennial College, Toronto; **Julie David**, Normandale Community College; **Russell Smiley**, Normandale Community College; **Marvin Schade**, Western Carolina University; **Linda Rankin**, Idaho State University; **Lesley Rennis**, Borough of Manhattan Community College; **Susan Hovey**, College of Southern Nevada–Charleston; **Greg Harris**, Polk College, and **Loren Toussaint**, Luther College.

I also owe a debt of gratitude to the University of Houston-Victoria (UHV) for granting me a sabbatical to conceptualize and develop this project as well as giving me the time and resources I needed for a head start in chapter writing. I want to thank UHV's dean of Arts and Sciences Jeffrey DiLeo for his support and encouragement in pursuing this endeavor, Academic Center Director of Academic and Career Services Sandra Heinhold for the many hours she dedicated reading the chapter drafts and offering her writing expertise suggestions, and Interlibrary Loan Assistants Lou Ellen Callarman and Shirley Parkan for their gracious assistance locating and forwarding to me the innumerable interlibrary loan books and journal articles I requested.

I would like to acknowledge two sterling psychologists whose mentorship and guidance during my early career gave me the experience and training I needed to set me on this pathway, Robert Gatchel, who coauthored the first nonedited book in the field of health psychology in the 1980s, and Edward Charlesworth, who around the same time coauthored a popular press book on stress management that has an amazing timeless quality.

Last, I want to express my deepest appreciation to my wife Cindy for her enduring patience and support as her husband sat transfixed in a state of flow in front of a computer screen for countless hours writing this book. I am grateful to her for the sacrifices she made in the interest of carving out a space for the development of this book.

As you now turn the pages of this book I hope you find its reading informative and enjoyable! Upon concluding the book I welcome any comments and suggestions you may have. Your feedback is valuable to me and will guide me when I update the next edition. You can best contact me at my e-mail address of harringtonr@uhv.edu.

—Rick Harrington

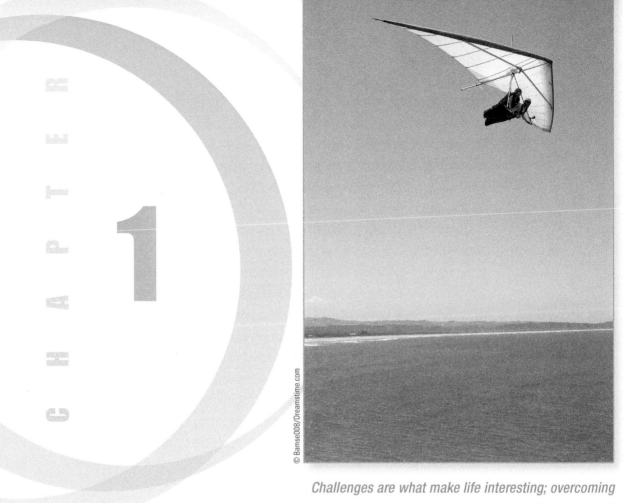

Challenges are what make life interesting; overcoming them is what makes life meaningful.

~Joshua J. Marine

CHAPTER 1

STRESS AND HEALTH

"John, it's your turn to give your presentation to the class," the instructor announced. At that moment, John felt the frenzied flight of butterflies in his stomach. As he rose from his seat to approach the lecture stand positioned at the front of the classroom, he was alarmed to feel his legs go slightly wobbly before they regained their strength. He moved haltingly to the stand where his shaky hands placed his notes into position. Looking up he surveyed the faces of his classmates, wondering if they would mentally render him a harsh verdict if his speech was not up to their standards. Worse, what if he inadvertently said something foolish or embarrassing during his talk? How would he recover such a loss of face with his peers and the instructor? On top of that, the final grade of "A" he hoped for was dependent on giving a good presentation. What grade would he receive if he didn't deliver a sterling performance? Spying the first word of his notes through his now tunneled vision, he took a deep breath and felt an unexpected dryness of throat and tightness in his lungs. As he exhaled and croaked out his first words in an unfamiliar crackling voice, he felt an alarming frustration that a frog now seemed to reside in his voice box.

What is wrong with John? Is he about to come down with a cold, the flu, or some other illness? Actually, nothing is wrong with John. Like many people, John has a fear of public speaking and he is experiencing the phenomenon known as stress. In this context, we can see that the word *stress* is a generic term that can be substituted for words like *apprehension, fear,* or *anxiety* though in other contexts stress could refer to any one of a host of different emotions like irritation, embarrassment, or grief. And stress is not just limited to emotional experiences but also encompasses the physiological (e.g., John's butterflies), behavioral (e.g., John's hesitant movement to the lecture stand), and cognitive (e.g., John's worrisome thoughts about how his performance will be perceived). Because *stress* is such a general word, what does it really mean?

Although the word *stress* today is intuitively understood by most people, its precise definition is generally elusive. Nevertheless, it is commonplace to regard stress as undesirable and harmful to one's health and well-being. Some authors (Hinkle, 1973; Newton, 1995) trace the use of the term *stress* back to the 17th century as a concept that denotes hardship. Others (e.g., Lazarus,

1993) allude to Robert Hooke's use of the word in the same century as a possible source of the concept. Hooke proposed a principle known today as Hooke's law to explain mechanical elasticity and noted how a structure like a bridge can be made to endure heavy loads when *stress* places a strain on it. Later, the concept was used as a model for the human body that must also endure wear and tear of everyday life.

Of course we know that, unlike a mechanical structure, the human body is a living dynamic organism that has an amazing capacity to adapt to the demands of its environment. As we observed with John's experience, concepts of stress and adaptation generally have biological underpinnings that include physiological components of stress reactions. For example, Walter Cannon's (1932) term **homeostasis** refers to the biological self-regulation process that enables an organism to adapt to life's demands. A healthy person under normal circumstances who experiences a stressor has a spike in physiological activity followed by a homeostatic return to baseline. Cannon's **fight-or-flight** reaction to a stressor, such as a physical threat, is an example of how one's body responds with physiological activation to protect itself through either fighting the threat or fleeing from it. Once the threat subsides, the body's homeostatic mechanisms work to return its biological systems to their normal prethreat levels.

What if the fight-or-flight reactions are frequent and excessive and the homeostatic mechanisms are overtaxed by exposure to chronic stressors? Can this lead to health problems? The idea that chronic stressors can be detrimental to one's health was formalized by the stress research pioneer Hans Selye (1956a), who proposed a three-stage model of chronic stress called the **general adaptation syndrome (GAS)**.

According to Selye, the first stage is the alarm stage. John was in the alarm stage when he gave his presentation. Let us now fast-forward and look at John over the ensuing decades and assume that he experiences many ongoing and difficult stressors such as job losses, financial problems, and a string of divorces. What could happen to John if he were to go through the three stages of the GAS eventually? Following the alarm stage John would enter the second stage, the resistance stage, in which his body would continue to mobilize its resources to deal with stressors until it begins to experience a depletion of physical reserves. John's ongoing struggle with stress would eventually lead him to experience lowered resistance to the effects of stress and to develop physical symptoms (e.g., heart palpitations or episodes of chest pains). Finally, if there is no relief from stress, John would enter the exhaustion stage where over time his body's systems would break down as they exhaust their biological resources. During this final stage John may ultimately develop an illness from stress that could in some cases lead to an early death (e.g., heart disease leading to a fatal heart attack). The fight-or-flight and GAS models are revisited in more depth later in this chapter. However, let us next think about other ways to conceptualize stress. For example, can you think of a time when stress was a positive experience?

homeostasis: the biological self-regulation process that enables an organism to adapt to life's demands.

fight-or-flight: Cannon's term for the body's physiological activation response when it prepares to fight off or flee from a threat.

general adaptation syndrome (GAS): Selye's three stage model of the effects of chronic stress.

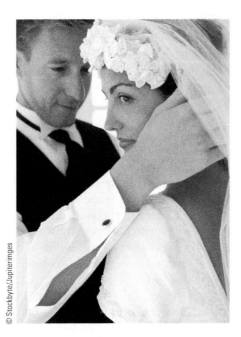

Even some positive events such as marriage are considered stressful according to Holmes and Rahe (1967).

eustress: Selye's term for positive stress.

Contrary to what may be your initial impression of Selye's concept of stress, he did not believe that all stress was negative. In fact, he referred to negative stress as *distress* and coined the term *eustress* to refer to positive stress. Selye included being a bride or groom in a wedding ceremony, singing in a church choir, or participating in an amateur sport competition as examples of eustress. Usually, eustress is a type of stress that is a challenge in a way that is motivating, satisfying, or even enjoyable.

Taking into account both types of stress, Selye defined stress as *nonspecific* responses the body makes to demands (Selye, 1956b). Holmes and Rahe (1967), building upon Selye's view of stress, also allowed for both negative and positive stressors in their model of stress and define stressors as any major life events that require adjustment to one's normal living patterns. These events may be negative, such as in-law problems, or positive, such as marriage.

Holmes and Rahe (1967) created an instrument called the **Social Readjustment Rating Scale (SRRS)** to measure these life change events. On the SRRS, life change events range from a low of 10 points for events like "minor violations of the law" to a high of 100 points for "death of a spouse." In their model of stress, higher life change event scores for the last 6 months to a year indicate that a person has a greater likelihood of developing an illness (see Chapter 4). This idea spurred debate over whether stress is determined by objective life events or subjective appraisals of these events.

hassles: small irritants and pressures experienced in everyday life.

Richard Lazarus, one of the most influential stress theory and research trailblazers of our time came down on the side of subjective appraisals. Lazarus and his associates created scales designed to capture *perceived* everyday life difficulties or *hassles* rather than purely objective life events. **Hassles**

INSIGHT EXERCISE **1.1**

How much stress did you experience last year? Take the College Life Stress Inventory (Renner & Mackin, 1998) that is based on the SRRS but more updated and designed for college students.

The College Life Stress Inventory

Instructions: Copy the "stress rating" number into the last column for any life stress event that has happened to you in the last year and then add these scores.

Event	Stress Rating	Your Event Score
Being raped	100	
Finding out that you are HIV-positive	100	
Being accused of rape	98	
Death of a close friend	97	
Death of a close family member	96	
Contracting a sexually transmitted disease (other than AIDS)	94	
Concerns about being pregnant	91	
Finals week	90	
Concerns about your partner being pregnant	90	
Oversleeping for an exam	89	
Flunking a class	89	
Having a boyfriend or girlfriend cheat on you	85	
Ending a steady dating relationship	85	
Serious illness in a close friend or family member	85	
Financial difficulties	84	
Writing a major term paper	83	
Being caught cheating on a test	83	
Drunk driving	82	
Sense of overload in school or work	82	
Two exams in one day	80	
Cheating on your boyfriend or girlfriend	77	
Getting married	76	
Negative consequences of drinking or drug use	75	
Depression or crisis in your best friend	73	
Difficulties with parents	73	

(continued)

INSIGHT EXERCISE **1.1** (continued)

Event	Stress Rating	Your Event Score
Talking in front of a class	72	
Lack of sleep	69	
Change in housing situation (hassles, moves)	69	
Competing or performing in public	69	
Getting in a physical fight	66	
Difficulties with a roommate	66	
Job changes (applying, new job, work hassles)	65	
Declaring a major or concerns about future plans	65	
A class you hate	62	
Drinking or using drugs	61	
Confrontations with professors	60	
Starting a new semester	58	
Going on a first date	57	
Registration	55	
Maintaining a steady dating relationship	55	
Commuting to campus or work, or both	54	
Peer pressures	53	
Being away from home for the first time	53	
Getting sick	52	
Concerns about your appearance	52	
Getting straight A's	51	
A difficult class that you love	48	
Making new friends; getting along with friends	47	
Fraternity or sorority rush	47	
Falling asleep in class	40	
Attending an athletic event (e.g., football game)	20	
Your Total Score		

NOTE: Adapted from "A Life Stress Instrument for Classroom Use," by M. J. Renner and R. S. Mackin, 1998, Teaching of Psychology, 46–48. Copyright © Taylor & Francis, Inc. Used by permission.

Did you take the test? Note that the developers of the inventory found that in their sample of 247 students with a median age of 19 years, their average total life events stress score was 1,247. Student scores ranged from 182 to 2,571. If you scored high, did you have very many illnesses last year? If you scored low, did you have few illnesses? Based on your results, what do you think of the Holmes and Rahe model of stress and illness?

are the irritants and pressures we experience in everyday life. His group also
wanted a measure of everyday **uplifts,** our positive encounters and experiences—
a counterbalance to hassles.

Lazarus and his colleagues created a scale for hassles and another one for
uplifts (Kanner, Coyne, Schaefer, & Lazarus, 1981). Examples of hassles on
the Hassles Scale include *misplacing things, noise, filling out forms, too many
interruptions,* and *having to wait,* whereas uplifts on the Uplifts Scale include
engaging in a hobby, laughing, having fun, eating out, and *completing a task.*
The Lazarus group gave their scales to a middle-aged adult sample and reported that the sample's top three most frequent hassles in rank order were
concerns about weight, health of a family member, and *rising prices of common goods.* Uplifts were *relating well with your spouse or lover, relating well
with friends,* and *completing a task* (Kanner et al., 1981). Kanner and colleagues (1981, p. 4) cite the poetic writing of Charles Bukowski (1980) in
Shoelace to capture the idea of daily hassles.

> *It's not the large things that send a man to the madhouse . . .*
>
> *No, it's the continuing series of small tragedies that send a man to the
>   madhouse*
>
> *Not the death of his love*
>
> *but the shoelace that snaps*
>
> *with no time left.*

Later Lazarus and Folkman (1984) narrowed the focus from general perception to a process called **appraisal** using the cognitive mediational approach
advocated by Arnold (1960). Appraisal denotes that more than simply perceiving
the situation, we make a judgment about the relative significance of the event.
During the appraisal process, we evaluate the event as a threat or a challenge.
In other words, we evaluate it as either negative (a threat) or positive (a challenge).
This process is an ongoing transaction (a two-way process) between us and the
situation with cognitive appraisals filtering our perceptions.

Self-perceptions and judgments also are involved through our evaluating
our ability to cope or deal effectively with the threat or challenge. Appraisal
patterns are linked to particular emotional responses because each appraisal pattern has its own **core relational meaning** (Lazarus, 2001). That
is, depending on the meaning we give to the appraisal, there will be a different emotional response. For example, the core relational theme of *a demeaning offense against me and mine* underpins the emotion of anger; the
theme of *facing uncertain, existential threat* relates to the emotion of anxiety; and the theme of *making reasonable progress toward realization of a
goal* leads us to experience the emotion of happiness (Lazarus, 1993, 1998,
p. 356). Lazarus identified 15 different core relational themes and their con-
comitant emotions (Table 1.1).

Generally when we use the word *stress,* we are referring to what Selye
called *distress* and not what he called *eustress.* The word *stress* has been
used to refer to both the cause and the effect of upsetting events. For example, a person may say "I have had a lot of stress at my job lately," using the
word *stress* to mean pressure at the job that causes negative physiological

TABLE **1.1**   Lazarus's (1993) description of the core relational themes associated with 15 different emotions

Emotion	Core Relational Theme
Anger	A demeaning offense against me and mine
Anxiety	Facing uncertain, existential threat
Fright	An immediate, concrete, an overwhelming physical danger
Guilt	Having transgressed a moral imperative
Shame	Failing to live up to an ego-ideal
Sadness	Having experienced an irrevocable loss
Envy	Wanting what someone else has
Jealousy	Resenting a third party for the loss of, or a threat to, another's affection or favor
Disgust	Taking in or being too close to an indigestible object or (metaphorically speaking) idea
Happiness	Making reasonable progress toward the realization of a goal
Pride	Enhancement of one's ego-identity by taking credit for a valued object or achievement, either one's own or that of someone or group with whom one identifies
Relief	A distressing goal-incongruent condition that has changed for the better or gone away
Hope	Fearing for the worst but wanting better
Love	Desiring or participating in affection, usually but not necessarily reciprocated
Compassion	Being moved by another's suffering and wanting help

NOTE: Adapted from "Psychological Stress to the Emotions: A History of Changing Outlooks," by R. S. Lazarus, 1993, *Annual Review of Psychology, 44*, 1–21. Copyright © Annual Reviews Inc. Used by permission.

stress: the constellation of cognitive, emotional, physiological, and behavioral reactions the organism experiences as it transacts with perceived threats and challenges.

and psychological reactions. The same person could say "I have been stressing a lot lately," using the word *stress* to mean that person's reaction to pressures or strains. For clarification purposes, it is more precise to use the word **stressor** to refer to the cause and **stress** to refer to the effect of the stressor.

Keeping these various concepts of stress in mind and borrowing heavily from Lazarus, we can define stress in the following manner: *Stress* is the constellation of cognitive, emotional, physiological, and behavioral reactions the organism experiences as it transacts with perceived threats and challenges. These reactions have adaptive significance for the organism.

WHAT IS HEALTH?

biomedical model:
a traditional model of
health that assumes
health is primarily a
product of biological
factors.

**biopsychosocial
model:** a newer model
of health that assumes
health is a product of biological, psychological,
and social influences.

Traditional models of health such as the **biomedical model** focus primarily on biological factors that contribute to health, whereas newer models of health such as the **biopsychosocial model** (Engel, 1977, 1980) view health as a product of biological, *psychological*, and *social* influences. The biomedical model assumes that health and illness are dichotomous states. A person is either healthy or not healthy. This assumption contrasts with the biopsychosocial perspective that regards health states as being on a continuum from the very ill to the super well (Table 1.2). A well-trained marathoner who is healthy in all respects is in a different state of health than the sedentary smoker who is not ill.

The biomedical model also divides the mind and body into separate entities in accordance with Rene Decartes's mind-body dualism philosophy, whereas the biopsychosocial model views the mind and body as an interactive whole. **Psychosomatic medicine,** inspired by Sigmund Freud's idea that repressed memories and intrapsychic conflict can lead to somatic conversions expressed as physical symptoms broke ranks with the conventional medical

TABLE **1.2**   Similarities and differences between the biomedical model and the biopsychosocial model of health

Issue	Biomedical Model	Biopsychosocial Model
Causes of Illness	Physical. A linear model.	Physical, social, and psychological. An interactive model.
Responsibility for Illness	Individuals are passive victims of illness pathogens.	Because behavior and lifestyle can play a role, individuals are not necessarily passive victims.
Treatment of Illness	Physical treatments.	Physical, behavioral, and psychological treatments.
Responsibility for Treatment	Medical profession.	May be an interdisciplinary health care team as well as the patient.
Relationship between Health and Illness	Qualitative model. Either healthy or ill.	Quantitative model. Continuum between health and illness.
Relationship between Mind and Body	Mind and body are separate so treatment of diseases is focused on the body.	Mind and body are integrated and interact with each other in a holistic manner so treatment is focused on both.
Role of Psychology in Health and Illness	Illness has psychological consequences but not causes.	Psychological factors affect illness and are consequences of illness.

thinking of the time and became one of the first medical areas to challenge the mind-body duality aspect of the biomedical model.

As indicated previously, another difference between the two models is that the biomedical model focuses on illness as caused by physical agents (e.g., bacteria, viruses, etc.) often to the exclusion of other factors, whereas the biopsychosocial model sees illness as caused by social and psychological factors as well as the aforementioned physical agents. For example, a clinical depression may lead to a depressed immune system, which may in turn lead to increased vulnerability to illness. In the traditional biomedical model, the sick individual is in many ways seen as a victim of unfortunate circumstances. In the biopsychosocial model the sick person may be seen as a victim but may also be viewed as having contributed to the illness through engaging in unhealthy behaviors.

Out of these new understandings and concepts of health arose several new synergies, including the field of behavioral medicine, the specialization of health psychology, and the concept of wellness. **Behavioral medicine** is the field of study that applies elements of the behavioral sciences to illness prevention and treatment (Schwartz & Weiss, 1977). In practical terms, it uses a multidisciplinary approach including professionals from the medical field (e.g., preventive medicine specialists), registered dieticians, exercise physiologists, psychologists, health educators, or other professionals to assist those who wish to maximize their health goals through behavioral approaches to illness prevention. It also focuses on treatments of existing illnesses or health disorders with behavioral approaches using stand-alone interventions when appropriate or, more commonly, treatments that are designed to assist traditional medical approaches.

health psychology: a specialty area of psychology that uses the scientific and professional knowledge base of the discipline of psychology to promote and maintain health as well as to treat illnesses.

Health psychology is a specialty area of psychology that is focused on using the scientific and professional knowledge base of the discipline of psychology to promote and maintain health as well as to treat illnesses (Matarazzo, 1980). **Wellness** encompasses a global approach to health that not only includes stress management and emotional self-regulation, but also focuses on healthy living, including exercise and proper nutrition as well as activities that promote personal growth (Edlin & Golanty, 1992). These may include promoting physical, mental, emotional, and spiritual well-being. When working together as a harmonic whole, these four elements of wellness are believed to lead to the highest level of life satisfaction.

What then can we say is an appropriate definition of health? The World Health Organization (WHO) employs many of the elements discussed previously in its definition and defines **health** as "a state of complete physical, mental, and social well-being and not merely the absence of disease or infirmity" (WHO, 2011).

health: a positive physical, mental, and social state of well-being.

The goal then according to the more comprehensive approaches to health is to engage in behaviors and practices that achieve optimal levels of health within a continuum of health. In **stress management** terms, the goal is to work toward staying in an optimal zone of functioning and life satisfaction through the use of health-promoting strategies.

ANTONOVSKY'S SALUTOGENIC MODEL

salutogenic model:
Antonovsky's model of
health that proposes that
health resides on a con-
tinuum from an entro-
pic end to a salutary end;
how one manages stress
can move a person to-
ward either end of the
continuum.

Aaron Antonovsky (1979, 1987), a medical sociologist, developed an alternative model to the biomedical pathogenic disease model of health that he coined the **salutogenic model.** His salutogenic model uses the health continuum approach advocated by proponents of the biopsychosocial model rather than the diseased-healthy dichotomous model advocated by proponents of the biomedical model.

The salutogenic model's emphasis is on what people do right to facilitate health rather than on risk and pathogenic factors. It asks the following question: What are the underlying origins of health (i.e., salutogenesis) rather than what are the underlying origins of disease? Further underlying his model is the assumption that we are all subject to the laws of entropy, the second law of thermodynamics—that is, all ordered systems, including life forms, eventually become disordered and chaotic (e.g., an ice cube melting, an organism dying, wood rotting).

The question he asks is how can we maintain our healthy state given the constant pressure of entropic forces? He answers this question by focusing on the factors that move individuals away from entropy and toward the healthy (what he called *health-ease*) end of the continuum rather than on risk factors and pathogens that move them toward the unhealthy end (what he called *dis-ease*). Antonovsky does not reject the pathogenic model but rather sees his salutogenic model as complementary to it.

The salutogenic model does not view stressors as inherently pathogenic, but rather as factors that create tension. Depending on how the tension is managed, the outcome may move the person toward the entropic end of the continuum, have no effect, or move the person toward the salutary (i.e., beneficial to health) direction. Antonovsky considers stressors to be omnipresent. Thus, his model suggests that adaptation to our stress-filled environments involves finding inputs from resources that enable us to resist entropy or make order out of chaos (i.e., negative entropy resources). Such resources can be classified as our personal reserves (e.g., our sense of optimism), our social environment (e.g., our social relationships), and our physical environment (e.g., our physical resources like money and possessions). He called these inputs **generalized resistance resources (GRRs)**, which serve to reduce the pressure on us to move toward the negative end of the pole, the entropic direction, when encountering stressors.

**sense of coherence
(SOC):** one's worldview
according to Antonovsky
that is comprised of the
three integrated fac-
tors of comprehensibil-
ity, manageability, and
meaningfulness.

The GRRs are important in shaping our worldview, or what Antonovsky referred to as our **sense of coherence (SOC)**. Our SOC becomes a relatively stable component of our personality structure by late early adulthood. It is comprised of three integrated factors that are influenced by our life experiences referred to as *comprehensibility, manageability,* and *meaningfulness.*

Comprehensibility indicates the degree to which we can make *cognitive sense* of the stimuli we perceive. The more consistent and predictable our experiences have been, the more we can make sense of them and understand how to adapt to future similar stimuli. We can mentally make order out of chaos. After experiencing a trauma like a devastating hurricane, can we make sense out of our experience? Do we mentally understand what has happened to us and have a sense of what to do, or are we in a state of confusion and paralysis? If we understand and have a sense of what to do, we have comprehensibility.

Manageability refers to our ability to access internal and external coping resources and use them when we need them. The more success we have had in our experiential history of coping with demands, the stronger our sense of manageability. How do we manage and cope with the aftermath of the hurricane (e.g., cleanup, relocation, dealing with grief and loss)? These are questions that concern manageability.

Finally, **meaningfulness** alludes to our ability to *emotionally* make sense of demands and to perceive these demands as worthwhile investments of our energy as challenges rather than burdens. Antonovsky views meaningfulness as the most important component of the three, followed by comprehensibility and then manageability. Without meaningfulness, the other two can lead only to short-term benefits. Meaningfulness provides the fuel and motivation to consistently invest our energy in making sense of chaos and transforming our coping resources, our GRRs, into benefits. Is there a way that we can see a larger meaning and purpose in our losses from the hurricane that motivates us to move forward in spite of the devastation and despair we may feel? Can the meaning give us a sense of uplift in the face of adversity? If so, we are able to apply meaningfulness to our sense of coherence. Antonovsky (1987) then defines SOC as the following: "The sense of coherence is a global orientation that expresses the extent to which one has a pervasive, enduring though dynamic feeling of confidence that (1) the stimuli deriving from one's internal and external environments in the course of living are structured, predictable, and explicable; (2) the resources are available to one to meet the demands posed by these stimuli; and (3) these demands are challenges, worthy of investment and engagement" (p. 19).

In what ways do strong SOCs benefit our health? As discussed by Korotkov (1998), a strong SOC affects our physiological systems, our motivation to engage in health-promoting behaviors, and our appraisal and coping processes. A brain with a strong SOC is more likely to send appropriate signals to the nervous, endocrine, and immune systems to resist entropic forces in the face of demands or to recover more fully when stressed. In addition, persons with strong SOCs are more motivated to engage in health-promoting behaviors like physical exercise and avoid health-destructive behaviors like tobacco smoking.

Health-promoting behaviors make sense, and they are seen as worthwhile investments. Appraisal and coping processes are more effective for a person with a strong SOC than one with a weak SOC. Stimuli that are appraised as stressful can be made sense of and cognitively and emotionally defined by a person with a strong SOC, so that person can then use appropriate coping resources (GRRs) effectively. Thus, persons with strong SOCs are reinforced with tension reduction and salutary benefits that in turn continue to strengthen their SOCs, whereas those with weak SOCs are more like victims at the mercy of continued entropic forces.

Eriksson and Lindstrom (2005) reviewed 458 publications of the salutogenic model and 13 doctoral dissertations from 1992 to 2003 and concluded that SOC promotes resilience and positive health, including mental health. One study (Van der Hal-van Raalte, Van IJzendoorn, & Bakermans-Kranenburg,

INSIGHT EXERCISE 1.2

Take the Short Form of Antonovsky's (1987) Orientation to Life Questionnaire that measures sense of coherence (SOC).

The Short Form of the Orientation to Life Questionnaire (Antonovsky, 1987). The questionnaire measures sense of coherence (SOC).

Here is a series of questions relating to various aspects of our lives. Each question has seven possible answers, with numbers 1 and 7 being extreme answers. If the words under 1 are right for you, circle 1; if the words under 7 are right for you, circle 7. If you feel differently, circle the number which best expresses your feeling. Please give only one answer to each question.

1. Do you have the feeling that you don't really care about what goes on around you?

1	2	3	4	5	6	7

   very seldom   very often
   or never

2. Has it happened in the past that you were surprised by the behavior of people whom you thought you knew well?

1	2	3	4	5	6	7

   never   always
   happened   happened

3. Has it happened that people whom you counted on in the past disappointed you?

1	2	3	4	5	6	7

   never   always
   happened   happened

4. Until now your life has had:

1	2	3	4	5	6	7

   no clear goals or   very clear goals
   purpose at all   and purpose

5. Do you have the feeling that you're being treated unfairly?

1	2	3	4	5	6	7

   very often   very seldom
                    or never

6. Do you have the feeling that you are in an unfamiliar situation and don't know what to do?

1	2	3	4	5	6	7

   very often   very seldom
                    or never

7. Doing the things you do every day is:

1	2	3	4	5	6	7

   a source of deep   a source of pain
   pleasure and   and boredom
   satisfaction

(continued)

8. Do you have very mixed-up feelings and ideas?

     1   2   3   4   5   6   7
  very often   very seldom
                                or never

9. Does it happen that you have feelings inside you would rather not feel?

     1   2   3   4   5   6   7
  very often   very seldom
                                or never

10. Many people—even those with a strong character—sometimes feel like sad sacks (losers) in certain situations. How often have you felt this way in the past?

     1   2   3   4   5   6   7
  never   very often

11. When something happened, have you generally found that:

     1   2   3   4   5   6   7
  you overesti-   you won't
  mated or under-   succeed in over-
  estimated its   coming the
  importance   difficulties

12. How often do you have the feeling that there's little meaning in the things you do in your daily life?

     1   2   3   4   5   6   7
  very often   very seldom
                                or never

13. How often do you have feelings that you're not sure you can keep under control?

     1   2   3   4   5   6   7
  very often   very seldom
                                or never

Key: Comprehensibility: Items 2R, 6, 8, 9, 11
      Manageability: Items 3R, 5, 10R, 13
      Meaning: Items 1R, 4, 7R, 12

Items that have an R behind them need to be reverse scored. In other words a 1 is scored as a 7, a 2 is scored as a 6, a 3 is scored as a 5, a 4 remains a 4, a 5 is scored as a 3, a 6 is scored as a 2, and a 7 is scored as a 1.

Add up the scores for each component of the SOC after reverse scoring the appropriate items to determine your level of Comprehensibility, Manageability, and Meaning. Then sum the total to determine your level of Sense of Coherence (SOC).

NOTE: Adapted from "The Sense of Coherence Questionnaire" from Unraveling the Mystery of Health: How People Manage Stress and Stay Well, *by A. Antonovsky, 1987. San Francisco, CA: Jossey-Bass. Copyright © Jossey-Bass, Inc. Used by permission.*

Did you complete the questionnaire? Which of the three factors of the SOC—comprehensibility, manageability, or meaningfulness—did you score the highest? How do you think each of these factors influence your ability to cope with stress? How do you believe they influence your health?

2008) found that within a group of 203 child Holocaust survivors, having a strong SOC protects and buffers the survivors against posttraumatic stress even in old age compared to survivors with a weak SOC. The authors of the study suggest that "survivors with a strong sense of coherence may be less pre-occupied by the traumatic consequences of their Holocaust experiences. Through their strong sense of coherence, they may have made sense of the Holocaust survival—in retrospection—of their own active role in coping with the Holocaust" (Van der Kal-van Raalte et al., 2008, p. 1363).

THE IMPACT OF STRESS ON HEALTH AND PERFORMANCE

Stressors produce cognitive, emotional, physiological, and behavioral changes that can be detrimental to both our physical and psychological health. Examples of detrimental cognitive changes include worry, loss of concentration, memory loss, and inability to make decisions as well as other mental changes. Emotional changes may include apprehensiveness, anxiety, irritation, anger, sadness, shame, guilt, and depression.

Physiological reactions to stressors typically involve not only the central nervous system, but also the immune system, the autonomic nervous system, and the endocrine system. These reactions may include heart rate increases, blood pressure elevation, muscle tension, dry throat and mouth, trembling, teeth grinding, cold hands and feet, headaches, weakness, fatigue, and frequent illnesses. Changes due to stressors typically have negative effects on our relationships and on our work performance. Behavioral changes such as frequent arguing, poor work performance, overeating or undereating, and others usually set up vicious cycles that amplify stress reactions.

When we think about stressors, we often think of situations involving too much unwanted stimulation that lead to these excessive undesirable physiological and psychological reactions. We may think the answer is to re-duce or eliminate much of the unwanted stimuli. For example, a person living in a noisy big city environment may want to get away permanently to the peace and quiet of an isolated country cabin. This may help in the short run, but what about the long run? Unfortunately, this may not be the answer either because people who experience long periods of understimulation often become bored and unhappy. Most would not consider this to be a desirable state either. So what is the answer? Before we look for the answer let us first look at the workplace. In the workplace, what is the desired level of excitement for best performing our work tasks? According to the **Yerkes-Dodson Curve** (Yerkes & Dodson, 1908), we know that optimal task performance occurs at the midlevel of excitement or what has been referred to as diffuse physiological arousal. At low levels, for example when we are bored, perfor-mance levels are also low. At high levels, for example when we are experi-encing extreme stress, our performance levels suffer. Therefore, we need sufficient diffuse physiological arousal to rise to the challenge, but not so much as to become overwhelmed by it.

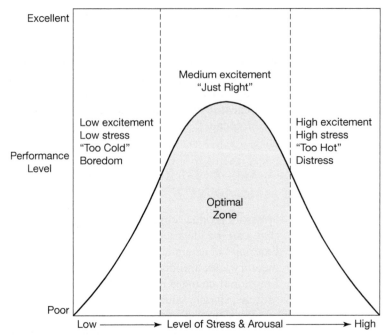

FIGURE **1.1** According to the Yerkes-Dodson curve, optimal performance occurs when we are at the midlevel of diffuse physiological arousal and excitement. It is like the Goldilocks theory of not wanting her bowl of porridge to be "too hot" or "too cold" but "just right."

The goal of stress management then is to maintain stress reactions within this optimal zone rather than adopting unrealistic goals such as totally eliminating stressors or stress reactions. People are most satisfied when they are neither understimulated nor overstimulated for extended periods. It is like the Goldilocks theory of not wanting her bowl of porridge to be "too hot" or "too cold" but "just right." We are most satisfied with the "just right" level of stimulation and diffuse physiological reaction (Figure 1.1).

THE IMPACT OF STRESS AND LIFESTYLE ON LONGEVITY

Eventually negative stressors can have an impact on life expectancy itself. Unhealthy behaviors and lifestyles, many related to stress, are believed to account for many premature deaths. For instance, in the United States smoking tobacco causes approximately 80% of the lung cancer deaths for women and 90% for men (National Cancer Institute, 2011). This is the bad news. The good news, however, at least in many parts of the world, is that people today who live healthy lifestyles can generally expect to live a long life.

For example, Yates, Djousse, Kurth, Buring, and Gaziano (2008, p. 284) conducted a prospective cohort study of 2,357 men participating in the Physician's Health Study with an average age of 72 and, beginning in 1981, tracked the subjects on a host of demographic, health, and lifestyle variables through the year 2006. They found that 41% of the men lived to the age of 90 or older. Lifestyle-related variables were found to have a large impact on longevity: "Smoking, diabetes, obesity and hypertension significantly reduced the likelihood of a 90-year life span, while regular vigorous exercise substantially improved it." Regular exercise alone accounted for a 30% reduction in mortality risk. Yates and her colleagues found that for a 70-year-old man who exercised 2 to 4 times a week, maintained normal blood pressure and weight, and did not have diabetes, there was a 54% likelihood of living to the age of 90. The authors concluded, "Thus, our results suggest that healthy lifestyle and risk management should be continued in elderly years to reduce mortality and disability" (p. 284). Because men have an average shorter lifespan than women, these results are heartening for women as well.

Concerning women and longevity, van Dam, Li, Spiegelman, Franco, and Hu (2008) found in a very large cohort of 77,782 women participating in the prospective Brigham and Women's Hospital-based Nurses Health Study since 1980, that as we know, lifestyle issues play a major role in women's longevity as well. These investigators determined that smoking accounted for 28% of deaths, eating an unhealthy diet 13%, being overweight 14%, and living a sedentary lifestyle 17%. They estimated that the combination of eating a healthy diet, not becoming overweight, never smoking, and maintaining a physically active lifestyle reduced mortality risk in women by 55%, thus promoting increased longevity.

What does living a healthy lifestyle have to do with managing stress? Stress and health is a two-way street. As you will see in subsequent chapters, when under stress, we are more prone to engage in adverse health behaviors such as smoking, drinking, or eating too much and paradoxically may experience disruptions in our ability to initiate or maintain health-protective behaviors such as eating healthy, engaging in regular physical activity, and using relaxation strategies. The result is we experience diminished health and well-being, which can in turn create a new set of stressors. It becomes a vicious cycle with stress contributing to poor health and poor health contributing to stress. The focus of this book is on lifestyle. The most effective way to manage stress is to manage lifestyle and complement it with specific stress-busting strategies. However, many components of a healthy lifestyle also serve a dual purpose of promoting health and longevity while attenuating the effects of stress. For example, regular physical exercise covered in Chapter 11 is an activity that is not only beneficial to our health as a lifestyle practice, but is also a powerful strategy for reducing the effects of stress.

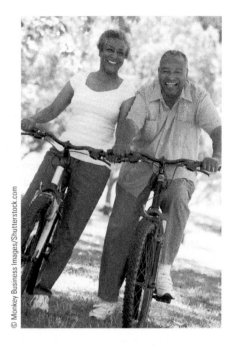

Living a healthy lifestyle including maintaining regular exercise promotes increased longevity in men and women.

THE PHYSIOLOGY OF STRESS

At the beginning of the chapter we looked at John's reaction to giving a presentation in front of his class and we saw that he had a number of prominent physiological reactions to stress. For example, he experienced butterflies in his stomach, his legs were wobbly, his hand trembled, his throat became dry, and his chest tightened. What do these reactions remind you of that we discussed earlier in the chapter? If you answered Cannon's fight-or-flight reaction you are correct. John's body was telling him to prepare for action, to hightail it out of there—the flight side of fight-or-flight. John's dilemma then was that he had a body hardwired for physical threats and activated for physical action in a way that was not appropriate to the psychological threats he currently faced. So he had to make the best of a body that in many ways was working against his best interests. Let us take a close look at Cannon's model and see how it applies to modern life.

Cannon's Fight-or-Flight Model

It is generally believed that Walter Cannon (1932) was the first to use the word *stress* as a psychological term. As we know, Cannon also introduced the concepts of *homeostasis* and the *fight-or-flight reaction*. Recall homeostasis is the tendency to maintain a balanced state. After a person experiences a stress reaction, like a spike in blood pressure, that person's blood pressure will normally return to its baseline due to homeostatic regulators in the body's physiological systems.

Stressors tend to evoke fight-or-flight reactions that affect a number of systems, including the autonomic nervous system. The **autonomic nervous system** is responsible for enervating the organ systems of the body, and with a few important exceptions (e.g., organs of the gastrointestinal system), its sympathetic branch is generally responsible for the arousal response of these organs. This **sympathetic nervous system** activation in concert with adrenal gland **catechol-amine** secretions such as **epinephrine** (known also as adrenaline) and **norepi-nephrine** (known also as noradrenaline) prime the body to physically fight off threats to safety or to flee from these threats through such activities as increasing cardiac output and blood pressure that transit additional blood to the brain and large muscles of the body where the blood is needed most acutely.

Also during the fight-or-flight response the adrenal glands release **gluco-corticoids** such as **cortisol** that help us rapidly facilitate the conversion of food stores such as proteins and fats in the body to glucose for ready energy. In a primitive state of nature, this has adaptive value in that it helps protect us from danger by making energy stores immediately available and ready where and when needed most. We will look at the physiological underpinnings of fight-or-flight in more detail in Chapter 3.

As Charlesworth and Nathan (2004) illustrate, the story of *fight-or-flight* often begins with a primitive human that they characterize as a *cave dweller* and the cave dweller's predator. With slight modifications, let us look at how the story unfolds. In the dawn of history the primitive human steps out of his cave and catches a glimpse of a large animal crouched in the brush. The prehistoric human's eyes grow wide and muscles tense upon realizing that the animal is a saber-toothed tiger. A split second fight-or-flight decision comes down on the fight side as the cave dweller lets loose a blood curdling yell at the tiger while simultaneously hurling a blunt stone. The tiger, startled by this display of aggressiveness, growls menacingly but then turns and disappears into the thicket. The fight-or-flight reaction prevented this cave dweller from becoming the tiger's next meal.

Let us next take a look at the primary physiological systems activated by the fight-or-flight response that saved this prehistoric human and helped modern humans like us live to read about its encounter.

> **Cardiovascular System**   The heart increases its rate of contraction and blood pressure spikes to circulate blood carrying oxygen and energy to the brain and large muscles of the body in preparation for action.
>
> **Muscular System**   The large muscles in the body tense as they also ready for action.
>
> **Gastrointestinal (GI) System**   The digestive process slows so that GI system blood that had been collecting energy can be quickly routed to the brain and muscles. Digesting food is not very adaptive when one is about to be eaten.
>
> **Respiratory System**   Breathing rate increases to oxygenate the large muscles of the body in preparation for action.
>
> **Dermal System**   The skin perspires to cool down the body and prevent overheating during action.
>
> **Hormonal System**   Hormones such as epinephrine, norepinephrine, and cortisol are secreted to stimulate the release of energy for action.
>
> **Sensory Systems**   Eyes dilate as vision and hearing become more acute to perceive the threat more acutely.

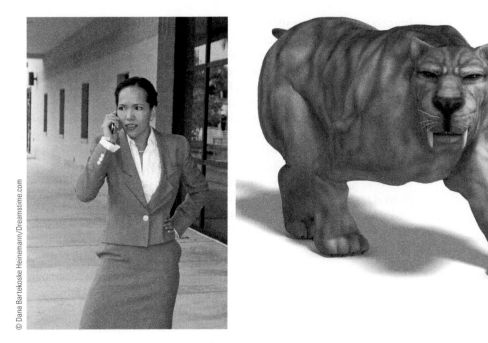

Today's stressors are primarily the saber-toothed tigers of our minds.

Though this pattern of physiological responses worked for our cave-dweller ancestors, we modern humans face a different set of stressors than saber-toothed tigers. These stressors are often intangible and complex though they represent the same threat in our minds as the saber-toothed tiger. They are the saber-toothed tigers of our minds.

Working to meet an important deadline can generate stress reactions as the deadline nears, such as a racing heart, excessive perspiration, or a slight queasiness in the stomach. These symptoms are all related to fight-or-flight but in this context, they have minimal adaptive value and may even be harmful to our overall health. Chronic stressors can lead to chronic activation of the body's fight-or-flight systems. The body's homeostatatic regulators may begin to fail in vulnerable systems. Eventually this can lead to hypertension, chronic headaches, sexual functioning problems, or a host of other chronic stress-related problems. To examine more closely how chronic stressors and the saber-toothed tiger of our minds can lead to these and other problems, let us take a more detailed look at Selye's GAS model.

Selye's General Adaptation Syndrome

As discussed earlier in the chapter, Hans Selye (1956a) used Cannon's ideas to develop a more systematic understanding of the physiology of stress. Examining Selye's research we know that he subjected rats to various physical stressors such as cold, heat, and toxic substances and measured their physiological responses. Based on these challenges to homeostasis, he determined through autopsies that his animals experienced common physiological patterns of change over time, such as reductions in the size of the thymus and lymph glands (used in the immune system), enlarged adrenal cortexes, and ulcerated stomachs. He described these physiological changes as *stress* reactions. They were characterized as **nonspecific responses** because they represented common patterns to a host of different stressors.

According to Selye, when the organism is first subjected to a threat from a stressor, the organism reacts with alarm by activating the adaptive fight-or-flight response. The resulting sympathetic nervous system activation and adrenal cortex hormonal secretions elevate the body's physiological arousal systems above the parameters of normal homeostasis, which results in the organism entering the first stage known as the **alarm stage.** Following an adaptive fight-or-flight reaction the homeostatic mechanisms return the body back to normal baseline. However, if the organism is subjected to repeated stressors, it must repeat the process.

With time and repetition, such as when the organism is subjected to chronic stressors, the systems at play begin to pay an increasing cost. This cost is known today as the **allostatic load** (Sterling & Eyer, 1988). The continual wear and tear and drawing of resources from the different systems of the body, including the immune system, can eventually propel the organism into Selye's second stage, which he called the **resistance stage.** Over a more extended time as the organism endures repeated exposure to stressors, the systems become so depleted that injury may result. Thus, the body experiences the final stage called the **exhaustion stage** where organ systems fail and possible death may ensue (Figure 1.2).

allostatic load: the cost the organism pays when subjected to chronic stressors.

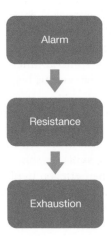

FIGURE **1.2**   Stages of Selye's General Adaptation Syndrome

According to Selye's general adaptation syndrome (GAS), chronic stress leads to an increasing allostatic load that over time can move an individual through all three stages of the GAS.

diathesis-stress model: illness results from environmental stressors having an adverse impact on an individual's most vulnerable biological systems.

Another biological model, the **diathesis-stress model,** also suggests that many illnesses may result from an interaction of biology and the environment. A person with a genetic predisposition to hypertension may develop essential hypertension if this person encounters sufficient chronic stressors. However, if that same person encounters few stressors throughout life, hypertension will never develop. This has sometimes been referred to as the *weak organ* model (Wiener, 1977). The organ or organ system that is most vulnerable is the one that will break down under chronic stress. In some ways this model is similar to Selye's GAS model, but it differs in that it postulates that each person will have a unique genetically predetermined organ system breakdown to chronic stress. Let us illustrate Selye's model and the diathesis-stress model by looking at Sarah. Sarah's parents are both taking high blood pressure medication and her mother has also been diagnosed with irritable bowel syndrome (IBS).

Sarah is a woman with bills to pay and a family to support who is working a job that asks more and more without providing requisite support. Each day her boss brings her a new stack of work, which causes a spike in her blood pressure and a knot in her stomach as she feels the pressure and strain of her boss's increasing demands. On the one hand she wants to lash out at her boss (the fight response) and on the other hand she wants to quit and find a new job (the flight response). She is in the alarm stage. However, given her family obligations and the uncertainties of finding a new and better job, she decides to endure the stressors. With time, her increased blood pressure and frequent abdominal discomfort from her repeated fight-or-flight responses begin to take their toll. Sarah's allostatic load is high as she enters the resistance stage.

As time wears on Sarah is eventually diagnosed with high blood pressure, essential hypertension. She has also developed GI problems with episodic bouts of abdominal pain and diarrhea. This final stage, the exhaustion stage, marks the breakdown of some of her homeostatic regulators and the loss of her once healthy state. According to the diathesis-stress model, Sarah's unique vulnerabilities were in the cardiovascular and GI systems. Therefore, when her systems began to fail due to chronic stress, these were the first ones to go.

Though Selye's model has intuitive appeal, it has its limitations. First, as a biological model, it does not address psychological processes such as cognitive appraisals of stressors and how they can uniquely affect one's perceptions and coping skills. Second, Selye claimed that there was universality to stressors and their effects. In other words, all stressors should have similar effects, but this is not accurate.

We now know that different types of stressors can produce different types of effects. For example, Mason (1971, 1975a, 1975b) concluded that physical stressors such as fasting and exercise have positive rather than negative effects as would be predicted by GAS. Further, Mason found that there are specific neuroendocrine patterns associated with different types of stressors. Likewise, Ax (1953) found different neuroendocrine patterns for fear and anger, with fear and adrenaline (i.e., epinephrine) being linked, yet anger was linked to a different hormone, noradrenaline (i.e., norepinephrine). Therefore, Selye's non-specific hypothesis may be overly general in explaining actual everyday responses to all stressors.

Cannon and Selye paved the way for research in fields like **psychoendocri-nology,** an area of study that examines the relationship between psychological processes and endocrine function. However, their models fall short of providing a comprehensive psychological model of stress. Most modern biological models of stress build on the work of Cannon and Selye by focusing on the measurement of stress reactions through catecholamine (i.e., epinephrine and norepinephrine) and cortisol excretions. For example, Marianne Frankenhaeuser and her col-leagues have shown that psychological stressors such as uncertainty and antici-pation (Frankenhaeuser & Rissler, 1970) can produce elevated catecholamine levels as can the experience of over- or understimulation (Frankenhaeuser, Nordheden, Myrsten, & Post, 1971). Her research team also found that feelings of distress are more closely related to the endocrine patterns of pituitary-adrenal activation, whereas feelings of alertness and of being ready for action are more closely related to endocrine patterns of sympathetic-adrenal activation (Lundberg & Frankenhaeuser, 1980). Such findings push the envelope of biological models to include psychological variables that illustrate how a variety of psychological stressors link to specific hormonal patterns.

The Psychology of Stress

Due to the limitations of the biological models of stress, researchers such as Arnold Lazarus and others sought to develop more comprehensive models of stress that incorporated the psychology of stress along with its biology. These more comprehensive views of stress rejected the notion that humans are simple stimulus-response biological organisms with stressor inputs producing pre-dictable biological outputs. Instead, they applied the theories and research findings of the field of cognitive psychology to explain how different individu-als have different reactions to the same stimulus based on their mental inter-pretations of the stimulus.

What some find stressful, others find exciting, and yet others may be unaf-fected. For example, driving over a high bridge is stressful to some people, some are excited by the sensation of the high view, and yet others do not seem to be affected in the least. What's the difference between these three groups? Cognitive theorists would say it is their interpretation of the event. Those who are stressed probably at some level, perhaps even unconsciously, are thinking that the height on the bridge they are experiencing is dangerous and could result in a fall, in-jury, or even death. Those who are excited are probably at some level thinking that it is a thrill to be able to see the vista from a bird's perspective. What about the indifferent group? They are likely thinking that the drive over the bridge is nothing special and might even be thinking about how they need to feed the cat when they get home. So each group applies a different type of cognitive filter to the stimulus and, as a result, interprets that stimulus differently. Such differ-ences help to explain why stress reactions to the same event vary from person to person. Lazarus's appraisal and coping model gives us more detail.

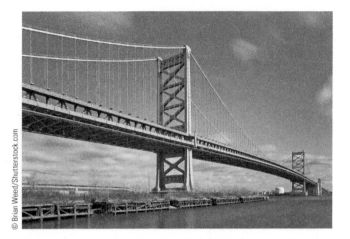

Imagine how you would feel if you were driving over this high bridge. Would you feel any stress? If so, would it be eustress or distress? What type of thoughts do you imagine you would have? How do these thoughts specifically relate to your feelings about driving over this high bridge?

Lazarus's Appraisal and Coping Model

Lazarus and Folkman (1984) proposed a three-process **cognitive model** of stress and coping consisting of what they labeled primary appraisal, secondary appraisal, and reappraisal. During **primary appraisal,** a person evaluates the present and potential harm or loss resulting from the stimulus event. Remember the saber-toothed tiger example? The cave dweller sees the tiger and immediately appraises the situation as potentially harmful. During **secondary appraisal,** the cave dweller evaluates coping resources. After evaluating the situation and seeing that a rock is available to throw at the tiger, the cave dweller employs that strategy. If the situation demands more coping resources than the person has available, that person will experience a sense of *threat*, which then leads to a stress reaction. **Reappraisal** occurs next when the person may change the meaning of the event to reduce stress reactions. For example, the cave dweller may evaluate the situation with the tiger as less dangerous than previously thought after throwing the rock at the tiger and seeing it flee. This reappraisal process helps the cave dweller manage subsequent stress reactions and return to homeostasis.

Although Lazarus chose to use the words *primary* and *secondary* to describe the appraisal process, he later expressed regret for using these terms because the terms implied that there is always a sequential process or that one (primary) is more important than the other (secondary). He notes that these meanings were not intended and that the process of appraisal is complex, continuous, and *transactive* (a two-way process) with the event. In primary appraisal the person asks, "Am I in trouble or being benefited, now or in the

primary appraisal: a judgment in Lazarus's model about the relative significance of an event regarding its potential benefit or harm-loss.

secondary appraisal: the judgment in Lazarus's model about how well one can deal or cope with a given stressful situation.

future, and in what way?" In secondary appraisal the person asks, "What if anything can be done about it?" (Lazarus & Folkman, 1984, p. 31).

Primary Appraisal   According to Lazarus, events can be appraised during primary appraisal in three possible ways. They can be seen as irrelevant, benign-positive, or stressful. If the event is seen as **irrelevant** because it has no implications for the person's overall health and well-being, then no response is required. For example, watching two people arguing loudly with each other on a nighttime television drama probably has no relevance to our lives, and so it would not be alarming to most of us. However, if they were arguing loudly in person in our living room, it would have relevance. Likewise, talking to a friend about the good weather outside would be **benign-positive** and would not merit a threat reaction. The overall emotional valence would be neutral or positive. Stressful reactions occur when the situation is judged as potentially involving harm-loss, threat, and/or challenge. **Harm-loss appraisals** are past or present oriented and result from appraisals of loss or damage that is happening or has already happened. The losses can be tangible such as loss of a loved one or a job, or psychological, such as loss of self-esteem.

Threat appraisals are future oriented. When the future suggests the possibility of harm or loss, the person will experience threat. With these appraisals, the person can anticipate future coping needs and prepare for the threat. In anticipating the future, when the coping abilities are self-assessed as meeting the demands of the situation, then the potential harm-loss appraisal will be seen as a challenge rather than a threat. **Challenge appraisals** see the potential for gain or growth. Whereas threat appraisals tend to evoke negative emotions such as anxiety, fear, and anger, challenge appraisals tends to evoke feelings of excitement, eagerness, and exhilaration. Threat and challenge appraisals may differ depending on the personal characteristics of the individual. For example, a person with low self-esteem may see a promotion as a threat, whereas someone with high self-esteem who has equal capabilities may see the same promotion as a challenge. Others may see the promotion as both a threat and a challenge because these two types of appraisals are not mutually exclusive. These appraisals are fluid and complex so that at one moment the event can be appraised as a challenge, yet in another moment a similar event can be appraised as a threat. For example, a person giving a speech may think that "all is going well, I am doing a great job" (a challenge appraisal) and in the next moment begin to doubt that things are going well and think, "I am really blowing it" (a threat appraisal) even though the audience reaction is the same in both moments.

Secondary Appraisal   The secondary appraisal process involves assessing how well we can deal or cope with a given situation. **Coping** refers to the effective use of resources and strategies to deal with internal or external demands (Coyne & Holroyd, 1982). Part of the coping assessment process involves estimating the

Coping: effectively using resources and strategies to deal with potentially harmful or stressful internal or external demands.

degree of **control** we have over the stressor. As you might assume, the less control we perceive we have over the stressor, the more stressful we perceive the event to be. This process is illustrated by the following experiment.

Corah and Boffa (1970) exposed research participants to bursts of loud noise. In one condition, participants were told that they could stop the loud noise at any time if they chose to do so; however, they were encouraged not to stop the noise. None attempted to stop the noise. This was the "I'm in control of the noise" condition because even though they did not stop the noise they believed they could stop it at any time. In the other condition, participants were not told that they could stop the noise, and they were given the same amount of noise stimulation as the other group. This was the "I'm not in control of the noise" condition because the participants did not think they could stop the noise. What were the results? As we might expect, the participants in this *uncontrollable* noise condition experienced a greater stress reaction than those in the controllable noise condition even though the amount of noise exposure in both groups was identical. So the perception of control is a key factor that influences our perception of the event and how much stress we will experience.

Bandura (1977, 1989) coined the term *self-efficacy,* a term related to perceived control, to refer to a belief in one's abilities and skills to bring about a successful outcome in a given situation (i.e., to control it). We might think of self-efficacy as similar to *self-confidence* except that unlike self-confidence, self-efficacy is target specific and pertains to a specific area of competence. For example, *academic self-efficacy* refers to how confident a person is about his or her ability to achieve academic success. The target in this case is academic.

Self-efficacy can be broken down into two component parts: outcome expectations and efficacy expectations. The term *outcome expectation* refers to our belief that a particular action will lead to a particular outcome. For example, an overweight person who wants to lose weight and has high outcome expectations may believe that reducing the amount of food eaten (i.e., reduce caloric intake) will lead to weight loss. The term *efficacy expectation* refers to the belief that the person can successfully execute the actions that lead to the desired outcome—that he or she can reduce the amount of food eaten. The overweight person with high outcome expectancy and high efficacy expectations believes that he or she can successfully reduce the amount of food eaten and that this will lead to success in losing weight. This person has a higher probability of success in a weight loss program than another overweight person with low self-efficacy. High self-efficacy also relates to secondary appraisal in that the person believes he or she has the coping resources to deal with the challenge (e.g., weight loss) and thus will be less stressed by it (Figure 1.3).

Stress Reappraisals   During the stress reappraisal phase of Lazarus's transaction model, the stressful situation is reappraised based on ongoing feedback from the situation along with the person's self-assessment of how well

self-efficacy: the belief in one's abilities and skills to bring about a successful outcome in a given situation.

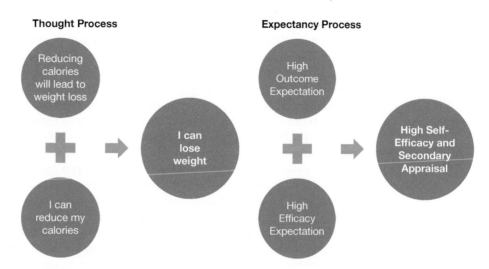

FIGURE 1.3   Weight Loss, Secondary Appraisal, and Self-Efficacy

High self-efficacy is related to high secondary appraisal. High self-efficacy is a result of having a high outcome expectation and a high efficacy expectation. People with high self-efficacy believe they have the coping resources to deal with a challenge like weight loss.

he or she is dealing with the situation. As Lazarus and Folkman (1984) note, "threat can be reappraised as unwarranted or, conversely, a benign appraisal may turn into one of threat, creating a succession of changing emotions and appraisals. A reappraisal is simply an appraisal that follows an earlier appraisal in the same encounter and modifies it. In essence, appraisal and reappraisal do not differ" (p. 38). Therefore, stress reappraisals are simply part of the ongoing pattern of the transactive appraisal chain to the particular stimulus event.

THE PROMISE OF POSITIVE PSYCHOLOGY

Stress research has paralleled the general thrust of the discipline of psychology in focusing on how to prevent and alleviate human problems and suffering. Thus, stress has been studied primarily with the aim of determining how it creates problems for us and how to prevent or manage these problems. However, as previously discussed, stress can also be viewed through a positive lens (e.g., eustress) with a focus on how it benefits us in different ways. For example, stressors can be perceived as challenges that prompt us to perform more optimally or grow psychologically.

Along this line there is burgeoning activity in an area of psychology with deep historical traditions (e.g., humanistic psychology) that has been somewhat dormant until more recently. This focus, called **positive psychology,** is a field of study that examines what goes right with us rather than what goes wrong. Martin E. P. Seligman, speaking in 1998 as the president of the American Psychological Association, urged psychologists to get back to their roots of focusing on psychological strengths rather than psychological problems. He called this focus *positive psychology*. In many ways Seligman's call for psychology mirrors that of Antonovky's for health. By studying the positive side of stress, we can learn its upside and apply it to our health and well-being. Positive psychology can be understood as a field with three related areas of study that include positive trait characteristics (e.g., virtues, strengths, talents, and values), positive subjective experiences (e.g., fulfillment, happiness, gratification, and satisfaction), and positive institutions (e.g., families, communities, schools, and organizations) (Peterson, 2006). It encompasses a wide range of themes but has a major focus on the study of the **good life.** Such a focus examines the elements that constitute a fulfilling life, a life well lived.

People who live the good life are often seen as those who have positive trait characteristics, positive social relationships, and positive life regulation capabilities (Compton, 2005). Positive trait characteristics may include, for example, having integrity, compassion, and courage. Positive social relationships are often seen as nurtured through love, altruism, forgiveness, and spirituality. Positive life regulation means persons can self-direct in ways that move them closer to their goals while uplifting others along the way. These elements are believed to contribute to a higher level of satisfaction and sense of well-being. However, as Peterson (2006, p. 7) notes, positive psychology is not just the study of "happiology."

Besides the study of happiness and well-being, positive psychology focuses on such themes as positive emotions (e.g., enjoyment and pleasure), optimism, flow and goal pursuit (often referred to a being "in the zone"), mindfulness (a type of present moment nonjudgmental awareness), love and relationships, meaning (e.g., resilience and thriving), and purposeful living (including religion and spirituality) among others.

So what then is the promise of positive psychology for understanding stress, health, and well-being? For most people it is simply not enough to be able to manage their stress well. As you will see in the next chapter, by managing our negative emotions without experiencing positive emotions we simply maintain a neutral state at best. If we want to live the good life, we also want to build on our good feelings and our sense of well-being. The field of positive psychology points the way. Therefore, when possible, we will look not only at the negative effects of stress, but also at the positive effects and how we can make "lemonade out of lemons" in pursuit of the good life. In addition, we will look at well-being and other areas of positive psychology and integrate them into the discussion of stress and health when viable. Chapter 2 expands on these themes and discusses them more fully.

CHAPTER SUMMARY AND CONCEPT REVIEW

- Over time models of stress have evolved from mechanistic, biological models to today's more complex cognitive transactional models.

- Walter Cannon introduced us to important biological concepts related to stress such as homeostasis and the fight-or-flight response.

- Hans Selye built upon Cannon's concepts to develop a three-stage model called the general adaptation syndrome that explains how chronic stress can adversely affect the organism.

- Selye also introduced the idea of positive stress, a concept that was later expanded on by Holmes and Rahe who developed their own model of stress as defined by objective life events.

- Richard Lazarus argued that focusing on subjective perceptions of stressors, especially at the day-to-day level, is more important than simply examining larger life events outside of their individual meaning contexts.

- Lazarus considered the appraisal patterns of individuals to be crucial to our understanding of the impact that a given stressor has on a given individual and included the concept of primary appraisals, secondary appraisals, and reappraisals.

- Traditional dichotomous models of health such as the biomedical model are less likely to include the effects of psychological variables such as psychological stress on physical states.

- The biopsychosocial model views health states along a continuum and includes causal behavioral and psychological variables along with traditional medical variables.

- Behavioral medicine, health psychology, the concept of wellness, and Antonovsky's salutogenic model subscribe to the biopsychosocial approach to understanding and promoting health.

- Antonovsky views stressors as omnipresent and possibly health promoting depending on how we adapt to them and how we use internal and external resources he called generalized resistance resources (GRRs).

- GRRs are important in shaping our worldview or what he referred to as our sense of coherence (SOC).

- Health and wellness are affected by stress responses that include cognitive, emotional, physiological, and behavioral changes.

- Though stress responses were adaptive for our distant ancestors, they can be maladaptive for modern humans.

- Managing our response to stress and engaging in an overall healthy lifestyle can increase our likelihood of living a long and healthy life.

- Positive psychology offers promise to our understanding of stress, health, and well-being.

- Besides the study of happiness and well-being, positive psychology focuses on such themes as positive emotions, optimism, flow and goal pursuit, mindfulness, love and relationships, meaning, and purposeful living.

- In this book we will look at how to live the good life and integrate other elements of positive psychology into the discussion of stress and health when viable.

CRITICAL THINKING QUESTIONS

1. Think of a time when you experienced eustress and another time when you encountered an uplift. How were they similar and different from each other? Which type of experience do you prefer? Why?

2. What is the difference between behavioral medicine and health psychology? How does the related concept of wellness fit into the biopsychosocial model of health?

3. What are some of the generalized resistance resources (GRRs) that you believe help you resist entropy? Can you think of any that have moved you toward the salutary end of Antonovsky's continuum? What are they and how do you think they were able to produce their salutary effects?

4. How is making a challenge appraisal more likely to result in the experience of eustress, whereas making a threat appraisal more likely to result in the experience of distress? What role does secondary appraisal play in the process of an experience of eustress or distress?

5. How does self-efficacy relate to Lazarus's appraisal and coping model? What role does the perception of control play?

KEY TERMS AND CONCEPTS

Alarm stage	Cardiovascular system	Dermal system	General adaptation syndrome (GAS)*
Allostatic load*	Catecholamines	Diathesis-stress model*	
Appraisal	Challenge appraisals	Distress	Generalized resistance resources (GRRs)
Autonomic nervous system	Cognitive model	Efficacy expectation	Glucocorticoids
Behavioral medicine	Comprehensibility	Epinephrine	Good life
	Control	Eustress*	Harm-loss appraisals
Benign-positive appraisals	Coping*	Exhaustion stage	Hassles*
Biomedical model*	Core relational meaning	Fight-or-flight*	Health*
Biopsychosocial model*	Cortisol	Gastrointestinal (GI) system	Health psychology*

Homeostasis*

Hormonal system

Irrelevant appraisals

Manageability

Meaningfulness

Muscular system

Nonspecific responses

Norepinephrine

Outcome expectations

Positive psychology*

Primary appraisal*

Psychoendocrinology*

Psychosomatic medicine

Reappraisal

Respiratory system

Resistance stage

Salutogenic model*

Secondary appraisal*

Self-efficacy*

Sense of coherence (SOC)*

Sensory systems

Social Readjustment Rating Scale (SRRS)

Stress*

Stress management

Stressor

Sympathetic nervous system

Threat appraisals

Uplifts*

Wellness

Yerkes-Dodson Curve

MEDIA RESOURCES

CENGAGE**brain**.com

Access an interactive eBook, chapter-specific interactive learning tools, including flashcards, quizzes, videos, and more in your Psychology CourseMate, accessed through CengageBrain.com.

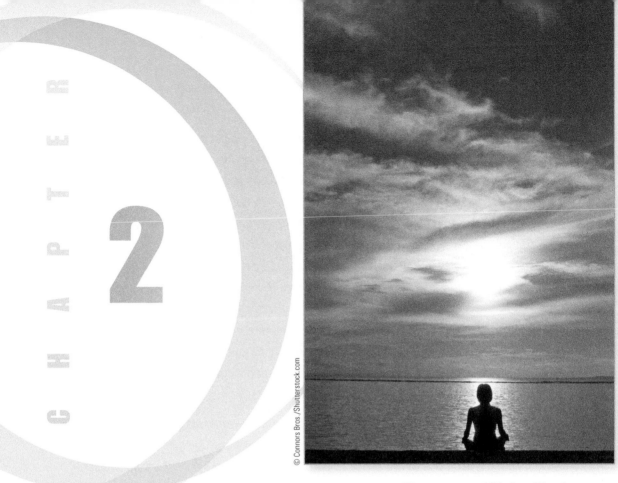

© Connors Bros./Shutterstock.com

2

The purpose of life is a life of purpose.

~Robert Byrne

Positive Psychology

Sonja Lyubomirsky (2007), one of the pioneer researchers in the field of happiness, recounts her experience interviewing a woman named Angela:

> "Angela is thirty-four and one of the happiest people that I ever interviewed. You wouldn't guess it, however, from all she's had to bear. When Angela was growing up in Southern California, her mother was emotionally and physically abusive to her, and her father did nothing to intervene. In addition to what she endured at home, she was overweight as a teenager and stigmatized at school. When Angela was in eleventh grade, her mother was diagnosed with breast cancer, and the physical abuse ended. However, the emotional abuse got only worse, until Angela couldn't stand it any longer and moved out to marry a man she'd only known for just three months. She and her husband moved up north and lived there for four years. Soon after the birth of their daughter, Ella, they divorced, and Angela moved back to California, where she still lives." (p. 28)

Given all that Angela has endured, why would she be one of the happiest people that Sonja Lyubomirsky has ever interviewed? Shouldn't she be one of the saddest, perhaps one of the most pessimistic and depressed persons Sonja Lyubomirsky ever interviewed?

> "Still, with all that has happened and all the challenges that have come to pass, Angela considers herself to be a very happy person. Her daughter Ella, to whom she is extremely close, brings her endless joy. . . . She has made many friends—indeed, formed a whole community of like-minded people—and they are a pleasure and support to her. She finds deep satisfaction in helping others heal from their own wounds and traumas, for as she reasons, 'It's virtually impossible to face one's shadows alone.'" (p. 29)

It is people like Angela who fortunately defy conventional logic that intrigue researchers in the burgeoning field of positive psychology. These researchers are drawn to those who successfully live the good life, especially those who overcome great adversity. As discussed in Chapter 1, **positive psychology** is the field of study that examines what people do right rather than what goes wrong. Not only is Angela happy in spite of the odds, but she must be doing something right to be one of the happiest people ever interviewed by one of the pioneering researchers of happiness. From studies of people like Angela, we learn a great deal about what we can do right to live a more fulfilling life. This chapter examines some of the major concepts and results of these findings. Many of these concepts relate directly or indirectly to stress and health. Others relate primarily to the topic of well-being. Together, stress, health, and well-being weave the tapestry of this book.

As discussed previously, positive psychology goes beyond the study of happiness and encompasses other aspects related to living an effective life such as the study of positive trait characteristics and subjective experiences as well as the role of supporting institutions. Before we explore some of these areas in more depth, let us first take a brief look at the history of positive psychology.

A Brief History of Positive Psychology

Western ideas related to today's positive psychology have deep roots. Many of the philosophical underpinnings of these ideas can be traced to the ancient Hebrews and Greeks around 2,500 years ago. The Hebrews and, later, many Christians followed what we now call the **divine command theory** of happiness that states that the path to happiness is to follow the commands of a supreme being. If one lives in accordance with divine laws and morals then one lives the good life. Today this influence is studied through research in religiosity, meaning, and spirituality and how these factors influence well-being.

The ancient Greeks during the Golden Age believed that the formula for the good life could be determined by logic and reason. Socrates (469–399 BCE) was the best known teacher of this approach. He believed in the Delphic motto, "Know thyself." Self-knowledge was the key to understanding *the good*, which then motivates virtuous behavior. This knowledge, he believed, had to be uncovered from timeless truths rather than emotions, sensory experiences, or perceptions. Plato (427–347 BCE), a student of Socrates, also distrusted sensory experiences to reveal the truth and believed that we have to look deeper within to find it. He objectively defined happiness as the love of "good and beautiful things" (Plato, 1999, p. 38). Aristotle (384–322 BCE), a student of Plato, continued the progression of his mentor's thinking and believed that the good life could be achieved by following the *golden mean,* the balance point between the extremes of life. He believed that *eudaimonia* (i.e., happiness possessed of true well-being) was not a goal to pursue but rather a by-product of living the virtuous life. In fact, he outlined basic virtues (e.g., courage, good temper, honor, etc.) that can lead to this outcome. As such, Aristotle's approach is referred to as the **virtue theory** of happiness. Today, this eudemonia theory of well-being is often contrasted with the more popular notion of happiness as **subjective well-being** determined by one's appraisal of life satisfaction and positive feelings. The idea of positive feelings, good moods, and pleasurable experiences leading to happiness embodies the **hedonic definition of happiness.**

Though the formalization of positive psychology as a field of study is fairly recent, behavioral scientists have studied positive topics for at least 100 years.

eudaimonia: Aristotle's concept of happiness possessed of true well-being that is a by-product of living the virtuous life.

subjective well-being: represents the concept that happiness is determined by one's appraisal of life satisfaction and positive feelings.

As Ed Diener (2009), another pioneer of positive psychology, notes, prior to the relatively recent emergence of the field of positive psychology, social psychologists were studying altruism, sociologists happiness, and counselors personality strengths. Diener (2009, p. 7) also credits individual pioneers in the field including "Don Clifton (who studied human strengths), George Vailant (who studies effective coping), Shelly Taylor (who studies health), Jane Piliavin (who studies helping and volunteerism), and Mihalyi Csikszentmihalyi (who studies flow and creativity)" as having worked in the area for decades.

It has only been more recently, however, that positive psychology has emerged as an integrated field of study. Former president of the American Psychological Association Martin E. P. Seligman (Seligman & Csikszentmihalyi, 2000) is credited with organizing and bringing together scholars in the late 1990s into the area he framed as *positive psychology*. Besides behavioral scientists, others who made important contributions to positive psychology before it was formalized as a distinct area are the humanistic psychologists including Carl Rogers and Abraham Maslow (e.g., self-actualization) and the existentialists including Viktor Frankl and Irwin Yalom (e.g., the search for life's meaning). Today the area of positive psychology is thriving thanks to Martin Seligman and others tilling and fertilizing the soil so that many seeds, some as old as written history, can be planted, nurtured, and harvested by those working in this burgeoning new field.

POSITIVE EMOTIONS

It is no surprise that the study of positive emotions attracted the attention of researchers in the area of positive psychology. However, what is surprising is that these emotions were largely neglected by investigators who, until the 1980s, focused almost exclusively on negative emotions. Why exclude positive emotions in favor of negative ones? There are a number of reasons. First, we associate negative emotions with problems and the focus of psychology has historically been, with good reason, on how to alleviate suffering and help those with problems. Second, there are fewer positive emotions than negative ones. For example, there appears to be "only one positive emotion for every three or four negative emotions" (Fredrickson, 1998, p. 301). Third, positive emotions seem less distinct from one another and more difficult to define operationally. For example, how do you sharply define *joy* or *bliss* so that they differentiate well from each other? Contrast that with how much easier it is to define *anger* or *anxiety* so that we can easily tell them apart. Fourth, in recent years, with the increased focus on how to live an effective life, there is a greater interest in the study of positive emotions. And last, we now know that strategies that support and sustain positive emotions can help those who experience problems like coping with stress and other difficulties.

When we examine the range of emotions, we can view them as residing on a continuum from the highly unpleasant on the negative end of the pole to the highly pleasant positive end. Though most experts in the field previously assumed that eliminating negative emotions would automatically lead to positive ones, we now know this is usually not the case. Negative and positive emotions are somewhat independent of each other and are only weakly inversely related.

For example, Watson and Naragon (2009) report that positive mood scale scores show only small negative correlations with measures of negative emotions (ranging from r = −.14 to −.21). As Watson and Naragon (2009, pp. 207–208) state, "over the past few decades, researchers have established that two largely independent factors—positive affect and negative affect—comprise the basic dimensions of emotional experience."

positive affect: pleasant emotions such as joy, love, and amusement.

Positive affect then refers to an experience of positive emotions and **negative affect** to an experience of negative emotions. Each appears to have different evolutionary and adaptive values. Whereas positive affect is approach oriented, moving the person toward situations or others that could yield pleasure and reward, negative affect is part of the withdrawal-oriented system designed to protect a person from threat, harm, or pain (e.g., fight-or-flight).

negative affect: unpleasant emotions such as sadness, anger, fear, and anxiety.

Fredrickson's Broaden-and-Build Model

broaden-and-build: Fredrickson's model that explains the adaptive and evolutionary value of our positive emotions.

Barbara Fredrickson (1998) proposed a *broaden-and-build* model to explain the adaptive and evolutionary value of our positive emotions. Whereas negative emotions tend to narrow our options, positive emotions tend to broaden them. These *specific action tendencies* of negative emotions (e.g., fight-or-flight) stand in contrast with the *nonspecific action tendencies* of positive affect. For example, it was not very adaptive for those primitive humans to ponder and contemplate a bevy of options for dealing with an approaching saber-toothed tiger unless they wanted to be the tiger's next lunch. Instead, their negative emotions helped them act quickly, sometimes without thinking, to either fight or flee the tiger.

Positive emotions, however, can evoke a wide range of options through broadening and building. By broadening what Fredrickson calls *thought-action repertoires* we are able to build personal resources. Thus, positive emotions evoke more flexible thoughts about actions we can take that in turn build resources (Figure 2.1). That is, we can think of lots of activities that give us pleasure and ponder them before we decide what potentially resource-building action to take (e.g., call a friend, go shopping, go out to dinner, take a walk, etc.). From this perspective, negative emotions lead to short-term survival gains through facilitating the employment of specific narrow options, and positive emotions lead to long-term survival through setting the stage for use of a general wide range of options. Also, it is not very adaptive for humans to continue to feel negative emotions once a threat subsides. So Fredrickson also suggests in her *undoing hypothesis* that positive emotions help us recover more quickly from detrimental effects of negative emotions. Why do we laugh sometimes immediately after a false startle—think of someone suddenly and unexpectedly tapping us on the shoulder from behind in a dark movie theater during a scary scene? Would we startle and then laugh? If we do, we laugh because the positive emotions help us relieve tension and regain our equilibrium. It is adaptive for humans to regain equilibrium once the tiger is gone, and then *broaden* attention to other people and resources to engender social support and resource sharing. Given that we humans are social beings, we would not last long in a cave or on the savannah if we had to fend for ourselves, alone against predators, famine, and diseases.

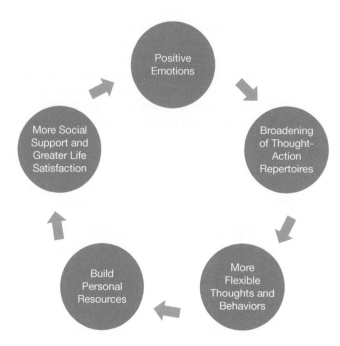

FIGURE **2.1**   Fredrickson's Broaden-and-Build Theory of Positive Emotions

In support of the *broaden hypothesis,* Cohn and Fredrickson (2009) point to visual attention studies that show that negative emotions are generally related to attention to details (a more narrowed focus), whereas positive emotions generally lead to a preference for viewing more global shapes (a broader focus).

Fredrickson and Branigan (2005) also found that when they induced positive, negative, or no emotions in experimental participants and asked them what they felt like doing *right now,* their positive-emotion participants listed more things they felt like doing (i.e., potential actions) than their neutral group, and their positive-emotion group's listing of things its participants felt like doing was more varied (a more broad focus). As predicted, the negative-emotion group participants listed fewer potential actions they were interested in doing than the neutral group.

In testing the *build hypothesis,* Fredrickson, Cohn, Coffey, Pek, and Finkel (2008) randomly assigned participants to either an experimental group or a waiting list control group (i.e., a group of participants who would later receive the experimental treatment who were placed on a waiting list). The experimental group participants were trained to experience daily positive emotions by engaging in loving-kindness meditation (see Chapter 14). The results indicated that the experience of daily positive emotions led the participants to improve their resources (e.g., more social support, increased purpose in life), which in turn led to greater life satisfaction.

Finally, in an examination of the *undoing hypothesis,* Fredrickson, Mancuso, Branigan, and Tugade (2000) provoked anxiety in their experimental participants and then showed them a film clip. In the conditions in which the film clips were designed to elicit positive emotions (amusement and contentment), cardiovascular responses recovered more quickly from anxiety than in the neutral film clip condition, thus suggesting that positive emotions do facilitate the undoing of the physiological effects of negative emotions. Therefore, it appears that there is at least some empirical support for Fredrickson's (1998) broaden-and-build model and her undoing hypothesis.

WELL-BEING

As discussed previously, the early thinkers and philosophers had different ways of conceptualizing the *good life* and what it entails. Today, as psychologists and other behavioral scientists study concepts such as happiness and well-being, they take these views and try to define them in ways that are amenable to scientific investigation. Two overlapping, though sometimes competing, views of well-being and happiness have emerged from the positive psychology literature. One is a subjective view and the other a more prescriptive view (see Kesebir & Diener, 2008, for discussion).

The first and most prevalent view among psychologists, the subjective view, is that happiness is defined as subjective well-being (Diener, 1984). For example, Sonja Lyubomirsky (2007, p. 32) states that she uses the terms *happiness,* which she defines as "the experience of joy, contentment, or positive well-being, combined with a sense that life is good, meaningful, and worthwhile," and *well-being* interchangeably. This *subjectivist* view suggests that each person knows best his or her level of happiness. Because there is no test tube objective measure of happiness we can use to determine a person's happiness levels accurately, we must then rely on the person's *subjective* appraisals. These appraisals can be measured by self-report tests. What do people base their subjective happiness appraisals on? They seem to rely on several factors. According to Kesibir and Diener (2008, p. 118), subjective well-being consists of the following general components: "These components include life satisfaction (global judgments of one's life), satisfaction with important life domains (satisfaction with one's work, health, marriage, etc.), positive affect (prevalence of positive emotions and moods), and low levels of negative affect (prevalence of unpleasant emotions and moods)."

life satisfaction: a global judgment about how good one's life is.

Remember Angela who reported being happy in spite of her many past difficulties? You might ask how she knows she is happy. According to the subjective well-being view, she uses at least three sources of information. One source is her global judgment about her life, her assessment of her **life satisfaction.** She asks herself if life is good. In her case, the answer was yes. Second, she looks at important domains in her life such as her relationship with her daughter Ella and her friends and subjectively assesses if things are going well. For her the answer was affirmative. And last, she asks if she generally feels good, that is, she has frequent positive affect coupled with infrequent negative affect. On balance, Angela's predominant affect is positive. Thus, overall Angela reports she is happy, and, therefore, we can say that she has a high level of subjective well-being.

The second and less prevalent view of the *good life* in the field of psychology, though arguably just as important, is prescriptive in that it specifies (i.e., prescribes) that certain factors must be present for a person to feel happiness and well-being. This view is less subjective and parallels Aristotle's *eudaimonic* perspective. Remember, Aristotle's theory stated that to live the *good life* a person must possess certain virtues. Hence, these virtues were the factors that must be present for us to experience happiness.

Today, Carol Ryff's model of **psychological well-being** (Ryff, 1989, 1995; Ryff & Singer, 1996) embodies the *eudaimonic* concept, but instead of virtues it substitutes dimensions of positive mental health. In her view a person must exhibit high levels of six dimensions of positive mental health in order to experience the highest levels of well-being. Ryff identified these six dimensions based on her understanding of classic theories of what determines good mental health along with research findings from personality, developmental, and clinical psychology. She named these dimensions *self-acceptance, positive relations with others, autonomy, environmental mastery, purpose in life,* and *personal growth*. Besides Ryff's psychological well-being model, there are a number of others that have a *eudaimonic* flavor such as Ryan and Deci's (2000) self-determination theory (see Chapter 9) and Seligman's (2002) theory of *signature strengths* (see Chapter 15).

Measurement of Subjective Well-Being

Most of the measures of happiness and subjective well-being are very straightforward and based on the idea that such a subjective phenomenon as happiness can be measured best by simply asking participants to report their subjective appraisals on a paper and pencil test. One measure that simply asks a person to rate his or her happiness on an 11-point scale is the Fordyce Emotions Questionnaire (Fordyce, 1988). This scale measures happiness as emotional well-being and has strong correlations with daily affect and life satisfaction (Diener, 1994).

Another very simple measure of happiness is the Subjective Happiness Scale (Lyubomirsky & Lepper, 1999). This scale has four items and uses a subjectivist approach to the measurement of happiness. The authors conducted 14 studies for a total of 2,732 participants to validate the scale.

Yet another scale that is used to measure one of the dimensions of subjective well-being is the 5-item Satisfaction with Life Scale (SWL) (Diener, Emmons, Larsen, & Griffin, 1985). As the name suggests, this scale measures life satisfaction. The popular SWL has respectable reliability and good construct validity (Pavot & Diener, 1993). Overall there are many self-report measures of happiness, subjective well-being, and other forms of well-being (e.g., psychological well-being) that have good reliability and validity

As Compton (2005) explains, all the self-report measures of happiness are based on two assumptions. The first is that the amount of happiness a person experiences can be quantified on a scale. And the second is that two people scoring the same number on the same scale have roughly equal levels of happiness. Thus, a carpenter in Nebraska who scores a 5 on the Subjective

INSIGHT EXERCISE **2.1**

You might find yourself wondering what happiness level you would mark on the Fordyce Emotions Questionnaire. Well, you will not have to wonder any longer. You now have an opportunity to take the questionnaire. When you are ready, go ahead and determine your level on the scale.

The Fordyce Emotions Questionnaire

Part 1 Directions: Use the list below to answer the following question: In general, how happy or unhappy do you usually feel? Check the *one* statement below that best describes *your average happiness*.

	10	Extremely happy (feeling ecstatic, joyous, fantastic!)
	9	Very happy (feeling really good, elated!)
	8	Pretty happy (spirits high, feeling good.)
	7	Mildly happy (feeling fairly good and somewhat cheerful.)
	6	Slightly happy (just above neutral.)
	5	Neutral (not particularly happy or unhappy.)
	4	Slightly unhappy (just a bit below neutral.)
	3	Mildly unhappy (just a little low.)
	2	Pretty unhappy (somewhat "blue," spirits down.)
	1	Very unhappy (depressed, spirits very low.)
	0	Extremely unhappy (utterly depressed, completely down.)

Part 2 Directions: Consider your emotions a moment further. *On the average,* what percent of the time do you feel happy? What percent of the time do you feel unhappy? What percent of the time do you feel neutral (neither happy nor unhappy)? Write down your best estimates, as well as you can, in the space below. Make sure the three figures add-up to equal 100%.

On the average:

The percent of time I feel happy   ___%

The percent of time I feel unhappy   ___%

The percent of time I feel neutral   ___%

                                   Total   **100%**

NOTE: Adapted from *A Review of Happiness Measures: A Sixty Second Index of Happiness and Mental Health,* by M. W. Fordyce, 1988, Social Indicators Research, 20, *255–281.* Copyright © M. W. Fordyce. Used by permission.

Did you complete the happiness scale? What did you think of it? Did your scores match what you expected? According to Seligman (2002), the average score for an adult American on the Fordyce Emotions Questionnaire is 6.92 with the average percentage of time feeling happy being 54.13%; feeling unhappy, 20.44%; and feeling neutral, 25.43%.

You may be curious about the SWL. If you would like to take it, the SWL is also available for you. The scoring and interpretation guide is provided with the scale. As you take this scale, notice any subtle differences between the concept of happiness as measured by the Fordyce Emotions Questionnaire and the concept of satisfaction with life as measured by the Satisfaction with Life Scale.

Satisfaction with Life Scale

Below are five statements that you may agree or disagree with. Using the 1–7 scale indicate your agreement with each item by placing the appropriate number on the line preceding that item. Please be open and honest in your responding.

7—Strongly agree

6—Agree

5—Slightly agree

4—Niether agree nor disagree

3—Slightly disagree

2—Disagree

1—Strongly disagree

	In most ways my life is close to ideal.
	The conditions of my life are excellent.
	I am satisfied with my life.
	So far I have gotten the important things I want in life.
	If I could live my life over, I would change almost nothing.

Scoring and interpretation of the scale

Add up your answers to the five items and use the following normative information to help in "interpretation":

5–9	Extremely dissatisfied with your life
10–14	Very dissatisfied with your life
15–19	Slightly dissatisfied with your life
20	About neutral
21–25	Somewhat satisfied with your life
26–30	Very satisfied with your life
31–35	Extremely satisfied with your life

NOTE: Scale adapted from "The Satisfaction with Life Scale," by E. Diener, R. A. Emmons, R. J. Larsen, and S. Griffin, 1985, Journal of Personality Assessment, 49, 71–75. *Used with permission. Scoring guide adapted from Subjective Well-Being: The Science of Happiness and Life Satisfaction, by E. Deiner, S. Oishi, and R. E. Lucas, 2009, in S. J. Lopez and C. R. Snyder (Eds.).* Oxford Handbook of Positive Psychology *(2nd ed., pp. 187–194). New York, NY: Oxford University Press. Used with permission.*

Happiness Scale should have the same level of happiness as an attorney in New Jersey who scores a 5. Because the concept of happiness is so subjective, when behavioral scientists first began researching the concept, they wondered whether these assumptions could be met. However, now that we have a good body of research findings addressing these questions, it does indeed appear as though these assumptions are generally valid. Validation can be determined by finding a general agreement between self-reports of happiness and other types of assessment such as judgments from friends and family about the subject's level of happiness (Diener, 1994; Sandvik, Diener, & Seidlitz, 1993).

What do self-report measures find? They find that the majority of people are happy (Myers, 2000; Myers & Diener, 1995). Though use of self-report measures is an important first step in the developmental progression of the science of the study of happiness and well-being, Ryff and her associates (2006) have urged researchers to develop valid non-self-report measures also including biologically based measures to further strengthen confidence in happiness research findings.

Happiness Set Point and Hedonic Adaptation

Happiness researchers generally share a popular assumption that we each have a happiness set point. The **happiness set point** concept is based on the well-known *weight set point* idea discussed in the weight loss literature (Stallone & Stunkard, 1991) (see Chapter 12). Think of how a thermostat works on an air conditioner and heater. The thermostat *sets the point* for the temperature so that when the ambient temperature gets too hot, the air conditioner blows to bring the temperature down to the *set point*. When it gets too cold, the heater blows to bring the temperature up to the *set point*. Likewise, when we lose too much weight, the *weight set point* model suggests our internal biological regulators try to bring our weight back up to its genetically determined weight set point, making it a struggle for us to keep the weight off without initiating and maintaining serious lifestyle changes. Similarly, when we are too happy or unhappy, our internal biological regulators eventually bring our happiness levels back to our genetically determined *happiness set point*. The set point is believed to be fixed, stable across time, and somewhat impervious to control, similar to a thermostat that is locked into position.

How did happiness researchers arrive at the assumption that we each have a happiness set point? They examined several lines of research including studies that show a large heritability influence for happiness, research that shows personality factors are often better predictors of happiness than circumstances, and studies that demonstrate good stability of subjective well-being across time even when circumstances change.

The first line of support, that there is a large heritability influence for happiness, was demonstrated by Lykken and Tellegen (1996) through examining identical twins at age 20 and then again at age 30 and finding that their well-being scores were very stable across time and consistent with each other. These researchers estimated that genetic variation accounts for between 44%

happiness set point: the idea that happiness levels are fixed, stable across time, and somewhat impervious to control.

and 52% of the variance of well-being. Based on these results and other findings, Lyubomirsky, Sheldon, and Schkade (2005) believe that the happiness set point probably determines about 50% of our long-term stable happiness levels.

The second line of support for the happiness set point assumption comes from findings that show well-being levels are very stable across our lifespan and some personality factors seem to contribute to this stability. For example, similar levels of stability in self-reports of subjective well-being were found over a 10-year period for people regardless of whether their income increased, decreased, or stayed the same (Diener, Sandvik, Seidlitz, & Diener, 1993). Further, people who go through many major life changes report the same level of stability in life satisfaction as people who undergo few life changes (Costa, McCrae, & Zonderman, 1987). These findings suggest that we are disposed to experience certain levels of well-being irrespective of our life circumstances.

This predisposition may be in large part due to personality factors. Researchers have primarily focused on two personality factors as consistent predictors of happiness and well-being. They are extraversion (e.g., warm, sociable) and neuroticism (e.g., anxious, depressed). On the average, extraverted individuals tend to score higher on self-report scales of happiness and well-being than their introverted counterparts, whereas neurotic individuals tend to score lower than their non-neurotic peers (Costa & McCrae, 1980; Harrington & Loffredo, 2001; Hayes & Joseph, 2003; McCrae & Costa, 1991) (see Chapter 6). In sum, personality usually trumps circumstances in determining long-term happiness levels.

The third source of information supporting the happiness set point idea concerns findings that changes in happiness due to circumstances tend to be temporary because we generally adjust fairly soon to our new circumstances. This idea, known as *hedonic adaptation,* is based on the concept that we are walking on a *hedonic treadmill* (Brickman & Campbell, 1971). Though our feet are moving, our happiness levels are not. Can you think of a time when you made a new purchase, say a new car, and were happier for awhile? Did that spike in happiness last for a long time? If not, why not? According to this concept, possessing the new car was fun and novel at first, but eventually your life driving the new car became your new normal as you experienced hedonic adaptation. This phenomenon relates to the concept in learning theory of **habituation** where the novelty of a new stimulus eventually wears off after repeated exposure—the stimulus gradually has less and less impact on you.

Have you ever wondered if you won the lottery, would your problems mostly go away, and you would be happy for the rest of your life? A classic study by Brickman, Coates, and Janoff-Bulman (1978) sought the answer to this question. They looked at lottery winners and paralyzed victims of accidents to investigate the effects of extreme changes in fortune, both positive and negative, and whether these changes would result in long-term changes in happiness. The investigators demonstrated hedonic adaptation for the lottery winners in finding that after winning the lottery (one participant won the

hedonic adaptation: the concept that happiness due to circumstances tends to be temporary because we generally adjust fairly soon to our new circumstances.

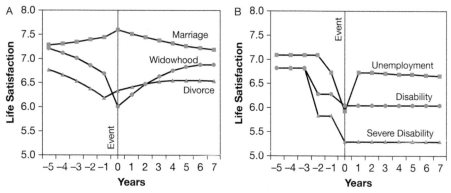

FIGURE **2.2**   Lucas's (2007b) findings suggest that hedonic adaptation is more likely to occur for marriage, widowhood, and divorce and is least likely to occur for disability and severe disability.   NOTE: Adapted from Long-Term Disability Is Associated with Lasting Changes in Subjective Well-Being: Evidence from Two Nationally Representative Longitudinal Studies, by R. E. Lucas, 2007b, *Journal of Personality and Social Psychology, 92,* 717–730. Copyright Association for Psychological Science. Used with permission.

lottery less than a month before the study was conducted, but the rest won it within a range of 1 month to a year and a half prior to the study), in spite of their good fortune, they astoundingly later had roughly the same levels of happiness as the nonwinner controls in the study. Further, those selected for the study because they were paralyzed with spinal cord injuries (for 1 month to 1 year prior to the study) reported happiness scores above the midlevel (neutral zone). Though this study is often cited as evidence for hedonic adaptation, it should be noted that the hedonic adaptation effect was most pronounced for the lottery winners and less so for those who were accident victims. In fact, even though time had passed for adaptation, the paralyzed participants still "rated themselves significantly less happy in general than controls" (Brickman et al., 1978, p. 924).

More recently Lucas (2007a, 2007b) examined archival data in a prospective research design of large representative panel studies (i.e., studies of cohorts of people who are followed across time) to examine the question of hedonic adaptation. Two panel studies, one with 40,000 people living in Germany and the other of 27,000 living in Great Britain, were assessed yearly for up to 14 to 21 years. He examined the extent to which people adapt to the life events of marriage, widowhood, divorce, unemployment, disability, and severe disability (Figure 2.2). As you can see on Figure 2.2, the level of hedonic adaptation, if any, depends on the nature of the life event. Whereas most people who married, experienced widowhood, or divorced eventually returned to their baseline level of subjective well-being, this same hedonic adaptation effect was not found for those who experienced unemployment or disability. The lack of hedonic adaptation was most pronounced for those with a severe disability. In fact, there was no rebound 7 years after their low point following their life-altering event.

Lucas does not believe that these findings refute the set point concept for happiness, but he does believe that contrary to the prevailing story concerning set points and adaptation, certain types of extreme life events can lead to lasting changes in happiness. As he states, the results "confirm that although happiness levels are moderately stable over time, this stability does not preclude large and lasting changes. Happiness levels do change, adaptation is not inevitable, and life events do matter" (Lucas, 2007a, p. 78).

There are, however, individual differences in how people respond to extreme negative events such as severe disability. In fact, many people are called **resilient** in that they "not only cope with the event, they often learn and are transformed by their experiences" (Dunn, Uswatte, & Elliot, 2009, p. 656). For example, Quale and Schanke (2010) found that the most common trajectory of adjustment in a rehabilitation setting to severe physical injury is a resilience trajectory, evident in 54% of the patients (average stay of 91 days) they studied, characterized by a low level of distress paired with a high level of positive affect at both admittance and discharge. These results support the contention of Bonanno (2004), based on his review of the relevant literature that most people confronted with life-threatening events or loss show healthy functioning and resilience. This is not to suggest that they did not experience some distress or grief, but rather that they display a healthy and timely trajectory of flexible adaptation following the event.

Those with disabilities who show resilience may also experience **positive growth** indicated by reduced anxiety and depression, enhanced well-being, and an uplifting of daily life satisfaction (Dunn et al., 2009) (see Chapter 3 for a discussion of posttraumatic growth). At-risk children who are resilient are said to exhibit "patterns of positive adaptation during or following significant adversity or risk" (Masten, Cutuli, Herbers, & Reed, 2009, p. 118). Their ability to bounce back from adversity and even **thrive** (i.e., to show vigorous growth or to flourish) are likely the result of these children possessing good adaptability to stress, good self-regulation, and personalities that enable effective problem solving (Masten et al., 2009).

In sum, though most people show hedonic adaptation relatively soon to most events, some extreme negative events may not be followed by significant upward hedonic adaptation during the same period. However, there are individual differences in this regard in that many youths and adults show an opposite pattern characterized by resiliency, positive growth, and thriving in the face of significant adversity. In fact, contrary to some of Lucas's (2007a, 2007b) findings, the resilience trajectory appears to be the most common way we respond to adversity.

Traits of Happy People

As discussed earlier, extraversion is a consistent trait characteristic associated with happy people. If you are an introvert, should you be worried? Does it mean that your happiness set point propels you toward unhappiness? Surveys consistently show that the majority of all people are happy (Myers, 2000; Myers & Diener, 1995), and that includes introverts. For example, Larsen and Kasimatis (1990) found that both introverted and extraverted

resilient: the ability to recover or respond positively to a negative event.

thrive: to flourish and show vigorous growth.

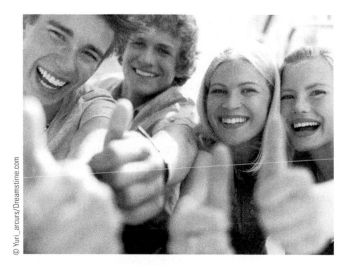

© Yuri_arcurs/Dreamstime.com

Studies consistently show that extraversion is the personality trait most closely associated with positive affect and happiness.

students rated themselves above the neutral level in happiness (as defined by pleasant mood) when they reported their daily mood states for a week—with extraverts reporting a slightly higher level. Thus, though there are many happy introverts, extraversion gives a person a slight advantage toward feeling happy. Why? There are many possibilities, but one common belief among researchers in the field is that extraversion, probably in part influenced by neurological structure, predisposes the extravert toward experiencing positive affect (see Chapter 6).

Even though extraverts are happier when alone or with others than introverts (Pavot, Diener, & Fujita, 1990), their positive affect is conducive to building and maintaining quality relationships that, in turn, can lead them to experience even more positive affect (see Fredrickson's 1998, broaden and build theory discussed earlier). Another trait, the trait of agreeableness, leads to more harmony in relationships and to higher levels of happiness (Malouff, Thorsteinsson, Schutte, Bhullar, & Rooke, 2010; Steel, Schmidt, & Schultz, 2008). A large recent meta-analytic review (a meta-analytic review combines and statistically averages findings from multiple studies) (Steel et al., 2008) found that the trait of agreeableness ranked second in happiness behind extraversion among the Big Five personality traits of neuroticism, extraversion, openness, conscientiousness, and agreeableness (Costa & McCrae, 1985, 1992) (see Chapter 6). Thus, extraversion and agreeableness seem to be traits that can boost happiness through their positive influence on social connections (see DeNeve & Cooper, 1998, for a review).

Interestingly also, meta-analytic reviews report that conscientiousness (self-disciplined, efficient) ranks number one as the Big Five trait with the strongest positive relation to *life satisfaction* (DeNeve & Cooper, 1998) or number two behind extraversion (Steel et al., 2008). Why would conscientious people be more satisfied with their lives? Perhaps it is due to their greater likelihood of achieving their goals than impulsive or undirected individuals (those with opposite trait characteristics). Further, the process of setting challenging goals and working steadily toward them can create *flow* experiences, a concept that is explored later, that lead to feelings of well-being (Csikszentmihalyi, 1990).

Also, as discussed earlier, neuroticism is a consistent negative predictor of happiness and well-being. Lahey (2009, p. 241) defines this trait as follows: "The personality trait of neuroticism refers to relatively stable tendencies to respond with negative emotions to threat, frustration, or loss." Individuals who score high in neuroticism are more prone to experience negative affect (e.g., anxiety, depression, anger, etc.), which, by definition, is associated with more unhappiness. Neuroticism is linked to many mental and physical disorders as well as to a poorer quality of life and possibly a shorter lifespan (Lahey, 2009). Often people who score high in neuroticism use ineffective problem-solving strategies such as rumination. Ruminators focus their attention on themselves and dwell on past problems and inadequacies while making negative self-evaluations (Lyubomirsky, Tucker, Caldwell, & Berg, 1999; Nolen-Hoeksema, 1991). This only serves to sustain negative feelings and perpetuate lower levels of subjective well-being.

Though the Big Five trait of openness to experience (adventurous, curious) sometimes positively correlates with subjective well-being, its effects are usually minimal and nonsignificant. When researchers measure the effect sizes for personality on subjective well-being they see a large overlap. For example, a recent metastudy (Steel et al., 2008) found that personality accounts for as high as 39% of the variance of subjective well-being.

What are the trait characteristics that define the *happiest* of happy people? Diener and Seligman (2002, p. 81) looked at those who scored in the top 10% of happiness in their sample of 222 undergraduates and found that they were "highly social," had strong social and romantic relationships, and "were more extraverted, more agreeable, and less neurotic." They further reported that "members of the happiest group experienced positive, but not ecstatic, feelings most of the time, and they reported occasional negative moods." Diener and Seligman's (2002) findings reinforce the general research observations of personality and trait characteristics associated with happiness and also show that even the happiest people still sometimes have bad moods.

Last, it should be noted that happy people are happy with themselves—they tend to have a positive self-esteem (Campbell, 1981). As Myers and Diener (1995, p. 14) noted, they are likely to endorse statements such as "I'm a lot of fun to be with" and "I have good ideas." Thus, self-acceptance and having a high positive self-regard appear to be important attributes associated with well-being.

Life Circumstances

As discussed earlier, happiness set point seems to account for about 50% of our long-term stable happiness, and life circumstances seem to play a minimal role. For example, Lyubomirsky, Sheldon, and Schkade (2005) estimate that life circumstances only account for about 10% of our long-term happiness

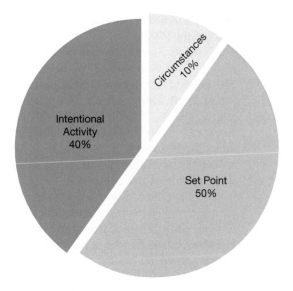

FIGURE **2.3** Sonja Lyubomirsky's estimate of what determines happiness: Life circumstances only account for 10% NOTE: Adapted from *The How of Happiness: A New Approach to Getting the Life You Want,* p. 20, by S. Lyubomirsky, 2007. New York, NY: Penguin Group. Copyright Sonja Lyubomirsky. Used with permission.

(Figure 2.3). They suggest that some circumstance variables may lead to temporary boosts in happiness, but that due to hedonic adaptation, these boosts will fade over time. Note that Lyubomirsky (2007) also believes that 40% of happiness levels are determined by intentional activities. These are discussed in Chapter 15.

In a review of the different types of influences on subjective well-being, Diener (1984) introduced the notion of **bottom-up theories of happiness** versus **top-down theories of happiness.** The bottom-up idea is predicated on life's circumstances influencing our happiness (i.e., the sum of our positive experiences)—all the things around us bubble up to affect our happiness levels. However, the top-down concept suggests that our happiness levels begin in ourselves, and as we look at our circumstances, we view them through our rosy or dark glasses. Given what you now know about happiness, which theory seems most valid, the bottom-up or the top-down theory of happiness?

Although it appears that the top-down theory accounts for most of our happiness levels (Diener, Suh, Lucas, & Smith, 1999; Lyubomirsky, 2001), we need also to be mindful that life circumstances may interact with top-down influences in a variety of ways (Headey, Veenhoven, & Wearing, 1991; Leonardi, Spazzafumo, Marcellini, & Gagliardi, 1999). For example, a person who values achievement (top-down) will be happier when getting promoted (bottom-up) than a person who does not care about getting ahead. It appears that only when we move toward goals that are in line with our motives (as opposed to moving toward goals that are not in line with our motives) that we have higher levels of circumstance-driven subjective well-being (Brunstein, Schultheiss, & Grassman, 1998).

Next let us look at some of the different circumstances—some of them out of our control—reviewed by Diener et al. (1999) of health, income, marriage, age, gender, intelligence, and education to see their relative influences on happiness levels. Does health have an influence on happiness? As discussed earlier (Lucas 2007a, 2007b), having a chronic severe disability can have a negative impact on happiness levels for long periods. There seems to be little hedonic adaptation for some. However, less severe health issues are more amenable to successful adaptation. Thus, when we are on the extreme end of Antonovsky's *dis*-ease side of the continuum (see Chapter 1) we are likely to have a lower level of happiness, but when we are on the *health*-ease side of the continuum we are not likely to experience added happiness. In other words, a person who is super healthy is not necessarily happier than a person who is just healthy. However, a person who is very unhealthy is generally less happy than a person who is somewhat unhealthy. It appears that good health is something we consider normal, so we seem to get no extra happiness bonus from good health though we get a lot of other benefits. Unfortunately, we do seem to get a happiness penalty from bad health.

What about the influence of money over happiness? Does money buy happiness? What do you think? Many research strategies have been employed to answer this question. These strategies used the following measures of money: the gross domestic products (GDPs) of different countries (Diener, Diener, & Diener, 1995), income levels (Diener et al., 1995; Myers, 2000), salary increases (Diener et al., 1993), and lottery winnings (Brickman et al., 1978) to name a few. One of the more interesting studies found that in spite of a steady increase in inflation-adjusted income from 1957 to 2002 in the United States, happiness levels stayed the same (Figure 2.4). The author of the study reported with irony that now "we are twice as rich and no happier" (Myers, 2000, p. 61).

When we review the results of the large number of studies on money and happiness, what is the take-away message? The message is not simple but is conditional. The results suggest that if a person is living in poverty and his or her basic needs for food, shelter, and safety are not being met, then receiving more money to provide for these basic needs can make an upward difference in happiness levels (Diener et al., 1999). However, the hedonic treadmill starts to take effect as income rises above this basic level.

The wealth of the country in which the person lives also seems to make a difference. As Diener et al. (1999, p. 288) noted, "wealthy people are only *somewhat happier* than poor people in rich nations, whereas wealthy nations appear *much happier* than poor ones." So overall, the *country's* wealth seems to set the conditions that determine how much influence its residents' *personal* wealth has on happiness. Seligman (2002, p. 53) also makes this point: "In very poor nations, where poverty threatens life itself, being rich does predict greater well-being. In wealthier nations, however, where almost everyone has a basic safety net, increases in wealth have negligible effects on personal happiness. In the United States, the very poor are lower in happiness, but once a person is just barely comfortable, added money adds little to no happiness."

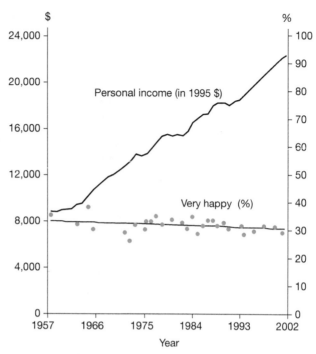

FIGURE **2.4**   Income and Percent of People Who Are Very Happy in the United States Over the Years

Even though income increased, the percentage of people who report they are very happy stayed the same.   NOTE: Income data from U.S. Commerce Department, Bureau of Census (1975) and Economic Indicators; happiness data from General Social Surveys, National Opinion Research Center, University of Chicago; data compiled by David G. Myers. From David Myers, Funds, Friends and Faith of Happy People, *American Psychologist, 55*(1), Figure 5, p. 61. Copyright 2000 by the American Psychological Association. Reprinted with permission.

Does marriage make a difference in overall happiness? Let us look at two conflicting sources of information. In the first, Myers (2000) reported that analyses of National Opinion Research Center General Social Survey data collected between 1976 and 1996 of 35,024 Americans revealed that nearly double the number of married adults (40%) stated they were *very happy* than never married adults (24%) (Figure 2.5). This seems to suggest that marriage leads to happiness. Do you agree?

However, before you reach this conclusion keep in mind that this study does not show us how marriage affects couples across time. Let us now look at a second source of information. Lucas, Clark, Georgellis, and Diener (2003) took data collected from 24,769 residents of Germany over a 15-year period. Within this group 1,761 were single and got married within the time of the study. The investigators were then able to track these individuals across time from before marriage to the wedding and thereafter.

The study revealed that on average most individuals got a very small boost in happiness levels after marriage, then adapted over about a 2-year

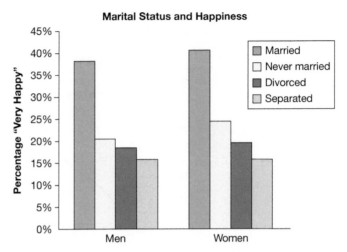

Marital Status and Happiness

FIGURE **2.5** National Opinion Research Center General Social Survey data collected between 1976 and 1996 of 35,024 Americans suggest that marriage leads to happiness. Is this an accurate assumption? NOTE: Adapted from The Funds, Friends, and Faith of Happy People, by David Myers, 2000, *American Psychologist, 55*(1), Figure 6, p. 63. Copyright 2000 by the American Psychological Association. Reprinted with permission.

period, and returned to their premarriage baselines (see Figure 2.2). Further, the study found support for the idea that "happy people are more likely to get and stay married" (p. 538). This finding probably accounts for some of the differences in overall happiness levels between married and unmarried individuals reported by Myers (2000). That is, happy people are more likely to get married than unhappy people, a self-selection process. The unhappy people who got married were more likely to divorce, again a self-selection process. So the unhappy divorced individuals dropping out of the married group would leave more happy folks in the married group. The greater number of happy people getting married plus the greater number of unhappy individuals not staying married contribute to an overall higher average level of happiness in the married group than the unmarried groups. This in turn can create a false overall impression that marriage generally causes happiness.

Lucas et al. (2003) also found that there are different trajectories for marriage with some people showing increasing levels of happiness, some decreasing levels, and others showing little change. The marriage partner's adaptation level seems to be based on his or her initial reaction to marriage, with the strongest positive or negative reactions to marriage leading to the lowest likelihood of returning to premarriage baseline levels for years to come. So if a person gets a big boost in happiness following marriage, there is a good chance that boost will persist. However, the norm is to get a very small boost from marriage followed by a gradual return to baseline.

Let us next look at the effects of age and gender on happiness. The effects of both appear to be negligible. Although general declines in health due to advanced aging may lead to reduced happiness, this can be offset by increased life satisfaction among older adults because these adults have had more time than their junior counterparts to realize many of their life goals (e.g., raising children, reaching career goals, and so forth). Gender seems to account for less than 1% of any differences in happiness (Fujita, Diener, & Sandvik, 1991). Women report that they feel all their emotions more intensely than men, so their more intense experiences of *both* positive and negative emotions balance their overall happiness levels to be roughly equal to those of men (Fujita et al., 1991).

What about intelligence and education? Surely they make a difference? Actually, studies have found that intelligence is not appreciably related to well-being (e.g., Watten, Syversen, & Myhrer, 1995) and that education is minimally if at all positively related to well-being at least in the United States (Witter, Okun, Stock, & Haring, 1984). When greater education is found to lead to greater happiness, it seems to be related more to indirect factors such as the fact that fewer educated workers live in poverty. You may be asking, "I thought income was not related to happiness?" Recall that living in poverty is linked to less happiness even though the correlation between overall income and happiness diminishes or becomes insignificant at higher income levels. Once the effects of income are statistically removed, there are no significant differences in happiness between the highly educated and those who have less education (Diener et al., 1993). Overall you can see why Lyubomirsky et al. (2005) estimate that life circumstances account for only 10% of the effects of stable long-term happiness levels.

OPTIMISM

I know that you have heard it before, the pessimist's creed—"I would rather be a pessimist than an optimist because when bad things happen I won't be disappointed and when good things happen I will be pleasantly surprised." Another justification you may have heard from pessimists is "I would rather be a pessimist than an optimist because I am a realist and I don't live with my head in the clouds." Do optimists see life through rose-colored glasses, unrealistically expecting the best? Are these people naïve or in denial? Which is the better life position to adopt, optimism or pessimism, to cope with life's inevitable frustrations, disappointments, and failures? Before we look at the evidence, let us first look at forms of optimism.

As defined by leading experts in the area, Carver, Scheier, Miller, and Fulford, "optimists are people who expect good things to happen; pessimists are people who expect bad things to happen" (2009, p. 303). **Dispositional optimism** is an enduring tendency to have global expectations of positive outcomes (Scheier & Carver, 1985, 1992). What we refer to as optimism can alternatively be seen as a type of **explanatory style** or a way in which people make causal inferences about why things happen to them (Peterson & Seligman, 1984). Optimists tend to see bad events as temporary, specific to the

dispositional optimism: an enduring tendency to have global expectations of positive outcomes.

situation, and caused by external factors (e.g., "We can chalk this one up to bad luck in this situation, but most of the time things go well."), whereas **pessimists** show the opposite pattern of seeing bad events as more enduring (e.g., "This problem is never going to go away."), global (e.g., "This always seems to happen to me."), and caused by internal factors (e.g., "If I were smarter this wouldn't have happened to me.") (Buchanan & Seligman, 1995).

Seligman proposed that whereas some people confronting stressors can learn to be helpless—known as **learned helplessness** (a passive state analogous to depressed states) (Peterson, Maier, & Seligman, 1993)—they also can develop the opposite, **learned optimism** (Seligman, 1990) (see Chapter 10). Persons in a state of learned helplessness believe that their efforts will not affect outcomes—they expect defeat—because they do not see a relationship between their efforts and results. However, people who learn optimism can begin to see connections between their efforts and outcomes, which then lead to a sense of hope.

With a few exceptions, the research evidence strongly suggests that dispositional optimism has advantages over pessimism for coping with stress and promoting subjective and physical well-being (see Carver et al., 2009 for a review). For example, presurgery optimism predicts higher quality of life and life satisfaction 8 months after coronary artery bypass surgery (Fitzgerald, Tennen, Affleck, & Pransky, 1993). A more recent meta-analysis (Solberg Nes & Segerstrom, 2006, p. 235) found that optimism leads to the use of more approach coping ("strategies aiming to eliminate, reduce, or manage stressors or emotions") and less avoidance coping ("seeking to ignore, avoid, or withdraw from stressors or emotions"), and this may lead to optimists' better adjustment to stressors. Further, dispositional optimists show less negative mood and biological inflammatory response to stress, "suggesting that optimism protects against the inflammatory effects of stress" (Brydon, Walker, Wawrzyniak, Chart, & Steptoe, 2009, p. 810). (See Chapter 4 for more discussion of the biological inflammatory response.)

Sarah Schneider (2001, p. 250) makes the case that *realistic optimism,* a form of optimism that does not "involve self-deception, or convincing oneself of desired beliefs without appropriate reality checks," is the preferred form. Realistic optimists have the following characteristics: (1) they give themselves and others the *benefit of the doubt;* (2) they *appreciate the moment;* (3) they seek *windows of opportunity;* and (4) they engage in *reality checks.* We will discuss the benefits of optimism more in Chapter 6.

learned helplessness: a passive state analogous to depressed states in which one's efforts are perceived as not affecting outcomes.

learned optimism: acquiring an ability to generally expect positive outcomes.

FLOW AND GOAL PURSUIT

Another important area of positive psychology concerns flow and goal pursuit. Have you ever been "in the zone"—that is, had the experience that you were so immersed in an activity that you lost awareness of everything else going on around you? Perhaps it was a time when you were playing a sport, dancing, or even rock climbing. During that activity, did time seem to fly by? Did you feel like being "in the zone" was a reward in and of itself? Did you feel like you had fully merged with the activity, become one with it? Like

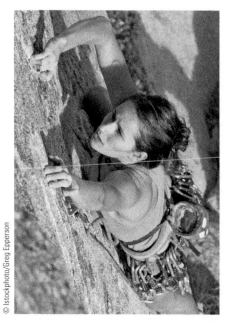

A rock climber in flow

water from a brook pouring into another clear stream, did you feel yourself merge and then flow with the stream of your activity? If so, you experienced what Mihaly Csikszentmihalyi (pronounced "cheeks sent me high") (1990) calls *flow*.

Though we tend to associate the phrase "being in the zone" with sports activities, the word *flow* extends to all types of activities that have these phenomenological properties. Csikszentmihalyi (1975) interviewed many people who experienced being fully engaged in their activities like dancers, chess players, rock climbers, and others, and based on his analysis of their common experiences, developed a model of what he first called autotelic experiences and later referred to simply as flow. **Flow** refers to "the experience of complete absorption in the present moment" (Nakamura & Csikszentmihalyi, 2009, p. 195).

flow: an experience of merging one's consciousness with an event in the present moment.

In order to increase your chances of entering flow, certain conditions must be present. These include:

- "perceived challenges, or opportunities for action, that stretch but do not overmatch existing skills;
- clear proximal goals and immediate feedback about the progress being made" (Nakamura & Csikszentmihalyi, 2009, p. 195).

The subjective state of flow includes the following elements:

- "intense and focused concentration on the present moment;
- merging of action and awareness;
- loss of reflective self-consciousness (i.e., loss of awareness of oneself as a social actor);

© Istockphoto/Greg Epperson

- a sense that one can control one's actions; that is, a sense that one can in principle deal with the situation because one knows how to respond to whatever happens next;

- distortion of temporal experience (typically, a sense that time has passed faster than normal);

- experience of the activity as intrinsically rewarding, such that often the end goal is just an excuse for the process" (Nakamura & Csikszentmihalyi, 2009, pp. 195–196).

Flow is *most* likely to occur when we engage in actions that push us toward the upper range of our capacities. We must be up for these challenges and feel some sense of mastery over them. If the actions we undertake are not challenging enough, however, we tend to experience boredom. On the other hand, if we feel overwhelmed by challenge, we are likely to experience anxiety instead of flow.

Why is the study of flow important? Flow gives us another perspective on how to live an effective life. For some, the setting of challenging goals and the process of moving toward them is what the good life is all about. In a study that randomly sampled self-reports (called the experience sampling method) of 78 adult workers throughout their day, Csikszentmihalyi and LeFevre (1989) were able to determine when people experience flow. They found that the majority of flow experiences reported were not when people were engaged in leisure activities, but rather when they were working. This was an apparent paradox because flow is associated with positive feelings and nonflow with negative feelings, yet when people were at work, many said they would rather be doing something else like a leisure activity. The authors suggested that cultural perceptions that work is not supposed to be enjoyable may undermine our ability to more fully appreciate our work-related positive experiences. Further, we may need our relaxation time, a period we look forward to, to recuperate from high-intensity work, even though low-intensity leisure time is not associated with as much flow. Thus, whereas engaging in activities that result in the experience of flow appears to be part of living an effective life, happiness and flow do not always go together.

Now, with over 30 years of research on flow, we have a much better understanding of its universality across cultures, gender, and age; in school, at work, and during leisure; and how it can lead to **optimal experiences**, that is, living life fully and in the moment (see Nakamura & Csikszentmihalyi, 2009, for a recent review of the flow research). We will briefly discuss more about flow in later chapters such as those dealing with job stress (see Chapter 9) and physical exercise (see Chapter 11).

Hope Theory

Hope theory was introduced by C. R. Snyder (1989) as a way to better understand how people move closer to their goals. In his formulation, **hope** is seen as a combination of cognitive pathways and agency. *Pathways* refer to the ability to envision one or more routes toward reaching a desired goal. And *agency* refers to the motivational trait-like perception that a wide range of goals will be pursued. Thus, "hopeful thinking requires *both* the perceived ability to generate routes to a goal *and* the perceived ability/determination to use those routes" (Rand & Cheavens, 2009).

Emotions are by-products of the endeavor of thinking about or moving toward one's goals and they serve as feedback regarding the perceived success or failure of the goal pursuit. Thus, people who perceive they are making good progress toward fulfilling their goals will have positive emotions, but those who perceive they are blocked or are making poor progress will feel negative emotions.

Some adults are more disposed to experience hope, and these people score high on the Trait Hope Scale (Snyder et al., 1991) though hope can also be measured as a temporary state by using the State Hope Scale (Snyder et al., 1996). Upon reviewing the research literature on hope theory, Rand and Cheavens (2009, p. 323) concluded that "higher hope corresponds with superior academic and athletic performance, greater physical and psychological well-being, and enhanced interpersonal relationships."

Hope seems very similar to optimism because both involve the prediction of a positive outcome. How then is it different? Bruininks and Malle (2005) sought to answer that question by more clearly differentiating the two concepts through asking their undergraduate study participants to define words such as *hope, optimism, want, desire, wish,* and *joy.* What they found, contrary to Snyder's definition of the construct, is that the *folk-conceptual* definition of hope is that of an *emotion,* whereas optimism is clearly viewed as *cognition.*

Further, based on their coding of the participant definitions provided, the two concepts are better differentiated along the two dimensions of *subjective likelihood* and *perceived control.* Along these dimensions optimism is associated with a higher subjective likelihood and more perceived control over a positive outcome than hope. For example, students can be optimistic about doing well on an exam after studying hard (high subjective likelihood and high perceived control) and also hope to win the lottery (low subjective likelihood and low perceived control). Hope has value in being a motivating emotion even in the face of long odds or to lift spirits when anticipating events that are not in our control. Conversely, it can motivate us to pursue unrealistic goals and needlessly expend valuable resources such as time, money, and energy toward futile endeavors. In these ways, it is similar to, though not exactly the same, as *wishing.*

MINDFULNESS AND SAVORING

The idea of actively cultivating conscious awareness and attention has roots in Buddhist traditions and is part of the practice of *mindfulness.* **Mindfulness** can be defined as "the state of being attentive and aware of what is taking place in the present" (Brown & Ryan, 2003, p. 822). A similar but slightly different definition of mindfulness is "awareness of the present with acceptance" (Siegel, 2010, p. 27).

Have you ever been on a road trip and found yourself several hours later when reaching your destination emerging from the blur of the drive to a more

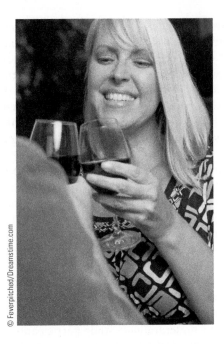

Think of a time when you engaged in savoring. What strategies did you use to bring a mindful awareness to your positive experience? How were you able to hold on to your savoring experience to prolong the enjoyment?

focused awareness of what you were doing? It is as though you were in a trance state while the car was moving only to awaken from the trance with sudden clarity and focus on reaching your destination. The trance-like state you were in during the drive was *mindlessness*—you were on autopilot—and the sharpened focused state at the end of the drive was *mindfulness*.

Mindfulness (Langer, 1989) is basically a type of conscious awareness. Some people are more disposed toward mindful states more often than others (trait mindfulness) though all of us can learn some voluntary control of mindfulness through practice, including the practice of mindfulness-based meditation (see Chapter 14). People who score high on trait mindfulness were shown through a series of studies (correlational, experimental, and quasi-experimental) conducted by Brown and Ryan (2003) to have an overall higher level of psychological well-being. High mindfulness participants tend to exhibit less depression, less anxiety, less negative affect, and more positive affect as well as to have a higher level of self-esteem than their low mindfulness counterparts. Brown and Ryan (2003) also note the results of their mindfulness-based clinical intervention, which showed that increased mindfulness was associated with less mood disturbance and stress in patients with cancer. For a more in-depth discussion on mindfulness, mindfulness meditation, and mindfulness interventions, see Chapter 14.

savoring: applying conscious awareness to enjoyment experiences.

A concept related to mindfulness is *savoring*. **Savoring** is about the process of applying mindful awareness to enjoyment experiences—that is, applying "a deliberate conscious attention to the experience of pleasure" (Bryant, 2003, p. 195). Although the idea of savoring has been around for centuries, Fred Bryant and Joseph Veroff (2006) were the first to investigate the positive benefits of savoring from a social sciences perspective (see Bryant, 1989). Whereas coping refers to our perceived control over negative emotions (e.g., fight-or-flight) among other things, savoring refers to our perceived control over positive emotions. Persons with a high capacity to savor are able to derive pleasure through anticipating positive experiences, appreciating the positive moments of these experiences when they happen, and reminiscing about them when they are over (Bryant, 2003). These people generally have a greater feeling of happiness (both intensity and frequency) and sense of life satisfaction; a higher self-esteem; higher levels of optimism and extraversion; and lower levels of neuroticism, depression, and guilt than those with a lower capacity for savoring (Bryant, 2003).

LOVE AND RELATIONSHIPS

When we think about our dreams, our hopes, and our aspirations of living the good life, we not only think about ourselves but also about other people and the meaningful roles they play in our lives. Recall Angela's story at the beginning of the chapter, who Sonja Lyubomirsky interviewed and considers one of the happiest persons she knows. What did Angela say about her life? She said that her daughter Ella "brings her endless joy," that Angela "made many friends" who "are a pleasure and support to her," and that "she finds deep satisfaction in helping others heal from their own wounds and traumas." In Angela's story we find many additional themes of positive psychology such as love, compassion, empathy, altruism, forgiveness, and gratitude. What do these themes have in common? They all serve to forge and strengthen social bonds and increase our closeness to one another. Like the study of the good life, these are universal themes with deep roots in culture, literature, poetry, art, music, religion, and philosophy that for the most part only in the recent past have been studied by social scientists.

By necessity, the discussion of these themes is brief in this chapter though many are reoccurring themes in subsequent chapters. As you might imagine, there are many theories of love, including the two-factor theory of love (Berscheid & Walster, 1978; Hatfield, 1988), love styles (Hendrick & Hendrick, 1986), and Sternberg's love triangle (Sternberg, 1986), to name a few. What each of these has in common is that they explore several dimensions or forms of love.

For example, the two-factor theory of love states that the primary elements of romantic love are passionate love and companionate love. Passionate love tends to predominate in the early stages of love and captures the "fall in love" component. Like someone who is staggering and "falling" from drinking too much alcohol, passionate love also has an unstable quality—the person is "intoxicated" with love. Companionate love predominates as the relationship matures. It is characterized by more stable, enduring friendship qualities.

Of course, there are many other forms of love besides romantic love. For example, there is the love a parent has for a child, such as Angela's love for her daughter Ella. Various forms of love seem to be involved in well-being and happiness. For example, one study (Hendrick & Hendrick, 2002) found that passionate love, friendship love, and relationship satisfaction were all positively correlated with happiness and that those who reported they were in love were happier than those who reported they were not.

Compassion is a feeling that we have when we witness suffering. According to Cassell (2009, p. 393), at its core, compassion "is a process of connecting by identifying with another person." He states that there are three conditions that are generally necessary for us to feel compassion: the troubles the other person is experiencing must be (1) serious; (2) not self-inflicted; and (3) we must be able to identify with the sufferer. This last condition relates to feelings of empathy for the sufferer. **Empathy** involves both identification and understanding and is believed to be the driving force for acts of **altruism**, the act of helping unselfishly. Altruistic people want to alleviate the suffering of persons they are helping. Though some believe that all behavior is motivated by self-interest, Daniel Batson demonstrated through over 30 experiments that pitted empathy-altruism acts of helping against egoistic (self-interest) motivated helping, that empathy-motivated altruism is a real phenomenon (Batson, Ahmad, & Lishner, 2009).

Forgiveness and gratitude research has expanded rapidly over the last decade. Both concepts link to positive well-being. **Forgiveness** is an act of giving up resentments toward those we perceive to have harmed us or another and letting go of claims for retribution or restitution. McCullough, Lindsey, Tabak, and van Oyen Witvliet (2009) note that forgiveness helps to restore relationships that are impaired by past aggression or conflict. Rather than engaging in an endless cycle of revenge and counter-revenge for perceived wrongs, forgiveness represents a prosocial tool for relationship restoration.

One study (Bono, McCullough, & Root, 2008) found that when people experienced normal fluctuations in forgiveness levels, elevated forgiveness was later followed by higher levels of psychological well-being in the form of greater positive affect and satisfaction with life and less negative affect and physical health symptoms. These findings suggest that elevated forgiveness may lead to increases in well-being. They also found evidence for a bidirectional relationship, suggesting that high well-being may lead to more forgiveness.

People with a greater tendency to forgive are generally more agreeable, more religious, less neurotic, less narcissistic (a trait associated with a sense of entitlement), and are better able to derive benefits from social support (McCullough et al., 2009). More forgiving personalities are less prone to exhibit hostility, anger, depression, and anxiety (Brown, 2003; Thompson et al., 2005).

Gratitude involves a feeling of appreciation for something good that another is responsible for bringing about. Those disposed to feel gratitude, like those disposed to forgive, are generally more agreeable, more religious, less neurotic, and less narcissistic (Watkins, Van Gelder, & Frias, 2009). Trait gratitude is an even stronger predictor of well-being and satisfaction with life than any of the Big Five traits (McCullough, Emmons, & Tsang, 2002; Wood, Joseph, & Maltby, 2008).

Interventions to increase gratitude include counting one's blessings (Emmons & McCullough, 2003; Froh, Sefick, & Emmons, 2008; Lyubomirsky, Sheldon, & Schakade, 2005) and writing a letter of gratitude to a benefactor (Seligman, Steen, Park, & Peterson, 2005). In each case participants who engaged in these acts showed increases in life satisfaction, well-being, or happiness, and letter writing also led to a decrease in depression along with an increase in happiness that persisted for up to at least a month.

Watkins et al. (2009) suggest that gratitude may benefit us through a number of different processes, including (1) enhancing our enjoyment of benefits because the benefits seem more special when they are perceived as gifts, (2) helping us focus attention on the good things in our life rather than what we are lacking because focusing on what we are lacking leads to envy and other negative emotions, (3) enhancing our social relationships because people like grateful people and give them more social rewards, (4) helping us cope better with difficult circumstances because we are able to focus more on the benefits of stressful experiences even though we are experiencing difficulties, and last (5) by enabling us to access more positive memories because encoding grateful memories gives us more favorable reflections on the past.

MEANING AND PURPOSEFUL LIVING

Why do we exist? What is our purpose in life? These age-old questions relate to our search for life's meaning. As you will recall from Chapter 1, Antonovsky's (1979, 1987) salutogenic model includes a *sense of coherence (SOC)* concept, and *meaningfulness* is the most important of SOC's three components (i.e., comprehensibility, manageability, and meaningfulness). Though there are many different definitions of the word *meaning*, Steger (2009, p. 682) defines **meaning in life** as "the extent to which people comprehend, make sense of, or see significance in their lives, accompanied by the degree to which they perceive themselves to have a purpose, mission, or overarching aim in life." From this definition we can see that meaning in life reflects both a cognitive component (comprehension) and a motivational component (purpose). And it is no coincidence that Antonovsky's SOC model also includes a similar cognitive component called *comprehensibility*. Purpose, the motivational component, relates to pursuing one's goals in accord with one's values. So purposeful living is living one's life in alignment with those values.

meaning in life: the larger understanding, significance, and purpose one sees in one's life.

Angela found happiness in spite of her past sufferings and disappointments because she created a meaningful life with purpose. Her personal meaning and purpose in life has its foundation in her relationships with her daughter Ella and friends. Steger (2009, p. 683) concludes that this is a common theme. He states that "across many studies, most people have indicated that relationships with others are the most important source of meaning in their lives."

As we can see, themes of comprehension, purpose, meaning, and coherence seem to interweave to form the complex patterns and fabric of our worldview that we can then apply not only to ourselves, but to others in our lives and to our relationships. From this worldview we gain a big picture perspective that promotes a better understanding of our place in the world and what we are meant to do with our lives. Numerous studies have documented that people who report that their lives have meaning or purpose find positive benefits including that they are happier, have a greater sense that they are in control of their lives, have less negative affect including depression and anxiety, have a greater sense of engagement at work without workaholism, are less

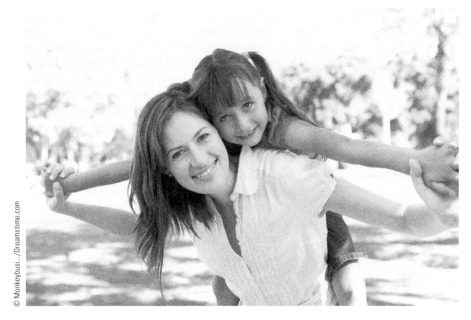

© Monkeybusi.../Dreamstime.com

Relationships are an important source of meaning in people's lives.

likely to engage in substance abuse, and overall report a greater level of life satisfaction and well-being (Steger, 2009).

No discussion of meaning and purpose would be complete without a discussion of spirituality and religion. **Spirituality** is defined as "a search for the sacred" (Pargament, 1999, p. 12), and **religion** refers to the practice of spirituality within the context of formal institutions. A person searching for the sacred has a desire for self-transcendence (i.e., going beyond one's normal self) or to form connections with a higher power, a divine being, or ultimate reality. Although the correlations tend to be modest, there is now a large body of research demonstrating that engaging in religious/spiritual endeavors is associated with higher levels of health and well-being.

In a review of the well-being research, Diener et al. (1999) concluded that subjective well-being is positively associated with how certain one is of one's religious beliefs and one's degree of participation in prayer and other devotional practices. They noted that participation in religion has psychological benefits such as, among other things, providing meaning and social support.

George, Larson, Koenig, and McCullough (2000) concluded from their review of the health and religiosity research that the practice of religion (e.g., attendance at religious services) was the strongest predictor of speed of recovery from illness or surgery, and that those who reported greater religiosity had lower rates of illness and had fewer deaths from heart attacks and cancer, which translated into an overall longer lifespan. In addition, they found that members of certain religious denominational groups tended to be healthier because their religions were more likely to promote healthier lifestyles and discourage behaviors that put health at risk (e.g., Mormons and Seventh Day Adventists).

spirituality: a search for self-transcendence or to form connections with a higher power, divine being, or ultimate reality.

A recent meta-analytic review (Chida, Steptoe, & Powell, 2009) that examined 69 prospective observational cohort studies found that religiosity/spirituality was associated with longer lifespans for initially healthy people but not for those who already had serious diseases when they entered the study. The beneficial effects for healthy people were especially pronounced for preventing early death due to cardiovascular disease. Reinforcing George et al.'s (2000) conclusion, the survival benefit appeared to be most strongly connected to participation in organizational activity such as church attendance. However, in part contrary to previous hypotheses, these researchers found that the benefit from religiosity/spirituality could not be explained by "behavioral factors (smoking, drinking, exercising, and socioeconomic status), negative affect, and social support" (Chida et al., 2009, p. 81). The authors suggested that religiosity/spirituality may enhance disease resistance perhaps through reducing sympathetic nervous system responsiveness to stress, but once a disease takes hold, it no longer has a positive effect on preventing early mortality.

Overall, then, the evidence is growing that engaging in religious/spiritual organizational activity confers positive effects on both health and well-being. Though the exact mechanisms for the health benefits have yet to be determined, the boost in well-being could be due to a number of factors including social support, meaning, and religious-oriented coping and practices (see Chapter 10).

CHAPTER SUMMARY AND CONCEPT REVIEW

- Positive psychology is the study of what people do right rather than what goes wrong.

- Western ideas related to positive psychology such as divine command theory, eudaimonia, and subjective well-being have deep roots and can be traced to the ancient Hebrews and Greeks.

- Fredrickson's broaden-and-build model and her undoing hypothesis explain that positive emotions have adaptive and evolutionary value by broadening our options and helping us build personal resources along with helping us recover more quickly from detrimental effects of negative emotions.

- Subjective well-being is determined by one's perceptions and emotions, whereas eudaimonic well-being is based on following certain practices or meeting particular needs.

- Some researchers believe that a happiness set point probably determines about 50% and life circumstances only 10% of our long-term stable happiness levels.

- Evidence for a happiness set point primarily comes from three lines—twin studies that show a large heritability influence for happiness, the remarkable stability of well-being levels across the lifespan, and the influence of hedonic adaptation.

- Happy people tend to be more extraverted, agreeable, conscientious, and social; they tend to have a higher self-esteem and are less neurotic than less happy people.

- The evidence strongly suggests that dispositional optimism, especially realistic optimism, has advantages over pessimism for coping with stress and in promoting subjective and physical well-being.

- The influence of happiness appears to be more top-down (e.g., determined by factors such as personality) rather than bottom-up (e.g., determined by factors such as circumstances).

- Money only appears to have a significant influence on happiness when a person is living in poverty or is living in a poor country.

- When pursuing a goal, having a flow experience is most likely when we engage in actions that push us toward the upper range of our capacities.

- Hope theory relates to goal pursuits with higher hope levels being associated with better academic and athletic performance, better interpersonal relationships, and positive health and well-being.

- Having high levels of mindfulness is associated with a host of positive health and well-being benefits; savoring also involves mindful attention.

- Love, compassion, empathy, and altruism are all important toward fostering and maintaining positive relationships.

- Forgiveness and gratitude are both associated with higher levels of positive affect, life satisfaction, well-being, and health.

- Meaning in life and purpose are important ingredients in happiness and well-being.

- Religiosity/spirituality is associated with positive well-being and longevity.

CRITICAL THINKING QUESTIONS

1. What can we learn from Fredrickson's broaden-and-build model and her undoing hypothesis about how to cope with stress? What do they tell us about the benefits of positive emotions in the coping process?

2. How do well-being issues relate to stress and health? If you were to map an optimal lifestyle and could only select three well-being practices, which would you select? Why?

3. Have you ever experienced flow? If so, how did you know? Was it a positive experience? Is flow an example of eustress or something entirely different? Explain.

4. Do you believe it is possible to change your happiness set point? If not, why not? Give your reasons. If so, what strategies would you use?

5. How do life meaning and purpose issues relate to stress and health? How do they affect your sense of optimism and perception control? How do they affect your experiences of compassion, forgiveness, and gratitude?

KEY TERMS AND CONCEPTS

Agency

Altruism

Bottom-up theories of happiness

Broaden-and-build*

Compassion

Dispositional optimism*

Divine command theory

Empathy

Eudaimonia*

Explanatory style

Flow*

Forgiveness

Gratitude

Habituation

Happiness

Happiness set point*

Hedonic adaptation*

Hedonic definition of happiness

Hedonic treadmill

Hope

Learned helplessness*

Learned optimism*

Life satisfaction*

Meaning in life*

Mindfulness

Negative affect*

Nonspecific action tendencies

Optimal experiences

Pathway

Pessimists

Positive affect*

Positive growth

Positive psychology

Psychological well-being*

Realistic optimism

Religion

Resiliency*

Savoring*

Specific action tendencies

Spirituality*

Subjective well-being*

Thought-action repertoires

Thrive*

Top-down theories of happiness

Undoing hypothesis

Virtue theory

MEDIA RESOURCES

CENGAGE **brain**.com

Access an interactive eBook, chapter-specific interactive learning tools, including flashcards, quizzes, videos and more in your Psychology CourseMate, accessed through CengageBrain.com.

3

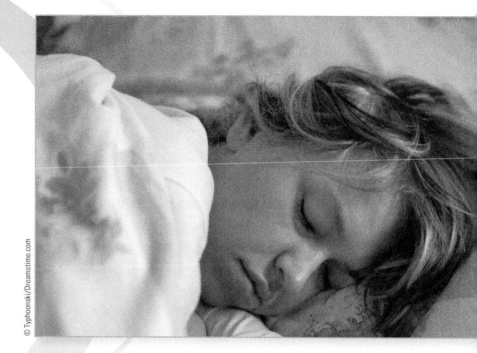

© Typhoonski/Dreamstime.com

Stress is when you wake up screaming and you realize you haven't even fallen asleep yet.

~UNKNOWN

STRESS AND THE NERVOUS SYSTEM

THE NERVOUS SYSTEM

STRESS AND THE ENDOCRINE SYSTEM

TRAUMATIC STRESS AND THE BRAIN

POSTTRAUMATIC GROWTH

It's late on a dark and wintry night and you have been drifting in and out of sleep beneath your warm wool blankets when a bang against your bedroom window awakens you. How does your brain respond to the bang? It first has to recognize the signal as important enough to wake you from your slumber. This process involves your brain's selectively attending to only meaningful stimuli, even during sleep.

Let's look at this attention process and what it involves. Every day we are constantly bombarded with visual (sight), auditory (sound), olfactory (smell), and tactile (touch) stimuli. If we did not use a selective attention screen, we would be so overloaded with processing stimuli that we would be unable to function. Therefore, our brain allocates attention through a gating process that allows in only meaningful stimuli and screens out the rest. So, for example, we are able to focus on what we are reading and block out extraneous visual and aural stimuli.

As we will soon discuss, your brain's thalamus selects which sensory information to send to your higher brain centers in the neocortex for further processing. The sound waves of the bang you heard are transduced (i.e., sound energy is converted to another form of energy) by your sense organs for hearing, and the transduced signal is then sent to your thalamus. Given that the bang is unusual and potentially threatening, its signal is important enough even in slumber to be sent through your sensory projection system for hearing from the auditory nucleus of the thalamus to the auditory region of the neocortex. The neocortex, which is associated with consciousness, in concert with regions of the hypothalamus and reticular formation, arouses you out of your slumber.

Your brain must interpret and organize stimulus information to make sense of it. This is part of the perception process. Your brain accesses and matches memories of similar events that were previously encoded by its hippocampus, such as memories of your neighbor's Siamese tomcat previously banging against your window late at night as it jumped up onto your outside window ledge.

Memory is a reconstruction, more like a painting than like a videotape playback. That is why memories can be altered through hypnosis or suggestive questioning methods. Our memories are shaped by our mood *states, our beliefs, our knowledge, and our expectations. Therefore, people who lived through the same event often share different memories and recollections of the event. For example, depressed individuals often recall the bad times, whereas happy people often recall the good times. Have you ever sat down with your brother, sister, or another loved one and recalled a birthday, wedding, or other event and had totally different recollections of who was present and the specific events that took place? These differences are not uncommon and are to be expected given the different ways we process and reconstruct our memories. Obviously, some individuals have more stressful memories of events than others even though they might have encountered the same set of stressors associated with the event. These memories then affect current experiences differently, depending on how the memories were encoded and recollected.*

When you hear the bang in the night, your higher cortical areas work quickly to access and integrate other relevant memories prompting you now to remember that a burglar was seen prowling your neighborhood in the late evenings. This is serious. Maybe it's not a cat but rather a cat burglar on the prowl.

Different brain areas, branches of your nervous and endocrine (i.e., hormonal) systems that are discussed more fully later in this chapter, are involved in your response. Suddenly your neocortex sends signals to your hypothalamus and limbic system to sound the alert. It's time for the fight-or-flight response.

Your hypothalamus sends an alarm signal down through the reticular formation to your brain stem and then to the organ systems of your body by way of the sympathetic branch of the autonomic nervous system to prepare you for action. It also activates your body further by sending signals to your endocrine system to stimulate your endocrine glands to release their fight-or-flight hormones such as the catecholamines epinephrine and norepinephrine.

Within seconds your heart rate, stroke volume, and blood pressure increase. Blood moves away from your skin and gastrointestinal (GI) system toward your brain and muscles. Your palms begin to sweat and your mind races as your brain becomes infused with new blood. In an instant you leap out of your cozy bed only to hear a cat growling at the window. Okay, no burglar, time to go back to sleep.

Some people have perceptual biases and are automatically inclined to think the worst. These individuals are likely to catastrophize when they perceive the stimulus event as potentially threatening. Thus, in this situation, the catastrophizing person will jump to the conclusion that a burglar made the noise and react with intense stress. Others may react with a bias in the opposite direction, minimizing the threat of the noise and automatically assuming that it must be the cat. These people may experience less immediate stress, but when a real threat like a burglar is present, they are slow to detect it. Later they will experience the stress of the consequences of their minimizing tendencies if their home is burglarized. Therefore, although the stimulus event may be the same for both the catastrophizer and the minimizer, their cognitions generated by their higher brain centers filter and ultimately determine their stress reactions.

Now it's time to try to get back to sleep. Your body's nervous and hormonal systems are revved up and now must use negative feedback loops to return to homeostasis. As your brain begins to shut down its fight-or-flight response and dampen arousal, in a graded fashion it shifts away from sympathetic activation to parasympathetic activation of your autonomic nervous system. Eventually, your body's systems return to their normal set points and sleep returns.

In your slumber you later float into a rapid eye movement (REM) dream state where you find yourself peering out a window only to see a saber-toothed Siamese cat looking lovingly back at you.

The alarm clock sounds off the next morning. Upon awakening you groggily climb out of your cozy bed and start your day with memories of a cold night and a cat that 100,000 years ago just might have been a lot bigger and a lot scarier than the actual cat at your window last night. Let's next take a closer look at the nervous system and its fight-or-flight response that saved our early ancestors from a cataclysmic demise.

THE NERVOUS SYSTEM

The human nervous system is complex and involves a myriad of structures and systems. Individuals who are versed in biology often find the discussion of the nervous system interesting and stimulating. However, others who are not biologically inclined may have the opposite reaction. If you are one of those whose eyes start to glaze over when reading about anatomy and physiology, you are not alone. However, there are good reasons to learn some basic biology when studying stress. As you know, stress and emotional reactions are intimately tied to physiological processes. To fully understand stress, you must have a basic understanding of some of the physiological structures and systems that are involved during stress. What follows is not intended to be a comprehensive survey of the anatomy of the nervous system, but rather an introduction to the crucial aspects of the nervous system that are related to stress. Gaining a better understanding of these physiological structures and systems provides you with the tools you need to enhance your learning of stress throughout the book. With that in mind, let us now take a closer look at the human nervous system.

The human nervous system (Figure 3.1) is divided into two main branches: the central nervous system (CNS) and the peripheral nervous system (PNS). The CNS includes the brain and the spinal cord. The PNS includes all the other neural pathways and is divided into two main branches: the somatic nervous system and the autonomic nervous system. The somatic nervous system innervates (i.e., supplies nerves to) the voluntary muscles of the body (i.e., the striated muscles like the biceps, quadriceps, etc.).

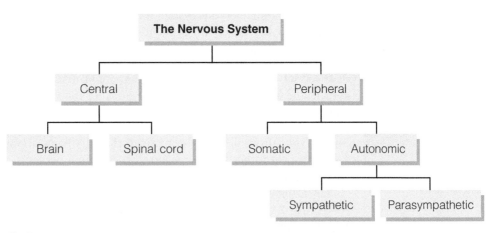

FIGURE **3.1**   The Human Nervous System

The central nervous system consists of the brain and spinal cord, and the peripheral nervous system consists of the nerves that cover the rest of the body (i.e., the periphery). The peripheral nervous system has somatic and autonomic subdivisions. The autonomic nervous system consists of the sympathetic and parasympathetic branches.   SOURCE: Garrett, *Brain and Behavior*, 2003, p. 76 (Wadsworth/Thompson Learning).

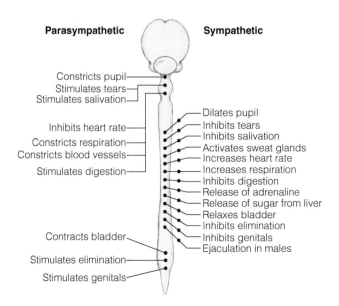

Parasympathetic — Sympathetic

Constricts pupil
Stimulates tears
Stimulates salivation

Inhibits heart rate
Constricts respiration
Constricts blood vessels
Stimulates digestion

Contracts bladder
Stimulates elimination
Stimulates genitals

Dilates pupil
Inhibits tears
Inhibits salivation
Activates sweat glands
Increases heart rate
Increases respiration
Inhibits digestion
Release of adrenaline
Release of sugar from liver
Relaxes bladder
Inhibits elimination
Inhibits genitals
Ejaculation in males

FIGURE **3.2**   The Two Branches of the Human Autonomic Nervous System: The Sympathetic Branch and the Parasympathetic Branch

Note that the spinal nerves of the sympathetic branch include the thoracic and lumbar regions (middle regions) of the spinal column. The parasympathetic branch's spinal nerves include the cranial and sacral regions (upper and lower regions). SOURCE: Garrett, *Brain and Behavior*, 2003, p. 78 (Wadsworth/Thompson Learning).

The autonomic nervous system innervates the organ systems of the body, the viscera. It has two main branches: the sympathetic and the parasympathetic. The sympathetic branch of the autonomic nervous system is what we most closely associate with the "fight-or-flight" reaction, like the one you experienced when you heard the bang in the night. Its spinal nerves include the thoracic and lumbar regions (middle regions) of the spinal column. The parasympathetic branch is associated with relaxation and restoration responses, the branch that was activated to shut down your fight-or-flight response and dampen your arousal once you realized that the bang at your window was caused by a cat rather than a cat burglar. Its spinal nerves include the cranial and sacral regions (upper and lower regions) (Figure 3.2).

The sympathetic and parasympathetic branches of the autonomic nervous system largely oppose one another in a smooth graded fashion. As one becomes more highly activated, the other is suppressed in a reciprocal manner.

Besides the two main branches, there is also a third, smaller branch of the autonomic nervous system that receives messages from the other two branches but can also function somewhat autonomously. This branch is called the enteric nervous system and it innervates the organs of digestion. For the purpose of our discussion, however, we will focus exclusively on the two main branches, the sympathetic and parasympathetic. Before we examine the autonomic nervous system and its sympathetic and parasympathetic branches, let us first take a closer look at the CNS.

Central Nervous System

The **central nervous system (CNS)** can be divided into the spinal cord and four major regions of the brain (Figure 3.3): the brain stem, the cerebellum, the diencephalon (i.e., the "between brain"), and the cerebral hemispheres. Of these neurosubstrate areas, the brain stem can be divided into the medulla, pons, and midbrain (i.e., mesencephalon). The diencephalon is subdivided into the thalamus and the hypothalamus. And the cerebral hemispheres, the largest area of the brain, are divided into the neocortex (otherwise known as the cerebral cortex, the convoluted gray outer covering of the brain) and its underlying white matter and the deeper structures of the basal ganglia, the amygdala, and the hippocampus.

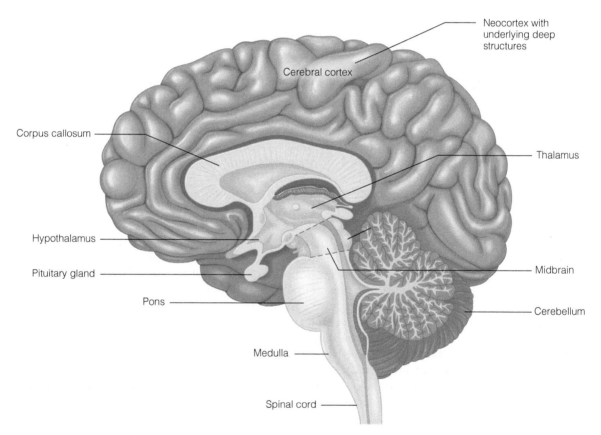

FIGURE **3.3** A Cross-Section of the Human Brain

Note that the **brain stem** consists of the medulla, the pons, and the midbrain; the **cerebellum** is a distinct area; the **diencephalon** consists of the thalamus and hypothalamus; and the **cerebral hemispheres** consist of the neocortex (cerebral cortex) and their underlying white matter and deeper structures (including the amygdala and hippocampus not shown here). SOURCE: Garrett, *Brain and Behavior*, 2003, p. 69 (Wadsworth/Thompson Learning).

Along with these regions, or parts of the brain, are particular systems and networks within the brain. Two of these are intimately tied into the fight-or-flight response: the reticular formation (RF) and the limbic system. The RF consists of nuclei (clusters of neurons) that run like a cable of fibers from the middle of the brain stem upward into the thalamus and hypothalamus. The limbic system consists mostly of the deep structure midline areas of the brain and includes the hypothalamus and parts of the cerebral hemispheres.

Let us next look at each of these areas and systems of the brain more closely. Before we do, it is important to remember that the brain has more than one functional region or pathway to achieve its ends. This capability is referred to as *parallel distributed processing* and is adaptive for our survival though it sometimes complicates our understanding of the role and function of the areas and systems of the brain. What follows is by necessity an abbreviated overview of our complex human neurological structures and systems relevant to our understanding of our physiological stress responses. For more detailed information refer to Kandel, Schwartz, and Jessell (2000) and Guyton and Hall (2006).

The Brain Stem   The **brain stem** (Figure 3.4) is responsible for many of the vegetative functions of the body (e.g., heartbeat, respiration, etc.) and consists of the medulla oblongata, which sits directly above the spinal cord; the pons, which sits above the medulla; and the midbrain, which lies rostral (toward the head end) to the pons.

The **medulla** of the brain stem contains vital life support centers that control autonomic processes such as heart rate, blood pressure, respiration, and digestion. This was the area of the brain responsible for increasing your heart rate, stroke volume, and blood pressure after you heard a bang at your window and perceived it as a potential threat. The **pons** (Latin for *bridge*) transmits information regarding the body's movement from the cerebral hemisphere to the region of the brain that fine-tunes and coordinates motor movement, the cerebellum (see Figure 3.3). Structures related to sleep and respiration also are found in the pons. Finally, the **midbrain** of the brain stem controls and coordinates many sensory and motor activities such as the auditory and visual systems as well as voluntary movement.

The **substantia nigra** in the brain stem's midbrain transmits important information to the basal ganglia, which is necessary for regulating voluntary motor movement. This midbrain area is unique in that it contains three of the brain's four major dopaminergic tracts. Its use of **dopamine** as a neurotransmitter contrasts with the more typical CNS use of the neurotransmitter norepinephrine. Dopamine in the brain is important for regulating motor movement. Also, dopamine is noteworthy because it is one of the "feel good" neurotransmitters of the brain that can elevate mood states and combat the effects of stress (see Chapters 6, 7, and 11).

The Diencephalon   The **diencephalon** region of the brain lies above (rostral to) the midbrain and contains the brain structures called the thalamus and the hypothalamus (see Figure 3.3). The **thalamus** of the diencephalon is located in

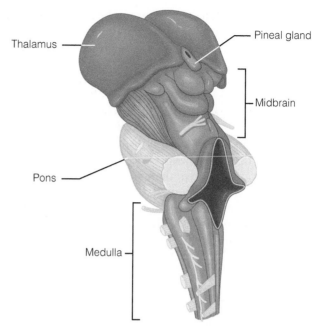

Thalamus

Pineal gland

Midbrain

Pons

Medulla

FIGURE **3.4**   The Human Brain Stem Connected to the Diencephalon's Thalamus

Note the major portions of the brain stem, starting from the bottom of the medulla extending from the spinal cord, to the pons, to the midbrain. From there it connects to the thalamus. The midbrain contains the substantia nigra, an area that is important in regulating voluntary motor movement. This midbrain area is unique in that it contains three of the brain's four major dopaminergic tracts.   SOURCE: Garrett, *Brain and Behavior,* 2003, p. 71 (Wadsworth/Thompson Learning).

the brain's central region and the diencephalon's hypothalamus sits below (ventral to) the thalamus.

The thalamus is an important sensory relay station that gates information from the sense organs (excluding olfactory) to the neocortex, the higher cortical regions of the brain associated with consciousness. When the thalamus opens the gate by increasing the **signal-to-noise ratio** or, in other words, by amplifying the signal to make it stand out against background noise, signal sensory information reaches conscious awareness in the higher center of the brain called the neocortex. For example, when you heard the bang against your window late during that wintry night, your thalamus opened a gate to allow the bang signal to get through to your neocortex because the bang represented a potential threat. At the same time your thalamus's gate blocked irrelevant sounds like the sound of your furnace fan blowing because it is not adaptive to wake up due to nonthreatening sounds. If your thalamus did not open its gate, you would have had no conscious awareness of the bang and would not have awakened. It is through this gating process that you were able to let in the meaningful stimulus of the bang and filter out and block from conscious awareness unimportant or insignificant stimuli.

sensory projection system: the circuit from a sense organ moving through the thalamus to its specific region in the neocortex responsible for the experience of sensation.

Each sensory system has a specific end point in the neocortex. The circuit from a sense organ moving through the thalamus to its specific region of the neocortex is called the **sensory projection system** for that sense. For example, from the ears through the auditory nucleus of the thalamus to the auditory projection area of the neocortex is the tract of the sensory projection system for hearing. The thalamus has a distinct nucleus for hearing, for vision, for taste, for the muscle senses, and for the skin senses that each relays its respective sensory information to its sensory projection target in the neocortex. Also, it is through the thalamus and its pain projection system to the neocortex that we experience the sensation of pain.

hypothalamus: region of the diencephalon that exerts control over fight-or-flight activities, fear and anger states, and a host of other functions.

The **hypothalamus** of the diencephalon consists of powerful nuclei that regulate, control, or are involved with most of the body's central and autonomic nervous system activities during the fight-or-flight reaction. This center for the fight-or-flight reaction became activated once you became consciously aware of the potential threat of the bang sound.

The hypothalamus exerts direct control over fight-or-flight activities during stress through influencing the brain stem to activate sympathetic responses of the viscera. It exerts indirect control through its connection to the master gland, the pituitary, to stimulate the endocrine system to facilitate a wide range of fight-or-flight responses. The hypothalamus is responsive to the neocortical command centers, including those involved with cognitions and emotional states, such as the frontal cortex (the outer covering of the brain behind the forehead). The primary emotional arousal states of fear linked to flight and anger linked to fight are strongly associated with the hypothalamus. Electrical stimulation of the posterior (back) region of the hypothalamus produces arousal like when you awakened from sleep after hearing the bang, whereas stimulation of the anterior (front) region and the adjacent basal forebrain region produces sleep (Roth & Roehrs, 2000).

Besides the fight-or-flight responses, the hypothalamus is involved in a host of other functions. For example, it is involved in normal homeostatic regulation of the body's autonomic systems through its influence over the brain stem. And it influences the hormonal systems through its neural connections with the posterior pituitary gland and through its use of biochemical peptide messengers, called releasing factors, to stimulate the anterior pituitary gland. Because of its rich supply of blood, the hypothalamus is able to monitor blood nutrient levels and body fluid volume. In this way it can influence our sensations of hunger or thirst, motivating us to eat or drink. On a general level it seems to be involved in the major motivational systems that we find rewarding. The hypothalamus also is involved in the homeostatic regulation of the body's core temperature by influencing the body's rate of metabolism. Furthermore, it regulates the body's circadian rhythms, the normal 24-hour hormonal and general biological cycle we experience (Amaral, 2000). Last, in addition to its homeostatic and motivational roles, the hypothalamus has influence over some of the skeletal motor functions (e.g., posture and locomotion).

The Cerebral Hemispheres   The two **cerebral hemispheres** connected by the corpus callosum (i.e., white matter in the center area that connects the two hemispheres and allows them to communicate with each other) (see Figure 3.3) consist of the neocortex, otherwise known as the cerebral cortex, and the white matter beneath it as well as the basal ganglia, the amygdala, and the hippocampus.

The six-layered **neocortex** is the highest center of the brain. The word *cortex* literally means "bark" and refers to the outside covering of an anatomical structure. This outside covering of neocortex gray matter is characterized by its wrinkles known as convolutions. The convolutions enable the brain to carry a greater surface area of cortex than would otherwise be physically possible. In fact, roughly two-thirds of the cortex is found within the folds of the convolutions (Shepherd, 1979). Due to the convolutions, the overall surface area of the cortex is surprisingly large at approximately 6.25 square feet (Mountcastle, 1979) given the relatively small surface area of the brain matter it covers. This means that the neocortex is able to house an enormous number of neurons. What does it do with all these neurons? It uses them for sensation, perception, emotion, movement, cognition, memory, organization, planning, language, and other processes, including other higher order functions associated with being human such as use of symbols and abstractions. This command center of the brain is associated with conscious awareness and what we typically think of as the *mind*. It is the area of your brain that became *consciously* aware of the bang and directed you to tend to the potential threat posed by the sound.

The basal ganglia of the cerebral hemispheres consist of four nuclei that are mediated primarily by the motor areas of the frontal cortex to control movement (DeLong, 2000). Though an important area, it is not vital to our understanding of our response to stress.

amygdala: region of the cerebral hemispheres and part of the limbic system responsible for mediating emotional responses, particularly fear and anxiety.

The **amygdala** of the cerebral hemispheres, however, is important to our understanding of our physiological and emotional responses to stress (Figure 3.5). It is part of the limbic system, which is discussed later, and is made of about 10 nuclei that are involved in mediating emotional responses, particularly fear and anxiety (Iverson, Kupfermann, & Kandell, 2000). How do we know this? We know this because people who have had their amygdala electrically stimulated report these emotional states. It is also involved in the social recognition of the fear state in the faces of others. Lesions of this area due to disease impair this emotion recognition ability. The amygdala also seems to participate in the process of storing memories about which stimuli should be approached and which to avoid. It seems to be involved in assessing threat stimuli and in emotional memory formation. Further, the amygdala participates in the process of classically conditioned fear responses where we learn to associate particular stimuli with fear or anxiety (see Iverson et al., 2000, for more discussion on the above findings).

hippocampus: region of the cerebral hemispheres involved in encoding declarative memories.

The **hippocampus,** named after the Greek word for seahorse because of its long curved shape structure (see Figure 3.5), has a more direct role in the memory process and is involved in encoding long-term memories of events that can be consciously discussed, termed **declarative memories.** It seems to have only an indirect role in the sensation and experience of emotion. The hippocampus appears to work with the amygdala in the fear conditioning process

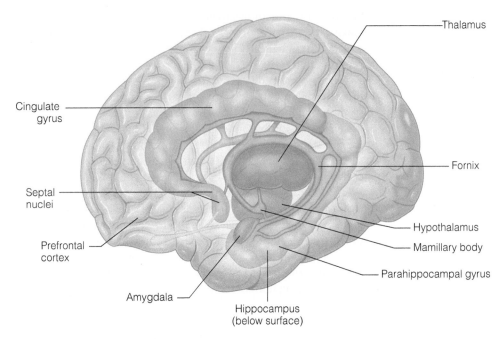

Cingulate gyrus

Septal nuclei

Prefrontal cortex

Amygdala

Thalamus

Fornix

Hypothalamus

Mamillary body

Parahippocampal gyrus

Hippocampus (below surface)

FIGURE **3.5**   The Limbic System Consists of Structures That Form a Ring Around the Inner Core of the Brain

This system is believed to be the brain's neural circuit for emotion. The limbic system includes the amygdala, hippocampus, thalamus, prefrontal cortex, parts of the hypothalamus, and other structures such as the cingulated gyrus.   SOURCE: Garrett, *Brain and Behavior*, 2003, p. 197 (Wadsworth/Thompson Learning).

by encoding context while the amygdala adds the emotion. Thus, seeing a poisonous snake behind glass in a zoo is a context that is not as frightening as seeing that same snake a few feet ahead of you on a hiking trail. It is the hippocampus that helps the amygdala put the threat significance of the snake in its proper situational context so that your amygdala adds fear to the experience of the snake on the trail but not to the experience of the snake in the zoo. Likewise, it is the hippocampus that helped you determine if the bang sound was dangerous enough to signal your amygdala to activate your fear emotions. Memories encoded by your hippocampus of your neighbor's Siamese tomcat previously banging against your window late at night as it jumped up onto your outside window ledge enabled you to eventually put the bang in a non-threatening context and resume your slumber.

The Reticular Formation   The **reticular formation (RF)** consists of a bundle of approximately 90 separate nuclei that run like a cord through the middle of the brain stem upward into the diencephalon. This network of neurons forms both ascending and descending pathways relaying important sensory and motor information between the brain and body. Sensory information from the

reticular formation (RF): a network of neurons through which the hypothalamus sends descending signals to the brain stem and the viscera to activate the fight-or-flight response; also serves as an ascending pathway of sensory information from the periphery to the thalamus.

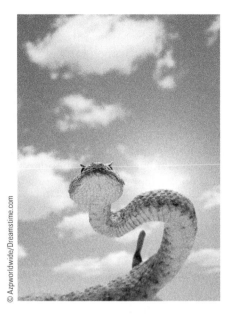

Your hippocampus helps your amygdala put the threat significance of this snake in its proper situational context as you encounter it on the hiking trail. As a result, your amygdala adds the fear to your experience, evoking the fight-or-flight response. If you saw this same snake in the zoo behind glass your hippocampus would signal your amygdala that there is no threat, so there is no need for the fight-or-flight response.

periphery is relayed in the brain's ascending pathway through the RF into the thalamus where it is gated to determine if it will be passed on to the neocortex as part of the sensory projection system. It is through the RF that the hypothalamus sends descending signals to the brain stem and the viscera to activate the autonomically mediated fight-or-flight response. The RF was also involved in rousing you from your slumber when you heard the loud noise at your window.

A small cluster of norepinephrine synthesizing cell bodies called the **locus ceruleus (LC)** residing in the dorsal brain stem region of the RF plays an important role in vigilance and arousal and is part of an ascending **arousal pathway system** that keeps the thalamus and cortex active in receiving and transmitting sensory information. This activation capability is especially important in facilitating the fight-or-flight response. Damage to the LC or other regions of the arousal system pathway that extends from the brain stem branching into the thalamus and hypothalamus can cause loss of consciousness. Overall then the RF plays an important role in transmitting arousal signals regarding stressful stimuli upward to the diencephalon and higher cortical areas as well as sending signals downward into the brain stem, viscera, and skeletal muscular system to activate the fight-or-flight response such as the one you had in response to the bang sound.

limbic system: the brain's neural circuit for emotion that includes the hippocampus, the thalamus, parts of the hypothalamus, the amygdala, the prefrontal cortex, and other structures such as the cingulated gyrus.

The Limbic System   The **limbic system** (see Figure 3.5) was first proposed by James Papez in 1937 and later extended by Paul MacLean (1949) as the brain's neural circuit for emotion. The system includes interconnected phylogenically primitive nuclei and parts of the neocortex that form a circle (a border or *limbus*) around the inner core of the brain. These structures include the hippocampus, the thalamus, parts of the hypothalamus, the amygdala, the prefrontal cortex, and other structures such as the cingulated gyrus (see Figure 3.5).

The **anterior cingulate** of the limbic system appears to play a major role in our emotional control system because of its extensive connections with the thalamus and its connections with other parts of the limbic system, including the amygdala and hypothalamus; it has been referred to as the "neurological hub of our affective control system" (Thompson & Thompson, 2007, p. 254). Current research suggests, however, that the hippocampus plays very little role in emotional states and that the amygdala plays an important mediating role between the areas of the brain involved with physiological expression of emotion and the conscious feeling of emotions (Kandel et al., 2000).

Lovallo (2005, p. 91) summarizes one of the adaptive roles of the limbic system in everyday life as one of appraising and reacting to potential danger: "The limbic system and its connections with the cortex help us form motivations to avoid things that are dangerous, approach and obtain things that are needed for survival, and remember motivationally relevant experiences for future reference. In cases of real or perceived danger, the limbic system, especially outputs from the amygdala, is responsible for integrating a state of fight-or-flight."

Thus, the limbic system played an important role in your fear response to the bang sound that you experienced when it seemed threatening, that is, before you were able to determine that the sound was made by your neighbor's Siamese tomcat.

The Peripheral Nervous System

The **peripheral nervous system** is comprised of both the somatic nervous system and the autonomic nervous system. The **somatic nervous system** innervates the **skeletal muscles** (striated muscles), the skin, and the sense organs. This bidirectional neural network transmits information from the brain to the periphery (the outer regions) and vice versa. The neural pathways that send signals from the brain to the periphery are called **efferent** and those that send signals from the periphery to the brain are called **afferent.**

In the somatic nervous system efferent pathways carry messages from the motor areas of the neocortex to the **striated** (red-colored) **muscles** to facilitate voluntary motor movement. Afferent pathways carry sensory information from the sense receptors to the sensory areas of the neocortex through the sensory projection systems. During the fight-or-flight response the brain sends messages through the efferent neurons to the striated muscles to tense in preparation for physical action. This is what happened when your brain directed your muscles to leap you out of your cozy bed in response to the bang sound. This is adaptive in the short run, but long term, as in many other conditions related to chronic stress, the mechanism can lead to health problems. For example, some people under chronic stress experience muscle tension-related headaches, neck or back pain, bruxism (teeth grinding), or other uncomfortable or painful skeletal muscle conditions related to chronic stimulation of the somatic nervous system (see Chapter 5).

The **autonomic nervous system** innervates the body's viscera generally through using both **preganglionic neurons** (those that exit the spinal cord) and **postganglionic neurons** (those that are stimulated by the preganglionic neurons). All preganglionic neurons use **acetylcholine** as their **neurotransmitter** as

norepinephrine: also known as noradrenaline, is a catecholamine hormone and neurotransmitter that excites the fight-or-flight systems.

do the postganglionic neurons of the parasympathetic branch. The great majority of the postganglionic neurons of the sympathetic branch use **norepinephrine** as their neurotransmitter.

The **viscera** consists of the organs, the ducts and glands, the **smooth muscles** (nonstriated muscles of the organs and blood vessels), and the blood vessels. Innervation of the viscera has both sensory and motor pathways. The sensory system of the viscera transmits information through the spinal cord and vagus nerve primarily to the brain stem and hypothalamus but not to the neocortex. Therefore, information about the ongoing state of our internal organs transmitted through this system typically does not reach consciousness. Likewise, the motor nerves in the autonomic nervous system originate in the brain stem and are homeostatically regulated without our awareness or voluntary input.

As discussed previously, the sympathetic branch of the autonomic nervous system is responsible for activating the fight-or-flight response, and the postganglionic neurons of this system have their effect on their visceral targets generally through the use of the neurotransmitter norepinephrine at the neuroeffector junction (e.g., the point where the neuron meets the organ). The targets of the autonomic nervous system's motor neurons include the smooth muscle cells as well as the **cardiac muscle** (heart muscle) and pacemaker cells (the specialized heart cells that create the heart's rhythms and therefore regulate its pace of contraction).

parasympathetic branch: the branch of the autonomic nervous system that damps down the fight-or-flight response and is responsible for the body's basal energy conservation and restoration state.

The **parasympathetic branch** of the autonomic nervous system is generally associated with the state of relaxation, and after a stressful encounter its activation serves to damp down the fight-or-flight response. As noted previously, the neurons of this system have their effect on their visceral targets through the use of the neurotransmitter acetylcholine. Most tissues of the viscera are innervated by both branches of the system. There are some exceptions; for example, the blood vessels and the adrenal medulla receive only sympathetic branch neurons.

Though it is common to think that only the sympathetic branch excites the organs (e.g., heart rate increase), that is a misconception. For example, it is the parasympathetic branch and not the sympathetic branch that excites the gastrointestinal system. The reason that some components of the viscera are excited by the sympathetic branch and others by the parasympathetic branch has to do with how the body's systems deal with threats to its survival. During normal resting nonstress periods it is more adaptive for the body to ingest food when needed, digest it, and store its energy. Without doing this, the body will not survive. However, during acute stress periods when there is imminent threat to survival, it is more adaptive to avoid ingesting food, stop digesting food previously ingested, and start mobilizing and expending energy; that is, to activate the fight-or-flight response. The parasympathetic branch supports the **basal energy conservation and restoration state,** and the sympathetic branch supports the **energy mobilization and expenditure state.**

Looking at it then from that perspective we see why the parasympathetic branch excites the salivary glands to make more saliva, the gut to alter the amount of its gastric secretions, the pancreas to increase secretion of gastric enzymes, the intestines to increase peristalsis (movement), and the bladder to constrict, all necessary for the intake and extraction of energy from solid food and from liquids. During the fight-or-flight response, the sympathetic branch damps down these gastrointestinal system responses. That is why a person may have a dry mouth and a queasy stomach, for example, before giving a big speech (remember John from Chapter 1 getting ready to give his presentation only to find butterflies in his stomach and a frog in his throat).

Also, from an adaptive perspective, the parasympathetic branch seems to be the gateway to reproduction and propagation in humans. For example, penile erection requires parasympathetic activation. Anxiety, which is primarily related to sympathetic activation, has an inhibiting effect on achieving and maintaining an erection. Although ejaculation is primarily sympathetic mediated, without an erection, it is unlikely that intercourse and pregnancy will occur. Therefore, the human body seems programmed to propagate more during nonstress periods, periods of abundance, and lower threats to survival. This makes sense for the primal environments of our distant ancestors because during these periods of abundance (i.e., low-stress periods) there was a greater likelihood of survival of their offspring that made our lives possible today. Let us focus next on the sympathetic branch and the fight-or-flight response.

Sympathetic branch activation during the fight-or-flight response results in increased dilation of the pupils for maximal visual access to threatening stimuli. Interestingly, our eyes also dilate when we see pleasurable stimuli, like potential mates, perhaps to maximize visual access also, though for obviously different reasons. The lungs experience bronchial dilation to maximize oxygen input into the bloodstream. The heart rate and **stroke volume** (the amount of blood ejected during the heart's contraction) increase while the blood vessels constrict, which has the net effect of cranking up the body's blood pressure to move blood more rapidly through the system so that it can oxygenate and fuel the brain and large muscles of the body more quickly. For example, the bang sound had a net effect of driving up your heart rate, stroke volume, and blood pressure.

The constriction of the blood vessels in the skin has a blanching effect so that the skin can look lighter or paler. In addition, the sweat glands become more active to cool down the body and keep it from overheating during action; that is why some people who are under stress experience sweaty and then later cold hands and feet. The adrenal medulla also receives stimulation during the fight-or-flight response, which prompts it to release epinephrine into the bloodstream, further exciting and maintaining the alarm response. A whole host of endocrine responses occur along with the epinephrine release, which we examine next.

sympathetic branch: the branch of the autonomic nervous system that is responsible for the fight-or-flight response and supports the energy mobilization and expenditure state.

STRESS AND THE ENDOCRINE SYSTEM

The **endocrine system** is a system of organs and glands that secrete **hormones** into our bloodstream that act as biochemical messengers to their respective target cells and organs. Upon reaching these targets, these hormonal messengers regulate activity of the cells they affect. Because the process requires the circulatory system to deliver the message to target cells, it is much slower than the almost instantaneous direct neural transmission to the target organs. However, once hormones reach their targets, their overall effect is sustained until these molecules are metabolized by the body. Whereas direct neural stimulation can be likened to the speed and shorter duration of a sprinter, hormonal action can be likened to the slower but longer term endurance of a long-distance runner.

Each has its advantages and disadvantages. During the fight-or-flight response the endocrine system and the sympathetic nervous system work as somewhat redundant systems to synergistically achieve a common outcome.

The Sympathetic-Adrenal-Medulla Axis

The primary command center for the endocrine's stress response is in the hypothalamus, and one of its primary target organs is the adrenal gland. By transmitting signals through the brain stem's nucleus of the solitary tract into preganglionic fibers of the sympathetic nervous system directly to the adrenal medulla, the paraventricular nucleus of the hypothalamus has a strong influence over this region of the adrenals. This **sympathetic-adrenal-medulla (SAM) axis** forms one of the primary systems of the fight-or-flight response.

The **adrenals** are cone-shaped glands that sit atop the kidneys. Each consists of an outer covering, the **adrenal cortex,** and an inner core called the **adrenal medulla.** Upon receiving neural stimulation, the adrenal medulla secretes the catecholamines epinephrine and norepinephrine. Because the adrenal medulla is stimulated by preganglionic fibers, it receives the neurotransmitter acetylcholine rather than norepinephrine that is typically secreted by postganglionic fibers in this system.

Epinephrine has a marked effect on the cardiovascular system, causing both an increase in heart rate and stroke volume as well as constriction of some blood vessels (the arterioles of the skin and abdominal viscera) and dilation of others (the arterioles of the skeletal muscles). The net effect is to shunt blood away from the outer periphery and digestive system and into the brain and large skeletal muscles. It also dilates the bronchi of the lungs to increase oxygen intake into the bloodstream. Epinephrine helps to stimulate the release of glucose (i.e., sugar) into the bloodstream from **glycogen** (long chains of glucose) stores in the liver and muscles and through a process called **gluconeogenesis** converts non-carbohydrate energy stores into **glucose** for use by the skeletal muscles. The net effect is an increase in the body's **metabolic rate** (the amount of energy expended by the body). In general, the hormone epinephrine has the same effect as the sympathetic nervous system on its target organs. For example, epinephrine injections given to treat severe allergic reactions can produce sympathetic pattern side effects such as a racing heart, nausea, sweating, tremors, headaches, and feelings of anxiety.

Norepinephrine has much the same effect as epinephrine on the body's systems. However, norepinephrine is released by the adrenal medulla in smaller amounts than epinephrine. The ratio of release is 1 to 5 of norepinephrine to epinephrine though this ratio may change under different conditions (Guyton & Hall, 2006). The effects of the *circulating hormone* norepinephrine last up to 10 times longer than the release of the *neurotransmitter* norepinephrine on the target cells by the sympathetic postganglionic fibers (Guyton & Hall, 2006). There is some research to indicate that epinephrine plays a much greater role in mental stressors such as mental arithmetic, and norepinephrine plays a greater role in physical stressors such as physical exercise (Ward et al., 1983). Also, epinephrine appears to be most closely associated with the emotional state of fear, and norepinephrine with anger (Ax, 1953). Although both epinephrine and norepinephrine have similar effects on the heart, the effect

sympathetic-adrenal-medulla (SAM) axis: a primary system of the fight-or-flight response that involves the hypothalamus commanding the sympathetic nervous system to stimulate the adrenal medulla to secrete the catecholamines epinephrine and norepinephrine.

adrenal cortex: the outer covering of the adrenal glands responsible for secreting corticosteroids.

adrenal medulla: the inner core of the adrenal glands responsible for secreting the catecholamines epinephrine and norepinephrine.

epinephrine: also known as adrenaline, is a catecholamine hormone secreted by the adrenal medulla that has a marked effect on the cardiovascular system, stimulates the release of glucose into the blood stream, and increases the body's metabolic rate.

is greater with epinephrine. Epinephrine also produces 5 to 10 times the acceleration of the body's metabolic rate compared to norepinephrine and is capable of more than doubling the body's normal rate (Guyton & Hall, 2006).

The Hypothalamic-Pituitary-Adrenal Axis

During the fight-or-flight response, the adrenal cortex is involved in a system referred to as the **hypothalamic-pituitary-adrenal (HPA) axis** (Figure 3.6). In this system the hypothalamus influences the adrenal cortex by way of the **pituitary gland,** the pea-sized master gland at the base of the brain. The pituitary gland, like the adrenal gland, is a structure with two glandular regions with separate functions. However, unlike the adrenal gland, which is divided into an inner and an outer region, the pituitary gland is divided into an anterior and a posterior region. The paraventricular nucleus of the hypothalamus responds to stressors in part by synthesizing and secreting peptide messengers called releasing factors that are released into the **pituitary portal system** of the **anterior pituitary.** These messengers stimulate the anterior pituitary to secrete beta-endorphin and adrenocorticotropic hormone (ACTH) into the bloodstream. **Beta-endorphin** is a natural opiate that has strong analgesic (pain-relieving) properties. In an imminent life-threatening struggle with a predator or competitor, pain from acute injury could debilitate a person and prevent him or her from escaping the threat. Therefore, it is more adaptive for a person's survival to have systems that temporarily inhibit pain until the person is safe from imminent threat. Beta-endorphin serves this purpose.

ACTH stimulates the adrenal cortex to release glucocorticoids, which play an important role in the fight-or-flight response. **Glucocorticoids** are a family of steroid compounds that were so named because of their effect of raising glucose levels in the bloodstream. The primary glucocorticoid secreted by the adrenal cortex is **cortisol** (known also as hydrocortisone), which accounts for over 95% of the effects on the body of this class of steroids (Guyton & Hall, 2006). Cortisol is needed by cells for normal cellular function. Like epinephrine, it affects metabolism through the process of gluconeogenesis. It also somewhat reduces glucose use at the cellular level. The combined effect of gluconeogenesis and reduced cellular use of glucose is to increase the overall glucose concentration in the bloodstream.

Cortisol also promotes the liberation of fatty acids from fat stores in a process known as **lipolysis** for use as a fuel source and increases concentrations of blood **amino acids** (protein-building blocks) in the bloodstream so they can be converted into glucose by the liver for muscle energy. This important steroid readies stress responses by increasing catecholamine synthesis at the neuronal level and by the adrenal medulla. It can sharpen memory functions of the hippocampus and increase sensitivity of the thalamus to sensory inputs.

In addition, cortisol reduces inflammation and plays a role through a **negative feedback loop** in regulating CNS excesses. This damping down action, however, can lead to the unwanted effect of a cortisol-mediated suppression of the immune system under conditions of chronic stress, discussed in more depth in Chapter 4. Along with psychological stressors, physical stressors such as intense heat and cold, surgical operations, and the experience of disease states all increase cortisol levels.

---

hypothalamic-pituitary-adrenal (HPA) axis: a primary system of the fight-or-flight response that involves the hypothalamus influencing the pituitary gland to secrete ACTH that in turn stimulates the adrenal cortex to release glucocorticoids.

ACTH: adrenocorticotropic hormone released by the anterior pituitary and responsible for stimulating the adrenal cortex to release glucocorticoids.

cortisol: the body's primary glucocorticoid secreted by the adrenal cortex during the fight-or-flight response that raises glucose levels in the bloodstream, increases catecholamine synthesis, and reduces inflammation.

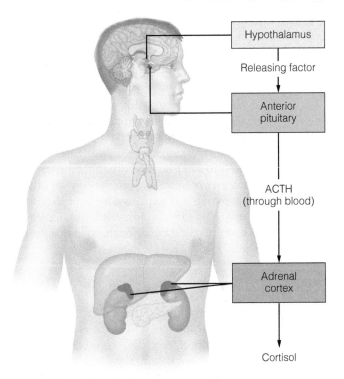

FIGURE **3.6** The Hypothalamic-Pituitary-Adrenal (HPA) Axis Network

The hypothalamus via the pituitary portal system of the anterior pituitary causes the release of ACTH, which stimulates the adrenal cortex to release cortisol, which through a process called gluconeogenesis increases the overall glucose concentration in the bloodstream and speeds metabolism.   SOURCE: Garrett, *Brain and Behavior*, 2003, p. 201 (Wadsworth/Thompson Learning).

The Thyroxine Axis

Because stress produces a demand on our biological systems, in order for the cells in the system to meet the demand, they must increase their fuel-burning capacity or metabolic rate. Most cells in the body depend on thyroxine, a thyroid gland hormone, to regulate their metabolic rate. **Thyroxine** is a strong hormone that can, with time and sufficient concentration levels, double basal metabolic rate. These increases in metabolic rate are more adaptive for dealing with more prolonged threats to survival than acute threats because there is a latent period of 2 to 3 days before thyroxine exerts its effect on cellular metabolism. However, once these changes begin to occur there is a progressive increase in metabolism until rates reach a peak and begin to level off after 10 to 12 days (Guyton & Hall, 2006).

Like the SAM and HPA axes, the action for the thyroxine axis begins with the hypothalamus. The paraventricular nucleus of the hypothalamus responds to the demands on our systems to increase metabolism by releasing a polypeptide messenger-releasing factor into the portal system of the anterior pituitary. This biochemical messenger prompts the anterior pituitary to release a compound called **thyroid-stimulating hormone (TSH)**. TSH then travels through the bloodstream to the **thyroid gland,** a gland shaped like a butterfly that sits just below the larynx (the Adam's apple is a good outer reference point for the larynx), prompting the release of thyroxine.

High levels of thyroxine can produce feelings of nervousness or anxiety, insomnia, increased heart rate, increased respiration leading to a sensation of shortness of breath, excessive sweating, diarrhea (due to increased gastric secretions and motility), and feelings of tiredness. The hormone can also amplify the effects of epinephrine, causing persons to experience more intense stress reactions to acute stressors than their normal reactions. Given its longevity and staying power relative to the majority of other stress-related hormones, the effects of thyroxine may explain why some individuals under chronic stress have difficulty returning to baseline levels once they leave a stressful environment. For example, some people have difficulty relaxing even during a 1- or 2-week vacation.

TRAUMATIC STRESS AND THE BRAIN

Sometimes stressors are much more severe than a loud bang in the night. The following section examines the effects of severe stressors on the brain. Examining the effects of traumatic stress can illustrate how the brain reacts to extreme stress and help us better understand how it functions following severe adversity.

What are traumatic stressors? **Traumatic stressors** are events such as combat; natural or human-made disasters; violent assault; sexual assault; kidnapping; torture; serious or life- threatening accidents; a life-threatening diagnosis; a close friend or relative dying suddenly and unexpectedly; being held captive perhaps as a prisoner of war (POW) or in a concentration camp; or other highly distressing experiences that can result in feelings of terror, extreme fright, or helplessness.

As is the case with all stressors, a person's reaction to severe stressors is individualistic and subjective, in part, because each person appraises the stressors through the lens of his or her own belief system or worldview. An encounter with traumatic stressors often poses a serious challenge to one's worldview. A person's **worldview** is a collection of assumptions and beliefs about oneself, others, and the world. Tedeschi and Calhoun (2004) liken an encounter with a traumatic stressor to an encounter with an earthquake in which "a psychologically seismic event can severely shake, threaten, or reduce to rubble many of the schematic structures that have guided understanding, decision making, and meaningfulness" (p. 5). Assumptions regarding safety and security are likely to be seriously disturbed or undermined and may result in a shattering or shakeup of a survivor's pretrauma worldview. How a person adapts to these challenges determines how transient or chronic the trauma reactions and symptoms may be.

Unfortunately for some, the reaction to traumatic stressors may result in the development of a **posttraumatic stress disorder (PTSD)**. PTSD is characterized by a number of symptoms including persistently reexperiencing the traumatic event, avoiding stimuli correlated with the traumatic event, experiencing a general response numbing, and having persistent increased arousal; the duration of

posttraumatic stress disorder (PTSD): a psychological disorder stemming from a reaction to traumatic stressors characterized by persistently reexperiencing the traumatic event, avoiding stimuli correlated with the event, experiencing a general response numbing, and having persistent increased arousal.

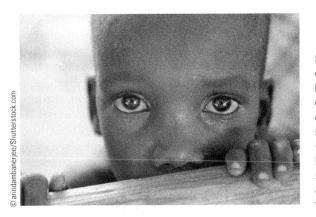

© arindambanerjee/Shutterstock.com

Surviving the magnitude 7.0 earthquake of 2010 in Haiti like this child did is the type of traumatic stressor that can produce posttraumatic stress disorder (PTSD). Other traumatic stressors have been likened to seismic events in that they can shake our worldviews.

the overall symptom pattern lasts at least a month, and there is distress or impairment in one or more primary areas of functioning (American Psychiatric Association, 2000).

What part of the brain appears to be most affected by PTSD? There is considerable evidence, including research from brain imaging studies, suggesting that the brain's limbic system is the area most affected because it functions abnormally in many people with PTSD (Handwerger & Shin, 2008). In particular, for people with PTSD, the limbic system's amygdala appears to overreact (i.e., hyperrespond), yet the anterior cingulated cortex (ACC) (a part of the cerebral cortex) and hippocampus appear to under-react (i.e., hyporespond) to certain stimuli.

Results of amygdala studies show that the higher the amygdala responsiveness to such stimuli, the higher the symptom severity for individuals with PTSD. In addition, both the ACC and the hippocampus show diminished size (Karl et al., 2006). Such abnormalities of limbic structures and functions help to explain some of the symptoms associated with PTSD, such as problems with memory, fear, anger, and hyperarousal. At this stage in the research, however, it is difficult to determine whether some of the structural abnormalities found are preexisting conditions that predispose a person to PTSD when exposed to traumatic stressors or whether these abnormalities are due to the PTSD—though there is twin study research suggesting that the smaller hippocampus volume may be a preexisting risk factor for PTSD (see Handwerger & Shin, 2008, for more discussion of the limbic system abnormalities and PTSD).

As discussed earlier in the chapter, the amygdala is involved in assessing threat stimuli, in emotional memory formation, and in conditioned fear responses. Remember, it adds the fear to the experience of seeing a stimulus like a poisonous snake on a hiking trail. Because the amygdala is more likely to be hyperresponsive for people with PTSD, this could account for their persistent increased arousal symptom patterns. Examples of arousal symptoms associated with PTSD include insomnia, poor concentration, hypervigilance (i.e., constantly being on the alert for threat or danger), angry outbursts and irritability, and an exaggerated startle response (i.e., becoming alarmed or jumpy when surprised suddenly).

The ACC and surrounding cortex function to process emotional information, to extinguish conditioned fear, and to regulate emotional responses. Therefore, retention of exaggerated fear responses to trauma-related stimuli beyond the period when these responses would normally fade or extinguish may be a function of the ACC's hyporesponsiveness.

Finally, as discussed earlier in the chapter, the hippocampus is involved in encoding declarative memories as well as working with the amygdala in the fear conditioning process by encoding context to threatening stimuli. A hyporesponsive hippocampus could account for some of the memory problems associated with PTSD such as experiencing recurring distressing memories of the trauma or flashbacks (e.g., feelings of reliving the trauma), exaggerated psychological and physiological responses to stimuli that symbolize or have similar characteristics to the traumatic stressors, and difficulties recalling significant aspects of the traumatic event. In other words, memory glitches and a reduced ability to contextualize benign stimuli that are correlated with the traumatic event (e.g., the sound of a car backfiring can be experienced with the same fear as the sound of a gun firing) could be the result of the hippocampus being underpowered.

Symptom improvement following therapy has been shown to be associated with reductions in amygdala activity and greater activation of the perigenual section of the ACC, the section associated with emotional information processing and response regulation (Felmingham et al., 2007). These results provide even more evidence of a causal pathway between abnormal limbic system activity and PTSD because in a reverse of the process, reducing PTSD results in reducing abnormal limbic system activity. Thus, the evidence appears compelling that exposure to traumatic stressors that results in PTSD adversely affects the limbic system.

POSTTRAUMATIC GROWTH

Is there anything positive that can result from encounters with traumatic stressors? As we have seen, unfortunate consequences such as developing PTSD can result from such encounters. No one would welcome a major earthquake, but if it does occur, can anything good come of it? Counter to our intuition, studies have found that seismic events in the form of traumatic stressors can ultimately result in some clearing of debris and subsequent building of stronger foundations and structures for our worldview and outlook on life.

Victor Frankl (1992, p. 116), founder of logotherapy—a form of existential psychotherapy, and a World War II concentration camp survivor, discussed finding meaning out of his suffering and tragedy and that of others who experienced the trauma of the concentration camp: "We must never forget that we may also find meaning in life even when confronted with a hopeless situation, when facing a fate that cannot be changed. For what matters then is to bear witness to the uniquely human potential at its best, which is to transform personal tragedy into a triumph—to turn one's predicament into a human achievement. When we are no longer able to change a situation—just think of an incurable disease such as inoperable cancer—we are challenged to change ourselves."

Frankl had experiences of personal meaning as he worked in a concentration camp when he thought about his wife who had been sent to another camp and put to her death without him knowing whether she survived or not.

> Another time we were at work in a trench. The dawn was grey around us; grey was the sky above; grey the snow in the pale light of dawn; grey the rags in which my fellow prisoners were clad, and grey their faces. I was again conversing silently with my wife, or perhaps I was struggling to find the *reason* for my sufferings, my slow dying. In a last violent protest against the hopelessness of imminent death, I sensed my spirit piercing through the enveloping gloom. I felt it transcend that hopeless, meaningless world, and from somewhere I heard a victorious "Yes" in answer to my question of the existence of an ultimate purpose. At that moment a light was lit in a distant farmhouse, which stood on the horizon as if painted there, in the midst of the miserable grey of a dawning in Bavaria. *"Et lux in tenebris lucet"*—and the light shineth in the darkness. For hours I stood hacking at the icy ground. The guard passed by, insulting me, and once again I communed with my beloved. More and more I felt that she was present, that she was with me; I had the feeling that I was able to touch her, able to stretch out my hand and grasp hers. The feeling was very strong: she was *there*. Then, at that very moment, a bird flew down silently and perched just in front of me, on the heap of soil which I had dug up from the ditch, and looked steadily at me. (pp. 51–52)

As Victor Frankl shows us, not everyone suffers from PTSD or other impairments in ability to function following trauma. In fact, only a minority develop PTSD (Charney, 2004). Some like Frankl may even have transcendent experiences or find meaning in suffering. In the days following the experience of psychological trauma, individuals may have at minimum subclinical symptoms or brief reactive symptoms (less intense or temporary symptoms than would be associated with PTSD), though they may have no long-term resulting functional impairment. In time, a certain percentage of people exposed to traumatic events ultimately experience positive changes (Ford, 2008). These individuals are said to have experienced **posttraumatic growth.**

posttraumatic growth: a positive response to trauma usually characterized by strengthening of relationships and development of more positive self and world views.

Posttraumatic growth is usually reported by trauma survivors who experience it as having three interrelated themes: (1) relationships are strengthened or enhanced, (2) self-views become more positive, and (3) worldviews or life philosophies are changed in positive directions (Linley & Joseph, 2004, 2008). For example, survivors may feel more compassion, altruism, and gratitude toward friends and family. They may have a greater sense of resiliency and personal strength along with a greater acceptance of their personal limitations. In addition, they may view life and their world with a greater sense of appreciation. In general posttraumatic growth seems to be associated with a perception that one has experienced a high level of threat or harm and has been able to exert some control over the traumatic events or outcomes.

Posttraumatic growth does not appear to be a mere polar opposite of PTSD, but rather a product of successful adaptation to trauma that may emerge independently from any point on the stress reaction continuum. Some describe the experience as having been given a second chance. There may be greater mindfulness of everyday experiences that had been taken for

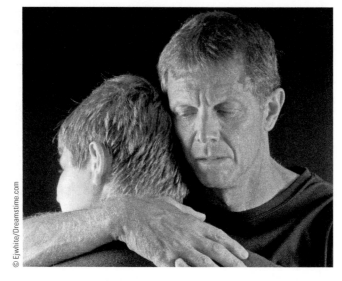

© Ejwhite/Dreamstime.com

Survivors of trauma may feel more compassion, altruism, and gratitude toward friends and family.

granted previously. Relationships and opportunities may be valued more highly. Individuals may report greater clarity of purpose, meaning, or direction in life.

Though the research on posttraumatic growth points toward some positive outcomes for those who experience traumatic events, there are a number of methodological issues that raise concerns about the validity of many of the posttraumatic growth studies. For example, Ford (2008) points out that the instruments used to measure posttraumatic growth involve self-report of retrospective recollections (retrospective memory is inherently unreliable) and that some of these paper and pencil measures only enable recording of positive outcomes. Thus, there may be biased recollections that lead to overreporting positive changes because the participants are not asked about negative changes.

Ford further expresses concern that alternative explanations for changes rather than trauma-induced growth may explain reported experiences such as feeling closer to friends and family more accurately. For example, the traumatic event may have caused significant others to offer more social support that in turn led to greater feelings of closeness rather than that the event caused the person suffering from trauma to grow in ways that led to greater closeness.

Finally, Ford notes that wishful thinking, positive reappraisals, or *positive illusions* may help a person cope by thinking that change and growth have occurred when they have not. **Positive illusions,** a term coined by Taylor and Brown (1988) to refer to unrealistic positive beliefs, may give a person a greater sense of control to cope with the negative impact of the trauma and may be adaptive short term but not result in actual growth.

In spite of these potential limitations, we should be mindful of the fact that this area of study is still relatively new and construct validity and methodological issues regarding posttraumatic growth still need to be sorted out. Nevertheless, the research findings show promising new directions for understanding the effects of traumatic stressors that had been previously understudied. Longitudinal studies with good baselines along with brain imaging research as has been used for studying PTSD would give new confidence to our understanding of how people may not only survive trauma but eventually grow and benefit from the experience, leading us to understand better Friedrich Nietzsche's quote—*what doesn't kill us makes us stronger.*

CHAPTER SUMMARY AND CONCEPT REVIEW

- There are two main branches of our nervous system: the central nervous system (CNS) and the peripheral nervous system (PNS).

- The CNS includes the brain and spinal cord, and the PNS includes all the other neural pathways that then divide into the somatic nervous system and the autonomic nervous system.

- The somatic nervous system innervates the skeletal muscles, the skin, and the sense organs, and the autonomic nervous system innervates the viscera.

- There are two main branches of the autonomic nervous system, the sympathetic and parasympathetic branches, which oppose each other in a graded fashion.

- The CNS can be divided into the spinal cord and four major regions of the brain that include the brain stem, the cerebellum, the diencephalon, and the cerebral hemispheres.

- There are also two major networks of the brain intimately tied to the fight-or-flight response: the reticular formation (RF) and the limbic system.

- The RF plays an important role in transmitting arousal signals regarding stressful stimuli upward to the diencephalon and higher cortical areas of the cerebral hemispheres as well as sending signals downward into the brain stem to the viscera and the skeletal muscular system to activate the fight-or-flight response.

- The limbic system, originally proposed as the brain neural circuit for emotion, helps to integrate the fight-or-flight experience.

- The endocrine system is a system of organs and glands that secrete hormones into our bloodstream that act as biochemical messengers to their respective target cells and organs.

- The primary command center for the endocrine's stress response is in the hypothalamus of the diencephalon, and one of its primary target organs is the adrenal gland.

- One axis of hypothalamic influence is the sympathetic-adrenal-medulla (SAM) axis whereby the hypothalamus controls the secretion of the catecholamines, epinephrine and norepinephrine, from the adrenal medulla.

- Another axis of hypothalamic influence, the hypothalamic-pituitary-adrenal (HPA) axis, involves the hypothalamus influencing the adrenal cortex via the pituitary gland to secrete glucocorticoids.

- A third major axis, the thyroxine axis, also begins with the hypothalamus, which in this case influences the release of the hormone thyroxine from the thyroid gland.

- For some, encounters with severe stressors can result in the development of a posttraumatic stress disorder (PTSD).

- PTSD is characterized by symptoms such as reexperiencing the traumatic event, avoiding stimuli associated with the event, experiencing a general response numbing, and having increased arousal.

- There is considerable evidence that the limbic system of the brain functions abnormally for many people with PTSD.

- Following a traumatic experience, some people may report positive changes prompted by the traumatic event in the form of posttraumatic growth.

- Posttraumatic growth is characterized by those who report it as a perception of having stronger or enhanced relationships, more positive self-views, and positive changes in worldviews following trauma.

CRITICAL THINKING QUESTIONS

1. What parts of the brain are most involved in the fight-or-flight response? What roles do the reticular formation and the limbic system play during fight or flight?

2. How are the sympathetic-adrenal-medulla axis and the hypothalamic-pituitary-adrenal axis similar? How are they different? How do they complement each other during the fight-or-flight reaction?

3. What hormones are involved during the fight-or-flight response? What role does each play? How does each help a person survive when threatened? How can these hormones released during chronic stress be detrimental to long-term survival?

4. What brain areas seem to be involved in posttraumatic stress disorder? How might they contribute to the symptoms of the disorder?

5. Why do you think some individuals experience posttraumatic growth in response to traumatic stressors and others do not? What factors might contribute to the development of posttraumatic stress disorder? How are these factors similar to or different from factors that may contribute to posttraumatic growth?

KEY TERMS AND CONCEPTS

Acetylcholine

ACTH*

Adrenal cortex*

Adrenal medulla*

Adrenals

Afferent

Amino acid

Amygdala*

Anterior cingulate

Anterior pituitary

Arousal pathway system

Autonomic nervous system

Basal energy conservation and restoration state

Beta-endorphin

Brain stem

Cardiac muscle

Central nervous system (CNS)

Cerebral hemispheres

Cortisol*

Declarative memory

Diencephalon

Dopamine

Efferent

Endocrine system

Energy mobilization and expenditure state

Epinephrine*

Glucocorticoids

Gluconeogenesis

Glucose

Glycogen

Hippocampus*

Hormones

Hypothalamic-pituitary-adrenal (HPA) axis*

Hypothalamus*

Limbic system*

Lipolysis

Locus ceruleus (LC)

Medulla

Metabolic rate

Midbrain

Mind

Negative feedback loop

Neocortex

Norepinephrine*

Neurotransmitter

Parasympathetic branch*

Peripheral nervous system

Pituitary gland

Pituitary portal system

Pons

Positive illusions

Postganglionic neurons

Posttraumatic growth*

Posttraumatic stress disorder (PTSD)*

Preganglionic neurons

Reticular formation (RF)*

Sensory projection system*

Skeletal muscles

Signal-to-noise ratio

Smooth muscles

Somatic nervous system

Striated muscles

Stroke volume

Substantia nigra

Sympathetic-adrenal-medulla (SAM) axis*

Sympathetic branch*

Thalamus

Thyroid gland

Thyroid-stimulating hormone (TSH)

Thyroxine

Traumatic stressors

Viscera

Worldview

MEDIA RESOURCES

CENGAGE brain.com

Access an interactive eBook, chapter-specific interactive learning tools, including flashcards, quizzes, videos, and more in your Psychology CourseMate, accessed through CengageBrain.com.

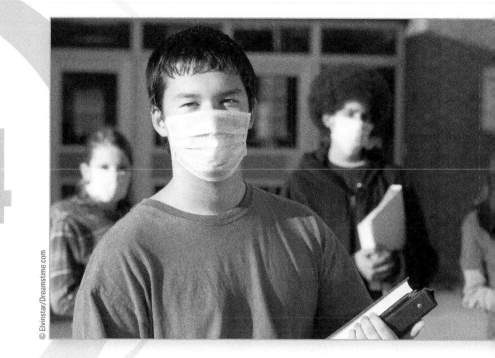

Pressure and stress is the common cold of the psyche

~ANDREW DENTON

STRESS, ILLNESS, AND THE IMMUNE SYSTEM

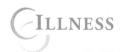

Nicole was facing the last stretch of her fall semester—college final exam time. As if on cue, she noticed a dreaded but familiar tickle in the back of her throat. "Oh, no—I don't need this—Not now!" she silently told herself. At a time when she wanted to be her best, she was instead starting to feel a little achy, tired, and muddle headed. Maybe she was just hitting the books too hard and pulling too many late nighters, she wondered. "By tomorrow morning all will be right with the world again if I just go to bed early and get a good night's sleep," she hoped.

Even with the early turn-in for the night, by the next morning, however, Nicole began to feel a steady trickle of watery mucus running down her nose and the back of her throat that wouldn't stop no matter how many times she blew her nose into her tissues. She looked down with disgust at the used tissues that were now starting to make quite a neat little pile. "Why me?" she thought. "I was doing pretty well with my stress." Before long she had the classic symptoms, the runny nose, the cough, the sneezing, the sore throat, and that spacey feeling that makes concentrating on her studies so hard. She just wanted to climb into bed and forget about her finals.

Nicole had told her mom and dad during the Thanksgiving holidays that she hoped she wouldn't catch it this year like last year and the year before, but sure enough she did. What did Nicole catch? Why do you think she caught it at this time of the year?

If you ask Nicole, she will tell you with absolute certainty that the stress of her upcoming final exams made her catch the common cold.

As with Nicole, many people believe there is a link between stress and illness. Each fall semester a certain number of college students, including Nicole, catch colds around the week of final exams. When asked, many will tell you that the stress of taking final exams led to their cold. Of course there is the matter of the pesky little virus, the cold virus and its role in the whole matter. So a more elaborate hypothesis Nicole might pose for her professors, friends, and family is that these viruses are more prevalent or more easily spread during times like the late fall, when there are more social gatherings like Thanksgiving. Nicole knows that the stressors of final exams do not actually infect her, but rather believes that these exams make her more vulnerable to the cold virus, that is, lower her resistance. Is this belief accurate?

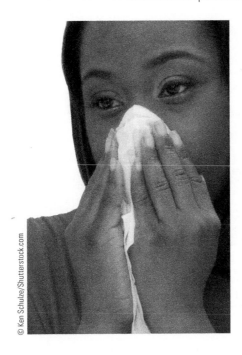

© Ken Schulze/Shutterstock.com

Many college students believe that the stress of taking exams makes them more susceptible to catching colds. What do you think?

Before we look for evidence of this linkage, let us first take a look at what an illness is. In the case of the common cold, Nicole must first be infected by a cold virus. A large percentage of these cold viruses are referred to as rhinoviruses, though other viruses can also cause a cold. There are over 200 varieties of the cold virus and any one of them can infect us.

Infection refers to an invasion of the body by a harmful microorganism—in Nicole's case the cold virus—that can create a pathological condition in the body's tissues and systems. This pathological condition usually has a recognized pattern of signs and symptoms and is referred to as a **disease.** For example, Nicole has the disease called the cold. Diseases may also be caused by other factors such as genetic defects (e.g., Duchenne muscular dystrophy) or environmental conditions (e.g., chronic obstructive pulmonary disease caused by cigarette smoking). **Illness** refers to the unhealthy state caused by the disease and **sickness** is a synonym for illness. Nicole's illness has the symptom pattern of her cold disease with a runny nose, sneezing, coughing, a sore throat, and tiredness. She is in an unhealthy state. She is sick.

Nicole's body has its own defense system against infections. Her body's system of organs, tissues, and cells is designed to protect her against infections and harmful substances and is referred to as her **immune system.** Therefore, in the case of the common cold, when Nicole becomes infected with the cold virus and cannot neutralize the virus sufficiently with her immune system, she contracts the disease and becomes ill.

The question we can ask then is the following: Can the stress of final exams really lead to sufficient weakening of her immune system to cause Nicole to catch a cold after exposure to a cold virus? Is Nicole on the right track with her hypothesis about stress and illness? What do you think?

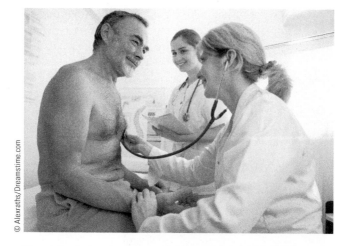

The sick role involves illness behaviors in which a person evaluates symptoms and seeks medical care and support from others. The secondary gains from additional care, attention, and sympathy received by the sick person can be rewarding.

Before we look at evidence for Nicole's hypothesis, let us next look at illness behavior because this phenomenon can affect our understanding of any evidence we examine. When people contract a disease and experience illness, they also show signs and symptoms of the disease, as Nicole does with her cold symptoms. These signs and symptoms usually prompt them to seek relief and sometimes medical care. Besides investing in boxes of tissues, Nicole next plans to go to the drugstore and buy some cold remedies. These might help her suppress some of her symptoms like her cough and runny nose. In addition, friends and family usually offer sympathy and other forms of social and emotional support. Later that evening Nicole will give her mom and dad a phone call and let them know about her sickness, knowing that they usually offer her empathy, kindly advice, and good wishes.

Ill people may take sick days or in other ways excuse themselves from their normal duties. Nicole would like a little sympathy from her friends also, and maybe her professors. She wonders if her professors would cut her some slack if they knew how bad she was feeling. The particular role Nicole and others adopt in these circumstances is called the **sick role**.

Like Nicole, those who adopt the sick role exhibit patterns of behavior referred to as **illness behavior** in which they evaluate symptoms, seek medical care, and ask for support from close others (Mechanic, 1966). Illness behavior is reinforced in this manner by those who find the additional attention, care, and relaxation of the demands of their normal duties rewarding. These rewards are referred to as **secondary gains**. As Nicole has learned, these secondary gains are some of the few silver linings that come with her illness.

Researchers studying the relationship between stress and illness know that it is important to sort out true illness from reports of illness made by those who seek secondary gains by reporting illnesses they do not have. This phenomenon and other measurement and report biases often confound efforts to determine the true nature of the relationship between stress and illness, making effective research strategies of paramount importance. How then can we best determine the answer to Nicole's hypothesis about the stress of final exams leading to her cold? What research strategies will give us the methods we need to find the answer? What strategy would you employ?

RESEARCH STRATEGIES FOR EXAMINING STRESS AND ILLNESS

One of the simplest and least costly methods you could use is the **retrospective research design** that asks research participants to recall past stressors and illnesses and then you record the information. If Nicole were in a retrospective study, you could ask her to tell you over a period of years how much stress she was experiencing each time she caught a cold. She would then search her mind for memories of her stressors and her bouts with colds and tell you that every year around the fall final exams, a period of high stress for her, she catches a cold.

Your next task is to determine if Nicole's report is accurate. How would you know? Could she have mistakenly remembered she had a cold at fall final exam time last year when in fact it was a few months before? The problem you now run into is that you cannot verify her memory. Because she has a belief that her cold happens around final exam time, could her belief be distorting her memory? You have probably wondered the same thing and concluded that her memories may be distorted or biased in some fashion, perhaps influenced by her beliefs, and you have no way to fact check with your retrospective method.

Remember, Nicole also enjoys secondary gains when she reports that she had been sick. Perhaps she feels motivated to report to you that she was sick to gain your sympathy when in fact she was not. If so, would that confound your results? As you must have determined, Nicole's secondary gains associated with the sick role could affect her recall and reporting and support a specious (an apparent though not real) appearance of a positive link between her stress and her illness.

What if Nicole has a personality where she is prone to exaggerate complaints about her psychological or physical health? Could that also confound your results? Indeed, as you may know, some personality characteristics such as neuroticism (see Chapter 6) can influence study participants to overreport recollections of illness symptoms or stress, thereby creating a false association between illness and stress.

Assuming that Nicole reports her connection to you between her stress levels and her colds, how do you know the direction of the relationship? In other words, how do you know if her stress contributed to her cold or that her cold contributed to her stress? Perhaps it is a two-way direction with each contributing to the other or perhaps it is just the case that Nicole's colds stress her and not the other way around. How would you know for sure?

In trying to answer these questions you could employ a stronger though logistically more costly and difficult strategy. You could use a **prospective research design,** known also as a longitudinal design, in which research participants are evaluated from day one of the research project on stress and illness variables and then tracked across a fixed period from baseline. If Nicole participates in this type of study, her stress levels are recorded prior to her catching the cold. So when she catches a cold, the stress data and cold data are already recorded in near real-time fashion, and memory confounds are less likely. You also are able to verify the timing to establish that her stress precedes her cold rather than the other way around. You do this by observing that she does not have a cold at baseline, she subsequently is under high stress around her final exam dates, and then she soon develops a cold.

In both retrospective and prospective designs, data can be collected that describe the relationship between stress and illness, but only in prospective studies can you examine the time element and verify that the stress preceded the illness rather than the other way around. Overall, the general quality of the data is higher with prospective designs, in part because the reporting of variables is less likely to be affected by memory distortions and biases. These distortions and biases are serious concerns in retrospective studies because most people like Nicole have illness cognitions and beliefs that affirm links between stress and illness that may cause them to inadvertently report accordingly.

Like the retrospective versus prospective approach, another important contrast in research methods is the correlational versus experimental strategy. **Correlational studies** (also called observational studies) describe the magnitude of covariation between stress and illness but do not give sufficient information to determine causation. In other words, they only give us information about the nature and strength of the relationship and not its causal relations. Correlation coefficients may be used to summarize the relationship between variables found in correlational studies.

Pearson Product Moment Correlation Coefficients are the most commonly reported correlations and are designated as r. They range from an anchor point of -1.0 to immediately below 0 for negative correlations, and from immediately above 0 to an anchor point of $+1.0$ for positive correlations. An $r = 0$ indicates the absence of a relationship. The absolute value of the correlation coefficient indicates the strength of the relationship and the sign indicates the nature of the relationship. For a **positive correlation** the higher the stress level, the greater the likelihood of illness, and for a **negative correlation** the higher the stress level, the lower the likelihood of illness. How about Nicole's stress-illness relationship? Is she hypothesizing a positive or a negative correlation? If you answered positive, you understand the concept.

As you will later see, stress and illness correlations found in self-report studies are often around $r = .30$. They are statistically significant in larger

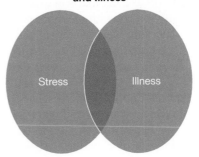

Overlapping Variance Between Stress and Illness

FIGURE **4.1** Interpreting Correlation Coefficients

An *r* = .30 for stress and illness means that 9% of the variance overlaps between stress and illness. In other words, 9% of the variance of illness can be accounted for by stress and vice versa.

---

sample sizes yet are relatively modest because they only account for 9% (.30 squared × 100) of the overlapping variance of stress and illness (Figure 4.1). Small statistically significant correlations are important for understanding relationships but they may not be that meaningful in the larger context of determining the magnitude of the effect on one's everyday living. So if only 9% of the total variance can be accounted for by stress in the stress and illness relationship, then that leaves 91% to be accounted for by other non-stress factors. This can make a difference in deciding strategies for preventing illness.

Let us say for hypothetical purposes that you establish that the relationship between stress and health does account for 9% of the variance and that you do not know exactly what accounts for the other 91%. If you had to pick one strategy for avoiding catching a cold during cold season between washing your hands frequently and engaging in better stress management, which would you choose? Perhaps you would choose hand washing because it would be easier to do and probably have a bigger payoff than the 9% strategy. Of course in real life—assuming you could determine that stress contributed to catching a cold after exposure to the cold virus through using the experimental method—you can do both, so the best approach would be to manage your stress *and* wash your hands frequently.

Experimental studies hold extraneous variables constant while manipulating other variables, the so-called **independent variables.** The outcome variables known as the **dependent variables** are then measured. If you want to measure the effects of stress on illness, what would be the independent variable? What would be the dependent variable? If you determined that stress is the independent variable and illness is the dependent variable in this context, then you identified the variables correctly.

Only the **experimental group** receives the manipulation. The **control group** serves as a comparison group. Often there is more than one experimental group and sometimes more than one control group. Following your strategy of trying to determine if stress contributes to illness, how could you do this experimentally?

Later, we will look at the work that Sheldon Cohen and his colleagues did in the early 1990s using experiments to determine if stress contributes to catching a cold. Then, if you thought of an experimental approach, you can check and see how closely your approach matches his (hint—you might have to infect your participants).

The results of a good experimental study can help explain a causal relationship. For example, they can give us information about the direction and magnitude of the causal relationship. In studying the stress-illness connection specifically, experimental studies can give us causal information that correlational research cannot. Experimental research is appropriate for addressing the following questions: Does stress cause illness? Does illness cause stress? Does a third variable cause both illness and stress? For example, Selye's (1956a) experimental studies discussed in Chapter 1 subjecting rats to various physical stressors such as cold, heat, and toxic substances determined that these stressors *caused* the animals to develop serious stress-related pathologies. Of course, these types of interventions would be unethical if conducted with humans so researchers must consider how to study the stress-illness relationship in ways that respect and do not harm their human research participants.

Let us now look at different types of research designs and see how each can contribute to our understanding of causal relationships. A type of study called a **cross-sectional design** observes several cohorts (groups with similar defining characteristics) by taking a snapshot of them at a given point in time, whereas **longitudinal designs** track cohorts over time taking multiple snapshots. Cross-sectional studies can tell us, for example, that sedentary individuals are more likely to have heart disease than their nonsedentary counterparts. However, they cannot tell us with certainty whether the cohort of sedentary individuals studied developed heart disease as a result of their sedentary lifestyle or whether they developed a sedentary lifestyle in response to their heart disease. Only longitudinal studies can provide the missing time element and tell us with certainty which came first, sedentary behavior or heart disease. Therefore, longitudinal studies are considered stronger for determining directions of influence of variables than cross-sectional studies.

In order to establish causality, three conditions must be present. First, if "A" is the causal variable under question, then "A" the cause and "B" the effect variables must be correlated. Second, "A" must precede "B" in time. Third, other potential causal variables, "C," must be ruled out. Cross-sectional studies are good for establishing that "A" and "B" are correlated; for example, that sedentary behavior and heart disease are related. Longitudinal studies are good for establishing that "A" precedes "B" in time; for example, that the participants in the study were sedentary *before* they developed heart disease. Good longitudinal (prospective) observational studies can even rule out other potential "C" variables statistically.

cross-sectional design: a study that observes cohorts at only one point in time.

longitudinal designs: a study in which cohorts are being tracked across time.

However, the best way to rule out "C" is through an experimental study where "C" variables are controlled. For example, healthy sedentary individuals can be randomly assigned to a group that begins an aerobic exercise program or to a nonexercise group. At the conclusion of the study 6 months later and at follow-up years later, heart disease levels can be measured. If the sedentary group has more evidence of heart disease than the aerobic exercise group, then the causal link between sedentary behavior and heart disease is more firmly established. The gold standard experimental study in medicine for determining these types of causal relationships is called a **randomized controlled trial** because participants are randomly assigned to groups and then the group that receives the intervention being tested (e.g., exercise) is compared to control groups. A randomized controlled trial has high **internal validity** because it is good at discerning causal relationships.

Whereas internal validity refers to how well the study establishes causal relationships, **external validity** refers to the generalizability of the results. High external validity means the study's findings generalize well to populations that have characteristics similar to the sample. Results of a research study that uses a large human sample tells us more about humans in general than results of a similar study with a small human sample or an animal study. For that reason, all other things being equal, the large human sample study is said to have higher external validity to human populations.

One study cannot match the potential generalizability of multiple studies statistically averaged together. When we average the results of a number of similar single studies of high methodological quality we can maximize both internal validity and external validity. It is important to note that if the studies being averaged have poor methodological quality, however, pooling them will not help. When multiple studies are combined and averaged and reported as one study, that report is known as a **meta-analytic study.**

Meta-analytic studies use statistical procedures that find the average **effect size,** an indicator of the strength of the relationship between the independent variables on the dependent variables. Effect sizes in meta-analytic studies are often reported as correlation coefficients though other statistics may be used instead. For r, a small effect size is in the range of .10, a medium effect size is around .30, and a large effect size is .50 or greater (Cohen, 1992). Effect sizes may also be reported as standard deviation units. As a general reference, consider that one-half a standard deviation unit is considered a medium effect size and one standard deviation unit is generally regarded as a high medium-to-large effect size.

Although there are some poor meta-analytic studies because of lax inclusion standards, in general, the investigators who conduct meta-analyses usually attempt to screen out poor methodological studies and include only the higher quality ones. Thus, we get relatively stable indicators of the effects of particular causal variables. When studying the relationship between stress and illness, as well as stress and health in general, the meta-analytic strategy gives us a great advantage in furthering our understanding. Therefore, special attention is given throughout this book to meta-analytic studies.

randomized controlled trial: the gold standard experimental study in medicine in which participants are randomly assigned to groups and then the group that receives the intervention being tested is compared to one or more control groups.

meta-analytic studies: also known as meta-analytic reviews; studies that use statistical procedures to determine average effect sizes of multiple studies.

effect size: an indicator of the strength of the relationship of the independent variable on the dependent variable.

TABLE **4.1**   Methodological Quality of Different Types of Studies

Weaker	Stronger
Retrospective—Lower internal validity	Prospective—Higher internal validity
Correlational—Lower internal validity	Experimental—Higher internal validity
Single Study—Lower external validity	Meta-analytic—Higher external validity

See Table 4.1 for an overview of the relative strengths of retrospective ver-sus prospective designs, correlational studies versus experimental studies, and single studies versus meta-analytic studies.

How you measure stress is an important issue also. Many instruments that purport to measure stress are paper-and-pencil self-report instruments such as the Social Readjustment Rating Scale (SRRS) that is discussed in the next section. Others may involve recording stressors or events by a third party either through paper-and-pencil recordings of behavior or events, audio or vi-sual recordings, or physiological recordings including invasive procedures such as drawing blood for a blood assay and noninvasive procedures such as measuring heart rate with external electrodes and a physiograph.

In all cases, the instruments used must be reliable to be useful. **Reliability** refers to consistency. If you step on a weight scale three times within a minute, assuming you made no changes (removed no clothing, drank no water, etc.), you should have pretty consistent weight readings if your scale is reliable. If your readings swing wildly by 5 or 10 pounds each time you step on the scale, you know you have an unreliable instrument. Without reliability, you have no chance for general accuracy. Thus, reliability is a precondition for **validity** (i.e., accuracy). We then assume that in any good study, the instruments used have acceptable reliability and validity. If they do not, then the results cannot be trusted and are of no use to you, just as the results of the wildly swinging weight scale are of no use to you.

Putting it all together, what strategies would you employ to determine the validity of Nicole's hypothesis that the stress of final exams contributes to her developing a cold?

THE LIFE EVENTS MODEL OF STRESS AND ILLNESS

Let us next look at early research that explored the stress and illness relation-ship. In the beginning stages of stress research Hans Selye (1956) demon-strated a relationship between chronic stressors and pathophysiological changes (i.e., the biological processes that underlie diseases or injuries) in ani-mals. In addition, clinicians historically reported anecdotal evidence of a rela-tionship between chronic stressors and the development of illness in humans. Therefore, the next step in investigating the stress-illness connection was to conduct formal human research in the area.

As you recall from Chapter 1, this led Holmes and Rahe (1967) to create an instrument called the **Social Readjustment Rating Scale (SRRS)** to determine if there is a predicted relationship between stress and illness in humans. The SRRS conceptualizes stressors as positive or negative life events that require adaptation or adjustment. In developing the instrument, each life event on the scale was assigned a number of **life change units (LCUs)** based on the mean participant ratings of their experiences with the events. After ranking the items, the highest ranked item, *Death of a spouse,* was given the top score of 100 and all subsequent items were scored in descending order of intensity. Most of the items on the resulting scale are low-to-moderate intensity stressors, examples of which include *Change in church activities, Change in eating habits,* and *Revision of personal habits.* In keeping with Selye's concept of negative and positive stress, some events are positive. An example is the seventh ranked event of *marriage.*

In a seminal prospective study, Rahe (1968) found that among 2,500 naval personnel, those with the highest scores on life change events for 6 months prior to their cruise had 90% more first illnesses during the first month of their cruise than those with the lowest life change event scores. In another classic study Holmes and Masuda (1974) examined data from a group of 88 physicians and discovered that when their score was over 300, over 70% reported illnesses the next year, but if their score was below 150, the majority of the physician participants reported that they were in relatively good health the subsequent year.

Over the ensuing years a number of criticisms were leveled against the SRRS including the charge that it is a simple checklist that does not include a number of relevant person and situation variables (Dohrenwend, Krasnoff, Askenasy & Dohrenwend, 1982; Dohrenwend, Raphael, Schwartz, Stueve, & Skodol, 1993). As a result, more than 20 additional stressful life event (SLE) checklist scales for adults were created to address some of these criticisms during the decades that followed (Scully, Tosi, & Banning, 2000). Nevertheless, reviewers of over 30 years of research on the SRRS concluded that despite the many criticisms of the instrument, the SRRS (with some minor updating) still remains a practical and robust tool for predicting stress-related symptoms, noting that "thirty years after its creation, the SRRS appears to be the instrument tool chosen most often by researchers" (Scully et al., 2000, p. 864). As a recent example illustrates, researchers (Kricker et al., 2009) employed an SRRS style checklist in a retrospective study of women diagnosed with breast cancer to discover to their surprise that the participants who experienced separation, divorce, or major tension in their intimate relationship one year prior to their cancer diagnosis had *smaller* rather than larger tumors when compared to their lower relationship-stress counterparts. They speculated that their surprising finding may be the result of high relationship-stress suppressing estrogen, a hormone associated with accelerating breast cancer tumor growth.

Although the SRRS and its variants continue to be popular, there are several problems with the SLE model as proposed by Holmes and Rahe (1967) that can confound some of the results. One is that many of the SLE studies supporting the model are based on retrospective self-reports. As discussed earlier, people often have difficulty remembering events accurately and may have memory distortions or biases when answering. This is especially true with ambiguous items (e.g., items such as *Revision of personal habits* and *Major change in social activities*) found on the original Holmes and Rahe checklist. Response bias is more likely to occur when distressed individuals are retrospectively searching for possible causes of their illnesses and interpreting ambiguous items as supportive of their illness beliefs.

Second, some of the items on SLE checklists overlap with physical illnesses because the items themselves refer to similar health-related events (e.g., items such as *Major personal injury or illness* and *Hospitalization*). Thus, this overlap embeds confounds of stress and illness in the self-report instrument itself that have to be teased out if there is any hope for an accurate measurement of the stress-illness relationship.

Last, the effects of negative affectivity or neuroticism levels of respondents may influence their responses because those who score high on measures of neuroticism on instruments like the NEO-PI (McCrae, 1982) (see Chapter 6) tend to report more health complaints than their low-scoring counterparts (Costa & McCrae, 1980; Tessler & Mechanic, 1978). These individuals may also endorse more SLEs that overlap with psychological disorders involving depression or anxiety (e.g., items such as *Major change in eating habits* or *Sexual difficulties*).

As an illustration of the issue of potential confounding of self-reported SLEs and health measures, note that Schroeder and Costa (1984) reported in a sample of 386 subjects a correlation of $r = .32$ between SLEs and self-reported illness, which is in keeping with other studies. However, when these same researchers removed the effects due to ambiguous items, health-related events, and neuroticism, they found that the *uncontaminated* correlation was an insignificant $r = .10$.

Does this mean then that there is not a meaningful correlation between SLEs and illness? Methodological problems with the Holmes and Rahe model and their scales have made it difficult to always establish firm and consistent meaningful relationships between life change events and illness. In addition, there is some evidence that the *positive* life stress events items on SLE scales do not contribute significantly to outcomes (Bhagat, McQuaid, Lindholm, & Segovis, 1985). However, as you will later see, there are a number of different strategies that researchers employ to understand the stress-illness relationship, including use of verified stressors such as loss of a loved one and use of hard measures (as opposed to soft ones like paper-and-pencil tests) through blood tests or other objectively verifiable means.

For example, a more recent study (Phillips et al., 2006) found no relationship between scores on a life events survey and antibody response to influenza vaccination in an elderly community sample. However, the investigators did find a negative relationship for this sample with bereavement. Bereaved participants had lower levels of antibody titers than nonbereaved, indicating a less robust immune response to the vaccination. So although there are some methodological issues associated with using Holmes and Rahe's model and their instruments, the basic concept of **negative life stress events** seems to have validity as it pertains to illness.

A slightly different model from the Holmes and Rahe checklist approach to life events stress is represented by the **Bedford College Life Events and Difficulties Schedule (LEDS)** (Brown & Harris, 1978). The LEDS requires training in its application and scoring and is used primarily with clinical populations such as

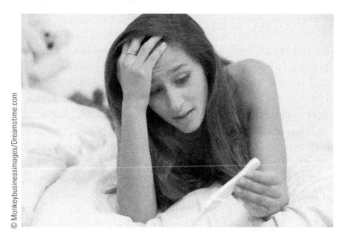

Context of the LEDS is important in determining the impact of the life event. An accidental pregnancy for a typical 13-year-old is a different context than an accidental pregnancy for a typical unmarried 18-year-old.

those with clinical depression (Lenze, Cyranowski, Thompson, Anderson, & Frank, 2008), bipolar disorder (Johnson et al., 2008), and forms of psychoses (Myin-Germeys, Krabbendam, Delespaul, & van Os, 2003).

Instead of using a self-report checklist, the LEDS uses a semistructured interview and a panel of trained raters to assess among other variables the degree of potential long-term *threat* of the life events noted by the participants within the *context* in which they occur. It is based on what a typical person in that situation would likely experience. For example, the context of an accidental pregnancy for a typical 13-year-old would be perceived as a higher long-term threat than that of an accidental pregnancy for a typical unmarried 18-year-old. Though threat is determined by its potential long-term negative implications, potential long-term positive aspects of the event can also be rated.

The LEDS is also used in health psychology applications but less frequently. For example, Ackerman et al. (2002) found that it could be used to determine that life event stress predicted exacerbation of multiple sclerosis symptoms. In another health psychology application, Phillips, Der, and Carroll (2008) were able to use health-related life events impact scores and event numbers from the LEDS in their prospective 17-year longitudinal study of 968 Scottish men and women to determine that stress strongly predicted **all-cause mortality** (i.e., death by all causes).

One disadvantage to the LEDS is that it requires training in conducting the semistructured interview and scoring the responses. In addition, it requires a panel to evaluate the responses and arrive at a consensus. Therefore, it is more expensive and time demanding than simple paper-and-pencil checklist measures. It also, like the SRRS, has some of the problems associated with collecting information based on retrospection. However, the LEDS is a good example of a gold standard approach to measuring life change events that can be used as an alternate to traditional paper-and-pencil self-report checklists.

DAILY HASSLES MODEL

As you recall from Chapter 1, Lazarus and his research group (Kanner, Coyne, Schaefer, & Lazarus, 1981) created an instrument to measure daily *hassles* and *uplifts* as an alternative to the life change events approach advocated by Holmes and Rahe. They were concerned that the SLE approach did not measure everyday chronic persistent stressors and contended that minor stressors or *hassles* that people experienced on a regular basis were better predictors of illness and other health problems than SLEs. That hassles items were more *proximal* measures of stress, they argued, than SLE items meant that they would have a more immediate impact on one's life and therefore were more likely to be reflected in somatic (i.e., physical) complaints.

In a multiple regression analysis (a multiple correlation technique) DeLongis, Coyne, Dakof, Folkman, and Lazarus (1982) found that hassles did predict somatic health and that the relationship was stronger than that of SLEs to health. The order of magnitude of the relationship was modest though statistically significant. There was, however, little support for uplifts as having any meaningful relationship to health. Perhaps somewhat overstated, Lazarus and his coauthor commented, "Our research findings have shown, in a regression-based comparison of life events and daily hassles, that hassles are far superior to life events in predicting psychological and somatic symptoms" (Lazarus & Folkman, 1984, p. 311).

Measures of daily hassles suffer from many of the same methodological problems as measures of SLEs. In addition, some of the hassles items overlap with SLE items. Hassles items also overlap significantly with symptoms of psychological disorders (Dohrenwend, Dohrenwend, Dodson, & Shrout, 1984). Hart (1999) found that neuroticism (see Chapter 6), a personality dimension that relates to psychological disorders, accounted for 29% to 40% of nonwork hassle score variance, demonstrating that personality factors also can confound results of hassles studies in the same way they can for SLE studies. These types of findings have led some researchers such as Evans, Johansson, and Rydstedt (1999) to abandon the use of self-report measures of hassles altogether and instead use independent behavioral observations to determine hassle events.

On the whole then, whereas measures of daily hassles show some improvements over measures of SLEs, the improvements are marginal. Today, researchers use hassles scales to measure the effects of daily stressors on a wide variety of health conditions including asthma (Kullowatz et al., 2008), fibromyalgia (Libby & Glenwick, 2010), and tension-type headache (Cathcart & Pritchard, 2008) to name a few. Often they use both measures of SLEs and those of daily hassles in their studies to determine the degree of external stress to which subjects were exposed. Why? Though studies indicate that these two measures overlap in what they measure, sophisticated statistical techniques such as path analysis and structural equation modeling have determined that they also each measure some separate aspects of stress on health outcomes (Aldwin, Levenson, Spiro, & Bosse, 1989; Zautra, Reich, & Guarnaccia, 1990).

LINKING STRESS, ILLNESS, AND THE IMMUNE SYSTEM

Conducting studies linking SLEs and hassles to somatic complaints and illnesses was a good first stage in the process of trying to address the stress-illness question in humans. However, these studies did not give sufficient insight into the "how" and "why" questions; in other words, what psychological and biological mechanisms are at play in the process?

Solomon and Moos (1964) were the first to publish the term **psychoneuroimmunology** (**PNI**) to refer to the study of the relationship among the psychological, neurological, and immunological interactions. Their introduction of the term was followed over a decade later by stress researcher Kenneth Pelletier, popularizing the idea in his 1977 book *Mind as Healer, Mind as Slayer*. Pelletier and Herzing (1988, p. 29) defined the then emerging interdisciplinary field of PNI as "the study of the intricate interaction of consciousness (psycho), brain and central nervous system (neuro), and the body's defense against external infection and internal aberrant cell division (immunology)."

As suggested by Pelletier (1977), stress plays a role in 50% to 80% of all illnesses and diseases. Given the magnitude of these estimates, it was incumbent on the relatively new field of PNI to explore the immunological links to stress and health in more depth. More recently, Segerstrom and Miller (2004) reported that numerous PNI stress and illness studies have now been conducted. At the time of their publication they noted that there were over 300 studies examining these links. Coe (2010, p. 182) also notes how far the field of PNI has traveled from its early days in the 1980s when the chair of his university's Department of Medicine remarked to him, "Oh, you work in that field of voodoo medicine." Today, three decades of research have confirmed PNI as an established discipline with a proven track record.

Before we examine that record, we need to first take a closer look at the structure and function of the human immune system. As with the discussion of the nervous system in Chapter 3, this coverage is not intended to be comprehensive. Rather we focus on the elements of the immune system that will give you the tools to better understand the linkage among stress, the immune system, and health.

The Human Immune System

The human immune system is designed to protect us from exogenous (outside) and endogenous (inside) toxins, substances, particles, cells, and organisms that pose a threat to our physical well-being. These threats to our health are referred to as **antigens**. Antigens are the cast of bad characters that we want to keep out of our biological systems because they are disruptive and often dangerous. Exogenous antigens include bacteria, viruses like the cold virus that infected Nicole, fungi, and other entities that could potentially become life threatening. Endogenous antigens involve our body's own cells that are infected with viruses or have mutated into tumor or cancer cells. The immune system is like a nation's federal law enforcement agency (e.g., the Federal Bureau of Investigation [FBI] in the United States) protecting its citizens and government against endogenous threats and the national armed services (e.g., the army, navy, air force, and marines) protecting citizens from exogenous threats. The various agencies and branches of the military each have specialized roles, and collectively they serve to defend the body of the nation against threats to its survival.

The Innate Immune System and the Adaptive Immune System Several layers of defense comprise our protective and immune systems. The first layer consists of our skin and mucous membranes. Most bacteria or viruses we contact are blocked by the skin from mounting an invasion. Those that manage to penetrate the skin are vigorously attacked. Did you know that pimples represent one outward manifestation of this process? Bacteria that penetrate the skin are ingested by white blood cells otherwise known as **leukocytes.** These defender cells soon die and help to form the resulting pus that fills the pimple. Thus, although we may look in the mirror and view any pimples we may have and their pus as unsightly or unhealthy, we can also see them in a positive light in that they show us that our immune system is performing its role of protecting us from unwanted invaders.

These first lines of defense consisting of our outer barriers such as the skin and early defenders are layers of the **innate protective system.** The innate protective system serves as an umbrella of protection. Its members are on constant patrol against threat (Figure 4.2). Agents of this **innate immune system,** also known as the natural immune system, have no memory of previous invaders and mount the same intensity of response each time they are threatened. This innate system contrasts with members of the **adaptive immune system,** also known as the acquired or specific immune system, that remembers past invaders and other bad characters (e.g., the FBI's 10 most wanted list) and can mount a vigorous response against specifically remembered offenders. Because the adaptive immune system takes 4 to 5 days to be activated against a novel invader, the innate immune system must defend us indiscriminately against threatening antigens in the meantime, using its quick reaction response capabilities that are often activated within minutes. Without the innate immune system defending us, we could very well die from infection waiting for the adaptive immune system to engage in battle.

Once engaged, however, the adaptive immune system is very effective at targeting and neutralizing the remaining invaders. Because it remembers the offenders, if they breach the system a second time, the members of the adaptive immune system can quickly neutralize the invader. The process is similar to combating computer viruses. Once a new virus is recognized on the web, a good computer antivirus programmer can write a script to prevent computers from becoming infected with it. Then subscribers download the script into their computer antivirus software as an update to ensure continued protection against that virus. Immunizations work in a similar fashion. For example, antigens from dead or weakened influenza viruses in a flu vaccine are injected and activate the adaptive immune system so that when we encounter live influenza viruses in the future, the live viruses are quickly recognized and neutralized by agents of our adaptive immune system because these agents now follow the new antivirus script.

Granulocytes, Monocytes, and Lymphocytes The innate immune system consists of phagocytic cells, natural killer (NK) cells, and various enzymes and serum proteins that are involved in the inflammation process. **Inflammation** is a response of the body to damaged tissue or infection characterized by swelling, pain, heat, and/or redness. The body's use of inflammation as a defense is like

innate immune system: also known as the natural immune system, this more primitive but rapid system consists of phagocytic cells, natural killer cells, and various enzymes and serum proteins that are involved in the inflammation process.

adaptive immune system: also known as the acquired or specific immune system, this slower but more advanced line of defense against antigens remembers past invaders and other antigens and consists of T-cytotoxic, T-helper, and B lymphocytes as well as immunoglobulins.

inflammation: an immune response of the body to damaged tissue or infection characterized by swelling, pain, heat, and/or redness.

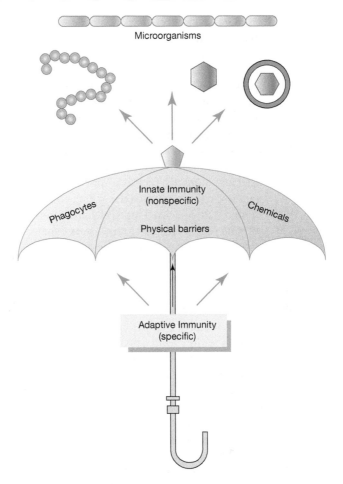

Microorganisms

Phagocytes

Innate Immunity
(nonspecific)

Physical barriers

Chemicals

Adaptive Immunity
(specific)

FIGURE **4.2**   Innate immunity and physical barriers like the skin serve to protect us against the threat of microorganisms and other pathogens in general ways. Adaptive immunity constitutes a second line of defense that is more specific and targeted.   SOURCE: Batzing, *Microbiology*, 1/E. © 2002 Brooks/Cole, a part of Cengage Learning, Inc. Reproduced by permission. www.cengage.com/permissions.

you taking a flame thrower to drive invaders out of your home. It is effective but you have to be careful about not setting your house on fire. If used too much or over a long enough period (e.g., chronic inflammation), you can cause more collateral damage to your house than to the invaders. Nicole's sore throat is a by-product of her inflammatory response to her invading cold viruses.

Our damaged cells and certain white blood cells release chemicals that are a call to action that mobilizes more white blood cells to the site. The first battle responders tend to be neutrophils and some monocytes. **Neutrophils** are the most common white blood cells (i.e., leukocytes), constituting over 50% of the total number. They are granular cells (i.e., cells with granules that contain digestive enzymes) called granulocytes that literally eat the antigens they attack. Cells like neutrophils that eat the antigens they attack are called **phagocytes** (*phagos* is Greek for "eat"). Phagocytes are like Pac Men from the vintage

phagocytes: cells of the immune system that eat the antigens they attack.

video game gobbling up any antigens they encounter. They are part of a primitive immunity system that is shared with lower order organisms, like the sponge, and provide a generalized response against pathogens within minutes to hours. Other white blood cell granulocytes include eosinophils and basophils. They are present in small numbers and are associated with inflammatory and allergic responses as well as other functions. **Monocytes** are mononuclear phagocytes (Pac Men) that become enlarged upon leaving the bloodstream and entering bodily tissue to then become **macrophages** (bigger Pac Men).

Another very important defender against the bad characters are the **natural killer (NK) cells,** which are lymphocytic cells programmed to recognize other cells that are "nonself" such as tumor cells and cells infected with viruses and to release cytotoxic (poisonous to the cell) chemicals that lyse (i.e., chemically degrade and destroy) these cells. These cells are important first defenders against endogenous threats such as tumors and cancers. They are like James Bond special agents that are licensed to carry specially designed poison dart weapons that neutralize domestic villains. Besides the NK cells, other lymphocytic cells include the T cells and B cells. Thus, T cells, B cells, and NK cells are referred to as **lymphocytes.**

An organ positioned above the heart, the thymus, develops mature **T cells** ("T" for thymus cells) from other immature bone marrow lymphoid stem cells. T cells include T-helper cells and T-cytotoxic cells. One variety of T-helper cells directs white blood cells to carry out cellular-mediated immunity, whereas another type of T-helper cells partners with B cells to produce humoral immunity. These two types of broad immune strategies each involving T-helper cells are discussed later, but let us first take a closer look at what T-helper cells are.

T-helper cells are immune cells that act to direct and amplify the immune response through the use of chemical messengers. They have no ability to engage in phagocytic or cytotoxic actions but can direct other cells to do so. You can think of T-helper cells as like sideline coaches of an American football team who call the plays but do not actually carry the football, tackle, block, or pass. They direct and coordinate both the offense and defense. Without them there would be no coordinated strategy, and the home team would be less likely to score or stop the opposing team from scoring. In battle, they are field marshals who direct the attack but do not actually engage in hand-to-hand combat.

A different type of T cell, the **T-cytotoxic cell,** does engage directly in the fight because like the NK cell, it is "licensed to kill." If you think of an NK cell as like the innate immune system's equivalent of a 007 lymphocyte, you could think of a T-cytotoxic cell as the adaptive immune system's 008 lymphocyte. The T-cytotoxic cells have a receptor known as **CD8** on their surface, which assists them in locking on to the targeted antigen; so all 008s carry this CD8 locking tool. They specialize in lysing unwanted cells with their own poison dart weapons, especially targeting the body's own cells that are infected with virus or otherwise compromised to become tumor or cancer cells (Figure 4.3).

All T cells contain receptors that recognize the targeted antigen, thus making them part of the adaptive immune system. T-helper cells have a molecule known as **CD4** on their surface that enables them to respond to the targeted antigen. It is important to note that, in a reverse of the normal process, the human immunodeficiency virus (HIV) attacks the CD4 T cells, which can then lead to an eventual compromise of the immune system against opportunistic

macrophages: monocytes of the innate immune system that become enlarged upon leaving the bloodstream and entering bodily tissue.

natural killer (NK) cells: lymphocytic cells of the innate immune system programmed to recognize other cells that are nonself such as tumor cells and cells infected with viruses, and to release cytotoxic chemicals that lyse these cells.

T cells: lymphocytic cells that develop in the thymus that are part of the adaptive immune system.

lymphocytes: a category of immune system cells that include the natural killer cells, the T cells, and the B cells.

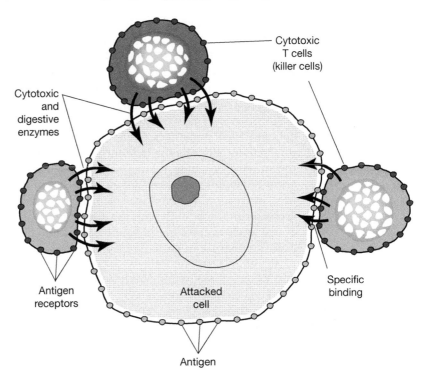

Cytotoxic
T cells
(killer cells)

Cytotoxic
and
digestive
enzymes

Antigen
receptors

Attacked
cell

Specific
binding

Antigen

FIGURE **4.3**   Action of Cytotoxic T Cells on a Targeted Cell

Like the James Bond-style NK cells of the innate immune system, these adaptive immune system 008s are "licensed to kill."   SOURCE: Guyton & Hall (2006), *Medical Physiology*, 11th ed., p. 448, Figure 34.8, Philadelphia: Elsevier Saunders. Reprinted with permission from Elsevier.

B cells: lymphocytic cells ("B" for bone marrow cells) of the adaptive immune system that produce antibodies.

immunoglobulins (Igs): also known as antibodies; soluble proteins produced by B cells that circulate in the bloodstream and bind to viruses and other antigens to neutralize them.

cellular mediated immunity: the defense strategy employed by the human immune system involving the natural killer cells, the granulocytes, the macrophages, and T cells inflaming, phagocytosing, and releasing toxic substances.

infections. With weakened and reduced numbers of T-helper cells to direct the counterattack to the opportunistic threats, a person infected with HIV can eventually develop an acquired immunodeficiency syndrome (AIDS).

The third category of lymphocytes, the **B cells** ("B" for bone marrow cells), produce **antibodies** called **immunoglobulins (Igs)**, which are soluble proteins that circulate in the bloodstream. These antibodies bind to viruses, rendering them incapable of invading the body's own cells. They may also neutralize targeted bacterial toxins. There are five kinds of antibodies: IgA, IgE, IgM, IgG, and IgD.

Cellular-Mediated Immunity (Th1) and Humoral Immunity (Th2) Strategies
The human immune system employs two major strategies, which can be called the one-two punch of cellular immunity and humoral immunity. The first punch, **cellular-mediated immunity** involves the NK cells, granulocytes (e.g., neutrophils), macrophages, and T cells quickly localizing to the site of injury or infection and in the process of inflammation either engulfing (phagocytosing—the Pac Man strategy) damaged endogenous cells along with invading exogenous antigens or releasing toxic substances (e.g., poison dart strategy) to harm them. This type of immunity is governed by a certain type of T cell known as a Type 1 T-helper (Th1) cell.

cytokines: chemical messenger molecules sometimes thought of as hormones of the immune system that stimulate immune responses.

Macrophages play a major role in triggering the immune system by releasing communication molecules called cytokines and stimulating the production of T-helper cells. The Type 1 T-helper (Th1) cells then partner with the macrophages to maximize their killing efficiency. The Th1 cells also produce cytokines that activate the NK cells and the cytotoxic T cells.

Cellular immunity **cytokines** stimulate other immune general responses as well such as inflammation, fever, and wound healing. These chemical messenger molecules, sometimes thought of as hormones of the immune system, are involved in mediating the inflammatory response. The homeostatic balance of the immune system is in large part dependent on the cytokines because some are proinflammatory (e.g., interleukin-6) and others are anti-inflammatory (e.g., interleukin-4). Cytokines include **interleukin, interferon,** and **tumor necrosis factor.** Most of the cold symptoms that Nicole experiences are due to elevated levels of cytokines that stimulate white blood cells into action but also cause an increase in nasal fluids; mucus; and general feelings of fatigue, achiness, loss of appetite, depression, and malaise. As Coe (2010) notes, it was PNI's groundbreaking research that established the significant role that cytokines play in inducing these symptoms and sickness behaviors like social withdrawal. Evidence comes from animal studies but also from, for example, patients with cancer who, when given interleukin-2 as a treatment to strengthen their immune responses, subsequently experienced malaise and depressive symptoms (Capuron, Ravaud, Miller, & Danzer, 2004).

humoral immunity: the second line strategy employed by the human immune system after cellular immunity involving Type 2 T-helper cells partnering with B cells to stimulate antibody production.

The second punch of the immune system's one-two punch, known as **humoral immunity** (refers to the body's noncellular fluid), is mediated by antibodies and has greater target precision but less speed. It may take several days for the humoral immunity system to build to maximum levels. The cells of this system are tailor made to have specific receptor sites that fit the molecular shape of the antigen. Therefore, these can only attack one specific type of invader. This type of immunity is most closely associated with the B cells. The B cells, antibodies, and a different type of T-helper cell, which is discussed shortly, form the primary components of the adaptive immune system.

Activating the humoral immunity strategy involves the Type 2 T-helper cells (Th2) partnering with B cells to stimulate antibody production (Figure 4.4). As discussed previously, this is a much slower process than cellular-mediated immunity, sometimes taking up to 7 days to reach full antibody immunity (Lovallo, 2005). It is no coincidence then that the average cold lasts about 7 days, long enough for the Th2 system to reach maximum strength. Th2 cells secrete a different set of cytokines to facilitate the humoral immunity response. For example, Th1 cells secrete interferon-γ, interleukin-2, and tumor necrosis factor-β; Th2 cells secrete cytokines such as interleukin-4, interleukin-10, and interlukin-13 (Elenkov, Iezzoni, Daly, Harris, & Chrousos, 2005).

On the whole, cytokines are involved in increasing immune cell replication, stimulating immune cells to attack antigens, promoting B cells to form antibodies, and assisting immune cells in recognizing future antigens they have already encountered. They can also signal the hypothalamus to "induce illness-related behaviors including sleep, reduced movement, and loss of appetite and sexual function" (Lovallo, 2005, p. 137).

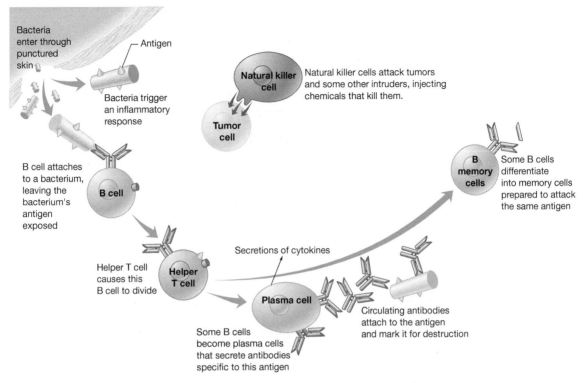

Bacteria enter through punctured skin

Antigen

Bacteria trigger an inflammatory response

Natural killer cells attack tumors and some other intruders, injecting chemicals that kill them.

Natural killer cell

Tumor cell

B cell attaches to a bacterium, leaving the bacterium's antigen exposed

B cell

B memory cells

Some B cells differentiate into memory cells prepared to attack the same antigen

Helper T cell causes this B cell to divide

Helper T cell

Secretions of cytokines

Circulating antibodies attach to the antigen and mark it for destruction

Plasma cell

Some B cells become plasma cells that secrete antibodies specific to this antigen

FIGURE **4.4**   Antibodies are produced in reaction to an exogenous threat such as bacteria. Note also, NK cells are especially adept at finding and attacking endogenous threats such as tumors.
SOURCE: KALAT, *Biological Psychology*, 10/E. © 2009 Wadsworth, a part of Cengage Learning, Inc. Reproduced by permission. www.cengage.com/permissions.

Th1 and Th2 cells inhibit each other's actions so that by the time the B cells are in full action the Th1 activities should be dampened (Table 4.2). A *dysregulated* immune system may involve chronic inflammation or autoimmune activity if the Th1 : Th2 ratio is chronically imbalanced. Therefore, a homeostatically balanced Th1/Th2 system is desired for good health.

The Immune System and Acute Stressors

The immune system of our distant human ancestors had adaptive value for them in being responsive to the many acute stressors that might have resulted in bodily injury. For example, the sight of a predatory animal like a tiger would likely induce an acute stress response that would activate the immune system in anticipation of a bite from that animal. In the event of a bite from the predator, the immune system's ability to mobilize itself to fight pathogens carried in the saliva of the predator was very important. Preventing infection and accelerating wound healing through a strong immune response had then and still has adaptive value.

As you will recall from Chapter 3, during the fight-or-flight response, the sympathetic-adrenal medulla (SAM) axis and the hypothalamic-pituitary-adrenal (HPA) axis are activated, resulting in the release of catecholamines and

TABLE **4.2** Immune System Elements, Branches, and Functions

Element of Immune System	Branch of Immune System	Function in Immune System
Neutrophils	Innate immune system	Inflames, phagocytic action
Eosinophils	Innate immune system	Inflames
Monocytes/Macrophages	Innate immune system	Inflames, phagocytic action
Natural Killer Cells	Innate immune system	Cellular (Th1), cytotoxic action
T-Cytotoxic Lymphocytes (CD8)	Adaptive immune system	Cellular (Th1), cytotoxic action
Th1-Helper Lymphocytes (CD4)	Adaptive immune system	Cellular (Th1), field marshals
Th2-Helper Lymphocytes (CD4)	Adaptive immune system	Humoral (Th2), field marshals
B Lymphocytes	Adaptive immune system	Humoral (Th2), stimulate Igs
Immunoglobulins (Igs)	Adaptive immune system	Humoral (Th2), antibody action

glucocorticoids. Catecholamines, especially norepinephrine, temporarily boost immunological activity (Dhabhar, 2009; Madden & Livnat, 1991). As Dhabhar (2009, p. 305) explains, within minutes of experiencing an acute stressor the catecholamine hormones arouse the leukocytes to exit their barracks and travel through the bloodstream—"As the stress response continues, activation of the HPA axis results in the release of glucocorticoid hormones which induce leukocytes to exit the blood and take position at potential 'battle stations' (such as the skin, lung, gastrointestinal and urinary-genital tracts, mucosal surfaces, and lymph nodes) in preparation for immune challenges which may be imposed by the actions of the stressor."

During physical exercise, **neuropeptides** such as **endorphins** also enhance the immune response. Therefore, acute transient stress responses that can involve fighting, fleeing, and possible injury result in the mobilization of the immune response. Following the acute stress response, cortisol plays a role through a negative feedback loop to damp down central nervous system excitement as part of the homeostatic system.

In a meta-analytic review looking at the effect size of 293 studies examining stress and the immune system published from 1960 to 2001, Segerstrom and Miller (2004, p. 617) found that "when stressors were acute and time-limited—that is, they generally followed the temporal parameters of fight-or-flight stress—there was evidence for adaptive redistribution of cells and preparation of the natural immune system for possible infection, injury, or both." For example, Coe (2010, p. 188) notes that during acute stress NK cell numbers (members of the natural/innate immunity system) "rise dramatically for 30–60 minutes, before showing a more sustained drop in peripheral blood."

Acute stressors are typically classified as lasting from minutes to hours, and they contrast with subchronic stressors that usually are defined as lasting days to less than 1 month and chronic stressors that last months to years. As we learn more about the role of time in the immune system's response to stress we can see more clearly how time relates to the upward or downward shift of different systems of immunity. In general, it appears that as stressors become more chronic, the body begins to switch away from the cellular-mediated immune system toward the humoral immune system. During acute (defined in minutes) stress, cellular immunity is regulated upward combined with specific humoral immunity regulated downward. As time exposed to stressors expands, there is a shift in the cytokine balance from Th1 (cellular) to Th2 (humoral) immunity. With sufficient time of exposure to the stressors, there is suppression of both cellular and humoral immunity.

The Immune System and Chronic Stressors

Chronic stressors, unlike acute stressors, generally have broad immunosuppressive effects as Herbert and Cohen (1993) and Zorilla et al. (2001) showed in their meta-analytic reviews of 36 and 82 studies, respectively. For example, whereas acute stress results in an increase in CD8 T cells (the 008s), chronic stress decreases their numbers (Rabin, 1999). Therefore, stressors seem to act as catalysts that lead to either stimulation of the immune system or its suppression, depending on the nature of the stressor, its intensity, and duration.

As noted earlier, the over- or underreaction of the immune system is referred to as **immune dysregulation.** Underreactions of the immune system can play a role in cancer and viral infections such as the common cold or flu and herpes outbreaks. Overreactions of the immune system are linked to allergies, arthritis, and lupus (see Chapter 5). In the case of allergies, the threat is exogenous (e.g., pollen), and for arthritis and lupus the threat is endogenous (e.g., one's own cells). A person can experience both underreaction and overreaction simultaneously because elements of each have different processes. For example, a person with a suppressed immune system to a cold virus and who is chronically stressed can succumb to the illness of the common cold while also experiencing a hay fever overreaction to pollen.

The hormones that seem to play the most important role in immunosuppression are the corticosteroids. For example, when the corticosteroid corticosterone is blocked in stressed laboratory animals, their immune systems are able to respond more effectively to viral infections (Hermann, Beck, & Sheridan, 1995). During periods of chronic stress, cortisol and its related glucocorticoids are generally elevated (Guyton & Hall, 2006).

Stress and Immunosuppression

One of the best ways to get a better understanding of the stress-health connection is to examine studies that show immunosuppressive effects of stress because suppressed immune systems are more vulnerable to infections, disease, and illness. Most of the stress-related immunosuppressive human studies fall into one of the following categories: exam stressors, large-scale disasters, chronic stress of long-term caregiving for loved ones with dementia, loss and bereavement, and viral challenges. Though these categories are important, they were not necessarily the focus of researchers because they are considered the most noteworthy, but rather because these stressors can be more readily objectively verified than many other types of stressors.

---

immune dysregulation: an impaired immune system that overreacts or underreacts to antigens.

Exam Stressors Exam stress, though not a long-term stress, is nevertheless a stress that can span many days. As Nicole experienced, the anticipatory stress leading up to exam dates includes more than just time spent taking exams. Therefore, this subchronic stressor seems to follow a pattern similar to chronic stressors more than acute stressors.

Let us look at the evidence that addresses the question of whether exam stress can lead to immunosuppression. First, we know that heightened sympathetic nervous system activity associated with taking exams can lead to increased levels of cortisol, which suppresses the immune system (Cacioppo et al., 2002; Glaser, Kutz, MacCallum, & Malarkey, 1995). Studies also indicate that students have higher levels of catecholamines, blood pressure, cortisol levels, and psychological distress on exam days (Herbert, Moore, de la Riva, & Watts, 1986; Sausen, Lovallo, Pincomb, & Wilson, 1992).

Second we know from a host of studies conducted by psychologist Janice Kiecolt-Glaser and physician Ronald Glaser and their colleagues that blood assays taken of medical students during their examination periods when compared to their baselines of 1 month earlier reveal evidence of immune suppression (Glaser et al., 1987; Glaser, Kiecolt-Glaser, Speicher, & Holliday, 1985; Kiecolt-Glaser et al., 1984). For example, Kiecolt-Glaser et al. (1984) found that the number of lymphocytes in their student participants decreased during exam periods compared to baseline and to a period after exams. More recently investigators confirmed that elevated anxiety associated with taking academic exams is associated with suppressed immune system functions, this time indicated by lower levels of the cytokine tumor necrosis factor alpha (Chandrashekara et al., 2007).

Can exam stress combined with suppressed immune systems then lead to more illnesses? It appears so. For example, in a classic study Glaser et al. (1987) found that medical student subjects reported more illness and had higher numbers of Epstein-Barr virus antibodies and lower levels of cytokine secretion and T-cell activation around exam days.

Large-Scale Disasters Large-scale disasters can be a source of chronic and intense stress. What immunological effects might we expect from such disasters? In a classic series of studies, Andrew Baum and his associates (Baum, 1990; McKinnon, Weisse, Reynolds, Bowles, & Baum, 1989) found that residents of the area surrounding Three-Mile Island experienced greater psychological distress than control subjects following the plant's 1979 emergency reactor shutdown due to a radiation leak. These residents also had higher urinary catecholamines and resting blood pressure. However, more dramatic was the evidence of the suppression of their immune systems, including lower levels of T cells, B cells, and NK cells as well as a higher number of herpes simplex virus. Baum also worked with colleagues after the devastating Hurricane Andrew in the United States to study community participants who were living in damaged neighborhoods and found that the more loss the survivors experienced, the lower their white blood cell counts (Ironson et al., 1997).

Long-Term Caregiving for Loved Ones with Dementia Providing long-term care for loved ones with dementia is stressful. In a meta-analysis of 23 studies

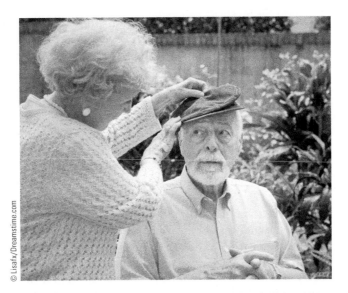

© Lisafx/Dreamstime.com

Long-term caregiving of a loved one with Alzheimer's disease can be stressful and result in immune system suppression for the caregiver.

conducted over a 38-year period of 1,594 caregivers of persons with dementia, Vitaliano, Zhang, and Scanlon (2003, p. 966) found that caregivers had higher chronic stress as evidenced by "a 23% higher level of stress hormones and a 15% lower level of antibody responses than did noncaregivers." Not only was the experience stressful, but it also resulted in immunosuppression. Individual studies illustrate these findings.

For example, Janice Kiecolt-Glaser, Malarkey, Cacioppo, and Glaser (1994) examined participants who were caregivers of their spouses who suffered from Alzheimer's disease and found that the caregivers who had low social support and high levels of distress also had more frequent respiratory tract infections and overall lower levels of cellular immunity. In addition, she and her associates (Kiecolt-Glaser, Marucha, Malarkey, Mercado, & Glaser, 1995) found that caregivers of relatives with dementia showed slower healing to a 3- to 5-mm punch biopsy wound than did their age-matched controls. Also, her research group (Kiecolt-Glaser, Dura, Speicher, Trask, & Glaser, 1991) determined that caregivers who had placed their loved one in an institution within the previous year were the ones who had the most negative immune changes.

More recently Kiecolt-Glaser collaborated on a project that found evidence that the chronic stress of giving long-term care to patients with Alzheimer's disease was "associated with altered T cell function and accelerated immune cell aging as suggested by excessive telomere loss" (Damjanovic et al., 2007, p. 4249). Telomeres are cellular chromosomal caps that can indicate how many rounds of cell division a cell has left. Shorter telomeres indicate a smaller number of rounds remaining and are a sign of a more aged cell. Thus, the telomere loss is one more example of the considerable body of evidence that long-term caregiving for loved ones with dementia can lead to suppression of the immune system.

Loss and Bereavement The loss of a spouse to separation, divorce, or more painfully to death is a very stressful event. Kiecolt-Glaser et al. (1988) discovered in their sample of 32 separated and divorced men that these men reported more distress and loneliness as well as more recent illnesses than did their matched married counterparts. In addition, the study participants had poorer values on their antibody titers to two herpes viruses. Those who initiated the breakup reported less distress and better health than noninitiators during their first year of postseparation. Also, they had lower antibody titers to the Epstein-Barr virus than noninitiators. These results suggest that the loss had a greater negative immunological impact on the separated and divorced men who experienced less control over the breakup process than those with more control.

Segerstrom and Miller (2004) presented immunosuppression evidence in their meta-analysis of bereavement studies in the form of a decrease in NK cytotoxicity. The NK cells of the subjects had decreased levels of effectiveness, which the authors believed was due to an increase in cortisol production in the bereaved. In addition, Phillips et al. (2006) found that their elderly bereaved (loss within the last year) study participants had a less robust response to influenza vaccination than their nonbereaved counterparts, suggesting some immune impairment within their bereaved sample.

Viral Infections A number of studies examine the effects of chronic stress on viral infections. The most common infections examined include the herpes simplex virus (HSV) and the Epstein-Barr virus (EBV), though studies also have looked at the common cold virus and immune responses to viral inoculations. Stress and HIV have been studied as well.

For chronic infections that have periods of dormancy followed by active phases (e.g., HSV and EBV), the presence of an increased titer of blood antibody levels for the virus suggests an immune response deficiency. This is counterintuitive because we are inclined to think that the higher level equals a more robust immune response. However, in the case of these viruses, the higher levels represent a failure of the innate immune system to suppress the viral activity, thus requiring more B lymphocytes to respond. Therefore, higher antibody levels mean a weaker immune system. In the case of viral inoculation, however, we can draw an opposite conclusion; that is, the more robust the antibody response, the stronger the immune system.

An initial active infection with **herpes simplex virus** (HSV) may involve an outbreak of a cold sore around the mouth (oral herpes) or around the genital area (genital herpes) that typically leads to a later dormant state followed once again by an active infectious state and so on in a cyclical manner. This reactivation, brought about by the endogenous latent HSV, may or may not result in the emergence of clinical symptoms. Even before research was conducted on a stress-HSV linkage, anecdotal evidence suggested that many people with HSV suspected from their own experiences that stress could trigger activation of oral or genital HSV infection symptoms. A body of research findings now supports this belief (Bonneau, 1994).

For example, in a prospective study by Kemeny, Cohen, Zegans, and Conant (1989) of 36 patients with recurrent HSV, researchers examined immune responses monthly over a 6-month period. Patients who reported high levels of stress had the lowest proportion of CD4 and CD8 T cells. Lower CD8 T-cell count was also associated with depressed mood, hostility, and anxiety. Depressed mood was in turn associated with higher reported rates of HSV infection reoccurrence. Another study (Pereira et al., 2003) determined that life stress as measured by a modified version of the Life Experiences Survey (LES), especially within the last 6 months, positively predicted the number of genital herpes recurrences in women with HIV. Additional evidence for the stress-HSV connection was found in the saliva of adolescents who had been physically abused or had a history of living in institutions prior to adoption, indicating higher HSV-specific antibody concentrations than normal controls (Shirtcliff, Coe, & Pollak, 2009).

The **Epstein-Barr virus (EBV)** is a virus within the herpes family that is associated with mononucleosis in adolescence and young adulthood. The virus is asymptomatically present in almost all adults by the age of 40. Through examining EBV antibody titers researchers can find evidence of EBV's activity level. For example, Cacioppo and his colleagues (2002) determined that elderly women who were high-stress reactors were found to have higher EBV antibody titers than those who were low-stress reactors. They found, as did Glaser et al. (1995), that EBV could be reactivated by corticosteroids that unfortunately seem to enhance replication of the EBV in infected cells. Thus, it appears that stress increases cortisol levels, which then activate EBV while simultaneously lowering the body's resistance to the virus.

Recall earlier being asked if you would think about a potential experimental research strategy for establishing that stress contributes to coming down with the common cold like Nicole contracted. Did you think of one? If so, what strategy did you select? You now have an opportunity to compare your idea to that of a group who actually used an experimental approach to answer this question.

Sheldon Cohen, Tyrell, and Smith (1991, 1993) conducted one of the most tightly controlled prospective experimental studies to date linking stress to a viral challenge. They divided their sample of 420 subjects into six groups, with one group, the control group, given nasal saline drops and the five experimental groups given nasal drops with a different respiratory/cold virus for each group. The subjects were quarantined for 2 days prior to viral exposure and 7 days after.

During the 2-day baseline period, subjects underwent a comprehensive medical exam, and they also completed questionnaires that measured life events stress, perceived stress, and degree of negative affect. Following viral exposure, the subjects were then observed over a 7-day period, and rates of respiratory infection and clinical colds were recorded. Infection was determined by either isolating the virus after challenge or by assessing virus-specific antibody serum. Clinical colds were diagnosed by a physician only if the clinical symptoms were present and there was evidence of infection.

The results indicated that the greater the stress levels as revealed by composite stress index scores from the three questionnaires, the greater the infection rates in the experimental groups and incidence of clinical colds. In other words, there was a dose-dependent relationship between the amount of stress experienced and the likelihood of infection and illness for those exposed to the cold virus, suggesting that higher doses of stress lead to a higher likelihood of illness.

In a later study Cohen and his associates (2002) examined the role that cortisol plays in the relationship between life stress and development of upper respiratory illness. In this prospective study the researchers gathered self-report data of negative major life events for the previous 12 months and physiological data including a measurement of cortisol levels following acute stress during a baseline period. Subjects were then tracked over a 12-week period. During the tracking period participants also completed a weekly 10-item stress scale. Participants were asked to report any cold or flu illnesses they contracted, and a nurse practitioner was asked to verify any illnesses reported.

Results indicated that weekly perceived stress and immune reactivity as determined by CD8 T cell numbers, NK cell numbers, and NK cell cytotoxicity were related to self-report of upper respiratory infections. Participants initially classified as low immune reactors were later more likely to report infections during high-stress weeks. Also, as predicted, participants who had the highest levels of cortisol following acute stress at baseline and who also had the highest levels of major negative life stress events at baseline were those who had the highest rates of illness during the 12-week period.

These results support the contention that negative life stress leads to immunosuppression in people who react to stress with high levels of cortisol because cortisol has a dampening effect on the immune system. However, for those who did not show high cortisol reactions, negative life stress had little or no relationship to incidence of upper respiratory illness. Therefore, as predicted, cortisol seems to be one of the primary mediators in the stress-illness causal relationship.

As discussed earlier, the **human immunodeficiency virus (HIV-1)** infects cells such as the CD4 helper T lymphocyte. This infection leads to a reduction in the number of CD4 T cells that can in turn result in an increase in opportunistic infections that the immune system would normally resist. Ultimately, the process can eventually lead to AIDS-defining conditions (Kemeny, 1994).

The chronic stress of having HIV can lead to higher cortisol levels, lower levels of lymphocytes, and an accelerated development to AIDS (Evans et al., 1997; Kemeny et al., 1995). Leserman et al. (1999) tracked 82 gay men with HIV infection who were asymptomatic for AIDS over a 5.5-year period and concluded that those who had more cumulative life event stress, more depressive symptoms, and less social support had the fastest progression to AIDS. His research group conducted another study (Leserman et al., 2002), a 9-year prospective study of 96 gay men with HIV infection, and replicated their finding of low social support, depression, and more life stress leading to a faster progression to AIDS. In addition, this investigative group found that for each one point increase in cumulative life stress, the risk of developing AIDS increased by 14% and increased by 50% for the equivalent (in point totals) of each moderately severe event. The risk of developing an AIDS clinical condition was even more dramatic with a two- to fivefold increase for each moderately severe event. Based on this and similar research findings, Cohen, Janicki-Deverts, and Miller (2007) conclude in their commentary in the prestigious *Journal of the American Medical Association* that the evidence does indeed establish an association between stress and HIV/AIDS.

At the beginning of the chapter we discussed the belief that Nicole has of the stress of taking final exams lowering her resistance to cold viruses and making her more susceptible to catching colds. Given what you have now read regarding exams and the immune system and stress and the cold virus, was Nicole right?

STRENGTHENING THE PROTECTIVE AND IMMUNE SYSTEMS

Assuming that Nicole was right, what can she do to strengthen her immune system against the cold virus and other infectious agents other than managing her stress better—though it is worth noting that meta-analytic studies have shown there is only modest evidence that stress management can modulate the immune system (Miller & Cohen, 2001)? Let us look at some behavioral strategies for strengthening the immune system.

1. Wash Hands   This may seem like an odd recommendation when we think about the immune system, but as you will recall, the skin is our outer protective layer that gives us a first line of immune defense against infectious agents. Hand washing serves to remove the virus, bacteria, or otherwise harmful pathogens from our hands so that we are less likely to self-infect through touching our nose, eyes, mouth, or other open areas of the body (Figure 4.5). This behavioral strategy serves as an outer immunity protection so that the pathogens do not breach our outer defenses and require action from our inner defenses.

To illustrate the benefit, a study by White, Kolble, Carlson, and Lipson (2005) found that college students living in residence halls reported washing their hands at a higher rate after being exposed to a hand hygiene message campaign and had fewer colds and flu illnesses than their control group counterparts. They also missed fewer classes and less work. So one simple commonsense approach Nicole can adopt is to wash her hands more frequently.

2. Get Immunized   According to the United States Centers for Disease Control and Prevention (2010a), adult immunizations are recommended for the following: tetanus, diphtheria, and pertussis (Td/Tdap) with a booster every 10 years; the human papillomavirus for females in the 19- to 26-year age group; varicella (chickenpox) for ages 19 and over; zoster (shingles) for ages 60 and over; and measles, mumps, and rubella for ages 19 to 49. In addition, if indicated by other risk factors for ages 50 and over, influenza for ages 50 and over and if indicated by other risk factors for ages 19 to 49; pneumococcal for ages 65 and over and if indicated by other risk factors for ages 19 to 64; hepatitis A if indicated by risk factors for ages 19 and over; hepatitis B if indicated by risk factors for ages 19 and over; and meningococcal if indicated by risk factors for ages 19 and over.

What about Nicole? Is there a vaccination for the cold virus? As of today there is not one, given the more than 200 varieties of cold viruses that would need to be covered. However, most of the immunizations that are available do give some protection against more harmful pathogens than the cold virus. So a good general illness prevention strategy for Nicole is to get immunized when appropriate.

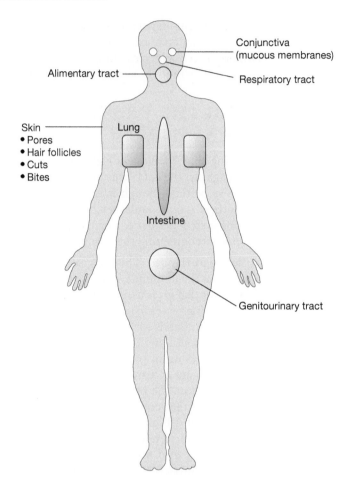

FIGURE **4.5** The Five Major Portals of Entry for Pathogens SOURCE: Batzing, *Microbiology*, 1/E. © 2002 Brooks/Cole, a part of Cengage Learning, Inc. Reproduced by permission. www.cengage.com/permissions.

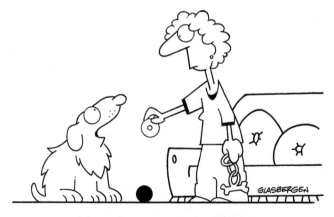

"I notice you always wash your hands after we play.
Frankly, I find that offensive."

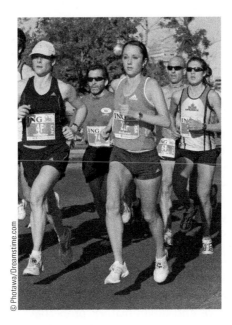

Exercise can boost the immune system if done in moderation. However, ironically, very high levels of exercise such as training heavily for and participating in a marathon can suppress the immune system.

3. Get Sufficient Sleep   Evidence is mounting that one of the restorative functions of sleep is to regulate the immune system. In a review of 20 years of discovery regarding human psychoneuroimmunology, one of the leading researchers in the field, Michael Irwin (2008), cites evidence that normal sleep consists of "increases in NK activity and a shift toward Th1/Th2 cytokine production" (p. 134). However, in people who have serious sleep disturbances, such as those who are under a lot of stress, these increases in NK activity and cytokine production are not present. Thus, good quality sleep is involved in maintaining immune competency. Irwin further notes that research, including his own, shows that even partial sleep loss results in reduced killer cell activity.

The good news is that persons can rebound back to normal immune activity upon making up sleep deficits if they address them soon enough. The bad news is that persons with chronic sleep problems and deficits will likely experience a persistent dysregulation of the immune system that can lead to increased disease risk and even risk of cardiac mortality.

Irwin suggests that chronic sleep loss also leads to a proinflammatory cytokine gene response associated with interleukin-6 (IL-6) production and expression that may account for increased cardiac mortality in patients with sleep disturbances (note that certain cardiovascular diseases such as coronary heart disease are associated with inflammation of the cardiovascular system—see Chapter 5). So when Nicole wants to climb into bed when she is sick with the cold, she is on the right track.

4. Physical Exercise   There are many benefits of physical exercise that are discussed in detail in Chapter 11. However, one benefit we will now discuss is an apparent strengthening of the immune system. Reviewers of the research in the area of exercise and the immune system (Rogers, Colbert, Greiner, Perkins, & Hursting, 2008) generally conclude that exercise seems to reduce inflammation and enhance macrophage and NK function. Regular moderate exercise (30- to 45-minute brisk walks) seems to be the most effective behavioral strategy for boosting the immune system. Too much exercise, however, can temporarily suppress immune function.

For example, Nieman (1995) reported that epidemiological data indicate that endurance athletes are at increased risk for developing infections like the cold and flu when training heavily for a marathon and for up to 2 weeks following the event. However, this same researcher and his colleagues found in a controlled study that a simple 30-minute brisk treadmill walk led to modest temporary beneficial changes in neutrophil and NK counts (Nieman, Henson, Austin, & Brown, 2005). So, when Nicole is well again, she would do well to put on that pair of walking shoes she has gathering dust in her closet and take a walk.

5. Eat Healthy Eating healthy is a good commonsense strategy that is covered in more depth in Chapter 12. The idea is to give your body the nutrition it needs to maintain and repair immune system cells. Foods that are high in antioxidants help to neutralize free radicals that can damage these and other cells in the body. For example, these include the pigment-rich berries like blueberries and strawberries. Other foods, such as those high in omega-3 fatty acids, appear to have anti-inflammatory properties, including certain fatty marine fish like salmon, particular nuts like walnuts, and seeds like ground flax seeds. Unfortunately, the nuts and seed sources only contain alpha-linolenic acid (ALA) and do not contain the more important eicosapentaeoic acid (EPA) and docosahexanoic acid (DHA) components of omega-3 that fish oils contain.

Foods rich in zinc also are beneficial to the immune system. Zinc supplementation reduces the likelihood of illnesses in the elderly and respiratory tract infections in children because zinc is used as an intracellular signal molecule by immune cells (Prasad, 2009). Foods rich in zinc include green peas, spinach, oysters, chicken, and asparagus.

Certain types of mushrooms show promise for their mild anti-inflammatory and beneficial immunomodulating effects (see Lull, Wichers, & Savelkoul, 2005, for a review). Green tea may also have antioxidant properties and potentiate the immune system (see Butt & Sultan, 2009, for a review).

In general the optimum strategy for Nicole is to provide her body with the micronutrients she needs to maintain a healthy immune system. As Bhaskaram (2002) notes, "several micronutrients such as vitamin A, beta-carotene, folic acid, vitamin B12, vitamin C, riboflavin, iron, zinc, and selenium have immunomodulating functions and thus influence susceptibility of a host of infectious diseases and the course and outcome of these diseases" (p. S40).

6. Seek Treatment for Clinical Depression Depression is covered in more detail in Chapter 7. It is now well documented that major depressive disorder is associated with many immunological changes (see Zorilla et al., 2001 for a comprehensive meta-analysis of more than 180 studies). As Irwin and Miller (2007, p. 375) discussed in their publication entitled "Depressive Disorders and Immunity: 20 Years of Progress and Discovery," during the last decade there has been mounting evidence of immunologic alterations associated with depression as part of a brain-immune reciprocal interaction pattern. They explain the process in the following way: "The experience of depression on the immune system is moderated by age, sex, socioeconomic status, life stress, physical activity and sleep. In turn, the central release of corticotrophin releasing hormone in depressed persons activates the hypothalamic pituitary axis and the sympathetic nervous system. For these efferent pathways, multiple aspects of the immune system are altered with evidence of immune suppression (e.g., decreases in lymphocyte responses), as well as inflammation. In turn, such immune changes have implications for infectious disease risk and the occurrence of inflammatory disorders." Hence, there is immunosuppression leading to potential infectious diseases as well as immune system inflammation leading to potential autoimmune disorders, cardiovascular disease, cancer, or more depression.

Should Nicole become clinically depressed, it would be in her best interest from a mental and a physical health standpoint to seek treatment. There are many effective treatments today for clinical depression, including pharmacologically based treatments and psychological treatments (see Chapter 7 for more information).

7. Avoid Known Immune System Suppressors   Another effective strategy for maintaining a healthy immune system is to avoid known immune system suppressors like cigarette smoke and excessive alcohol intake. NK cell activity, antibody responses, and functional capacity of leukocytes are all reduced in smokers in spite of the fact that they often have leukocytosis (a higher level of blood leukocytes that, in this case, is a by-product of smoking) (Sopori, 2002). Nicotine is the main immunosuppressive agent in cigarette smoke and is known to also adversely affect T cells. In addition to increased rates of cardiovascular disease, chronic obstructive pulmonary disease (COPD), and lung cancer, smokers are slower to heal from wounds (e.g., surgery) than nonsmokers. Luckily for Nicole, she is a nonsmoker.

The evidence is strong that alcohol (ethanol) has immunomodulatory effects. Moderate intake of alcohol attenuates the inflammatory response, whereas heavy use augments it. Alcoholics when defined as people who have eight or more drinks per day appear to have suppressed immune systems reflected by their higher rates of bacterial and viral infections (Goral, Karavitis, & Kovas, 2008). High levels of alcohol seem to alter cytokine production as well as create functional abnormalities in NK cells, T and B lymphocytes, and macrophages (Romeo et al., 2007). Further, alcohol seems to interfere with the ability of white blood cells to travel to sites of infection or injury.

As you may have heard, however, alcohol consumption can result in favorable health effects at low to moderate levels. People who drink low to moderate levels of alcohol (defined as one to three drinks per day) have lower mortality rates than those who drink no alcohol or who are heavy alcohol users (Goral et al., 2008). We can conclude that this is probably in part due to the drug's low-dose ability to reduce the inflammatory response, thereby lowering the risk of heart disease (Romeo et al., 2007). However, there is mounting evidence indicating that women drinking even a low to moderate level of alcohol have a small but increased risk of developing breast cancer (Goral et al., 2008). Given that the risks for low to moderate use of alcohol are mixed, it is best for Nicole to apply common sense and caution in deciding how much to drink, if at all. The evidence is clear, however, that she should avoid heavy daily drinking or binge drinking because, among other things, these behaviors lead to immunosuppression.

CHAPTER SUMMARY AND CONCEPT REVIEW

- The system of organs, tissues, and cells designed to protect the body against infections and harmful substances that can lead to illness is referred to as the immune system.

- Psychoneuroimmunology refers to the study of the relationship between the psychological, neurological, and immunological interactions.

- Prospective research designs have advantages over retrospective and cross-sectional designs in that they can verify when stress precedes illness.

- Experimental studies are better than correlational studies for determining causal relationships between stress and illness.

- Meta-analytic studies find the average effect sizes from multiple studies, thus increasing the external validity of the general findings.

- Reliability of measures is an important precondition for validity; it is necessary but not sufficient for establishing validity.

- Early researchers examining the relationship between stress and health focused mainly on self-reported stressful life events and daily hassles and later broadened to include more objectively verifiable measures of stressors because of problems associated with self-report measures.

- The human immune system can be divided into the innate immune system and the adaptive immune system.

- The innate immune system is involved in the inflammation process and includes phagocytic cells and natural killer cells.

- The adaptive immune system, a system that includes T-cytotoxic cells and B cells, remembers past invaders and can mount a vigorous response against specifically remembered offenders.

- One of the methods that immune cells use to communicate with each other is through chemical messengers called cytokines.

- Cellular-mediated immunity (Th1) quickly localizes to the site of injury or infection, and humoral immunity (Th2), mediated by antibodies, has greater target precision but less speed.

- A dysregulated immune system may involve chronic inflammation or autoimmune activity if the Th1 : Th2 ratio is chronically imbalanced.

- Acute transient stressors result in mobilization of the immune response; however, chronic stressors generally produce a broad immunosuppressive effect.

- The dampening of the immune system during chronic stress is believed to be, in large part, due to high levels of circulating cortisol.

- A significant body of research indicates immune system suppression for exam stress; large-scale disasters; loss of a spouse; response to viral challenge including herpes simplex, Epstein-Barr virus, HIV, and cold virus; and long-term caregiving by loved ones of persons with dementia.

- Recommendations for strengthening the immune system include hand washing, receiving appropriate immunizations, getting sufficient sleep, exercising in moderation, eating healthy, seeking treatment for clinical depression, and avoiding known immune system suppressors like cigarette smoke and too much alcohol.

CRITICAL THINKING QUESTIONS

1. If you were to conduct a study measuring the effects of stress on the development of cancer, what type of research method would you use? What would be the advantages and disadvantages of your method? How would you determine if stress played a role in the psychoneuroimmunological development of cancer?

2. What psychological factors like behaviors, emotions, and thoughts seem to influence the immune system? How do they exert their influence? Do you believe in the reverse process, that is, that the immune system can influence our behaviors, thoughts, and emotions? If so, how? What are the mechanisms?

3. How do you believe stress can dysregulate the immune system? What biological mechanisms seem to be involved?

4. What positive role does inflammation play in fighting infections? How does stress play a role in triggering the inflammatory response? Why is chronic inflammation considered unhealthy if inflammation is such a beneficial mechanism for fighting infection?

5. What are the top three strategies that you could employ to bolster your immune system against the effects of stress? Why did you select these three? How could you best implement these strategies?

KEY TERMS AND CONCEPTS

Adaptive immune system*

All cause mortality

Antibodies

Antigens

B cells*

Bedford College Life Events and Difficulties Schedule (LEDS)

CD4

CD8

Cellular-mediated immunity*

Control group

Correlational studies

Cross-sectional design*

Cytokines*

Dependent variable

Disease

Effect size*

Endorphins

Epstein-Barr virus (EBV)

Experimental group

Experimental studies

External validity

Herpes simplex virus (HSV)

Human immunodeficiency virus (HIV-1)

Humoral immunity*

Illness

Illness behavior

Immune dysregulation*

Immune system

Immunoglobulins (Igs)*

Independent variable

Infection

Inflammation*

Innate immune system*

Innate protective system

Interferon

Interleukin

Internal validity

Leukocytes

Life change units (LCUs)

Longitudinal designs*

Lymphocytes*

Macrophages*

Meta-analytic studies*

Monocytes

Natural killer (NK) cells*

Negative correlation

Negative life stress events

Neuropeptides

Neutrophils

Pearson Product
    Moment Correlation
    Coefficient

Phagocytes*

Positive correlation

Prospective research
    design

Psychoneuroimmunology
    (PNI)

Randomized controlled
    trials*

Reliability

Retrospective research
    design

Sickness

Sick role

Secondary gains

Social Readjustment
    Rating Scale
    (SRRS)

T cells*

T-cytotoxic cells

T-helper cells

Tumor necrosis
    factor

Validity

MEDIA RESOURCES

CENGAGE **brain**.com

Access an interactive eBook, chapter-specific
interactive learning tools, including flashcards,
quizzes, videos, and more in your Psychology
CourseMate, accessed through CengageBrain.com.

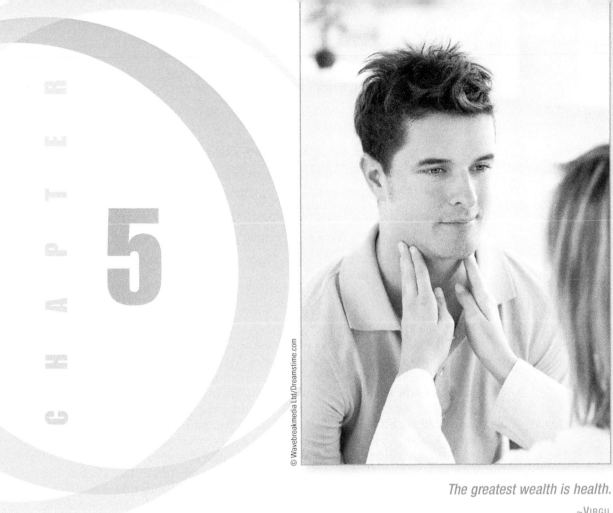

© Wavebreakmedia Ltd/Dreamstime.com

The greatest wealth is health.

~VIRGIL

CHAPTER

5

THE IMPACT OF STRESS ON HEALTH CONDITIONS

THE STRONG EVIDENCE

THE MIXED EVIDENCE

THE WEAK EVIDENCE

Marty had a history of periodic health problems. When he was younger he would experience excruciating headaches on and off. His doctor ran a series of tests only to come up empty. "It could be stress," his doctor told him. Then there was a period when Marty found himself at odds with some of his coworkers. He dreaded going to work each day. Like clockwork, he had bouts of diarrhea before heading off to work each morning. Once again after undergoing some diagnostic tests, his doctor told him, "It could be stress." Now, Marty has just been told by his physician that he has the beginning stages of thyroid cancer. Marty wondered, "Could it be stress? Why me? Why now?"

The question many like Marty ask is what role does stress play in causing health conditions and diseases. Most health conditions and diseases seem to be adversely affected by stress. Stress may or may not have contributed to the cause of these conditions, but in most cases there is good evidence that it exacerbates them. In addition, the exacerbation of symptoms associated with these conditions often creates more distress in the sufferer, which leads to a vicious cycle. Further, the stress and impairment of the health condition may lead to less sleep and detrimental changes in health behaviors such as engaging in less physical activity, using substances like alcohol and nicotine to self-medicate, or engaging in poor dietary habits that may also exacerbate symptoms. In some cases, such as in the sudden death phenomenon, stress may lead to a life cut short.

This chapter examines evidence of the adverse effects of stress on many health conditions that have attracted the attention of psychologists. Some of these conditions are considered **functional syndromes** because they are health conditions with no detectable organic cause.

The word *functional* often carries an unwarranted negative connotation, suggesting that somehow the symptoms are imagined or not real. Some estimates suggest that primary care physicians can medically explain only 16% of the symptoms that patients report (Kroenke & Mangelsdorff, 1989). Because there is no known organic cause of functional health conditions, stress is often suspected as a causal or contributing agent. An example of a functional condition covered in this chapter is irritable bowel syndrome (IBS), a gastrointestinal system condition.

Other conditions covered are long suspected of having a stress component associated with their onset or exacerbation even though underlying pathophysiological mechanisms can explain their symptom patterns once the disease unfolds. These conditions include the autoimmune conditions of systemic lupus erythematosus, rheumatoid arthritis, and Crohn's disease as well as the mucosal inflammatory disorders of asthma, allergic rhinitis, and atopic dermatitis.

In addition, cardiovascular disease and cancer, two other potentially stress influenced diseases, receive a lot of attention from stress researchers because they are so prevalent and life threatening.

The sections in this chapter are organized according to the strength of the evidence with health conditions supported by strong evidence for stress as a contributing agent to their etiology being discussed first, followed by those where the evidence is mixed, and then last the health conditions where the evidence is weak.

THE STRONG EVIDENCE

Cardiovascular Disease

Rhonda, a 56-year-old African American real estate agent, was showing a two-story home to one of her clients when a vague sense that something was not right with her began to take hold. She wondered if perhaps she had been under too much stress lately or simply hadn't been getting enough sleep as waves of fatigue began to sweep over her. By the time she walked her client upstairs to show him the home's extra bedrooms, she started feeling a nagging pain in her jaw accompanied by nausea and dizziness. She was now sweating profusely and beads of perspiration began to dot her forehead. What was happening?

She was confused as she struggled to sit down on the bare floor to regain her composure. Luckily for Rhonda, her client was a physician who recognized her symptoms immediately, called 911, and administered emergency treatment.

Rhonda recovered, but like many women, she had not recognized the signs of a heart attack because they sometimes differ from the classic male symptoms that we usually hear about. She was surprised to learn that more women die of heart disease than any other cause, including cancer, and that the statistics show a higher number of women than men die from heart disease, a supposed men's disease. Rhonda also discovered that although African Americans have a higher rate of hypertension, they have a slightly lower rate of diagnosed coronary heart disease than White Americans. However, they are more likely to die from the disease than White Americans, a disturbing statistic (American Heart Association, 2010).

Humberto's story was more common for both males and females (in spite of the atypical symptom pattern found in a large percentage of women like Rhonda). He was enjoying an outdoor South Texas backyard barbecue with his friends and family when he soon felt his left arm tingling. He sat his plate down on the picnic table, and then the full force of his symptoms hit him with a crushing pain in his chest below his sternum (breastbone). He later described the sensation as an elephant sitting on his chest. With such a heavy weight on his chest he found it hard to breathe. His breathing became increasingly labored and his skin

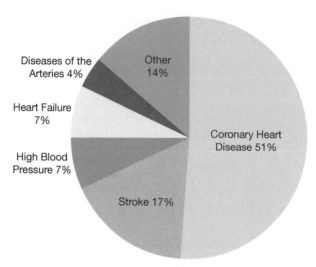

FIGURE **5.1** Deaths from Different Types of Cardiovascular Diseases in the United States in 2006

The primary cause of death from cardiovascular disease in the United States by a wide margin is coronary heart disease. SOURCE: American Heart Association (2010). *Heart disease and stroke statistics-2010 update.* Dallas, Texas: American Heart Association.

turned ashen. His left arm hurt, too, before becoming numb. He felt sick to his stomach. Droplets of cold sweat covered his body.

Before he collapsed, Humberto was able to tell his guests that he thought he was having a heart attack. They quickly called for help. Because Humberto had the classic signs of a heart attack, he was able to recognize his condition and seek immediate help that saved his life.

Humberto later learned that contrary to what he experienced, Hispanic Americans are less likely to have coronary heart disease than non-Hispanic White Americans and as he experienced, they are less likely to die from it (American Heart Association, 2010). Rhonda and Humberto are the lucky ones; they are among the survivors rather than among those who do not survive a heart attack. Cardiovascular disease includes coronary heart disease like that experienced by Rhonda and Humberto, stroke, and hypertension as well as other heart and vascular health conditions. It is the primary cause of death worldwide.

According to the American Heart Association (2010), 51% of cardiovascular disease deaths are from coronary heart disease, 17% from stroke, 7%, from heart failure, 7% from high blood pressure, and other causes constitute the remainder (Figure 5.1). By far the largest category of cardiovascular-related death causes is coronary heart disease.

coronary heart disease (CHD): also known as coronary artery disease; a progressive degenerative inflammatory disease involving atherosclerosis of the heart's arteries.

Coronary Heart Disease   Cardiovascular disease dominated by **coronary heart disease (CHD)** (i.e., coronary artery disease [CAD]), is the leading cause of death in the United States for both men and women, eclipsing cancer (Figure 5.2)

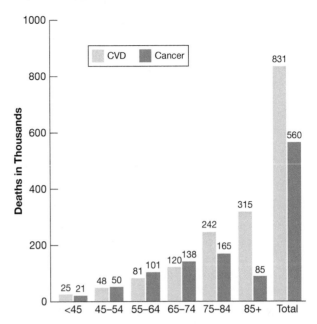

FIGURE **5.2** Cardiovascular Disease Deaths vs. Cancer Deaths by Age in the United States in 2006

As can be seen, the death rates from cardiovascular disease begin to far surpass those from cancer beginning around age 75. SOURCE: American Heart Association (2010). *Heart disease and stroke statistics-2010 update.* Dallas, Texas: American Heart Association.

even though the mortality rates have steadily declined since the mid-1960s (Figure 5.3) (American Heart Association, 2010).

CHD is a progressive degenerative inflammatory disease that involves coronary **atherosclerosis.** The atherosclerosis process is believed to be the body's way of responding to injury of the interior walls of the affected arteries. The inner lining of the vascular wall, the *intima*, is composed of endothelial cells. These cells form a type of "Teflon lining" that prevents other cells from sticking to them (Granato, 2008). However, with sufficient irritation or injury, these endothelial cells become compromised. For example, smoking cigarettes is analogous to taking sandpaper and sanding the Teflon lining so that circulating cells and compounds in the bloodstream can adhere to and penetrate the vascular walls. Other sources of injury may be stress reactions, high blood pressure, chronically high circulating blood sugar levels due to diabetes, chronic inflammation, or a chronic bacterial infection of the arteries. It is the latter two conditions that flossing our teeth may help to reduce, thereby reducing the likelihood of heart disease—reduced bacterial infection of the gums leads to reduced general bacterial infection and inflammation of the vasculature (Larkin, 2002).

Irritation or injury stimulates the inflammatory response and calls the white blood cells, the leukocytes, to action. Leukocytes called monocytes are attracted to vascular adhesion molecules on the endothelial cells and penetrate

atherosclerosis: a progressive degenerative arterial disease characterized by a narrowing of blood flow through affected arteries due to the formation of arterial fibrous plaque layers.

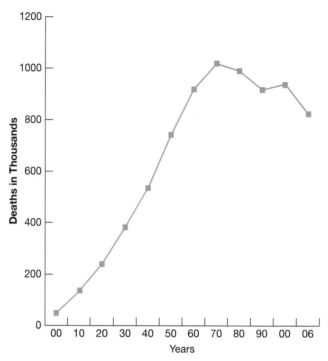

FIGURE **5.3** Deaths from Cardiovascular Disease in the United States from 1900 to 2006

The trend in deaths from cardiovascular disease in the United States increased steadily from 1900 until around the mid-1960s and then began trending downward.

SOURCE: American Heart Association (2010). *Heart disease and stroke statistics-2010 update.* Dallas, Texas: American Heart Association.

the vascular wall. Once inside, these monocytes transform into macrophages (see Chapter 3) that eat modified low-density lipoprotein (LDL), otherwise known as "bad cholesterol." It is noteworthy that the more LDL particles circulating in the bloodstream, the greater the likelihood that some will penetrate the endothelial lining. That is why it is important to keep LDL levels within normal limits. As Granato (2008, p. 14) explains, these particles tend to congregate on the endothelium "like condensation on a shower door."

As these now cholesterol-laden macrophages grow they turn into foam cells. These very large fatty foam cells stimulate smooth muscle cells from the middle layer of the arterial wall to migrate to and congregate at the site. As a result, an atherosclerotic plaque forms inside the vascular wall, a type of intra-arterial pimple that consists of cholesterol-laden foam cells, smooth muscle cells, and other debris (Granato, 2008). The coronary artery has essentially been remodeled by the plaque, which causes it to enlarge and weaken. The plaque is now like a slow-growing volcano with a fibrous cap that could erupt if it becomes unstable (Figure 5.4).

Chronic inflammatory immune responses attract platelets (small disc-shaped cells that clump together to coagulate and plug bleeding sites), lipids (fats), and

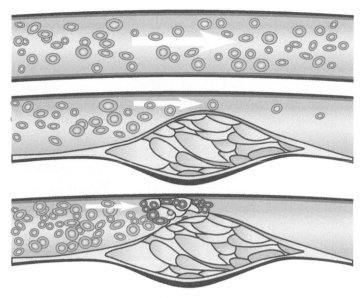

FIGURE **5.4**   An Atherosclerotic Plaque Forms Inside the Vascular Wall of the Coronary Artery, a Type of Intra-Arterial Pimple That Consists of Cholesterol-Laden Foam Cells, Smooth Muscle Cells, and Other Debris

The coronary artery has essentially been remodeled by the plaque, causing the bulge in the arterial wall and partial to total occlusion of blood flow to the heart.

Diamondimages/Dreamstime.com

leukocytes to the affected site to build on the plaque. As plaque layers build, a gradual narrowing of the affected arteries occurs. With time, the fibrous plaque hardens further through mixing with other blood components like calcium, resulting in a lack of flexibility of the arterial wall. The hardened and partially occluded artery is then no longer able to expand to allow sufficient blood to flow to the heart muscle when blood pressure increases. **Arteriosclerosis** refers to this "hardening" of the arteries. Atherosclerosis is a form of arteriosclerosis.

In the advanced stages of the disease, proinflammatory cytokines may promote plaque instability. This stage is believed to be a particularly dangerous time: A cardiac event may occur when an unstable plaque ruptures (the volcano erupts) and a blood clot (thrombosis) forms to staunch the bleeding. Blood clots may further restrict or block oxygenated blood from reaching the heart.

Evidence of the role of cytokines in this process comes from findings that elevated levels of the proinflammatory cytokines interleukin-6 and tumor necrosis factor alpha are associated with cardiac events and death in patients with acute coronary syndromes; elevated levels of tumor necrosis factor alpha are associated with a threefold risk of a recurrent myocardial infarction (MI) or death due to a coronary event (Biasucci et al., 1999; Ridker et al., 2000). The ratio of anti-inflammatory-to-proinflammatory cytokines appears to be especially predictive of acute MI (Biswas, Ghoshal, Mandal, & Mandal, 2010). In addition, these cardiac events are often associated with higher levels

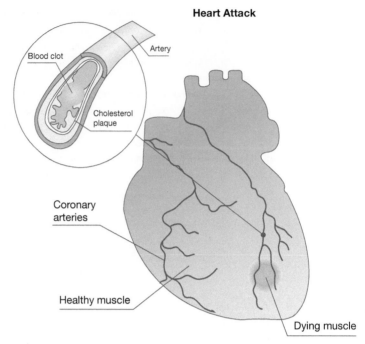

FIGURE 5.5 The Coronary Atherosclerotic Plaque Ruptures, Causing a Thrombus
The thrombus (i.e., blood clot) blocks oxygenated blood from reaching the heart, resulting in a heart attack and potential death of the cardiac muscle affected if not treated in time.　© P6m5/Dreamstime.com

myocardial infarction (MI): also known as a heart attack; when the heart has insufficient blood supply usually due to occlusion of a coronary artery which results in cardiac tissue death.

angina pectoris: severe chest pain resulting from the heart receiving inadequate oxygen.

sudden cardiac death (SCD): cardiac arrest that occurs very shortly after symptom onset that results in death.

of serum albumin and C-reactive protein (CRP), which are nonspecific markers of systemic inflammation (Benton et al., 2010; Danesh et al., 2004).

Have you ever wondered why taking a daily baby aspirin is recommended for heart health? You have probably figured it out already. Baby aspirin works as both an anti-inflammatory and anticlotting agent (it blocks an enzyme that helps platelets aggregate) (Harvard Men's Health Watch, 2010). The downside to the use of daily aspirin is that it can increase the chance of bleeding in the gastrointestinal tract, so baby aspirin is the minimum effective low-risk dose.

In the advanced stages of atherosclerosis, heart muscle deprived of oxygen develops **ischemia** (too little blood flow), which can in turn lead to angina or myocardial tissue death. A **myocardial infarction (MI),** known also as a heart attack, may be the ultimate result (Figure 5.5). There are typically three forms of clinical symptoms presentation. These include **angina pectoris,** or chest pain; an **acute coronary syndrome (ACS),** in the form of an MI; or **sudden cardiac death (SCD),** which is cardiac arrest that occurs very shortly after symptom onset that results in death (see Kop & Cohen, 2007, and Steptoe & Brydon, 2007, for a more detailed discussion of the CHD disease process and the role of the immune system).

The Effects of Stress on Blood Pressure Acute stress can cause spikes in blood pressure, and chronic stress can prevent elevated blood pressure from recovering to its normal homeostatic levels; chronic stress may also drive inflammatory responses (Chida & Hamer, 2008; Dimsdale, 2008). In addition, blood pressure spikes may cause tiny tears in the inner arterial walls that need to be patched by cholesterol-laden plaques. An example of the connection between stress and blood pressure was demonstrated in a study (Sausen, Lovallo, Pincomb, & Wilson, 1992) that found higher blood pressure activity the day before and during a student examination period, suggesting that the stress of anticipating an exam and the stress of taking an exam elevated blood pressure. Similarly, higher blood pressure was found in male Hispanic immigrant farm workers in the United States when they experienced increased stress due to perceived discrimination (McClure et al., 2010).

Essential hypertension (HTN), known most simply as *high blood pressure*, is a chronic condition with no known organic cause that is characterized by systolic blood pressure (SBP), the top number when blood pressure is reported, of 140 mm Hg or higher or diastolic blood pressure (DBP), the bottom number when blood pressure is reported, of 90 mm Hg or higher. This condition is related to increased risk of MI, congestive heart failure, stroke, and peripheral vascular disease because it can result in structural changes in the blood vessels and the heart.

Hypertensives are documented to have higher levels of circulating catecholamines, suggesting overall higher sympathetic nervous system reactivity to stressors (Goldstein, 1983). In their meta-analytic review of behavioral stress and hypertension, Fredrikson and Matthews (1990, p. 36) determined that individuals with HTN show "exaggerated blood pressure responses to all stressors" irrespective of their psychological elements. Thus, it appears that individuals with HTN display hormonal changes and blood pressure changes indicative of exaggerated physiological reactions to stress. Further, after reviewing the relevant research in the field, Steptoe (2000, p. 274) concluded that "research on psychosocial aspects of hypertension has reached a stage where secure conclusions can be drawn. The pooling of evidence from epidemiological, naturalistic, and experimental studies indicates that both psychological characteristics and chronic stressors in the environment contribute to the development of raised blood pressure and risk of hypertension."

Cholesterol and Stress Stress is commonly believed to be associated with high levels of circulating cholesterol. In a classic study, Friedman, Rosenman, and Carroll (1958) found that tax accountants had higher levels of serum cholesterol in the 2 weeks prior to the United States federal income tax deadline. Subsequent results are not as clear-cut, however. McCann et al. (1999) found in a study of 173 tax attorneys that their plasma cortisol, triglyceride, and apolipoprotein B levels were higher during tax deadline periods though the subjects' LDL, high-density lipoprotein (HDL), and total cholesterol levels were unaffected. Another study by Schwartz, Schmitt, Ketterer, and Trask (1999) replicated earlier results of a negative relationship between emotional distress and total cholesterol that, counter to intuition, high levels of emotional

essential hypertension (HTN): also known as high blood pressure; a chronic condition with no known organic cause that is characterized by systolic blood pressure of 140 mm Hg or higher or diastolic blood pressure of 90 mm Hg or higher.

distress are associated with low levels of total serum cholesterol. More recently investigators failed to find a predicted relationship between serum lipids and work stress in a 22-month longitudinal study of 1,137 healthy participants (Shirom, Melamed, Rogowski, Shapria, & Berliner, 2009).

Does that mean, then, that stress management strategies are likely to be ineffective in reducing cholesterol levels? A large multisite intervention study (Daubenmier et al., 2007) of 869 patients with CHD found that participation in a 3-month stress management program that was part of a combined multicomponent lifestyle intervention program led to reductions of total cholesterol/HDL in men participants with CHD and lowered levels of triglycerides in men and women participants with CHD. Therefore, at least in men with CHD and to a certain extent women with CHD, stress management appeared to reduce their lipid levels. It appears, however, that studies have been inconclusive regarding the nature of the complicated relationship between stress and serum lipid levels.

Sudden Cardiac Death   SCD is due to a cardiac event that leads to an abrupt loss of consciousness shortly after the onset of the event. SCD is more likely to occur in individuals with preexisting coronary and vascular diseases, such as those with CAD, angina pectoris, and HTN, but may also occur in individuals with no evidence of coronary disease (Morse, Martin, & Moshonov, 1992). Engel (1971) was the first scientific investigator to search newspaper accounts of people who had died of sudden death and draw a common thread of stress. He found that the primary categories of stress-related SCD were "personal danger or threat of injury," "the collapse or death of a close person," and "acute grief." An example of *danger or threat* was illustrated in the following newspaper account reported in his article: "A 61-year-old man shouted at boys who had been throwing stones at him and then collapsed when he went into a nearby store to phone the police" (p. 776). Engel cited the following example to represent the category of the *death of a close person*. "A 71-year-old woman arrived by ambulance at the emergency room accompanying her 61-year-old sister who was pronounced dead on arrival. The patient collapsed at the instant of receiving the news. An electrocardiogram showed AV dissociation or nodal rhythm with retrograde conduction, left bundle block and myocardial damage. Shortly she developed ventricular fibrillation and died" (p. 774).

Acute grief is seen in the following newspaper story quoted in Engel's article: "A 52-year-old man had been in close contact with his physician during his wife's terminal illness with lung cancer. Examination, including electrocardiogram, 6 months before her death showed no evidence of coronary disease. He died suddenly of a massive myocardial infarction the day after his wife's funeral" (p. 774).

Kamarck and Jennings (1991) reported in their review of five available retrospective studies of life stress and SCD that the informants across all studies reported an increase in life stress hours to months before the onset of SCD. There are many cases of SCD following the experience of a high level of stress or an intense emotional reaction. In their review of the literature, Morse et al. (1992) concluded that individuals prone to SCD were more likely to have suffered a recent major loss, be highly anxious or hostile, and/or be socially isolated. They reported that "the mechanisms for actual death can vary, but most likely pathways are: (1) excessive epinephrine release, which leads to either ventricular fibrillations or coronary artery spasm; and (2) sympathetic/parasympathetic overload leading to sinus bradycardia, which, in turn, can develop into either vertricular tachycardia, arrhythmias, and fibrillations or hypotensive shock, with resultant insufficient circulation to the heart and brain" (p. 40).

The impact of major acute stressors, such as earthquakes, can also precipitate SCD. For example, Leor, Poole, and Kloner (1996) reported upon examining death records from the Los Angeles County coroner's office that the emotional stress associated with the Los Angeles-area Northridge earthquake may have precipitated a higher number of sudden deaths due to cardiac events. Prior to the day of the earthquake the average number of SCDs was 4.6, but on the day of the earthquake the number was 24 SCDs. They stated that 16 of the 24 SCDs had reported chest pain within the first hour following the initial tremor. Heart attack death rates doubled in Israeli cities targeted by Iraqi Scud missiles during Operation Desert Storm (Kark, Goldman, & Epstein, 1995). Similarly, during World Cup soccer, researchers determined that "viewing a stressful soccer match more than doubles the risk of an acute cardiovascular event" (Wilbert-Lampen et al., 2008, p. 475).

The Role of Emotion   **Anger** and **hostility** may play a role in acute MIs or lethal arrhythmias. As Futterman (2002) explains, anger increases catecholamine levels, blood pressure, heart rate, the likelihood of vasospasms, as well as platelet aggregation, thus making it more likely that there will be a disruption of vulnerable areas of plaque resulting in occlusive ischemia followed by an MI or SCD. Futterman (2002, p. 575) also points out that, "emotional or psychological stress, specifically anger or hostility, are significant and independent risk factors in ischemic heart disease and can precipitate an acute myocardial infarction (MI) or lethal arrhythmias." A recent meta-analysis also concluded that "anger and hostility are associated with CHD outcomes both in healthy and CHD populations" (Chida & Steptoe, 2009, p. 936). Trait anger is associated with both an increased risk for HTN and CHD in men (Player, King, Mainous, & Geesey, 2007) although anxiety may be a better CHD predictor than anger or hostility for women (Consedine, Magai, & Chin, 2004). See Chapter 6 for a more in-depth discussion of these risk factors.

A recent meta-analysis of 28 studies confirmed that depression also is an independent risk factor for cardiovascular disease (Van der Kooy et al., 2007). Lett et al. (2004), based on their review of relevant studies, concluded that depression increases the risk of developing CAD by between 1.5 and 2 times and increases the risk of cardiac death in those with CAD by between 1.5 and 2.5 times. Robles, Glaser, and Kiecolt-Glaser (2005, p. 111) suggest that proinflammatory cytokines, especially interleukin-6 (IL-6), are "directly stimulated by chronic stress and depression," and "that a key pathway through which chronic stress and depression influence health outcomes involves proinflammatory cytokines."

One of the most saddening and severe stressors a parent can experience, the death of one's child, was found in a prospective study of bereaved parents to increase their risk of MI long term (at a 6-year follow-up) (Li, Hansen, Mortensen, & Olsen, 2002).

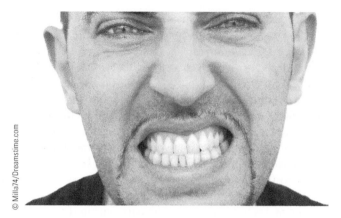

Anger and hostility are associated with increased risk of coronary heart disease.

In general, so-called negative emotions such as anger, hostility, anxiety, and sadness, the distress emotions, seem to be those most closely associated with CHD.

Stress and Cardiovascular Disease   Dong et al. (2004) conducted a retrospective cohort study of 17,337 adults and found that adverse childhood experiences (e.g., family dysfunction, neglect, abuse) increased the risk of developing adult ischemic heart disease by 1.3- to 1.7-fold in a dose-dependent way; in other words, the more adverse childhood experiences, the greater the risk of ischemic heart disease. They also found, as have others, that ischemic heart disease was associated with increased risk of anger and depressed affect. The authors suggested that "the chain of events begins with childhood exposure to abuse, neglect, and household dysfunction, which lead to the development of unpleasant affective states, depression and anger/hostility, as a result of the long-term effect of physiological response to stress. Attempts to cope with these stresses may also lead to the adoption of risk behaviors such as smoking, overeating, and physical activity" (p. 1765).

Out-of-hospital cardiac arrests were determined to be more common on Mondays than any other day of the week, suggesting that the stress of going to work after the weekend may be a possible trigger (Gruska et al., 2005). The stress and circadian rhythm changes associated with long-term (6 or more years) shift work also can lead to increased risk of CHD, as was demonstrated in a large-scale study of 79,109 female nurses (Kawachi et al., 1995).

Among workers in general, the mix of job strain, low job control, and low social support is related to **coronary vascular disease (CVD)** (Niaura & Goldstein, 1992). In a review of research on work stress and cardiovascular disease, Landsbergis and his colleagues (2001) concluded that the psychological stress of having a low degree of control, known as **low decision latitude** (see Chapter 9), was the most consistent predictor of CVD. They cited as support for their conclusion studies such as Haynes and Feinleib's (1980) Framingham Heart Study that found clerical workers to be twice as likely as white-collar workers (e.g., managers) to have heart disease. A more recent meta-analysis of 14 prospective cohort studies of a combined 83,014 employees suggested that work stress was associated with an overall increased risk of CHD by 50% (Kivimaki et al., 2006). Having a low socioeconomic status (SES) is another stress factor associated with increased CHD risk because individuals with low SES are more likely to engage in a pattern of adverse health behaviors such as smoking, eating a higher fat diet, and infrequent exercise (Govil, Weidner, Merritt-Worden, & Ornish, 2009).

Earlier we discussed the major categories of newspaper accounts of sudden death reported by Engel. However, to round out the discussion, one of the minor categories of his newspaper clippings with a twist also should be discussed. This one dealt with excitement of a positive nature. As an example, Engel included the following account in his article: "A 56-year-old man collapsed and died while receiving congratulations for scoring his first hole-in-one" (p. 777).

Therefore, extreme excitement, even when positive, can trigger SCD. Could this be an example of *eustress* rather than *distress* causing a lethal outcome? In a review of the SCD trigger events literature from 1970 to 2004, Strike and Steptoe (2005) concluded that the primary behavioral and emotional trigger events were emotional stress, including anger and extreme excitement, and physical exertion in the nonfit, and that many of the symptoms occurred within 1 to 2 hours after the trigger event.

Prevention Strategies   The news, however, is not all bad. Though genetics plays a role, at least 90% of the risk of heart attack can be modified by lifestyle changes according to Yusuf and colleagues' (2004) INTERHEART study of 15,152 cases of acute MI and 14,820 controls from 52 countries. This finding is true for people of all ethnic group categories measured in their study (defined as Europeans, Chinese, South Asians, Black Africans, Arabs, and Latin Americans). The INTERHEART study is the largest global study to date to measure risk of MI. Based on the study's findings, let us examine recommendations for reducing risk according to the nine modifiable risk factors studied.

1. Do Not Smoke   The INTERHEART study found that smoking results in a 36% increase in risk for an acute MI. No amount of smoking is safe. The American Heart Association (2010) estimates that smoking cuts short a male smoker's life by 13.2 years and that of female smokers by 14.5 years.

2. Eat Fruits and Vegetables   Eating a variety of fruits and vegetables lowers the risk of CHD by 30% (Yusuf et al., 2004). The phytochemicals (bioactive plant chemicals) found in these foods may cleanse the body's cells and help to neutralize damage. In addition, fruits and vegetables may help to keep weight, blood pressure, and cholesterol in check. An optimal diet for preventing CHD is one that has nonhydrogenated unsaturated fats as the primary source of fat (see Chapter 12), whole grains, many fruits and vegetables, and sufficient omega-3 fatty acids (Hu & Willett, 2002).

3. Exercise More   Physical exercise can strengthen the heart muscle, lower blood pressure, help with weight management, reduce the risk of diabetes, and preserve muscle mass (see Chapter 11). The INTERHEART study found that combining the actions of breathing clean air (i.e., not smoking), eating a variety of fruits and vegetables, and exercising can lower relative risk of having an MI by 80%.

4. Lower Cholesterol   The key to controlling cholesterol is to keep LDL levels low and HDL (the "good cholesterol") levels high. HDL repackages and transports excess cholesterol to the liver so that it can be eliminated in bile. It is the "antidote to toxic LDL" (Granato, 2008, p. 36). Eating foods low in saturated fats can help reduce LDL levels. Exercising, stopping smoking, losing weight if overweight, and consuming moderate levels of alcohol (1 to 2 drinks per day) can lower LDL levels and raise HDL levels. Eating foods high in omega-3 fatty acids, increasing soluble fiber through eating a variety of fruits and vegetables, and increasing monounsaturated fats (e.g., olive oil) in the diet can increase HDL levels (see Chapter 12 for a more complete discussion of dietary fats and cholesterol). If these measures are insufficient, a physician may prescribe one of the cholesterol lowering drugs that reduces LDL levels.

5. Control Obesity   Obesity increases the risk of diabetes, HTN, and high cholesterol. Abdominal (around the waist region) obesity is a particularly dangerous risk for CHD.

6. Prevent Diabetes   Diabetes, a disorder of metabolism that results in high circulating levels of glucose in the bloodstream following digestion, dramatically increases the risk and severity of CHD. High blood glucose levels can damage the blood vessel walls over time and initiate the atherosclerotic process. Maintaining a regular exercise program and keeping weight in check will help prevent type 2 diabetes. Having metabolic syndrome increases the risk of developing both heart disease and type 2 diabetes. The National Cholesterol Education Program (2002) defines metabolic syndrome as consisting of at least three of the following conditions: high waist circumference, triglycerides, blood pressure, and fasting blood glucose levels, or low levels of HDL (Table 5.1).

7. Manage Stress   Given what you have previously read, it goes without saying that managing stress is an important strategy for reducing risk of CHD. See the next section, Coping with Coronary Heart Disease, for more discussion on the benefits of stress management for the prevention of recurrent heart attacks.

8. Prevent High Blood Pressure   As discussed previously, high blood pressure may damage the lining of the arterial wall, initiating the CHD process. Engaging in regular physical exercise, maintaining optimal weight, and reducing salt intake may help to maintain normal blood pressure. If HTN develops, it should be treated before it does too much damage. Though behavioral treatments for HTN have shown some modest results (see Linden & Moseley, 2006, for a review), in general they are not as potent as pharmacological strategies (e.g., Perez, Linden, Perry, Puil, & Wright, 2009) and should at this stage be regarded with some skepticism given the poor methodological quality of many of the studies purporting to demonstrate effectiveness (see Dickinson et al., 2008, for a review). There are a number of effective blood pressure medications for managing HTN.

9. Alcohol   Moderate alcohol (1 to 2 drinks) intake actually decreases the chance of CHD. This could be due to its ability to reduce inflammation and raise

TABLE **5.1** Conditions Associated with Metabolic Syndrome

The National Cholesterol Education Program (2002) defines metabolic syndrome as consisting of at least three of the following conditions: high waist circumference, high triglycerides, high blood pressure, high fasting blood glucose levels, or low levels of high-density lipoprotein. Metabolic syndrome increases the risk of developing both heart disease and Type 2 diabetes.

Traits and Medical Conditions	Definition
Elevated waist circumference	Waist measurement of • 40 inches or more in men • 35 inches or more in women
Elevated levels of triglycerides	• 150 mg/dL or higher or • Taking medication for elevated triglyceride levels
Low levels of HDL (good) cholesterol	• Below 40 mg/dL in men • Below 50 mg/dL in women or • Taking medication for low HDL cholesterol levels
Elevated blood pressure levels	• 130 mm Hg or higher for systolic blood pressure or • 85 mm Hg or higher for diastolic blood pressure or • Taking medication for elevated blood pressure levels
Elevated fasting blood glucose levels	• 100 mg/dL or higher or • Taking medication for elevated blood glucose levels

Source: Grundy, S.M. et al. (2005). Diagnosis and Management of the Metabolic Syndrome: An American Heart Association/National Heart, Lung, and Blood Institute Scientific Statement. *Circulation*, 112:2735–2752.

Note: Other definitions of similar conditions have been developed by the American Association of Clinical Endocrinologists, the International Diabetes Federation, and the World Health Organization.

HDL levels while somewhat lowering LDL levels. Alcohol also has the ability to counteract blood-clotting tendencies. However, recommending alcohol use as a CHD prevention strategy is controversial because of cultural or religious proscriptions, not to mention the possibility of increasing the risk of alcohol abuse. So good judgment should always be employed when thinking about using alcohol as a prevention strategy. In general, the American Heart Association (2011) advises that if you do not already drink alcohol, you should not start.

Yusuf et al. (2004, p. 950) ultimately narrow their focus onto a few risk factors to lower the chance of developing CHD determined by the INTERHEART study as they conclude, "Therefore, smoking avoidance, increased consumption of fruits and vegetables, and moderate activity (along with lipid lowering) should be the cornerstone of prevention of coronary heart disease in all populations worldwide."

Coping with Coronary Heart Disease   Most people assume that they will not have a heart attack, so when they do, they may be shocked and even traumatized. As a result, some begin to have problems with anxiety, fearing a reoccurrence that may lead to disability or death. The loss of health and/or of confidence in a regularly beating heart, also can lead to depression. Anxiety and depression are common by-products of the heart event experience, and counseling may be beneficial for understanding and coping with the disease and its psychological corollaries (Carney & Freedland, 2007).

In addition, cardiac rehabilitation programs may yield beneficial results physically and psychologically (Bellg, 2008; Harlapur, Abraham, & Shimbo, 2010). These programs often use a broad behavioral medicine strategy that has multiple components. For example, the Daubenmier et al. (2007) study discussed previously employed a Multisite Cardiac Lifestyle Intervention Program over a course of 3 months to evaluate the independent effects of exercise, low-fat eating, and stress management in a group of 869 nonsmoking patients with CHD. These investigators found overall significant coronary risk reduction. When they teased out the component parts they discovered that exercise was related to lower total cholesterol; stress management to weight loss, reduced triglycerides, and lowered hostility; and low-fat eating to weight loss, lower total cholesterol, and lower HDL levels. In addition, the research group discovered independent, interactive, and additive benefits for each of these strategies. An earlier meta-analysis of 37 studies found that psychoeducational programs for patients with CHD resulted in a 34% reduction in cardiac mortality and a 29% reduction in the likelihood of having another MI (Dusseldorp, van Elderen, Maes, Meulman, & Kraaij, 1999).

Blumenthal et al. (2005) demonstrated that exercise and stress management were more effective at reducing emotional distress and cardiovascular risk markers than medical care alone for a group of 134 patients with stable ischemic heart disease in their randomized controlled trial study. However, one review (Rees, Bennett, West, Davey, & Ebrahim, 2004) of 36 trials for a total of 12,841 patients concluded that stress management alone showed no strong evidence for reducing cardiac mortality even though it was associated with a reduction of nonfatal MIs. The authors also expressed concern about the poor quality of many of the studies examined. Further, they saw a tendency toward publication bias of favorable studies. As a result, they expressed skepticism about the validity of some of the results that showed beneficial outcomes for stress management. Evidence for the use of exercise-based rehabilitation programs for CHD is more supportive. And, on average, these programs result in a 31% reduction in cardiac-related mortality for those with CHD (Joliffe et al., 2001).

In a classic study conducted by Dean Ornish and his associates (1990) that helped to overturn the conventional wisdom of the day that CHD was irreversible through lifestyle changes, diet modification programs associated with low-fat vegetarian eating combined with smoking cessation, exercise, and stress management were determined not only to reduce the risk of recurring MI but also to actually reverse the CHD process as measured by average percent diameter coronary artery stenosis (narrowing). These findings have been replicated by his group (Ornish et al., 1998) in patients who maintained these lifestyle changes for 5 years with even more improvement of CHD at

5 years (a 7.9% relative improvement) than had occurred in the 1-year interval (a 4.5% relative improvement) measured in the previous study. This compares to the control group that showed a 5.4% relative worsening at 1 year and a 27.7% relative worsening at 5 years. In addition, the control group experienced twice as many cardiac events (as experienced on an average per patient basis) than their counterparts who made the sustained lifestyle changes.

Unfortunately, a more recent study failed to replicate the reversal of cardiac artery narrowing, but it did find other benefits such as reduced cardiovascular risk factors and lower rates of angina with the Ornish program (Aldana et al., 2007).

Skeletal Muscle Conditions

Robert had been looking forward to his first date with Heather all week. It had taken all his courage to ask her out because he thought she was definitely out of his league. However, as the days counted down to Saturday night, he could feel the tension in his body grow, turning his neck, shoulders, and back muscles into hard knots. By Saturday morning, he woke up with a stiff neck and felt a dull, pounding pain radiating though his head and out his eyes. He popped a few aspirin and waited, but they didn't make a dent. In fact, his headache got worse.

Robert had wanted to make a good impression on Heather, but he knew he wouldn't be good company with a head pain like this. He gave her a quick call, apologized for having to cancel his date, then climbed into bed and put a cold compress over his eyes. "Oh well," he thought, "maybe I'll ask her out again next month or, on second thought, maybe not."

Does Robert have a brain tumor? No, but without a confirmed diagnosis, it is always prudent to see a physician to rule out the possibility of organic causes. However, in this case we know what Robert has. What do you think? He has a regular garden variety headache called a tension-type headache.

The human body has three types of muscles: the skeletal muscles, the heart or cardiac muscles, and the smooth muscles. The **skeletal muscles,** the muscles of the body attached to bone, also are known as the striated muscles because of their shape and color, and as the voluntary muscles because we have control over their contractions except during reflex actions. These muscles contrast with the **heart muscles,** which are responsible for the heart's contractions, and the **smooth muscles** such as those found in the gastrointestinal tract, which are responsible for gastric motility, and in the walls of the arteries. The skeletal muscles are often measured in psychophysiological research with an **electromyograph (EMG).** Tension-type headaches (TTH), bruxism, and temporomandibular pain and dysfunction syndrome (TMPDS) are all conditions associated with tension of the skeletal muscles.

tension-type headache (TTH): the most common type of headache, characterized by head pain that often has corollary pain in the neck, back, or other related muscle areas.

migraine headaches: head pain believed to be neurovascular in origin that is typically felt more on one side of the head and may be accompanied by feelings of nausea and auras such as unusual lights and odors.

Tension-Type Headache   The most common type of headache is the **tension-type headache (TTH).** This type of headache, formerly known simply as tension headache, was renamed TTH in 1988 by the International Headache Society. TTH accounts for the vast majority of all headaches (Rasmussen, Jensen, Schroll, & Olesen, 1991) and is characterized by head pain that often has corollary pain in the neck, back, or other related muscle areas. It is different from **migraine headaches.**

Migraines are believed to be neurovascular in origin and are experienced more frequently by women than men. They are typically felt more on one side of the head. These painful headaches (i.e., migraines) may be accompanied by feelings of nausea and auras such as unusual lights or odors. It is a common belief that headaches, especially TTHs, are stress related. But does the research support this belief? Research suggests that TTHs are related to **proximal** (i.e., near term) **stressors** and that development of migraine headache patterns are related to **distal** (i.e., distant term) **stressors.** For example, Benedittis and Lorenzetti (1992) found that study participants with chronic headache reported higher numbers of daily hassles (i.e., indicators of proximal stress) than control participants but not more major life events (i.e., indicators of distal stress). Their patients with TTH reported a higher incidence of daily hassles than their patients with migraine.

proximal stressors: stressors that occurred in the more recent past.

distal stressors: stressors that occurred in the more distant past.

Ficek and Wittrock (1995) also discovered that study participants with TTH reported more daily hassle stress than their headache-free counterparts. Likewise, Venable, Carlson, and Wilson (2001) found that study participants with TTH reported increased levels of psychological distress compared to controls' levels. In addition, Armstrong, Wittrock, and Robinson (2006) presented evidence that patients with TTH seem to have more difficulty than controls in coping subjectively with aversive stimulation.

A recent laboratory study by Cathcart, Petkov, Winefield, Lushington, and Rolan (2010) found that 91% of participants who had a history of suffering from TTH developed a headache after being exposed to an hour-long stressful mental task, but only 4% of healthy controls developed a headache. Other test runs of pain thresholds and muscle tenderness indicated that the participants with TTH were generally more pain sensitive than controls, suggesting a possible mechanism for their vulnerability to TTH.

In a long-term longitudinal cohort study, Waldie (2001) examined childhood headache patterns and found that headache sufferers who reported experiencing more stress during adolescence were more likely as adults to have a migraine diagnosis than a TTH diagnosis. She concluded that this finding supports the claim that the initial onset of migraine headache is related to distal stress. Recent reviewers also confirm that "there is evidence that a stressful time period might precipitate the onset of migraine attacks in a patient who has not had them before, but who may be predisposed to develop clinical migraine by genetic factors" (Sauro & Becker, 2009, p. 1381).

Bruxism and the Temporomandibular Pain and Dysfunction Syndrome

Amanda was under a lot of stress. Her marriage was falling apart, her work was demanding, and her three young children whom she loved dearly were, as she said, "driving her crazy." Amanda's husband noticed that she clenched her jaw repeatedly when she was on the receiving end of one of their frequent arguments. After each restless night of sleep, she awoke with a sore jaw and sensitive teeth.

On her next visit to the dentist, Amanda was told she had bruxism and possibly TMPDS. "What is bruxism?" she asked, recoiling from the strange exotic name of the disorder. "Bruxism," her dentist told her, "is teeth grinding." If she continued at this pace, her dentist warned, she would grind the enamel off her teeth and wear them down to nubs. Her dentist prescribed stress management and a device called a night guard to wear while sleeping to protect her teeth from further damage.

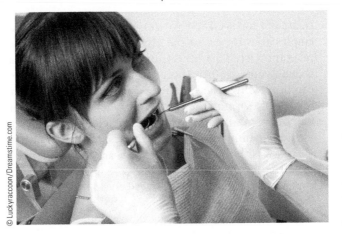

Bruxism and temporomandibular pain and dysfunction syndrome (TMPDS) are most likely to be diagnosed by dentists.

© Luckyraccoon/Dreamstime.com

temporomandibular pain and dysfunction syndrome (TMPDS): a syndrome characterized by myofascial pain, particularly in the temporomandibular joint and the muscles involved in chewing.

bruxism: involuntary habit of excessive teeth clenching or grinding that can lead to abrasive wear on the teeth, headaches, and/or temporomandibular pain and dysfunction syndrome.

Both bruxism and **temporomandibular pain and dysfunction syndrome (TMPDS)** are disorders that dentists, among health care professionals, are most likely to see.

Bruxism is defined as an involuntary habit of excessive teeth clenching or grinding that can lead to abrasive wear on the teeth, headaches, and/or TMPDS. Both TMPDS and bruxism seem to be stress related. TMPDS is characterized by myofascial pain, particularly in the temporomandibular (TM) joint (the joint used to open and close our jaw) and the muscles involved in mastication (i.e., chewing). The TM joint may emit clicking or popping sounds during movement, and there may also be deviations in jaw movement. Ruth Moulton (1955) was the first to propose that the habit of teeth grinding along with TM joint problems may be a misguided attempt to reduce inner tension that inadvertently creates a vicious cycle of muscle spasm followed by pain and then, once again, spasm.

In a review of the literature concerning TMPDS and bruxism, Biondi and Picardi (1993) reported that there is a body of evidence supporting the contention that stress and bruxism are related. Examples of supportive research include a study (Rugh & Solberg, 1975) that found that nocturnal bruxism is more common after stressful days. Bruxing behavior is reported in response to anticipatory stress as well (Funch & Gale, 1980). A recent study (Giraki et al., 2010) confirms through examination of the wear patterns on bruxism monitoring devices worn by participants during sleep for five consecutive nights that bruxism is related to self-reported stress including daily stress and work stress.

Likewise, TMPDS appears to be mediated by stress and is related to hyperactivity and spasms of the masticatory muscles (Scott & Lundeen, 1980). Schumann, Zeiner, and Nebrich (1988) discovered that, as hypothesized, patients with TMPDS had higher muscle tension (as measured by electromyography activity) in the masticatory muscles during resting baselines and during stressful mental activity. Such results suggest a strong link between stress and bruxism as well as between stress and TMPDS.

Prevention and Behavioral Treatment Strategies for Skeletal Muscle Conditions
Fumal and Schoenen (2008) reviewed the research on TTH and concluded that preventive therapy is generally not effective. However, acute behavioral

treatment for specific episodes of TTH can be effective. In fact, there is good empirical evidence for the effectiveness of EMG biofeedback combined with relaxation (see Chapter 14 for more discussion). The authors also found that, though cognitive-behavioral stress management approaches (see Chapter 10) can be effective, they are most successful when combined with biofeedback or relaxation. Overall they recommended the combination of drug therapies (e.g., ibuprofen or aspirin) and nonpharmacological approaches (e.g., stress management relaxation or physical therapies) for the treatment of TTH.

As was the case with Amanda, an oral appliance like a night guard is the most frequent treatment for bruxism or TMPDS though there has been some controversy regarding its effectiveness for the treatment of musculoskeletal facial pain (Marbach & Raphael, 1997). Flor and Birbaumer's (1993) study of 57 patients with chronic back pain and 21 with TMPDS found that EMG biofeedback was more effective following treatment and at a 6- and 24-month follow-up than cognitive-behavioral treatment or a conservative medical treatment for reducing chronic musculoskeletal pain.

So the most likely effective behavioral treatment for TMPDS is to use a combination of an oral dental occlusion appliance like a night guard to protect the teeth from excessive wear and EMG biofeedback to reduce jaw tension and pain.

Atopic Disorders—Asthma, Allergic Rhinitis, and Atopic Dermatitis

> Rodney was just 5 years old and had been playing outside running and throwing snowballs at his older brother when he started coughing, wheezing, and gasping for air. This had never happened to him before and was very scary. Rodney was having his first asthma attack. Since that day and his subsequent diagnosis, Rodney has lived his life following an asthma action plan. As an adult, he now keeps an asthma diary, measures his peak expiratory flow (PEF) with a peak flowmeter, and takes oral medication and another medication in the form of a corticosteroid inhaler to control his lung inflammation. He also has an emergency plan for what to do if his asthma attack becomes too severe.

atopic disorders: health disorders characterized by biological hypersensitivity and inflammation such as asthma, allergic rhinitis, atopic dermatitis, and conjunctivitis.

Atopic disorders like Rodney's asthma are characterized by a biological hypersensitivity and inflammation. These mucosal inflammatory disorders are believed to be due to a dysregulation of the immune system whereby it overresponds to certain exogenous antigens. The atopic category includes asthma, allergic rhinitis (i.e., hay fever), atopic dermatitis (e.g., some forms of eczema), and conjunctivitis (e.g., allergy form of pink eye). Let us examine the effects of stress on atopic disorders, focusing primarily on asthma, allergic rhinitis, and atopic dermatitis.

Asthma is a chronic condition that has acute phases in which the respiratory system becomes inflamed and bronchial airways constrict. The acute phases may be triggered by one of many allergens, changes in air temperature or moisture, exertion, or other factors.

In a recent meta-analysis by Chida, Hamer, and Steptoe (2008) of 34 studies examining the relationship between atopic disorders (over 90% of which were the atopic disease of asthma) and psychosocial factors, the investigators determined that the psychosocial factors of early stress exposure, psychological distress, and low social support were related significantly to the future onset of atopic disorders and their clinical course. The conclusion that early psychosocial factors relate to the later development of atopic disorders is very important and the first of its kind. They also found support for a bidirectional relationship in which the presence of an atopic disorder is related significantly to psychological distress and vice versa.

Rona, Smeeton, Amigo, and Vargas (2007) were able to rule out the possibility that distress leads to overreporting of asthma symptoms, and they confirmed the association between psychological distress and asthma symptoms. It is likely then that there is a positive feedback loop between asthma and stress whereby the asthma attacks create distress, which, in turn, precipitates more attacks.

Prevention and Behavioral Treatment Strategies   There are a number of primary prevention strategies for allergy and allergic asthma (one form of asthma) outlined by the World Allergy Organization and the World Health Organization (Asher et al., 2004). These include avoiding tobacco smoke, especially during pregnancy and early childhood, and eliminating it from the workplace; reducing indoor air pollution; minimizing exposure of at-risk young children to inhalant allergies like dust mites, cockroaches, and furry animals; preventing or eliminating exposure to highly irritating or sensitizing agents in occupational settings; minimizing exposure to damp housing conditions; and breastfeeding infants exclusively until the age of 4 to 6 months (breast milk may contain some protective factors).

One strategy for managing asthma once it develops involves avoiding triggers. Triggers are different for each person and can include cold air; exercise; irritants like cigarette smoke or perfume; certain medications like aspirin; certain foods like peanuts or food additives like sulfites; or allergens like dust mites, mold, animals, and pollens.

Some evidence suggests that writing about stressful events has benefits for patients with chronic illness, including those with asthma. For example, Smyth,

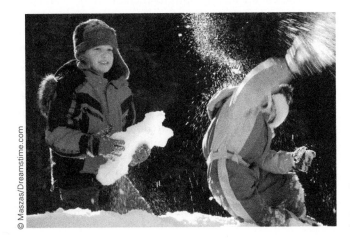

© Maszas/Dreamstime.com

For those with asthma, attacks can be triggered by exercise or cold air.

Stone, Hurewitz, and Kaell (1999) conducted a randomized controlled trial of patients with asthma and rheumatoid arthritis and asked them to write about their stressful life experiences or about neutral topics. Patients with asthma who wrote about their stress showed significant lung function improvements at a 4-month follow-up, whereas those who wrote about neutral topics showed no improvements. Likewise, patients with rheumatoid arthritis showed improvements of overall disease activity at follow-up, but only if they were writing about their stress experiences and not about a neutral subject.

Hockemeyer and Smyth (2002) also found improvements in lung function for young adults with asthma using a manual-based self-administered 4-week stress management treatment as compared to a matched placebo intervention control group. The workbook exercises consisted of writing about stressful experiences, doing cognitive-behavioral work, and following audio guidelines played on a cassette for deep breathing and relaxation. Curiously, though lung function improved in the workbook group, members of this group did not perceive stress levels improving as a result of the exercises. The authors speculated that relaxation and breathing exercises may promote diaphragmatic breathing (a form of deep breathing) that could benefit those with asthma. In addition writing about stress events may help people better make sense of their troubles, which, in turn, may promote healthier psychological and physiological functioning.

> Shelly always dreaded this time of year, hay fever season. It was especially bad when the winds kicked up and the trees and grasses released their pollen. No matter how careful she was, some of these little irritants seemed to find their way into her nose to torment her, causing her to sneeze, get congested, have red watery eyes, and generally feel bad. Shelly has hay fever or what physicians refer to as allergic rhinitis.

allergic rhinitis (AR): also known as hay fever; involves allergic reactions to certain pollens, dust particles, or airborne chemicals.

In a review article concerning **allergic rhinitis (AR),** Mosges and Klimek (2007) noted that AR is most common in children and affects 20% to 30% of the world's population. They also expressed concern that over 90% of those diagnosed with AR suffer from moderate to severe symptoms.

AR sufferers have allergic reactions to certain pollens, dust particles, or airborne chemicals. Symptoms include itchy, watery, or burning eyes; nasal congestion; loss of smell or runny nose; stuffy head; headaches over the paranasal area (alongside the nose); blunted taste; an itchy roof of the mouth; dry cough; sore throat; drainage down the back of the throat; itchy ears; or a full or plugged feeling in the ears (Johnson, Harrington, & Perz, 2004).

What role, if any, does stress play in the development of this allergic condition? One large-scale survey study done in Finland of over 10,000 first-year university students reported that subjects who had been diagnosed with allergic rhinitis or asthma were more likely to have experienced stressful life events such as death of a family member or parental or personal conflicts at some point in their life than nonatopic subjects (Kilpelainen, Koskenvuo, Helenius, & Terho, 2002). The effect was stronger for allergic rhinitis than asthma but not found for atopic dermatitis. Because this was a retrospective study, we must be somewhat cautious in interpreting the results, but when viewed in concert with Chida and colleagues' (2008) meta-analytic conclusions discussed earlier, it lends support to the idea that risk for developing allergic rhinitis may also be related to early stress exposure.

A recent experiment conducted by Jan Kiecolt-Glaser and her colleagues (2009) found that people with seasonal allergies in a high-stress condition (giving a videotaped 5-minute speech to an audience then performing 5 minutes of mental arithmetic followed by watching their videotaped speech and math performances) had a resulting welt from an allergen prick test that was magnified by their anxiety. The anxiety experienced by the stressful experience was also associated with increased interleukin-6 production, a proinflammatory cytokine. Thus, acute stress appears to exacerbate the hay fever allergic response.

> Phillip had a skin condition he was embarrassed about. It was especially embarrassing when his condition appeared on his face and he had to go to work, especially because he worked in a kiosk in a shopping mall and dealt with lots of people. When he got it on his arms or legs, it was easier to hide. It would start with an unbearable itching sensation somewhere on his skin, then develop into a patch of rash that became inflamed, scaly, and dry. Phillip had a form of eczema that his doctors called atopic dermatitis.

Atopic dermatitis is characterized by a hypersensitivity of the skin to particular foods or environmental allergens that results in the skin becoming inflamed, feeling itchy, and perhaps scaling or flaking.

What role does stress play in atopic dermatitis? In a normal immune system Th1 and Th2 immunity are in proper balance (see Chapter 4). However, in eczema, there is too much Th2 relative to Th1. Upon reviewing the allergy literature, Hashizume and Takigawa (2006) concluded that acute stressors that chronically and repeatedly raise the anxiety levels of patients with atopic dermatitis lead to a worsening of allergic symptoms by dysregulating the immune system through enhancing Th2 responses. This model of stress-induced dysregulation toward Th2 immunity can be applied to all the atopic disorders. In a review by Marshall and Agarwal (2000, p. 241), the authors suggested "that chronic stress does not simply suppress the immune system, but induces a shift in the type-1/type-2 cytokine balance toward a predominant type-2 cytokine response. Such a change would favor the inflammatory milieu characteristic of asthma and allergic diseases."

Coping Strategies   At present, most coping strategies recommended for those with hay fever involve avoidance. The same is true for those with skin allergies. The general idea is to avoid allergens or minimize indoor allergen counts. For example, when working outdoors, hay fever sufferers are advised to wear a filter mask during peak seasons and times, to wash their clothes that might contain allergens after going outside, to wash their hair before going to bed, and to keep their windows closed.

Medications like antihistamines also are used to control allergic responses for those with hay fever or skin allergies. Atopic dermatitis can be managed through good skin care, including providing skin hydration for eczema, limiting allergen and irritant exposure, and controlling itchiness and inflammation through oral or topical medications (e.g., corticosteroids).

Some strategies for controlling eczema involve suppressing the entire immune system (both Th1 and Th2) or, in a more precisely targeted fashion, selectively boosting Th1 and/or suppressing Th2 (Nasir & Burgess, 2005).

THE MIXED EVIDENCE

Cancer

Diana had turned 40 this last year. She knew that reaching 40 meant she should get her first mammogram.

Just routine, she thought, as her radiology technician placed her left breast in position between two plastic plates in preparation for the x-rays. When she was done she didn't give it a second thought because she had no family history of breast cancer.

However, later that week she was on the phone with her physician asking, "What do you mean when you say the test found an abnormality?" Her doctor explained that it could be cancer or it could be benign and recommended further testing.

Again, not to worry she told herself, because after looking at statistics online, she learned that mammograms often have false positives—that is, the test sometimes wrongly suggests cancer. She agreed to a fine-needle aspiration where the area of concern is numbed and a needle is inserted to extract suspicious cells.

The results came in. Diana looked with disbelief at her doctor as he told her she had a malignancy. After getting over the initial shock of her diagnosis and going through her treatment, Diana realized she was one of the fortunate ones who received a diagnosis when the cancer was localized. She had a good chance of becoming one of the 98% who survive to the 5-year benchmark and beyond because she had testing that caught the cancer at its early stage (American Cancer Society, 2010).

cancer: an umbrella category of around 200 diseases involving endogenous abnormal cells developing, proliferating, and then invading the body's healthy tissues.

Cancer is a term used to describe a category of around 200 diseases in which endogenous abnormal cells develop, proliferate, and then invade the body's healthy tissues. The death rates for cancer vary by type with lung cancer being the leading cause of cancer death for both men and women (Figures 5.6 and 5.7). There is a widespread belief that stress can lead to susceptibility to cancer. However, at the present time, the evidence for this belief is mixed.

Supportive studies include one by Scherg and Blohmke (1988). These authors conducted a retrospective study of 508 German women who were born before World War II and who were diagnosed with cancer (40% had breast cancer). Compared to controls, they found a dose-response relationship between the number of traumatic WW II experiences the women had and cancer risk; that is, the greater the number of traumas experienced, the greater the cancer risk. In addition, they found that those who had lost a mother in childhood to death and those who had lost a spouse through divorce, separation, or death had a greater risk for cancer.

In a review of the literature relating stress and cancer, Levenson and Bemis (1991) reported that a number of studies have revealed an increased number of life-event stressors prior to developing cervical, pancreatic, gastric,

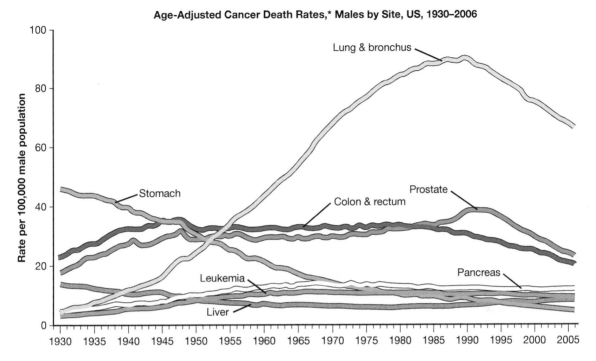

Age-Adjusted Cancer Death Rates,* Males by Site, US, 1930–2006

*Per 100,000 age adjusted to the 2000 US standard population.

FIGURE **5.6**   Though declining, lung cancer continues to be the leading cause of cancer death among men, followed by prostate and colon cancer.   SOURCE: American Cancer Society (2010), *Cancer facts and figures 2010.* Atlanta, GA: American Cancer Society, p. 2. www.cancer.org/acs/groups/content/ @nho/documents/document/acspc-024113.pdf.

lung, and breast cancer. They also discussed a possible mechanism for these results as immunosuppression of the natural killer (NK) cells, cells that are specifically involved in cancer surveillance. These cells, they noted, vary in activity with stress in noncancer as well as breast cancer research subjects. However, they cautioned against making direct causal links between psychosocial factors and cancer until more methodologically rigorous studies are conducted. Levenson and Bemis concluded that there is more evidence for a linkage between stress and cancer progression than stress and cancer onset.

One review (McKenna, Zevon, Corn, & Rounds, 1999) found a *moderate* association between stress and the development of breast cancer in a meta-analysis of 46 studies examining psychosocial factors and the development of breast cancer. Factors such as history of stressful life experiences, experience of loss and separation, and use of denial- or repression-based coping strategies were all related to breast cancer onset.

However, in a similar meta-analysis of 29 studies, Petticrew, Fraser, and Regan (1999) concluded that whereas analysis of their larger study's sample found that adverse life events were twice as likely to be reported by patients with breast cancer than by controls, when poorer quality studies were eliminated

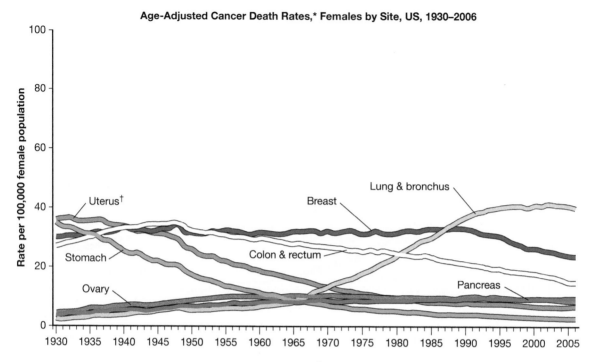

Age-Adjusted Cancer Death Rates,* Females by Site, US, 1930–2006

*Per 100,000 age adjusted to the 2000 US standard population. †Rates are uterine cervix and uterine corpus combined.

FIGURE **5.7**   Lung cancer is the leading cause of cancer death among women, followed by breast and colon cancer.   SOURCE: American Cancer Society (2010), *Cancer facts and figures 2010.* Atlanta, GA: American Cancer Society, p. 3. http://www.cancer.org/acs/groups/content/@nho/documents/document/acspc-024113.pdf.

from their analysis, there did not appear to be a causal relationship between these variables. Likewise, Butow et al. (2000) reviewed the studies that examined the relationship between psychosocial factors and development of breast cancer and found that "few well-designed studies report any association between life events and breast cancer, the exception being two small studies using the Life Events and Difficulties Schedule (LEDS) reporting an association between severely threatening events and breast cancer" (p. 169). They concluded that the overall empirical evidence of a link is weak. Similarly, Duijts, Zeegers, and Borne (2003) concluded from their more recent meta-analysis of breast cancer studies conducted between 1966 and 2002 that their findings "do not support an overall association between stressful life events and breast cancer risk" (p. 1023). Current research findings continue to confirm that at most there is only a "weak association between life stress and losses in adulthood and breast cancer risk" (Eskelinen & Ollonen, 2010, p. 899).

Researchers also have discovered a positive relationship between stressful events such as foot-shock and subsequent tumor growth in animals such as mice (Sklar & Anisman, 1980). However, as discussed by Levenson and Bemis (1991),

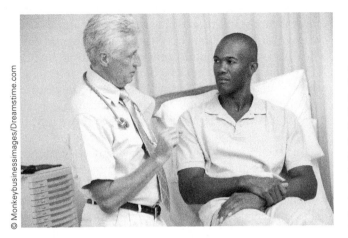

African American men have double the risk of developing prostate cancer and dying from it than other American men, making prostate cancer screening all the more important for men of this ethnic group.

it is difficult to generalize from mice to humans regarding this issue for several reasons. These rodent strains have been bred specifically to develop cancers from viruses, a process that is uncommon in humans, occurring in only 2% to 3% of known human cancers. In addition, when these animals are exposed to carcinogens, it is typically at very high doses, which does not match the chronic low-dose exposure that humans with cancer may have had in the real-life environment.

Prevention Strategies Cancer prevention strategies focus primarily on screening for cancer, practicing sun safety, eating healthy foods, losing weight, exercising, and avoiding tobacco smoke and environmental carcinogens (Paharia, 2008). A more recent addition is the use of the human papillomavirus (HPV) vaccine for females age 11 to 18 for prevention of cervical cancer. Cancer screenings are recommended routinely for breast cancer; cervical cancer; colon and rectal cancer; oral cancer; skin cancer; and prostate cancer depending on gender, age, and risk. Along with gender and age, ethnicity also may play a role in cancer risk. For example, African American men have double the risk of developing prostate cancer and dying from it than other American men (American Cancer Society [ACS], 2010).

Sun safety involves protecting the skin from harmful ultraviolet rays with proper shade, fabric, or sunscreen. According to the ACS (2010), cancer of the skin is more prevalent than any other type of cancer, accounting for almost 50% of the cancers diagnosed in the United States. Eating healthy and maintaining a healthy weight reduces cancer risk. The overweight and obese are more likely to have higher levels of hormones such as estrogen and insulin that can potentially foster cancer cell growth. A diet high in fruits and vegetables (at least 5 servings a day); low in processed and red meats; with whole grains instead of processed grains; and with limited, if any, alcohol intake (for women 1 drink per day and for men 2 drinks per day maximum) is recommended by the ACS (2011a). The ACS also recommends between 30 and 60 minutes of exercise for a minimum of 5 days a week. Regular exercise reduces the risk of breast cancer by as much as 30% and colon cancer by up to 40% (Lee, 2003).

Smoking tobacco increases cancer risk considerably, especially lung cancer, one of the most life-threatening cancers. Breathing secondhand smoke also increases risk of lung cancer. Other environmental carcinogens to be avoided when possible include air pollution; radiation; some infectious agents (e.g., HPV); and certain chemicals like benzene, arsenic, formaldehyde, lead, and asbestos among others. Estimates based on the research evidence suggest that smoking cessation combined with consuming a healthy diet would prevent over 50% of the current cancer incidence (Bowen & Boehmer, 2010).

Coping Strategies   Upon receiving a diagnosis of cancer, patients naturally often feel distress or anguish. Much of the distress results from worries about disfigurement, disability, or death. The intensity and frequency of the distress varies according to many factors, including the type of cancer diagnosed. For example, a higher percentage of those diagnosed with lung cancer report high levels of distress than those diagnosed with cancer with a better prognosis, such as breast, prostate, or colon cancer (Zabora, BrintzenhofeSzoc, Curbow, & Hooker, 2001).

Psychological interventions for people diagnosed with cancer usually focus on decreasing anxiety and any depression they may experience (Jacobsen & Jim, 2008). Although there is a widespread belief that cancer is associated with depression, at best it is only slightly more prevalent in patients diagnosed with cancer than in general medical patients; and unlike CHD, which has a strong depression link, depression does not appear to cause or accelerate cancer's progression (Simon, Palmer, & Coyne, 2007).

There is a growing body of literature exploring the potential for using psychological interventions (e.g., psychotherapy) to improve longevity in cancer survivors. Spiegel and his colleagues are the most vocal advocates of this hypothesis (Spiegel, 2002; Spiegel, Bloom, Kraemer, & Gottheil, 1989; Spiegel & Giese-Davis, 2003). However, the primary studies that support their position have confounds that, if removed, could lead to the alternative conclusion that the benefits experienced by patients with cancer were due to receiving more intensive medical care and better medical surveillance than to the psychological interventions (Coyne, Stefanek, & Palmer, 2007; Palmer & Coyne, 2004). Statistical problems also may have led to erroneous conclusions in some supportive studies (Simon et al., 2007).

A hopeful more recent study found that psychological interventions based on mindfulness-based stress reduction approaches (see Chapter 14) can reduce stress, cortisol levels, systolic blood pressure, and Th1 proinflammatory cytokines in outpatients with breast and prostate cancer immediately after the intervention and at a 1-year follow-up (Carlson, Speca, Faris, & Patel, 2007). Along the same line, McGregor and her colleagues (2004) found that cognitive-behavioral stress management increased immune function (improved lymphocyte proliferation) in a group of women with early-stage breast cancer. They noted that these immune system changes at a 3-month follow-up were preceded by an increase in positive emotions due to finding some benefit out of their breast cancer experience. The participants had apparently positively reframed their cancer experience, which may then have led to more positive emotions and an enhanced immune system (recall posttraumatic growth from Chapter 3).

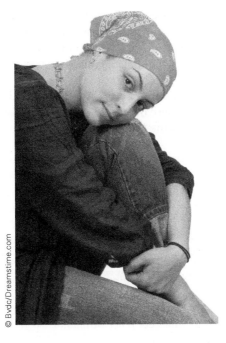

Mindfulness-based stress reduction approaches have been found to reduce stress, cortisol levels, systolic blood pressure, and Th1 proinflammatory cytokines in outpatients with breast and prostate cancer.

© Bvdc/Dreamstime.com

Dean Ornish, who you will recall conducted pioneer lifestyle change research in the area of CHD, more recently also conducted similar research in the area of cancer. Ornish and his associates (2005) compared two groups of men diagnosed with early-stage prostate cancer who, under the supervision of their oncologists, decided to monitor their cancer's progression rather than seek conventional treatment. Using a random assignment procedure, 49 patients were placed in a control group where they continued their normal lifestyles and 41 were placed in an experimental group where they engaged in an intensive lifestyle change program that involved eating a vegetarian low-fat diet, taking nutritional supplements, practicing stress management, and participating in a support group. During the study the patients' prostate-specific antigen (PSA) levels were monitored to determine potential cancer activity and tumor growth. As a result of PSA and/or magnetic resonance imaging testing, six members of the control group ultimately elected to drop out of the study and receive conventional treatment (surgery, chemotherapy, and radiotherapy).

At the conclusion of the study's 12-month interval, the remaining members of the control group saw their cancer worsen an average of 6% as reflected by their PSA levels. However, *none* of the 41 patients in the lifestyle change group elected to seek conventional treatment because their average PSA levels *decreased* by 4%, suggesting that their cancerous tumors were regressing.

In addition, laboratory testing revealed an impressive finding, that is, blood from the lifestyle change group was almost *eight times* more effective at inhibiting cultured laboratory prostate cancer cell growth than blood from the control group. Thus, Ornish and his colleagues concluded that intensive lifestyle changes may slow the progression of prostate cancer.

In sum, there continues to be suggestive evidence that psychological interventions and lifestyle changes can lead to immune system and health-enhancing improvements in patients with cancer. At this stage of the research, although there is hopeful evidence, we can only speculate as to whether these changes will ultimately lead to a longer life for patients with cancer.

THE WEAK EVIDENCE

Gastrointestinal System Conditions

Fred was finding it harder and harder to drink his daily cups of coffee or even eat anything with tomato sauce on it, like his favorite meal, spaghetti and meat sauce. When he did, his stomach almost always got upset. Actually, it got worse than upset. He would feel a burning sensation in his insides above his bellybutton and described it as like having one of those movie space-alien monster babies gnawing on his stomach trying to get out. This didn't feel like indigestion even though he sometimes got relief with antacids. What's wrong he wondered? This isn't normal.

When Fred finally went to a gastroenterologist, he received the diagnosis. Fred had a peptic ulcer.

"I-B what?" Nadia asked. "IBS," her doctor repeated. "In fact, you have what is known as alternating IBS, the most common pattern of irritable bowel syndrome, and one that occurs in about 50% of cases. Alternating IBS," her doctor explained, "is where your bowel patterns alternate between constipation and diarrhea." "What's the cause?" she asked. "It is a functional disorder that often has triggers but no known cause," her doctor replied. Although she didn't like that answer, she felt some consolation in at least knowing there was a diagnosis for her condition. Nadia wondered why she would get these cramps in her abdomen and have diarrhea all day long after going several days with no bowel movements at all. Sometimes she passed thin ribbon-like stools or other stools she called "rabbit pellets." This had been going on for far too long and now maybe she could get some relief she thought.

The gastrointestinal (GI) system in humans is designed to ingest and digest food. It consists of the upper GI tract, the lower GI tract, and the accessory organs. The upper GI tract involves the mouth, pharynx, esophagus, and stomach, and the lower GI tract consists of the small intestine and the large intestine, of which a section of the latter includes the colon. Accessory organs are organs that aid in digestion and include the liver, gallbladder, and pancreas (Figure 5.8).

Two of the GI system conditions that popular wisdom suggests are most closely associated with stress are peptic ulcers and IBS. However, what do the research studies show? Does stress cause ulcers? How about IBS?

peptic ulcers: erosions in the lining of the esophagus, stomach, or duodenum.

Peptic Ulcers   **Peptic ulcers** are erosions in the lining of the esophagus, stomach, or duodenum (upper small intestine). For many years these ulcers were

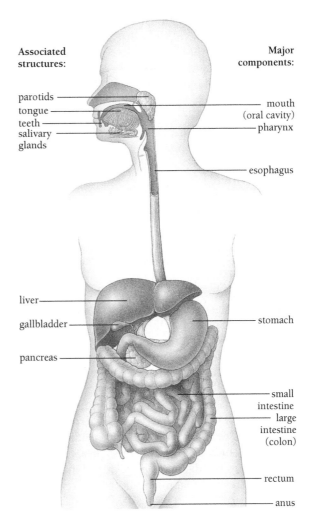

FIGURE **5.8**   Upper and Lower GI Tract and Accessory Organs

The upper GI tract involves the mouth, pharynx, esophagus, and stomach, and the lower GI tract consists of the small intestine and the large intestine, of which a section of the latter includes the colon. Accessory organs are organs that aid in digestion and include the liver, gallbladder, and pancreas.   SOURCE: BRANNON/FEIST, *Health Psychology*, 6/E. © 2007 Wadsworth, a part of Cengage Learning, Inc. Reproduced by permission. www.cengage.com/permissions.

Helicobacter pylori (H. pylori) **bacteria**: bacterial microorganisms that are usually benign but can sometimes inflame the mucosal layer of the stomach or duodenum, leading to the development of an ulcer.

widely believed to be caused by stress, diet, or other lifestyle issues. However, during the past 20 years the pathogenic focus has been primarily on infection with the *Helicobacter pylori (H. pylori)* **bacteria**. These bacteria, which are usually benign, can sometimes inflame the mucosal layer of the stomach or duodenum, leading to the development of an ulcer.

In a review of studies examining the relationship between stress and peptic ulcers, Jones (2006, p. 407) concluded that "at present there is no definitive study proving a causal relationship between psychological stress and the development of ulcer disease." However, he also noted that between 5% and 20% of those who have peptic ulcers do not have *H. pylori* bacteria present or evidence of any other recognized organic etiology such as use of **nonsteroidal anti-inflammatory drugs** (**NSAIDs**) (e.g., aspirin). Therefore, he argues that there may be at least a small percentage of those with peptic ulcers who have symptoms caused by psychosocial factors. Further methodologically controlled studies need to be conducted, however, to make more definitive determinations.

irritable bowel syndrome (IBS): a functional disorder characterized by episodes of pain or tenderness along with bowel disruptions in the form of diarrhea and/or constipation.

functional disorder: a health condition with a diagnosable pattern that has no known organic cause.

Irritable Bowel Syndrome **Irritable bowel syndrome** (**IBS**) is a **functional disorder,** that is, a disorder of no known organic cause. It is characterized by episodes of abdominal pain or tenderness along with bowel disruptions in the form of diarrhea and or constipation. It is sometimes called "spastic colon" though it is different from colitis, which is a more serious inflammatory bowel disease. IBS is more common in females and affects as many as 10% of adults (Talley & Spiller, 2002).

Most patients with IBS believe that stress plays a role in their symptoms, but the causal relationship is somewhat unclear (Blanchard et al., 2008). Tally and Spiller (2002) contend that chronic, rather than acute, stressors account for most of the impact of stress on the onset and persistence of IBS symptoms.

However, in a large-scale prospective study of over 200 patients with IBS, Blanchard and his colleagues (2008, p. 127) found "little support for a causal model" of stress, though they did find that patients with IBS reported more frequent hassles than their nonill controls.

Hertig, Cain, Jarrett, Burr, and Heitkemper (2007) discovered that the 187 women with IBS they studied reported more frequent and higher severity of retrospective stress, greater daily stress when tracked across approximately a 1-month period, and more psychological distress than did controls. Stress was significantly positively correlated with the severity of abdominal discomfort in women with IBS across groups but not day-to-day changes in abdominal discomfort within groups. Controlling for anxiety and depression eliminated most of the relationship between stress and the severity of abdominal discomfort in participants with IBS. Though it is clear that the participants with IBS were more distressed than their counterparts with no IBS, the relationship between stress, distress, and symptoms appears to be complex. Some of the complexity, the authors suggest, is that illness behavior may contribute to perpetuation of the disorder through a process, whereby those with IBS react to their GI symptoms with distress that in turn exacerbates their symptoms.

Searle and Bennett (2001) reviewed a decade of literature between 1990 and 2000 that included 14 papers on a related though more serious condition called **inflammatory bowel disease** (**IBD**). Whereas IBS is a functional disease that eludes detection with traditional testing, IBD always has visible inflammation of the intestinal lining that is seen through x-ray or colonoscopy (Salt & Neimark, 2002). IBD is a broad term that incorporates both **Crohn's disease** (**CD**) and **ulcerative colitis** (**UC**).

Though two distinct diseases, CD and UC are chronic diseases that have episodic overlapping symptoms that vary in severity such as stomach pain, diarrhea (often bloody), weight loss, and tiredness. CD is an autoimmune disease; the immune system attacks the GI system, leading to GI symptoms. There also may be swollen joints, skin rash, and eye inflammation. UC also is a serious IBD that is characterized by GI symptoms and ulcers of the colon. The authors of the review, Searle and Bennett (2001), concluded that "there is a considerable body of research literature examining the impact of psychological stress on the aetiology and course of IBD" (p. 122). Results of the review point to daily hassles being more significantly associated with IBD symptoms than major life events. They suggested that daily hassle stress exacerbates IBD symptoms, which, in turn, create psychological distress.

However, though stress may play a role in exacerbating symptoms, Maunder and Levenstein (2008) concluded from their more recent review of IBD that "evidence of a contribution of stress to disease onset is very weak" (p. 247).

Coping Strategies   Peptic ulcers can be cured in a relatively short time, often in 2 to 4 weeks. Treatment varies depending on the cause. Ulcers caused by the *H. pylori* bacteria are usually treated with antibiotics to kill the bacteria. The antibiotics are usually combined with a stomach acid–reducing medication to aid healing. Behavioral changes such as quitting smoking and reducing or eliminating alcohol or caffeine consumption may help the healing process. Ulcers caused by using NSAIDs can be treated by discontinuing their use. Surgery may be required in some severe cases.

Treatment for IBS is complicated and generally focuses on managing the symptoms. One approach is to identify the specific triggers like certain foods, caffeine, stress, and so on and then avoid or minimize them. If stress is a trigger, then attending a stress management program may be beneficial. General lifestyle changes to improve health may be recommended such as getting regular exercise or quitting smoking. Medications that manage the symptoms may be taken as needed. Unfortunately, most of the studies conducted to date assessing treatments for IBS have poor methodological quality. However, there is some scattered evidence of the clinical effectiveness of a variety of different interventions (Akehurst & Kaltenthaler, 2001).

Treatment for IBD is individually tailored and may involve use of medications, smoking cessation, dietary changes, counseling, and sometimes surgery. Due to methodological problems of the few studies assessing psychological interventions to reduce stress and their apparent weak or negative outcomes, stress management approaches should be used only for individuals with IBD with known stress vulnerabilities (Maunder & Levenstein, 2008).

Systemic Autoimmune Disorders

Maria found herself lying in the grass looking up at the face of a paramedic leaning over her. She had passed out while taking a morning walk in the neighborhood park and a stranger had called for help. Maria had been having strange, unaccounted-for symptoms of muscle and joint pain, heavy fatigue, heart palpitations, mouth sores, and fever that came and went. Though she knew that her body was screaming out to her, she could never seem to get to the bottom of what her body was trying to tell her. Lately, she had been depressed and anxious, and she thought that maybe if she did some exercise it would lift her spirits and calm her down. When she awoke, however, she was confused and couldn't quite remember why she was walking in the first place.

By the time Maria was admitted to the ER, her doctor noticed a butterfly-shaped rash covering her cheeks and bridge of her nose, the telltale sign. Her doctor explained to Maria that she probably had lupus, an autoimmune disease. Lupus, the ER doctor stated, occurs more frequently in women, African Americans, Latinos, American Indians, and Asians than in men and Caucasians (Centers for Disease Control and Prevention, 2011b).

systemic autoim-
mune disorders: disorders characterized by the immune system broadly attacking the body's own cells and tissues.

In **systemic autoimmune disorders,** the body's immune system mistakenly attacks its own cells and tissues. The immune system is dysregulated in that it fails to recognize *self* from *other.* As discussed in Chapter 4, immune dysregulation is an under- or overreaction of the immune system to exogenous or endogenous threats. In autoimmune disorders, the immune dysregulation is an example of an overreaction against mistaken endogenous threats. Overreactions of the immune system are believed to play a role in transplant tissue rejection and in well-known autoimmune diseases such as lupus erythematosus and rheumatoid arthritis. A number of studies examined the effects of stress on systemic lupus erythematosus and on rheumatoid arthritis. Let us next look at their findings.

Systemic Lupus Erythematosus   **Systemic lupus erythematosus (SLE)** is a relatively rare chronic multisystemic autoimmune disease whereby the body's antibodies target its own organs and tissues. Symptoms vary widely and may include fatigue, fever, skin rash, weight loss, various inflammation responses, and lowered resistance to infections. Individuals with SLE may also experience secondary psychological issues such as cognitive deficits, acute states of confusion, and mood disorders.

As far back as the mid-1950s, Selwyn Brody concluded after studying 42 patients with lupus that "stress plays a part in the precipitation, recurrence, and exacerbation of the disease" (Brody, 1956, p. 44). However, more recently, after reviewing the SLE and stress studies done from 1990 to 2006, Bricou et al. (2006, p. 283) surmised that "stress as a causal factor is not proved, but it seems to act as an exacerbating factor in disease activity and to have an impact on the quality of life."

A number of studies revealed that daily stress seems to have a bigger impact than life-event stress on exacerbation of self-reported symptoms of those with SLE. For example, in a prospective study of patients with SLE given daily evaluations over an average of 1.6 months, a group of researchers found that daily stress was more strongly related than major life events to the exacerbation of SLE symptoms (Adams, Dammers, Saia, Brantly, & Gaydos, 1994). Likewise, Peralta-Ramirez, Jimenez-Alonso, Godoy-Garcia, and Perez-Garcia (2004) examined daily stress for 6 months in a group of patients with SLE and found that daily stress, rather than stressful life events, best predicted symptom severity as perceived by their subjects.

Bricou et al. (2006) also commented that a couple of studies reported that patients with SLE differed from controls in their immune responses to stressors. This suggests that patients with SLE may have a dysfunctional immune system response to stress. They also reviewed retrospective studies that tried to examine the role that stress played in the origin of the disease and found them to be methodologically inadequate. Therefore, Bricou and his colleagues suggested that one cannot draw conclusions at this time about the role that stressors may play in the onset of the disease. The authors concluded that the reviewed studies suggest that stress has the biggest impact on quality of life for those with SLE and, to a lesser extent, plays a role in ongoing disease activity.

Coping Strategies   Medications often are used to control lupus symptoms. These may include NSAIDs to reduce pain and inflammation or corticosteroids to reduce inflammation and regulate immune system activity. More aggressive immunosuppressive drugs may be used to manage severe cases. Curiously, antimalarial drugs are sometimes effective though the disease has no relationship to malaria. Use of sun block is recommended to reduce the likelihood of rash outbreaks. Lifestyle changes such as incorporating a diet high in fish oil and low in saturated fats, smoking cessation, and stress avoidance also may be recommended (Ioannou & Isenberg, 2002). Cognitive-behavioral therapy (see Chapter 10) may reduce depression, anxiety, and somatic symptoms although it does not seem to reduce disease activity (Navarrete-Navarrete et al., 2010) Though idiosyncratic in its clinical presentation and often a challenge for physicians to formulate a successful treatment plan, the prognosis for SLE management has improved considerably over the last several decades due primarily to the increased availability of an array of pharmacological agents (Ioannou & Isenberg, 2002).

Rheumatoid Arthritis

> Mark described it as a war within his body. He had been suffering from this inner battle fatigue for years. Each morning it would take him an hour or more to work through his morning stiffness and loosen his joints. His joints were tender, painful, and swollen. As if that wasn't enough, he often had fatigue, weakness, a low-grade fever, and a general feeling of being sick with the flu, only he wasn't. Sometimes he got these strange bumps under his skin on his elbows.

Although women are more likely to have this condition than men (Centers for Disease Control and Prevention, 2011a), Mark's gender did not protect him against this autoimmune disease. Mark's immune system is in a constant war with his own body, particularly the joints in his body. Mark has rheumatoid arthritis.

Rheumatoid arthritis (RA) is a chronic autoimmune disorder characterized by inflammation of and sometimes damage to the joints and surrounding tissues. It also may involve other organs of the body. The inflammation can lead to pain and limitations in joint function. Clinical observations have long suggested a relationship between RA and stress though early studies found contradictory results when appropriate controls were applied.

A review of the findings by Koehler (1985) prompted the author to explore three possible pathogenic models of the stress-RA causal relationship. The first model posits that stress leads to more muscle tension that in turn affects the joints. Koehler found no evidence for this model. The second model states that stress-related hormonal changes lead to inflammation of the joints. Though this model is possible, Koehler argued that increase in stress usually results in increased cortisol, which should reduce, rather than increase, inflammation. A third model suggests a direct causal linkage between stress and the immune system. For example, he notes that direct sympathetic nervous system stimulation of immune system organs such as the spleen and thymus could affect inflammation without necessarily elevating cortisol levels.

Affleck, Tennen, Urrows, and Higgins (1994) used a prospective daily design to examine the relationship between stress and RA over a 75-day period. These researchers discovered that participants with RA who reported higher levels of negative life change stress for the 6-month period prior to the study also reported higher pain levels in their daily diaries the day after a high level of undesirable events. Further, in the study the participants with RA with the most active inflammatory disease showed a more pronounced positive relationship between reported daily stressors and same- and next-day pain. Finally, subjects with RA who reported less social support also reported greater levels of next-day mood disturbance following a daily stressor. These results suggest that vulnerabilities to the effects of daily stressors such as having a higher level of negative life change stress, having a more active inflammatory disease, and experiencing less social support all exacerbate the impact of daily stressors on the pain and mood state experienced by the person suffering from RA.

Are there direct biological markers that demonstrate the relationship between acute stress and inflammatory responses? Yes. Steptoe, Hamer, and Chida (2007) conducted a meta-analysis of 30 laboratory studies and found robust effects for higher levels of interleukin-6 (IL-6), interleukin-1β (IL-1β), and marginal effects for CRP following acute stress. Each of these has been used as a biological marker for proinflammatory responses. In fact, they noted that studies support the use of these inflammatory markers to predict future CHD and mortality. Thus, Straub and Kalden (2009, p. 114) contend that "stress in patients with chronic inflammatory diseases such as rheumatoid arthritis (RA) stimulates proinflammatory mechanisms."

A recent groundbreaking study (Dube et al., 2009) of 15,357 adult health maintenance organization members is the first of its kind to find that retrospective self-reports of childhood traumatic stress are positively associated with a greater likelihood of being hospitalized with a diagnosis of an autoimmune disease such as RA decades later. Because childhood trauma was recently found to be associated with the inflammatory marker CRP in adults two decades later (Danese, Pariante, Caspi, Taylor, & Poulton, 2007), it is plausible that proinflammatory activity initially triggered by childhood stress could partially explain the mechanism for developing adult RA. Although the

RA diagnoses and hospitalizations were objectively verified, the childhood traumatic stress could not be verified due to the retrospective nature of the study. Therefore, as in all retrospective studies, some caution in interpreting the results is advised.

Nevertheless, there is strong evidence that acute stress often leads to circulating inflammatory agents and is associated with flare-ups of RA. Also, there is now very limited emerging evidence linking childhood stress to adult RA though more studies are needed before evidence-based conclusions supporting the link can be drawn.

Coping Strategies   As with the management of SLE, pharmacological approaches may include use of NSAIDs or corticosteroids. There also is a class of medications called disease-modifying antirheumatic drugs (DMARDs) that can be used to alter the course of the disease. Surgical approaches (e.g., joint surgery) also may be indicated.

Behavioral approaches include stress management, cognitive-behavioral therapy, and self-management approaches. For example, Parker et al. (1995) found that patients with RA in a stress management group showed "improvements on measures of helplessness, self-efficacy, coping, pain, and health status" (p. 1807). These results were still present at a 15-month follow-up. Evers, Kraaimaat, van Riel, and de Jong (2002) found that patients with relatively early RA who received tailored cognitive-behavioral therapy showed reduced fatigue, depression, and helplessness following treatment and at a 6-month follow-up. These patients also reported using more posttreatment active coping strategies to deal with stress.

After reviewing lay-led (as opposed to doctor or nurse led) self-management education programs for those suffering from chronic conditions like RA, the authors of the review (Foster, Taylor, Eldridge, Ramsay, & Griffiths, 2007) concluded that these programs can lead to short-term small improvements in self-rated health, self-efficacy, and frequency of aerobic exercise. Though there were modest improvements in pain, fatigue, depression, and disability, these were not seen as clinically meaningful.

CHAPTER SUMMARY AND CONCEPT REVIEW

- Stress may play a causal role in the development of some health conditions, and in other conditions it appears to play no causal role yet contributes to the exacerbation of symptoms.

- Stress-induced spikes in blood pressure can begin the process of coronary heart disease (CHD) with periods of sustained high blood pressure increasing the risk of developing essential hypertension.

- Chronic distress emotions as well as depression are demonstrated risk factors for CHD.

- Sudden cardiac death often occurs after the presence of a traumatic stressor.

- Prevention of CHD includes lifestyle changes such as not smoking, eating fruits and vegetables, exercising, lowering cholesterol, controlling obesity, preventing diabetes, managing stress, preventing high blood pressure, and using alcohol in moderation if at all.

- Evidence suggests that tension-type headache (TTH) onset, a skeletal muscle condition, is related to proximal stressors, and migraine headache, a neurovascular condition, to distal stressors.

- Stress management strategies that include electromyograph (EMG) biofeedback along with use of appropriate medications are often effective for managing TTH.

- Stress is strongly linked to both bruxism and temporomandibular pain and dysfunction syndrome (TMPDS).

- The combination use of a dental occlusion appliance and EMG biofeedback is the most likely effective behavioral treatment for bruxism and TMPDS.

- Evidence suggests that early stress exposure, psychological distress, and low social support are related to the later onset of atopic disorders and to their symptom expression.

- Effective coping strategies for those with asthma involve avoiding triggers, writing about stressful events, and managing stress.

- Strategies for dealing with hay fever and skin allergies include avoiding allergens or other triggers when feasible.

- There is more evidence for a link between stress and cancer progression than stress and cancer onset.

- Cancer prevention strategies include screening for cancer, practicing sun safety, eating healthy foods, exercising, and avoiding tobacco smoke and environmental carcinogens.

- Peptic ulcers are more closely linked to bacterial infection than stress and can be cured with appropriate medication or with surgery.

- Irritable bowel syndrome (IBS) and inflammatory bowel disease (IBD) probably are not caused by stress but are exacerbated by daily stressors.

- Treatment of IBS focuses on managing the symptoms by avoiding triggers, making healthy lifestyle changes, and using appropriate medications when needed.

- Treatment of IBD is individually tailored and may involve use of medications, smoking cessation, dietary changes, counseling, and sometimes surgery.

- Stress as a cause of the autoimmune diseases of systemic lupus erythematosus (SLE) or rheumatoid arthritis (RA) has not been demonstrated.

- Daily stressors seem to play a role in exacerbating symptoms and reducing quality of life for SLE and RA.

- Lifestyle changes such as using sun block, making dietary changes, ceasing smoking, and avoiding stress may be recommended for managing the symptoms of SLE.

- Behavioral approaches to RA that are often effective include stress management and cognitive-behavioral therapy.

CRITICAL THINKING QUESTIONS

1. Which health conditions seem to be at least partially driven by inflammatory processes? How does stress-related inflammation play a role in each?

2. How can acute stressors lead to sudden cardiac death? How is this process similar or different from the chronic stress linked to CHD? What are the similarities and differences in the likely mechanisms?

3. Evaluate the current state of the research on the relationship between cancer and stress. Why do you believe there are conflicting results? Where does the evidence seem to be the strongest? Where is it the weakest?

4. Why do you believe the stress causal evidence is weak for some of the health conditions discussed and strong for others? Is it that the research designs have not yet uncovered stress-illness links in some conditions yet will in the future? If not, why not? If so, what research strategies could investigators use to best determine a hidden link?

5. Of the different health conditions discussed, which one do you believe you are most vulnerable to experiencing? What three prevention strategies can you employ to minimize your risk? If you are already experiencing one of these health conditions, what lifestyle or behavioral strategies can you use to cope with the condition most effectively?

KEY TERMS AND CONCEPTS

Acute coronary syndrome (ACS)

Allergic rhinitis (AR)*

Anger

Angina pectoris*

Arteriosclerosis

Asthma

Atherosclerosis*

Atopic dermatitis

Atopic disorders*

Bruxism*

Cancer*

Coronary heart disease (CHD)*

Coronary vascular disease (CVD)

Crohn's disease (CD)

Distal stressors*

Electromyograph (EMG)

Essential hypertension (HTN)*

Functional disorder*

Functional syndrome

Heart muscles

Helicobacter pylori (H. pylori) bacteria*

Hostility

Inflammatory bowel disease (IBD)

Irritable bowel syndrome (IBS)*

Ischemia

Low decision latitude

Migraine headaches*

Myocardial infarction (MI)*

Nonsteroidal anti-inflammatory drugs (NSAIDs)

Peptic ulcers*

Proximal stressors*

Rheumatoid arthritis (RA)

Skeletal muscles

Smooth
   muscles

Sudden cardiac
   death (SCD)*

Systemic autoimmune
   disorders*

Systemic lupus
   erythematosus (SLE)

Temporomandibular
   pain and dysfunction
   syndrome
   (TMPDS)*

Tension-type
   headache (TTH)*

Ulcerative
   colitis (UC)

MEDIA RESOURCES

CENGAGE**brain**

Access an interactive eBook, chapter-specific interactive learning tools, including flashcards, quizzes,
videos, and more in your Psychology CourseMate,
accessed through CengageBrain.com.

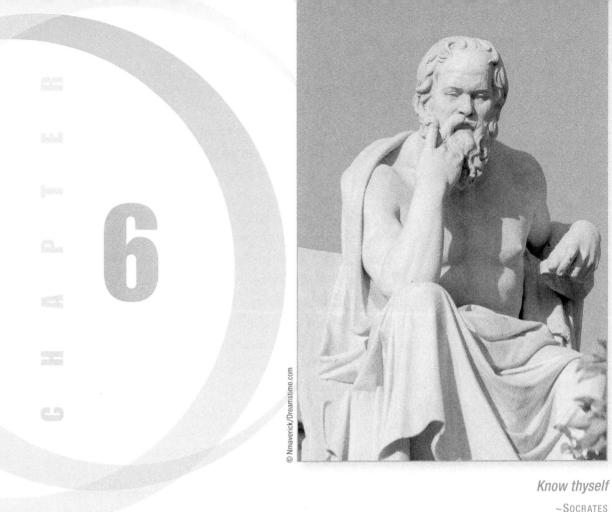

© Nnaverick/Dreamstime.com

Know thyself

~SOCRATES

PERSONALITY AND STRESS

MODELS OF PERSONALITY, STRESS, AND HEALTH

WHAT IS PERSONALITY?

STRESS AND HEALTH PERSONALITY VULNERABILITY FACTORS

STRESS AND HEALTH PROTECTIVE PERSONALITY FACTORS

● INSIGHT EXERCISE 6.1
What Is Your Locus of Control?

Much to everybody's surprise, Alicia and Claudia started out as best friends. Why the surprise? Though we all know that sometimes opposites attract, it's still surprising when two best friends have such contrasting personalities. Alicia is highly extraverted and is very warm and friendly with almost everyone she meets. Claudia, on the other hand, is socially inhibited and comes across as reserved and aloof.

Whether things go Alicia's way or not, she always seems to have a cheerful disposition and is optimistic and hopeful about the future. She believes in herself and thinks she can deal well with most stressful situations. On the other hand, Claudia worries a great deal, is often grumpy or mad when things don't go well, and feels a sense of despair and hopelessness when she encounters even the least setback.

Alicia is very creative and imaginative and enjoys variety in life, whereas Claudia prefers things to stay the same, to be predictable and routine. Even ordering a meal in a restaurant, Alicia is game to try new dishes, but Claudia always orders the same item on the menu. In addition, Alicia is very conscientious about her work and life, a very responsible person, whereas Claudia cuts a few corners and sometimes puts her commitments on the back burner.

One time Alicia and Claudia had plans to go out to lunch together and Alicia forgot. This was not like her, but Alicia was so busy with clients she inadvertently double-booked her lunch appointment and went out to lunch with her work associate Monica instead. Alicia was a "go-getter" and would often continue working on projects with coworkers through lunch. As fate would have it, Alicia and Claudia ran into each other at the restaurant, and, Alicia, suddenly realizing what had happened, expressed her embarrassment and immediately apologized to Claudia. Instead of understanding, Claudia walked away in a huff and later even refused to answer Alicia's phone calls or apologetic texts and e-mails.

Although Alicia forgave Claudia many times for various things, Claudia was not inclined to do the same for Alicia. Instead, Claudia ruminated about the slight in the morning when she got up, during the day, at night, and when she lay in bed before falling into a fitful sleep. She got angry and depressed, and because of her hurt feelings, she wanted Alicia to feel hurt also. Claudia thought, "This always happens to me," "I guess I'm just cursed or something," "How could she do this to me?" "She needs some pay-back for what she did."

One evening after fuming for hours about the slight, Claudia reached her boiling point. She sent an angry e-mail to Alicia, accusing her of being selfish, insensitive, and careless. In her e-mail she said that no true friend would treat her so badly. Though stung by the e-mail, Alicia felt compassion for Claudia and sent her another apologetic e-mail only to be rebuked.

After several attempts at repairing their relationship, Alicia decided it was time to move on. In her heart she forgave Claudia for sending such a hurtful e-mail and was grateful for the good times they had shared. She and Monica struck up a friendship and became best friends. They shared many good times and good feelings together. On the other hand, Claudia continued to have conflicts with many of the people she worked with and felt lonely and isolated. Most of her days were filled with worries, sadness, or irritations of one sort or the other.

As we can see, Claudia's personality traits leave her vulnerable to stress and stand in contrast to Alicia's personality traits, which protect her from stress. Claudia would score high on measures of neuroticism because she experiences a great deal of negative affect and very little positive affect. However, Alicia, with more of the protective factors in her constitution, would score low on neuroticism. Alicia has predominately positive affect with very little negative affect. Claudia is socially inhibited, one of the personality traits that, when combined with negative affectivity, define the Type D personality (D for distress), which is discussed later. These characteristics contrast with Alicia's more social and extraverted personality traits that are associated with higher levels of well-being.

Notice also some other dispositional characteristics that contrast the two former friends discussed in Chapter 2 on the topic of positive psychology. Have you thought of them? You have probably noticed that whereas Alicia is more optimistic, hopeful, forgiving, grateful, and resilient, Claudia shows the opposite trait characteristics. In addition, Alicia has a high self-esteem and Claudia has a low one. Finally, Alicia has what is known as an internal locus of control, whereas Claudia has an external locus of control. The locus of control concept is discussed in more depth later in this chapter. However, for now keep in mind that it refers to a belief that one has control over one's destiny (internal locus of control—Alicia) or a belief that one's destiny is controlled by others (external locus of control—Claudia).

MODELS OF PERSONALITY, STRESS, AND HEALTH

There are several models that explain the relationships among personality, stress, and health, including biological predisposition models, health behavior models, and moderation models. Perhaps the most basic model is the **biological predisposition model.** This model stipulates that genetic or constitutional (i.e., general biological makeup) factors influence a person's physiological, emotional, behavioral, and cognitive response to stress. A person with biological vulnerabilities is more likely to develop impaired health in response to stress, but personality plays no causal role. Personality is simply a reflection of underlying biological predispositions or temperaments. Thus, in biological predisposition models, how a person responds to stress is largely biologically determined. For example, according to this model Claudia's biological predisposition to experience an exaggerated stress response explains her neuroticism but her neuroticism does not explain her exaggerated stress response because neuroticism has no causal influence on her stress.

Health-related behavior models focus on how personality factors influence health-related behaviors, which, in turn, have important future consequences for health and well-being. Certain personality factors predispose us to engage in more health protective behaviors and others to engage in more health risk behaviors. For example, Booth-Kewley and Vickers (1994) found that people who scored high on the Big Five factors of extraversion, agreeableness, and conscientiousness and low in neuroticism were more likely to engage in health protective behaviors associated with wellness (e.g., exercise, healthy eating, etc.), but those who scored high in openness were more likely to engage in health harming behaviors such as substance use. They reported that "the correlations of Conscientiousness with health behavior were substantial, accounting for as much as 29% of the variance in the health behavior scales" (p. 288). Some health protective or health harming behaviors are motivated by a desire to cope with stress. Therefore, in this model, personality influences our stress-motivated health behaviors in the positive or negative direction, which, in turn, increases our chance of developing improved health or impaired health.

moderation models: assume that personality or other factors are intervening variables between stress and health and can serve as an intensifier of stress or a buffer that reduces the impact of stressors.

Moderation models assume that personality influences the strength or direction of the relationship between stress and health. Personality is an intervening variable between stress and health and can serve as an intensifier of stress or as a **buffer** that reduces the impact of stressors. Thus, when a person encounters a potentially stressful situation, that individual's personality influences how he or she will appraise and then cope with the event. This in turn will affect that person's physiological, emotional, behavioral, and cognitive responses, which will then increase or decrease susceptibility to illness (Schneiderman, Ironson, & Siegel, 2005). For example, according to this model Claudia's pessimism leaves her vulnerable to stress, whereas Amanda's optimism protects her from the effects of stress.

Further, interpersonal factors may play a role whereby personality predisposes persons to intensify or reduce interpersonal stressors in a transactive fashion (a two-way direction) (Bolger & Schilling, 1991; Bolger & Zuckerman, 1995). For example, individuals low in the Big Five's agreeableness and high in neuroticism will likely transact with others in ways that bring about more interpersonal conflict experiences (a stress-enhancing event) and less social support (a stress-reducing resource) during times of stress. This process was illustrated when Claudia's personality traits of neuroticism and low agreeableness predisposed her to relate to Amanda in a way that compounded Claudia's stress and reduced her social support. The cumulative effect of the original plus added transactive stressors then disposes the person toward illness. This process is illustrated in more detail later in this chapter when we discuss the *neurotic cascade*.

In sum, according to the biological predisposition model, biology may play a role in reaction to stress and in the expression of personality, but personality plays no direct role in response to stress or to health outcomes. In contrast, the health-related behaviors model suggests that personality influences the likelihood of engaging in stress-motivated, health-related behaviors. Engaging in health-harming or health-protective behaviors in turn influences the subsequent likelihood of negative or positive health outcomes. Finally, the moderation models view personality as influencing how we respond to stress with some personality characteristics increasing health risk and others decreasing risk. If there is a transactive quality to interpersonal stressors, stress levels may be reduced or magnified, or additional stressors may be added and resources subtracted depending on how the personality dispositions unfold with respect to the person precipitating or managing the interpersonal conflict.

What Is Personality?

Personality refers to the overall enduring pattern of thoughts, emotions, and behaviors that define an individual. It may be influenced by underlying physiological processes reflected in temperament as well as by past experiences. **Temperament** is "the biologically based foundation of personality, including such characteristic patterns of behavior as emotionality, activity, and sociability" (Cloninger, 2008, p. 260).

traits: also known as dispositions; the particular characteristics or structural elements of personality that predispose a person to respond in certain ways.

Personality **traits** refer to particular characteristics or structural elements of personality that predispose a person to respond in certain ways. For example, Alicia's warm, extraverted, and friendly characteristics are all traits of her personality that predispose her to be more socially engaging. Whereas **states** are considered more temporary internal phenomena, traits are considered more enduring and stable personality characteristics. By way of example, when Claudia feels mad at Alicia because of Alicia's perceived slight of her, Claudia is experiencing state anger at that moment. However, Claudia's general tendency to feel angry when things do not go her way can be considered *trait* anger. Sometimes traits are referred to as **dispositions** because they imply that persons are inclined or *disposed* toward particular experiences or expressions of personality.

Gordon Allport's (1937) book, *Personality: A Psychological Interpretation*, broke new ground in establishing trait theory as a legitimate scientific endeavor. He viewed traits as important structural elements to understanding personality. Allport's early work laid the foundation for other important contributors to the personality trait field such as Raymond Cattell and Hans Eysenck. Although Allport rejected the use of what was then a relatively new statistical technique called factor analysis to determine the major domains of personality, Cattell preferred this rigorous statistical approach and readily adopted its use to better map these domains.

Factor analysis uses multiple correlations to determine which of the measured elements cluster together. The elements that cluster together form a factor that is named for the common theme that the elements in the cluster possess. For example, if words like *reticent, timid, bashful, modest, demure, self-conscious,* and *reserved* form a statistical cluster, then this cluster, known as a factor, can be labeled *shyness* because shyness is the construct or theme that the factor appears to represent.

Based on his factor analyses, Cattell proposed that there are 16 distinct correlated factors or what he referred to as *source traits* (because they each presumably tapped into the one underlying *source* of all personality characteristics) that constitute each person's personality. He developed the **Sixteen Personality Factor (16 PF) Questionnaire** to measure these dimensions (Cattell & Eber, 1962).

Eysenck's PEN Model

Eysenck, a contemporary of Cattell, also employed factor analysis, although he disagreed with Cattell's use of correlated factors and preferred instead to use uncorrelated factors to map the personality. As a result, he employed a statistical technique of rotating his factors so that they were highly independent (sometimes called *orthogonal*) of each other. In doing so, he found substantially fewer factors. Instead of 16 correlated factors, he discovered 3 superfactors that are referred to as **the Big Three** *supertraits* or *personality types.*

Personality types are qualitative categories of personality within a particular domain that define the person according to the construct's characteristics. For example, the Type A person is defined according to the construct characteristics of being hard driving and competitive and having an exaggerated sense of time urgency, and the Type B person is defined as having the opposite set of characteristics. Most *types* are dichotomous in that a person fits into one of two categories. For example, a person is either Type A or Type B, but not both. This contrasts with the idea of personality traits as continuous variables along different dimensions reflected in varying degrees of the trait. Note that even though Eysenck sometimes referred to his three supertraits as personality types, he actually regarded them as continuous variables. For example, the instrument that Eysenck developed to measure the supertraits, the Eysenck Personality Inventory, scores along a continuum reflecting gradations of each supertrait. However, for the sake of convenience, it is often easier to say that someone either is an extravert or an introvert rather than say that the person has a high level of, for example, the trait of extraversion. True types are discussed in more depth later in this chapter (e.g., Type A).

The three supertraits in Eysenck's model are *psychoticism, extraversion-introversion,* and *neuroticism* (Eysenck, 1967, 1990; Eysenck & Eysenck, 1985). Together they are referred to as **Eysenck's PEN** (psychoticism, extraversion, and neuroticism) **model.** Eysenck discovered that his first superfactor has trait

Eysenck's PEN model: Eysenck's three supertraits of psychoticism, extraversion, and neuroticism that define an individual's personality.

characteristics that overlap with traits exhibited by individuals who are psychotic or who exhibit antisocial behavior, so he named it *psychoticism*. This was an unfortunate choice of a label because it unintentionally implies that all people who score high on the supertrait of psychoticism have a clinical psychosis (i.e., impaired reality testing combined with other clinical features), which usually is not the case.

Although people diagnosed with psychoses do tend to score high on this supertrait, so do creative nonpsychotic individuals. Instead of measuring a clinical condition, the **psychoticism** factor seems to reflect more broadly those traits often associated with nonconformity or social deviance. Most of the characteristics it reflects have negative connotations such as *aggressive, cold, egocentric, impersonal, impulsive, antisocial,* and *unempathic,* although at least a few have positive or neutral connotations such as *creative* and *tough-minded.* The social deviancy observed in many individuals with high psychoticism may have biological underpinnings reflected in lower cortical arousal because people scoring high in psychoticism tend to show a higher interest in violent material and more quickly desensitize to violent imagery (Bruggemann & Barry, 2002).

Due in part to the unfortunate choice of the label for the psychoticism dimension and its lack of clarity, this supertrait is typically not used as much in today's personality research though extraversion-introversion and neuroticism are constructs that are still popular. Eysenck's concept of **extraversion** embodies the generally positively connoted traits of *sociable, lively, active, assertive, sensation-seeking, carefree, dominant, surgent,* and *venturesome.* **Introverts** possess the inverse of these traits.

Neuroticism traits are generally seen as undesirable even to those who score high on this superfactor, and include characteristics such as *anxious, depressed, guilt feelings, low self-esteem, tense, irrational, shy, moody,* and *emotional.* Being in touch with our emotional side is usually beneficial, although we could probably do without frequent experiences of being tense, irrational, or moody. See Table 6.1 for Eysenck sample questions used to assess neuroticism.

Eysenck (1967) believed that his PEN supertraits were outward manifestations of underlying biological differences or temperaments. His biological differences hypotheses stimulated a wealth of research examining the physiological underpinnings of extraversion, introversion, and neuroticism, in particular. According to the temperament aspect of Eysenck's model, environmental stimulation leads to arousal of the nervous system. Some people require more stimulation and others less to reach an optimal zone of functioning.

Eysenck proposed that extraverts have a greater capacity for stimulation than introverts, including stimulating social encounters. In order to prevent overstimulation, introverts often withdraw from or avoid social situations that would otherwise overstimulate their nervous systems. Thus, the introvert's optimal zone of functioning (e.g., Yerkes-Dodson curve, see Chapter 1) is at a slightly lower level of arousal than extraverts, and both introverts and extraverts seek out environments that support their optimal levels.

Eysenck proposed that the ascending reticular activating system (otherwise known as the ascending reticular formation, see Chapter 3), one of the brain's systems responsible for arousal, accounts for the biologically driven differences between extraverts and introverts. He hypothesized that the higher

extraversion: one of the Big Three and Big Five traits; attributes include being warm, friendly, social, active, and passionate.

neuroticism: one of the Big Three and Big Five traits characterized by a disposition to experience emotional lability, a general sense of vulnerability, and negative affect.

TABLE **6.1**   Sample questions by Eysenck that assess neuroticism

1.	Do you sometimes feel happy, sometimes depressed, without any apparent reason?
2.	Does your mind often wander while you are trying to concentrate?
3.	Are you inclined to be moody?
4.	Are you frequently "lost in thought" even when you are supposed to be taking part in a conversation?
5.	Are you sometimes bubbling over with energy and sometimes very sluggish?
6.	Are your feelings rather easily hurt?
7.	Do you get attacks of shaking or trembling?
8.	Are you an irritable person?
9.	Are you troubled with feelings of inferiority?
10.	Do you suffer from sleeplessness?

SOURCE: H.J. Eysenck, *Eysenck on Extraversion*, p. 33, New York: John Wiley & Sons, 1973. Used by permission of John Wiley & Sons, Inc.

level of arousal from the ascending reticular activating system for introverts is revealed in introverts exhibiting greater cortical arousal than extraverts.

Are introverts more physiologically aroused than extraverts? What does the research suggest? Over 1,000 studies have been conducted testing this hypothesis in one form or another over the past 50 years. For example, in the *lemon drop test,* researchers discovered that extreme introverts secreted copious amounts of saliva when lemon juice drops were placed on their tongues compared to extreme extraverts who showed only minimal increases in salivation (Deary, Ramsey, Wilson, & Raid, 1988; Eysenck, 1990). Research findings indicate that even pupillary responses differ with introverts' pupils constricting faster than extraverts' when a bright light is shown onto their eyes, suggesting higher arousal to the light stimulus and a higher need to reduce stimulation (Holmes, 1967). Under certain conditions, brain wave responses to auditory stimuli also indicate more reactivity in introverts than extraverts, possibly emanating from the brain stem (Swickert & Gilliland, 1998).

Although the results of this large body of empirical research examining the introversion-extraversion differences in arousal have been inconsistent sometimes, there is modest evidence that introverts do seem to have a lower threshold for low-to-moderate levels of stimulation than extraverts, but only during certain periods of the 24-hour diurinal cycle (e.g., in the morning when cortical arousal differences between introverts and extraverts are found to be more pronounced). There also is considerable research supporting the idea that extraverts seek out more stimulating environments, especially social environments, than introverts. However, whether the reticular activating system is the area of the brain most responsible for these differences, as proposed by Eysenck, remains an unresolved question.

J. A. Gray's (1987) **reinforcement sensitivity theory** based on animal research builds on Eysenck's biological model and proposes two functionally independent motivational systems that have a bearing on our understanding of underlying temperament factors driving extraversion and neuroticism (note that his current model also proposes a third system not directly relevant to this discussion). Gray's two systems are the **behavioral approach system (BAS)** that is sensitive to reward and fueled by the dopamine areas and circuits of the brain, and the opposing **behavioral inhibition system (BIS)** that is sensitive to punishment or nonreward and is driven by the norepinephrine systems of the brain.

The BAS motivates us to approach potentially rewarding situations or stimuli, whereas the BIS inhibits action and is associated with avoidance behavior. Thus, persons high in BAS sensitivity show exaggerated positive affect (e.g., happiness) to rewards, and persons high in BIS sensitivity show exaggerated negative affect (e.g., anxiety) to aversive stimuli. For example, a daily event diary study found that participants with greater BAS sensitivity (as measured by a self-report instrument designed to measure levels of BAS and BIS) record more positive affect throughout their days, yet those with greater BIS sensitivity report more daily negative affect (Gable, Reis, & Elliot, 2000).

Recent versions of Gray's theory link extraverts' higher levels of positive affect to the BAS. For example, reviewers of the ties between the dopaminergic systems (associated with feeling good) and extraversion conclude that there is a strong connection between the two (Depue & Collins, 1999; Wacker, Chavanon, & Stemmler, 2006). A more dominant BAS could account for extraverts' higher well-being scores than introverts because extraverts are more likely to find all positive experiences more rewarding, including positive social experiences. In contrast, as you would expect, some research findings show that those with low BAS sensitivity are more prone to depression (Harmon-Jones & Allen, 1997). So in simple terms, high BAS sensitivity equals more positive affect and low BAS sensitivity equals less positive affect.

Just as the trait of extraversion is linked to the BAS, the trait of neuroticism is linked to the BIS. High levels of neuroticism are associated with greater BIS sensitivity, and this may account for the predominant negative affect experienced by individuals with high neuroticism. Thus, the higher BIS sensitivity of individuals with neuroticism explains their greater negative response to stressors or other stimuli they find threatening or punishing.

According to Eysenck, those scoring high in neuroticism have overreactive limbic systems. Gray (1987) proposed that the amygdala of the limbic system, the area of the brain associated with assessing threat, plays an important role in the BIS. An overreactive amygdala prompts heightened vigilance and anxiety in response to perceived threats. (Recall the evidence from Chapter 3 of hyperresponsive amygdalas associated with posttraumatic stress disorder [PTSD].)

Individuals with high neuroticism exhibit a lower tolerance for stress and, in particular, *aversive* stimuli. Thus, according to Eysenck, they are more likely to perceive threat and become *emotionally* aroused than those who score low on neuroticism. In his review of the neuroticism research, Lahey (2009, p. 246) concludes that there is "mounting evidence" that individuals with high neuroticism "respond with negative emotions more frequently and intensely when they experience stressful life events."

---

behavioral approach system (BAS): the system in Gray's reinforcement sensitivity theory that is sensitive to reward and fueled by the dopamine areas and circuits of the brain.

behavioral inhibition system (BIS): the system in Gray's reinforcement sensitivity theory that is sensitive to punishment or nonreward and is driven by the norepinephrine systems of the brain.

The Big Five

Today, the most widely accepted model of broad personality traits is **the Big Five,** also known as the **Five Factor Model (FFM).** This model, based on the results of factor analyses of everyday words used to describe personality characteristics, as the name implies, proposes that there are a total of five relatively independent factors that make up the entire personality. Paul Costa, Jr. and Robert McCrae are the two pioneers in the field most closely associated with the model. They developed a popular self-report instrument designed to measure the Big Five called the NEO-PI (Costa & McCrae, 1985, 1992).

NEO stands for the three personality factors used in the first version of the instrument of neuroticism (N), extraversion (E), and openness (O); PI stands for personality inventory. The last two factors of conscientiousness (C) and agreeableness (A) were subsequently added to complete the Big Five. A useful mnemonic for remembering the Big Five is OCEAN (openness, conscientiousness, extraversion, agreeableness, and neuroticism)—though the factors are usually presented in the order of NEOCA, it is fine to mix the order of the factors because order does not imply importance. See Table 6.2 for a

Five Factor Model (FFM): also known as the Big Five; the five relatively independent factors of neuroticism, extraversion, openness, conscientiousness, and agreeableness.

TABLE **6.2** The Big Five Factor Dimensions

Factor	Description of High Scorer	Description of Low Scorer
Extraversion (E)	Talkative Passionate Active Dominant Sociable	Quiet Unfeeling Passive
Agreeableness (A)	Good-natured Soft-hearted Trusting	Irritable Ruthless Suspicious
Neuroticism (N)	Worrying Emotional Vulnerable Anxious	Calm Unemotional Hardy Self-controlled Sense of well-being
Openness (O)	Creative Imaginative Prefers variety	Uncreative Down-to-earth Prefers routine
Conscientiousness (C)	Conscientious Hardworking Ambitious Responsible	Negligent Lazy Aimless Irresponsible

SOURCE: Cloninger (2008), *Theories of Personality: Understanding Persons.* Pearson/Prentice Hall.

TABLE **6.3**   Facets of the Big Five Factor dimensions as measured by the NEO-PI-R

Factor	Facets
Extraversion (E)	Warmth Gregariousness Assertiveness Activity Excitement-seeking Positive emotions
Agreeableness (A)	Trust Straightforwardness Altruism Compliance Modesty Tender-mindedness
Neuroticism (N)	Anxiety Hostility Depression Self-consciousness Impulsiveness Vulnerability
Openness (O)	Fantasy Aesthetics Feelings Actions Ideas Values
Conscientiousness (C)	Competence Order Dutifulness Achievement striving Self-discipline Deliberation

SOURCE: Cloninger (2008), *Theories of Personality: Understanding Persons*. Pearson/Prentice Hall.

listing of the Big Five factors of personality and the major characteristics of high and low scorers for each factor.

There also are subcomponents of each factor, labeled *facets,* that are separately measured using the NEO-PI. See Table 6.3 for a listing of the facets for each factor of the NEO-PI.

As you can see from the tables, those who score high on extraversion display many of the personality characteristics attributed to Alicia, such as warm, friendly, and social. As discussed earlier and in Chapter 2, extraverts have a disposition to experience more positive affect. Other characteristics associated with extraversion include being more active and passionate, suggesting that they bring a lot of energy to their endeavors. Due to Claudia's social inhibition tendencies, she would score low on extraversion.

agreeableness: one of the Big Five traits with soft-hearted, trusting, and good-natured characteristics.

Next, looking at the trait characteristics for **agreeableness,** it is fair to say that Alicia would score high given her generally good-natured, soft-hearted, and trusting personality, whereas Claudia would score low given her suspicious, distrusting nature, and her general tendency toward irritability.

As discussed previously, Claudia also would score high on neuroticism given her disposition to experience negative affect, such as worry, anxiety, hostility, and depression, as well as her general sense of vulnerability. However, Alicia is calmer and shows less emotional lability (i.e., reactivity) and more self-control, reflecting a low score for neuroticism.

openness: also known as openness to experience; one of the Big Five traits associated with being creative, imaginative, and enjoying variety.

Alicia would score high on **openness** given that she is creative and imaginative and enjoys variety, though Claudia would score low on this factor given her penchant for keeping things the same and following routines.

conscientiousness: one of the Big Five traits with characteristics such as ambitious, responsible, and hardworking.

Finally, with Alicia's hardworking, ambitious, and responsible nature, she would score high on **conscientiousness,** whereas Claudia's tendencies to cut corners, not return phone calls, and give her commitments a low priority indicate that she would score low on this dimension. The NEO-PI-R (revised version) or the short version called the NEO Five Factor Inventory (NEO-FFI) that measure these Big Five factors are popular self-report instruments used in research to evaluate stress and well-being personality correlates.

STRESS AND HEALTH PERSONALITY VULNERABILITY FACTORS

Neuroticism

Psychoneurosis, Stress, and Physical Symptoms

In the early part of the 20th century **psychosomatic medicine** broke new ground in linking psychological health to physical conditions. It was inspired by Freud's view that physical symptoms known as somatic conversions were a result of underlying psychological dynamics such as repressed memories or intrapsychic conflict. In this early model, when different components of the psyche are in conflict with each other due to a *psychoneurosis* (a term no longer in use for a type of neurosis characterized by emotional conflict), a physical symptom can emerge. For example, a soldier who is terrified of combat may develop a hysterical blindness. The blindness is a compromise between parts of the soldier's personality that fear combat and parts that feel duty bound to enter into combat. Thus, with the development of a disabling condition (i.e., the symptom), the soldier can be excused from combat while still preserving a sense of honor. Though the cases of hysterical blindness seen in Freud's day were usually temporary—once a soldier was well out of harm's way the disability often mysteriously disappeared—other, more enduring physical illnesses were later believed to be caused by similar conflict processes.

Franz Alexander (1950), a psychoanalyst (i.e., of the Freudian school), proposed a view that psychosomatic illnesses developed from emotional conflicts. For example, Alexander described a case of a 23-year-old university student with a duodenal ulcer who was conflicted between wanting to become emotionally involved with a woman yet not wanting the involvement because unconsciously such a relationship would indicate to him that he was weak and dependent like he felt with his mother. Accordingly, the stress of this conflict led to gastric hypersecretions, which, in turn, led to the development of his ulcer. As Alexander (1950, p. 112) stated, "ulcers usually develop in personalities with a deep-seated neurotic conflict which in itself calls for psychoanalytic treatment." Although the psychosomatic conflict theory was popular during the Golden Age of psychoanalysis, supportive evidence has not been found for Alexander's theory that psychological conflicts are the root causes of stress-related health conditions.

Neuroticism as a Broad Trait Personality Construct   The psychoanalytic idea of psychological conflicts being expressed as symptoms (either psychological or physical) played an important role in Freud's theory of **neurosis,** a construct that was widely accepted by mainstream American psychiatry until the latter part of the 20th century. The original *Diagnostic and Statistical Manual* **(DSM),** a manual developed by psychiatrists to guide psychiatric diagnoses, published in 1952 by the American Psychiatric Association and the next edition published in 1968 included neurosis as a condition that typically involved anxiety or depression and contrasted with psychosis because there is no impaired reality testing (e.g., hallucinations, delusions, etc.) in neurosis.

Although eventually dropped as a diagnostic category by the third version of the DSM in 1987 as the psychoanalytic paradigm began to lose favor, the term *neuroticism* survives today within mainstream personality research in its nonpsychodynamic form discussed earlier (e.g., Eysenk's PEN model, the Big Five). As Lahey (2009, p. 241) explains in his review of the contemporary research in neuroticism, "although *neuroticism* has its roots in Freudian theory, and the ancient philosophical and medical traditions on which psychodynamic models are based, the modern conception of neuroticism is unrelated to such theories as unconscious conflict."

As discussed earlier, neuroticism as measured by the NEO-PI includes trait descriptors such as *anxious, depressed, guilt feelings, low self-esteem, tense, irrational, shy, moody,* and *emotional.* When we examine the different broad personality vulnerability factors, neuroticism appears, by a large order of magnitude, to confer the most stress, health, and well-being risk. For example, Lahey's (2009, p. 245) review concludes that neuroticism "predicts shorter, less happy, less healthy, and less successful lives to a meaningful extent."

The Neurotic Cascade   Why do individuals with high neuroticism report more frequent and intense negative affect in their everyday lives? Why do they have a tendency to "make mountains out of mole hills" as Claudia did with Alicia? Why do small everyday stressors often elicit the same dramatic over-the-top responses as big stressors? According to Suls and Martin (2005), the answer lies in understanding how they experience the **neurotic cascade.** The

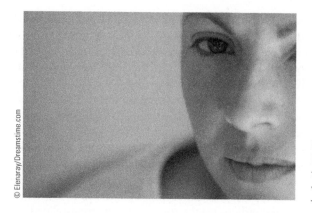

Neuroticism appears to be a Big Five factor that confers the most stress, health, and well-being risk.

neurotic cascade involves five distinct, though interrelated, processes they labeled: (1) *Hyperreactivity*, (2) *Differential Exposure*, (3) *Differential Appraisal*, (4) *Mood Spillover*, and (5) *The Sting of Familiar Problems*. Each mechanism in the cascade serves to reinforce the other as each prompts a series of unfortunate yet somewhat predictable set of interlocking events. Let us examine the elements of the cascade briefly and see how they apply to Claudia.

1. Hyperreactivity As discussed earlier, theories presented by Eysenck and also Gray propose that there are biological reasons why those with high neuroticism traits exhibit negatively oriented emotional hyperreactivity toward stressors. Both theories suggest that specific areas of the brain are responsible (i.e., the limbic system—Eysenck—or the amygdala within the limbic system—Gray). Further, Gray's theory suggests that one of the primary motivators for individuals with high neuroticism is the brain mechanism that is more responsive to punishment, the BIS. Thus, according to these models, Claudia is more likely to react to stressors with excessive negative affect because she is biologically predisposed to do so through areas of the brain that support a more sensitive or dominant BIS.

2. Differential Exposure Those who score higher in neuroticism often set up scenarios that lead them to experience more hassles or negative life events than they would otherwise experience. Social transactions within these scenarios lead to unwanted stressors. For example, Claudia's reaction to Alicia's forgetting their lunch engagement led Claudia to miss lunch, ruminate for many hours, write an angry e-mail, rebuff Alicia's attempts at repairing their friendship, and ultimately to lose a close friend. Each of these events adds additional unnecessary hassles or negative life change experiences to the original one. In this case, Claudia also lost the important social support resource of a good friend—leaving her even more vulnerable to the effects of stress.

3. Differential Appraisal Individuals with high neuroticism are more likely to appraise situations negatively even when the situations are nonthreatening (high primary appraisal) and to lack confidence in their ability to use personal resources to cope with or gain mastery over these situations (low secondary appraisal). For example, Claudia appraised Alicia's forgetfulness as a personal affront—she assumed that Alicia must not value her or their friendship—a harm-loss appraisal. In addition, she chose to avoid attempts to work through their differences in favor of ruminating. Her thoughts of "This always happens to me" and "I guess I'm just cursed or something" suggest a predominance of helplessness-oriented secondary appraisals.

4. Mood Spillover High neuroticism often leads to rumination that then leads to negative emotions or even depressive states well beyond the event. Ruminators recycle old hurts and grievances so that they have trouble recovering following a stressful interpersonal encounter. As we know, Claudia ruminated and stayed trapped in her own negative self-defeating spiral, whereas Alicia was able to break free and establish a new and healthier relationship with Monica.

5. The Sting of Familiar Problems Have you ever noticed how a fly gets trapped in a window as it tries repeatedly to move through the glass barrier? It fails to escape because it can see only one solution, which it tries over and over and over again. Unfortunately, for many people like Claudia who lack psychological flexibility, failed solutions are applied repeatedly in spite of their proven ineffectiveness. Individuals with high neuroticism often have distorted reasoning and impaired decision-making processes that hinder their ability to access or use appropriate coping strategies. When they become aware that their issues and problems reoccur, rather than try new solutions, they view these repeated patterns as validating their sense of helplessness and pessimism. For example, Claudia recognized that difficulties with relationships often happen with her, but her cognitions conveyed helplessness and despair when she thought that she was "just cursed or something" instead of thinking, "maybe I ought to try a different approach."

The following study illustrates this ineffective coping strategy. A meta-analysis (Conner-Smith & Flachsbart, 2007) of 165 samples that included 33,094 participants found that individuals who score high in neuroticism are more likely to use broad disengagement coping strategies like wishful thinking ($r = .35$) or withdrawal ($r = .29$) and to a lesser extent denial ($r = .18$) or avoidance ($r = .13$) as well as to use drugs and alcohol for coping ($r = .28$)—strategies that the authors suggested may lead to short-term gains in stress relief but with long-term costs. Although Claudia did not use drugs and alcohol to cope, she did employ some of the broad disengagement strategies examined in this study such as withdrawal and avoidance. In her case, however, she had few, if any, short-term gains, though certainly some long-term costs.

Neuroticism, Well-Being, Mental Health, and Relationship Satisfaction As discussed in Chapter 2, high neuroticism is consistently and robustly negatively associated with subjective well-being. In a recent large meta-analytic study of 347 samples that included published articles, unpublished dissertations, and other unpublished data (to control for publication bias) representing 2,142 correlation coefficients and 122,588 participants, Steel, Schmidt, and Shultz (2008) found a large negative effect size for neuroticism with happiness ($r = -.46$), indicating that higher neuroticism was associated with greater unhappiness. They also found a large positive effect size for neuroticism with negative affect

TABLE **6.4**   Meta-analytic effect sizes of affect and subjective well-being for the Big Five Factor dimensions found by Steel et al. (2008).

Construct	K	n	r̄
Neuroticism			
Happiness	6	621	−.46
Life satisfaction	36	9,277	−.38
Positive affect	57	11,788	−.30
Negative affect	73	16,764	.54
Extraversion			
Happiness	6	829	.49
Life satisfaction	35	10,528	.28
Positive affect	53	12,898	.44
Negative affect	49	11,569	−.18
Openness to Experience			
Happiness	5	779	.13
Life satisfaction	26	9,075	.03
Positive affect	27	7,340	.20
Negative affect	26	8,008	−.02
Agreeableness			
Happiness	4	441	.30
Life satisfaction	22	7,459	.14
Positive affect	23	6,040	.12
Negative affect	27	7,306	−.20
Conscientiousness			
Happiness	4	441	.25
Life satisfaction	25	6,685	.22
Positive affect	24	5,976	.27
Negative affect	28	7,749	−.20

NOTE: K refers to the number of studies, n means number of participants, and r̄ is the average effect size.

SOURCE: Steel, P., Schmidt, J., & Shultz, J. (2008), Refining the relationship between personality and subjective well-being, *Psychological Bulletin*, 134, 138–161. Reproduced with permission via Copyright Clearance Center, Inc.

($r = .54$) and moderate to large negative effect sizes for neuroticism with positive affect ($r = −.30$) and with life satisfaction ($r = −.38$) (Table 6.4). Thus, individuals with high neuroticism report that they have high levels of negative affect and low levels of positive affect, happiness, and life satisfaction.

People with high neuroticism also appear to be at greater risk for developing psychological disorders than those with low neuroticism. For example, Jylha and Isometsa (2006, p. 281) found in a random general population sample of 441 Finnish subjects that "neuroticism is strongly associated with depressive and anxiety symptoms." In fact, they reported a correlation of $r = .71$ for neuroticism with depression and $r = .69$ for neuroticism with anxiety. They also reported a significant correlation between neuroticism and self-reported lifetime mental disorder of $r = .30$. Such findings may be in part a reflection of the ineffective stress coping abilities of people who score high in neuroticism.

Given these findings, it is no surprise that many studies have associated high scores on neuroticism with a greater likelihood of developing an *internalizing disorder* such as a mood disorder (e.g., major depression) or an anxiety disorder (e.g., generalized anxiety disorder). **Internalizing disorders** are those characterized by an inward expression of pathology, whereas **externalizing disorders** (e.g., substance abuse or dependence, antisocial personality disorder) are evidenced by an outward expression of pathology (Krueger, 1999).

Although personal distress and impaired functioning are hallmarks of clinical disorders, some research findings point to greater *personal distress* being more closely linked to internalizing disorders, whereas greater social and occupational *impairment* being more closely connected to externalizing disorders (e.g., alcohol dependence) (Howell & Watson, 2008). In a meta-analysis (Malouff, Thorsteinsson, & Schutte, 2005, p. 101) examining the five-factor model of personality and symptoms of clinical disorders from 33 studies, the primary pattern found for those with clinical disorders "was high Neuroticism, low Conscientiousness, low Agreeableness, and low Extraversion." The researchers reported large effect sizes for mood disorders (e.g., depression) and anxiety disorders as well as a few other disorders (i.e., somatoform disorders, schizophrenia, and eating disorders). However, these same researchers determined that externalizing disorders deviated from this profile in that these disorders revealed a pattern of low neuroticism and high extraversion.

A meta-analytic study by Saulsman and Page (2004) of **personality disorders** (an enduring personality pattern associated with distress or impairment) and the Big Five found that the personality disorder categories that were more distress oriented (e.g., Avoidant, Dependent, Borderline, Paranoid, and Schizotypal) had stronger associations with neuroticism than those that were not. The highest effect sizes were in the medium range, so the effects were not as strong as those found for clinical disorders such as mood and anxiety disorders.

In addition, Lahey (2009, p. 242) concluded in his review of the neuroticism research that, although items that measure the construct of neuroticism overlap with criteria used to diagnose disorders such as depression, "a number of longitudinal studies have controlled for shared items and concurrent depressive states and still found significant associations between the construct of neuroticism and measures of depression."

Thus, there is strong evidence that neuroticism is robustly associated with anxiety and depression symptoms and clinical disorders known as the internalizing disorders, such as anxiety disorders and mood disorders, and to a lesser extent the distress-oriented personality disorders. The effect is not merely an artifact of overlapping constructs, but rather a reflection of independent risk factors.

Neuroticism is also negatively implicated in studies of intimate relationship satisfaction. In a meta-analysis of 19 studies for a total of 3,848 participants, Malouff, Thorseinsson, Schutte, Bhullar, and Rooke (2010) found that high neuroticism was the most significant predictor of the Big Five for intimate partner relationship dissatisfaction ($r = .22$). The most favorable pattern for intimate partner relationship satisfaction was low neuroticism combined with high levels of the Big Five traits of extraversion, agreeableness, and conscientiousness. There were no differences found between men and women or between married and nonmarried participants in their study. Even though the effect sizes found by Malouff and his associates were modest (in the range of small to medium) and causality could not be determined from the study, the authors speculated that high neuroticism probably leads to more partner criticisms and to defensiveness that would then contribute to relationship dissatisfaction.

Similarly, Gattis, Berns, Simpson, and Christensen (2004) reported from their study of 132 distressed couples and 48 nondistressed couples that the Big Five pattern most closely associated with marital dissatisfaction was high neuroticism, low agreeableness, and low conscientiousness. Consequently, it seems that there is at least a modest effect for neuroticism playing a role in intimate relationship partner dissatisfaction.

Neuroticism and Physical Health In the early stages of investigating the relationship between neuroticism and physical health, Costa and McCrae (1987) cautioned that individuals who score high in neuroticism are more likely to overreport or exaggerate somatic complaints and that researchers should be wary of potential measurement artifacts (false positives) when exploring the neuroticism health-risk link. Many of the studies indicating a neuroticism-health link used *soft* measures of health (i.e., self-reports) rather than *hard* measures (i.e., results of biological tests). Even assessing degree of angina, a traditional medical measure, because it relies on the patient's reporting of chest pain, can be exaggerated. Likewise, *hard* measures such as biological laboratory tests can occasionally produce erroneous results if not performed properly. One *hard* measure, however, that is beyond dispute is mortality.

Over the years an increasing body of empirical findings has emerged from researchers who examined neuroticism as a health risk for early mortality, a standard that Costa and McCrae (1987) held as the highest benchmark to validate the neuroticism-health link. The emerging pattern is currently mixed, reflecting a split with the largest body of studies showing that neuroticism predicts early mortality and the remainder (still a substantial portion of the whole) showing that neuroticism is either unrelated to longevity or may even be protective of health (a small minority of studies).

A study by Shipley, Weiss, Der, Taylor, and Deary (2007) of a large community-based sample with a long follow-up period is illustrative of the findings of a neuroticism health-risk connection. Their prospective study used the Eysenck Personality Inventory (EPI) to measure neuroticism and looked at a large United Kingdom cohort of 5,424 residents over a 21-year period. After statistically controlling for other relevant health risk factors (e.g., smoking, alcohol consumption, exercise, initial health variables like blood pressure, respiratory function, and body mass index) and social and demographic factors (age, gender, education, occupation), the investigators determined that each standard deviation increase in neuroticism led to a 10% greater risk of death from cardiovascular disease.

Another illustrative study conducted by Wilson and his colleagues (2005) used four items from the Neuroticism scale of the NEO-FFI to measure neuroticism in their cohort of 6,158 Chicago residents 65 years of age or older, and examined them over a 6-year period. They found that after statistically adjusting for age, gender, race/ethnicity, and education, those scoring in the top 90th percentile or higher of neuroticism had a 33% greater risk of dying from all causes than those scoring in the bottom 10th percentile.

Contrary findings, however, were reported by Weiss and Costa (2005) in a 5-year cohort study of 1,076 *frail* participants ages 65 to 100 using the NEO-FFI that found evidence that neuroticism was protective. Some of these inconsistencies in the neuroticism-mortality findings may relate to methodological differences, the way neuroticism was measured, and characteristics of the participants.

Should new research decidedly favor neuroticism as an early mortality risk, then one of the likely mechanisms for early mortality would be neuroticism's relationship to stress-related physiological reactivity. Although the evidence here is also mixed, there are a number of studies that suggest that individuals high in neuroticism experience greater activation of the sympathetic nervous system in response to stressors (Lahey, 2009).

Another plausible explanation of neuroticism as a health vulnerability factor is that individuals with high neuroticism may be more prone to engage in certain behaviors that have an adverse impact on their health. We will next look at meta-analytic evidence that individuals with high neuroticism have a greater probability of engaging in health risk behaviors such as using alcohol, smoking tobacco, and being involved in occupational setting accidents.

In a meta-analysis of 20 studies that included 7,886 participants, Malouff, Thorsteinsson, Rooke, and Schutte (2007) found a small effect size for high neuroticism, low agreeableness, and low conscientiousness as predictors of alcohol involvement with alcohol problems and diagnoses showing stronger associations to neuroticism. The authors suggested that the profile pattern of high neuroticism, low agreeableness, and low conscientiousness fits a *low self-control pattern* associated with "emotional distress and hostile, uncooperative, irresponsible, and careless behavior" (p. 285).

Previously Malouff, Thorsteinsson, and Schutte (2006) had identified a similar profile pattern in their meta-analysis of nine studies of 4,730 tobacco smokers that also found a small effect size. Malouff and his colleagues' two substance use meta-analytic studies are corroborated by Conner-Smith and Flachsbart's (2007) meta-analytic study discussed earlier that indicated that persons with high neuroticism are more inclined to use drugs and alcohol to cope with stress.

Besides engaging in health risk behaviors such as smoking and problem use of alcohol, neuroticism seems to be associated with an increased risk for occupational accidents. For example, Clarke and Robertson (2005) conducted a meta-analysis of 47 studies and found a small effect size for high neuroticism being linked to occupational accidents, yet not to nonoccupational accidents. Why high neuroticism was associated with greater occupational accidents was not investigated in this study nor was the negative finding for a nonoccupational-accidents–neuroticism link. It does appear, however, that individuals with high neuroticism were engaging in behaviors that put them at greater risk for potentially injurious workplace mishaps because the accident measures reported in this study represent *hard* outcomes.

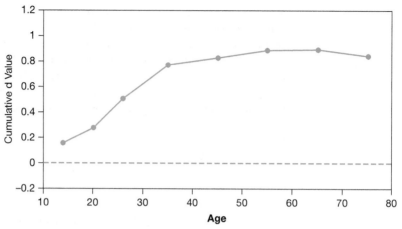

FIGURE **6.1** Emotional Stability Across the Lifespan

Average standardized mean-level change reported by Roberts and Mroczek (2008).

SOURCE: Roberts & Mroczek (2008), Personality trait change in adulthood, *Current Directions in Psychological Science*, 17; 1, 31–35. Copyright © 2008 by Sage Publications. Reprinted by permission of SAGE Publications.

Therefore, there is meta-analytic evidence that neuroticism modestly increases the risk of adverse health consequences through engaging in certain types of health risk or harming behaviors. These health risk behaviors may account for some of the findings of early mortality for persons with high levels of neuroticism.

Overall, then, it appears that high neuroticism found in people like Claudia is associated with a higher level of negative affect such as anxiety and depression; a lower level of positive affect, happiness, and life satisfaction; a greater use of disengagement coping; a greater chance of developing a clinical disorder (especially an internalizing disorder) or a personality disorder (especially a distress-related disorder); more intimate relationship dissatisfaction; a greater probability of engaging in health-harming behaviors such as tobacco smoking and problem alcohol use; a greater likelihood of being involved in an occupational accident; and perhaps a greater risk for early mortality, although the neuroticism-mortality link is not firmly established.

Although these findings are very concerning, there is some room for optimism. For example, the trait called *emotional stability,* which is the trait at the opposite end of the neuroticism dimension, shows steady increases across our lifespan (Figure 6.1) (as do traits such as *warmth, self-control*, and *confidence*) until it levels off in late adulthood (Roberts & Mroczek, 2008). These findings suggest then that the personality trait of neuroticism would in turn gradually lessen over the lifespan—good news for those who suffer some of the pitfalls of neuroticism.

The Type A Behavior Pattern

In the 1950s, two cardiologists named Myer Friedman and Ray Rosenman (1974) made the observation that many of their patients had *hurry sickness*. They wondered if the hurried behavior patterns that these *tense* individuals displayed were related to the development of coronary heart disease (CHD). The duo captured the behavior pattern they often saw in their patients of an exaggerated sense of time urgency, competitiveness, and an inordinate drive in a construct they called the **Type A** behavior pattern. Later definitions of Type A also included negative affectivity qualities "such as irritation, hostility, and increased potential for anger" (Rosenman, 1990, p. 2). Friedman and Rosenman called those who showed the opposite pattern, the more relaxed and easy going types, **Type B.**

Type A: a behavior pattern characterized by an exaggerated sense of time urgency, competitiveness, hostility, and an inordinate drive that Friedman and Rosenman proposed as a predictor of coronary heart disease.

The Type A behavior pattern, they posited, could be evaluated through using an assessment tool the two developed, called the Structured Interview. The Structured Interview was administered by trained examiners who recorded interviews that were later evaluated for Type A qualities such as rapid-accelerated speech with loud punctuated words or phrases, nervous movements (e.g., jaw clenching), exaggerated gesticulation when talking (e.g., fist pounding), and other indicators of the *hurried* and *tense* pattern. Later, a self-report instrument called the Jenkins Activity Survey (Jenkins, Zyzanski, & Rosenman, 1979) also was developed to measure the pattern.

In their landmark prospective study known as the Western Collaborative Group Study, Rosenman et al. (1964) assessed 3,411 men, medically evaluated and determined free of CHD, to determine their type. The investigators then tracked the participants for 8½ years. What did they find? They found that Type As were twice as likely to develop CHD as Type Bs—a finding made more remarkable because it held firm after statistically adjusting for other risk variables (Rosenman et al., 1975).

A number of other studies also identified a significant link between Type A and CHD in both men and women (see Rosenman, 1993, for a review). At the time, these were groundbreaking findings and represented a paradigm shift toward legitimizing personality variables as medical risk factors for CHD. Over the decades that followed, the impact of this early study and others, along with the subsequent publicity surrounding them, was sufficient to popularize the concept in the mind of the general public.

However, although Type A is still well accepted in popular culture, by the 1980s researchers began to doubt the validity of the construct when a series of prospective studies failed to show the expected Type A-CHD relationship—the most prominent being a large-scale clinical trial called the Multiple Risk Factor Intervention Trial (MRFIT) that detected no relationship between Type A and CHD (Shekelle et al., 1985). Myrteck's (2001) meta-analysis of prospective Type A studies published between 1966 and 1998 reinforced the point in revealing a near-zero effect size.

Such findings led researchers in the area to search for reasons for replication failures. For example, the self-report instrument that assesses behavior patterns indirectly, the Jenkins Activity Survey, was determined to be a much weaker predictor of CHD than the Structured Interview that assesses behavior directly, and was believed to be responsible for some of the inconsistent findings (Davis & Cowles, 1985). Eventually, however, investigators began to dissect the components of the construct and look for more potent CHD predictors that could be considered the *toxic core* of Type A.

Redford Williams and his associates (1980) were among the first to seriously explore *hostility* as a toxic core component. Using a subscale of the

Minnesota Multiphasic Personality Inventory designed to measure hostility, called the Cook-Medley Scale, they reported a finding that scores on this scale were more robust predictors of coronary atherosclerosis than Type A. A few years later Shekelle, Gale, Ostfeld, and Oglesby (1983) published findings of a much larger prospective study, the Western Electric Study, that stated that high hostility (top 20%) as measured by the Cook-Medley Scale was related to a 42% greater risk of death than low hostility (bottom 20%).

Subsequent researchers discovered that hostility was also associated with higher levels of proinflammatory cytokines such as tumor necrosis factor (TNF)-α that are implicated in cardiovascular disease (Suarez, Lewis, & Kuhn, 2002) (see Chapter 5), thereby suggesting a potential mechanism for hostility's pathogenic effect on the cardiovascular system.

The health risk effects of various types of anger expression were also examined. For example, Dembroski, MacDougall, Williams, Haney, and Blumenthal (1985, p. 230) found that *anger-in,* an anger expression style associated with anger suppression that they described as "an unwillingness in a variety of circumstances to express frustration-induced hostility and/or anger overtly," was positively associated with severity of angina symptoms and frequency of myocardial infarctions (MIs). Corroborating evidence also was found for suppressed anger as a health risk factor for CHD in a number of other studies—moderate anger expression was indicated as optimal (Eng, Fitzmaurice, Kubzansky, Rimm, & Kawachi, 2003; Harburg, Julius, Kaciroti, Gleiberman, & Schork, 2003).

hostility: an attitudinal disposition of cynicism, suspicion, and resentment toward others.

Although hostility and anger are overlapping constructs, Suls and Bunde (2005, p. 283) point out that **hostility** refers to "cynical attitudes about others," whereas **anger** involves "feelings of being treated unjustly and is accompanied by subjective arousal"; "**anger expression** refers to tendencies to be verbally or physically antagonistic." Thus, hostility refers to an *attitude,* anger refers to a *feeling,* and anger expression refers to *behaviors.* Over the ensuing decades, they noted, hostility, anger, anger expression, as well as depression (see Chapter 5) and anxiety have all been linked to CHD. In addition, they pointed out that these risk variables amount to three overlapping negative affectivity dimensions of *anger-hostility, depression,* and *anxiety* that, in spite of their linkage to CHD, have also at times produced mixed or even negative results as CHD predictors. Some of the negative results may stem from the differences in the way these negative affectivity constructs have been defined and measured.

The anger-hostility dimension of negative affectivity receives a lot of attention as a documented *acute* risk factor for cardiac events (see Chapter 5), though there are questions regarding the form (hostility, anger, anger expression) and degree of risk it confers as a *long-term* risk factor for heart disease. Prior to Chida and Steptoe's (2009) recent review, which is discussed next, of the anger-hostility long-term risk for CHD, previous reviews had been inconclusive (e.g., Myrteck, 2001).

Chida and Steptoe (2009, p. 936) performed a meta-analysis that included newer studies published that were not included in previous inconclusive reviews and, based on their results, concluded definitively that "anger and hostility are associated with CHD outcomes both in healthy and CHD populations." They reported that the effects were slightly higher for patients with CHD than for those who were healthy at baseline, suggesting that anger episodes might lead to an acceleration of the progression of CHD. They also found "that the harmful effects of anger and hostility on CHD events in a healthy population was greater in men than women, suggesting that men are more responsive to anger and hostility factors in relation to CHD" (Chida & Steptoe, 2009, p. 943). This dovetails with findings that healthy men participants show a greater anger–hostility-related cardiovascular response to stressors than women (Chida & Hamer, 2008). In fact, some investigators have contended, based on their research findings, that anxiety, rather than hostility, is a better predictor of cardiovascular disease in women (Consedine, Magai, & Chin, 2004).

The type of anger expression as a gender-related risk factor for CHD has also been explored recently. Davidson and Mostofsky (2010) coded interviews of 785 men and women participants according to the following anger expression styles: (1) *constructive anger expression*—assertively discussing why they are upset with the person toward whom they feel anger in an attempt to resolve the situation while considering that person's point of view; (2) *destructive anger justification*—blaming others for their anger and expressing self-justification and desire for vindication; and (3) *destructive anger rumination*—holding grudges, brooding, and discussing their anger repetitiously in a way that magnifies their animosity. Their prospective study found that constructive anger seemed to have a protective effect for CHD in men but not women, whereas *destructive anger justification* increased CHD risk for both men and women.

To summarize the findings then for Type A and its *toxic core* elements, the current state of the research evidence suggests that the Type A behavior pattern as a global construct is at best a weak CHD risk predictor, but hostility and particular forms of anger expression (e.g., suppressed anger and destructive anger justification), especially in men, are more robust predictors. There is preliminary evidence that suggests that constructive anger expression in men is protective of CHD. More quality prospective research needs to be conducted about the relationship between anger-hostility and CHD, and anxiety and CHD in women before we have a clearer picture of women's toxic core CHD risk factors. Hostility may inconsistently predict CHD in women though it is a weaker predictor than for men. Later we will examine a study of women with a massive sample size that determined that hostility did not predict CHD in women, but that it did predict cancer-related death and death from all causes. Destructive anger justification may be as toxic for women as men for CHD, though more studies are needed in this area before we can be entirely confident of these results.

A recent personality construct has emerged as a possible replacement for Type A, called the Type D (distressed) personality. Type D appears to be a predictor for a *poor prognosis* in patients with heart disease (Denollet, Sys, & Brutsaert, 1995). To date, prospective studies have yet to be conducted testing Type D's ability to predict future CHD in healthy participants.

Type D: a distressed personality type that has high negative affectivity and social inhibition; the construct was proposed as an indicator of a poor prognosis for patients with heart disease.

Johan Denollet and his associates (1995) introduced **Type D** and defined it as a personality type that has high negative affectivity (NA) and high social inhibition (SI)—remember, Claudia has these traits. A Type D person is similar to an introverted neurotic. However, although NA and neuroticism are overlapping constructs, they are not identical—likewise for SI and introversion.

TABLE **6.5**   The DS14 Used to Assess Type D

DS14
Makes contact easily when meeting people[a]
Makes a fuss about details
Often talks to strangers[a]
Often feels unhappy
Easily irritated
Is inhibited in social interactions
Takes a gloomy view of things
Has difficulties starting a conversation
Often in a bad mood
Is a closed kind of person
Tends to keep others at a distance
Tends to worry a lot
Tends to be down in the dumps
Does not find things to talk about

NOTE: The "a" represents a reverse scored item. In other words, not endorsing this item adds points to the Type D score.

SOURCE: Kupper, N., & Denollet, J. (2007), Type D personality as a prognostic factor in heart disease: Assessment and mediating mechanisms, *Journal of Personality Assessment*, 89, 265–276. Reproduced with permission of Taylor & Francis; permission conveyed through Copyright Clearance Center, Inc.

In a review of the nascent research findings in this area, Kupper and Denollet (2007, p. 266) reported that "between 26% and 53% of cardiac patients can be classified as Type D." They further determined that Type D is highly correlated with hostility, cynicism, inward and outward expression of anger, physical aggression, anxiety, and depression. Overall, individuals with this personality type have a greater tendency to feel negative emotions and to inhibit their expression in social interactions.

The DS14 is a 14-item scale that measures Type D status. Its item of *Often in a bad mood* is illustrative of NA and *Is a closed type of person* is a representative item for SI (Kupper & Denollet, 2007) (Table 6.5).

Clearly much of the construct overlaps with risk factors that are already established such as anger-hostility, depression, and anxiety. In addition, Denollet and his associates (1995), the originators of the construct, to date have conducted most of the supportive research. Therefore, more research needs to be done by other investigators to corroborate the Denollet group's findings before the construct can gain more ground in the scientific community.

Finally, as Smith and MacKenzie (2008, p. 450) remarked in their negative critique of the Type D construct, "this model implies that the combination of negative affectivity and social inhibition provides unique prognostic information, yet the incremental effect of the statistical interaction of these traits is not tested." It is not without irony then that even though we have moved further through the alphabet in a linear fashion, we have come full circle from Type A to Type D in our search for the silver bullet of a personality type that robustly predicts CHD.

STRESS AND HEALTH PROTECTIVE PERSONALITY FACTORS

Conscientiousness

Among the Big Five, research findings are steadily converging on conscientiousness as the most health protective. Individuals with high conscientiousness like Alicia are generally self-disciplined, responsible, hard-working, persistent, and well-organized. They are highly disposed to follow rules and norms, to exhibit good impulse control, and to plan and then follow through with goal-directed behavior (John & Srivastava, 1999).

Meta-analytic studies indicate that high levels of conscientiousness are associated with less negative and more positive affect and greater subjective well-being (Steel et al., 2008), a lower incidence of clinical or personality disorders (Malouff et al., 2005; Saulsman & Page, 2004), less problem alcohol use (Malouff et al., 2007), less tobacco use (Malouff et al., 2006), more satisfying intimate relationships (Malouff et al., 2010), and greater academic achievement (Trapmann, Hell, Hirn, & Schuler, 2007). Given these qualities, it should be no surprise then that this broad trait domain has emerged as the most important of the Big Five for positively predicting health and longevity. However, because past researchers have focused primarily on health risk rather than health protective personality factors, and the construct of conscientiousness as a broad personality dimension is relatively new, the body of

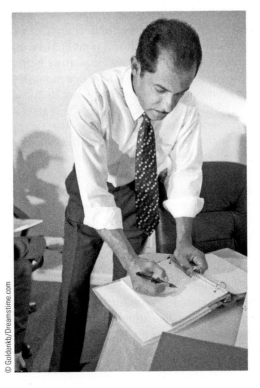

© Goldenkb/Dreamstime.com

People who score high in conscientiousness are generally self-disciplined, responsible, hard-working, persistent, and well-organized. Evidence suggests high conscientiousness is health protective.

research findings in this area is still somewhat small compared to that for neuroticism and extraversion.

One of the first major studies to find a positive role for conscientiousness in longevity was a study done by Freidman and his associates (1993) when they examined longitudinal archival data collected for the landmark Terman Life Cycle Study. Lewis Terman (the creator of the Stanford-Binet Intelligence Test) and his colleagues began the now famous Terman Life Cycle Study in 1922 by selecting more than 1,500 intellectually bright children, later named the "Termites," who were at the time around 11 years old. The researchers collected baseline data from the Termites on a host of psychosocial variables and then assessed the cohort participants periodically for the rest of their lives.

Friedman et al. (1993) were given access in 1986 to comb through the massive data sets collected by Terman's group. The mean age of the Termites by that time was 76. Friedman's group culled parent and teacher trait and activity ratings of the Termites taken at the 1922 baseline and were able to use these data to derive six trait dimension scores for each participant that they called (1) *Conscientiousness-Social Dependability,* (2) *High Motivation-Self-Esteem,* (3) *Cheerfulness-Humor,* (4) *Sociability,* (5) *High Energy-Activity,* and (6) *Permanency of Moods.* The investigators proposed that their *Conscientiousness-Social Dependability* Scale was a proxy for the Big Five conscientiousness factor and that their *Sociability* Scale was similar to extraversion. It should be noted that a later study coauthored by Friedman (Martin & Friedman, 2000) validated the use of their Conscientiousness-Social Dependability Scale as a substitute for the Big Five conscientiousness factor when they determined that these two scale scores strongly correlated.

Using a statistical program called a survival analysis and another called a logistic regression analysis, the researchers were able to, for the first time, document that personality in childhood predicted longevity across the lifespan. Only one personality variable, however, strongly predicted survival, and that was the trait of conscientiousness-social dependability. Their results indicated that someone scoring in the bottom quarter in conscientiousness had a 35% greater chance of dying before the age of 70 than someone scoring in the top quarter of conscientiousness. Contrary to their expectation, sociability was not associated with longevity. Only conscientiousness seemed to have a protective effect for health.

Why would conscientiousness have a protective health effect? One strong possibility based on the findings discussed earlier in this chapter is that individuals high in conscientiousness are more likely to engage in health protective behaviors and avoid health risk and harming behaviors. Recall the Booth-Kewley and Vickers (1994) study that found up to 29% of the variance of correlations between the Big Five factors and health behaviors was accounted for by conscientiousness.

Bogg and Roberts (2004) conducted a meta-analysis of scores from conscientiousness-related personality scales and health-related behaviors for 194 studies (including 10% unpublished studies and dissertations to guard against publication biases). The authors of the study found that participants who were high in conscientiousness were less likely to engage in negative health-related behaviors. The highest negative effect sizes were found for *drug use, excessive alcohol use, risky driving,* and *violence.* More modest negative effect sizes were found for *tobacco use, risky sex, unhealthy eating,* and *suicide.* A very weak positive effect was found for engaging in the positive health-related behavior of *activity.* Thus, there is considerable evidence that conscientious persons are less likely to engage in health-harming behaviors, but not as much evidence in this meta-analytic study, unlike the Booth-Kewley and Vickers (1994) single study finding, that they are more likely to engage in health-enhancing behaviors.

Kern and Friedman (2008) recently conducted a meta-analysis of 20 independent samples for a total of 8,942 participants from six different countries as Friedman continued his exploration of the effects of conscientiousness on longevity. What did they find? After conducting the analysis they determined that the overall effect size was $r = .11$. On the whole, then, their findings show that people with high conscientiousness live longer. The authors noted that this effect may seem modest but that the practical significance of the effect is comparable to or greater than other important epidemiological or medical effects. For example, a coronary bypass surgery 5-year survival effect size is 0.08 (Myer et al., 2001). They also point out that whereas much of the health protective effect may be from health behavior variables, several studies indicate that the effect is still present, though to a lesser extent, when statistically controlling for these variables. This raises the possibility that biological or moderator variables also may play a role in the protective effect.

One of these moderator variables may be everyday mindfulness. Recall from Chapter 2 that mindfulness involves a type of present moment awareness and acceptance and is associated with a number of salutary benefits (see also Chapter 14). A recent meta-analysis of 32 samples by Giluk (2009) found that of the Big Five, conscientiousness showed the strongest positive relationship ($r = .32$) and neuroticism showed the strongest negative relationship ($r = -.45$) to mindfulness. The overlap between mindfulness and conscientiousness is reflected in characteristics such as self-discipline and self-regulation. In contrast, high neuroticism is associated with poor self-regulation, especially with regard to stress reactivity.

Another intriguing recent study, this one conducted by O'Cleirigh, Ironson, Weiss, and Costa (2007), examined 119 participants positive for HIV over a 1-year time span to determine the relationship between conscientiousness and the progression of their disease. The investigators measured disease progression by assessing CD4 T-cell count and viral load at baseline and at a 1-year follow-up. After controlling for other relevant variables (e.g., medications, demographic factors, and baseline disease status), they found that "conscientiousness predicted significant increases in CD4 number and significant decreases in viral load at 1 year" (p. 473). Their follow-up at the 4-year period found that openness and extraversion were also related to slower disease progression (Ironson, O'Cleirigh, Weiss, Schneiderman, & Costa, 2008).

In their initial study, O'Cleirigh et al. (2007) found that although high conscientiousness was associated with greater medication adherence, this medication use variable did not statistically explain the effect, and neither did the lower rates of depression or greater use of active coping for the participants with high conscientiousness. The investigators did find a weak effect for *perceived stress* as a mediator, suggesting a possible biological underpinning of the hypothalamic-pituitary-adrenal (HPA) axis. Thus, if individuals with high conscientiousness perceive less stress they may have less HPA activation, leading to less immune system suppression than their counterparts with low conscientiousness.

In sum, high conscientiousness found in people like Alicia appears to be protective of health and modestly associated with increased longevity. The longevity increase for conscientiousness is likely due to a combination of factors including less participation in health risk and harming behaviors, greater engagement in health-promoting behaviors, greater mindfulness and self-regulation, and use of more adaptive stress appraisal processes.

Extraversion, Openness to Experience, and Agreeableness

If conscientiousness is the champion of health and longevity, extraversion is the champion of good feelings and happiness. Of the Big Five, extraversion consistently rates number one in both positive affect and subjective well-being (Steel et al., 2008). Why? Recall earlier in this chapter how Gray's theory links extraverts' higher levels of positive affect to the BAS that is sensitive to reward and is fueled by the dopamine circuits of the brain (the reward centers). In a related fashion extraverts may be better at savoring positive experiences and keeping their good moods going longer (Hemenover, 2003). They also seem to be less deterred by punishment (Pearce-McCall & Newman, 1986) and less affected by negative social encounters than introverts (Graziano, Feldesman, & Rahe, 1985). Thus, overall, extraverts appear to be more responsive to reward, less responsive to punishment, experience higher levels of positive affect for longer periods, and on the whole report higher levels of well-being than introverts. Do these differences give them an advantage in longevity?

Unlike conscientiousness, large-scale prospective community-based mortality studies have yielded inconsistent results. For example, the Wilson et al. (2005) study of Chicago residents discussed earlier ascertained that those who scored in the top 10% for extraversion had a 21% less mortality risk than those who scored in the bottom 10%. However, Nakaya et al. (2006, p. 149) concluded from their study of Danish residents that "no significant association was found between extraversion and risk of death from all causes nor of cancer-related death." Shipley et al. (2007) found a higher risk of death from cardiovascular disease for extraverts between the ages of 40 and 59 years in their United Kingdom cohort but a lower risk for extraverts for respiratory disease in all age groups. They could not explain such inconsistent findings and attributed them to chance.

If longevity is not an established benefit, then what are some of the benefits of extraversion besides increased well-being? As discussed earlier, a large meta-analytic study indicates that high extraversion is associated with greater satisfaction in intimate relationships (Malouff et al., 2010). It may also confer some protective effect against developing an internalizing psychological disorder, though this good news is tempered by the bad news that it seems to be a risk factor for developing an externalizing disorder (Malouff et al., 2005).

One area that is beginning to emerge that shows a more consistent benefit for high extraversion is posttraumatic growth (see Chapter 3), though more longitudinal studies are needed in the area. For example, in a retrospective cross-sectional study of residents of Spain following the March 11, 2004, Madrid train bombings, the study's authors (Val & Linley, 2006) reported that extraversion is positively related to posttraumatic growth and that neuroticism is negatively related. In a different study, Sheikh (2004) also found that extraversion significantly predicted posttraumatic growth ($r = .25$) for participants with heart disease who were in cardiac rehabilitation programs or cardiac support groups, and that the growth could not be statistically attributed to greater social support for extraverts.

Furthermore, extraversion and conscientiousness seem to be the Big Five traits most closely associated with *resilience*. For example, Campbell-Sills, Cohan, and Stein (2006) found in a sample of college students that resilience was positively related to extraversion and conscientiousness and negatively related to neuroticism. They hypothesized that extraverts' positive affective style contributes to their greater ability to broaden and build (Fredrickson, 1998) (see Chapter 2) during times of stress. This capacity then leads them to build their social resources networks and more flexibly deal with adversity (recall how Alicia made a new friend after losing an old one). In keeping with Fredrickson's model, they also suggested that positive affect additionally helps extraverts recover more quickly from the physiological effects of stress. Campbell-Sills et al. (2006) discerned that the higher resilience found in individuals with high conscientiousness was fully explained in their statistical analysis by these hard workers' tendency to use task-oriented coping during times of stress.

What are the benefits of scoring high in openness? A very small body of research findings suggests that elements of the Big Five's openness to experience may have some health protective effects. For example, Jonassaint et al. (2007) administered the NEO-PI to 977 patients with coronary artery disease (CAD) coronary catheterization and followed them prospectively over a 15-year period. Consistent with other studies, they found that openness to experience did not predict all-cause mortality. However, the two openness facets of *Feelings* and *Actions* were positively associated with greater longevity even after controlling for other relevant variables. Interpreting the facets suggests that those participants with greater *emotional awareness* and higher levels of *curiosity* lived longer. These qualities may be related to a more flexible coping style in dealing with stressors such as their cardiovascular disease.

What are the benefits of scoring high in agreeableness? Very few studies have examined the relationship between the Big Five's agreeableness and longevity, and those that have, with one notable exception, have not found significant results. The exception is the Weiss and Costa (2005) study discussed earlier, an outlier that examined older frail participants and found high neuroticism, conscientiousness, and agreeableness to positively predict longevity. Also as discussed previously, high levels of agreeableness were reported in a meta-analysis to be favorable for intimate partner relationship satisfaction along with low neuroticism and high levels of extraversion and conscientiousness (Malouff et al., 2010). So, as one would expect, its beneficial stress effects are most likely constrained to the interpersonal domain.

Dispositional Optimism

Dispositional optimists like Alicia have a personality style that expects positive outcomes. As Seligman (2002, p. 24), a prominent optimism researcher, notes: "Optimists . . . have a strength that allows them to interpret their setbacks as surmountable, particular to a single problem, and resulting from temporary circumstances or other people. Pessimists, I have found over the last two decades, are up to eight times more likely to become depressed when bad events happen; they do worse in school, sports, and most jobs than their talents augur; they have worse physical health and shorter lives; they have rockier interpersonal relations . . . ."

Numerous studies over the last several decades report positive health benefits for dispositional optimism though some do not. However, until recently, no meta-analytic study had been conducted that enabled a quantitative review of the findings. This changed when Rasmussen, Scheier, and Greenhouse (2009) examined 83 published studies that included both the dispositional view of optimism and the explanatory style view (see Chapter 2). The authors of the meta-analytic review reported that they found an overall mean effect size for the relationship between optimism and health to be in the small to moderate range (effect size = .17). This may seem modest, but like the small effect size for conscientiousness, it is very meaningful from a health and epidemiological standpoint. The type of optimism construct measured, whether it was dispositional optimism or the explanatory style view, did not significantly differ in effect size. The subjective health measures showed a higher effect size than objective measures, however, lending more credence to the strategy of using objectively verifiable health measures when possible.

Individual studies illustrate findings of a protective health effect for optimism. For example, for 15 years, Giltay, Kamphuis, Kalmijn, Zitman, and Kromhout (2006) followed a group of 545 older Dutch men who were initially free of cardiovascular disease. During that time 187 died of cardiovascular disease. They found at follow-up that those scoring in the top third in dispositional optimism had a 55% lower risk of cardiovascular death than those in the bottom third, even after statistically adjusting for other health-related predictor variables.

In a study published in the prestigious medical journal *Circulation,* Tindle and her colleagues (2009) reported results from the Women's Health Initiative study (the same study that found a health risk for certain forms of hormone replacement therapy) of 97,253 postmenopausal women that focused on the connection between optimism and health as well as cynical hostility (a subscale of the *Cook-Medley Scale*) and health—cynical hostility is believed to be even more pernicious than general hostility. This was the largest sample to date that examined these variables. Based on medical screenings, the women were assessed as free of clinical cardiovascular disease and cancer at the onset of the study and tracked for 8 years. What did they find?

Those scoring in the top quarter in optimism had a reduced hazard adjusted risk of 16% for MI, 30% for CHD-related mortality, and 14% for death from any cause when compared to those scoring in the bottom quarter. They also discovered that the positive effect was particularly pronounced for

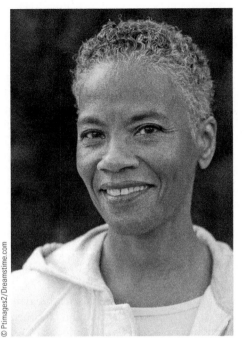

According to results from the Women's Health Initiative study, postmenopausal optimistic Black women showed a more pronounced protective effect against cancer-related mortality and mortality from all causes.

optimistic Black women, who showed a reduced hazard adjusted risk of 44% for cancer-related death and 33% for death from any cause.

The investigators further determined that high levels of cynical hostility increased the adjusted hazard risk for cancer by 23% and for all causes of death by 16%, but it did not increase risk for CHD after adjustment. These results lend support to the findings discussed earlier in this chapter that hostility may not be a robust predictor of cardiovascular disease in women (Consedine et al., 2004) but it nevertheless is a general health risk for them.

Highly cynical hostile Black women exhibited a more pronounced and astoundingly high increased adjusted risk effect of 142% for mortality from cancer and 62% for death by all causes. The authors of the study noted that, overall, the Black women in their sample had a higher level of cynical hostility than the White women. They speculated that this could be a by-product of coping with discrimination. More about the stress and health effects of living with prejudice and discrimination is discussed in Chapter 8. Overall, then, the protective effects for optimism and the harmful effects for cynical hostility were more exaggerated for Black women.

Why does dispositional optimism appear to have a protective health effect? What are the underlying mechanisms and pathways involved in the optimism-disease-protection link? These have yet to be determined. However, Carver and Connor-Smith (2010, p. 679) point out that "meta-analyses link optimism, extraversion, conscientiousness, and openness to more engagement coping; neuroticism to more disengagement coping; and optimism, conscientiousness, and agreeableness to less disengagement coping." **Engagement coping,** which deals

engagement coping: the stressor or the emotions it evokes are dealt with directly.

directly with the stressor or the emotions it evokes, is more effective at mitigating the effects of stress than **disengagement coping** that involves escape and avoidance (see Chapter 10). Therefore, optimists may be more effective at coping with stress. In keeping with their propensity to use engagement coping, they also may be more willing to use the health care system rather than avoid it when confronting health risk symptoms. Similarly, they may be more likely to engage in more positive health-related behaviors as an active engagement preventive strategy.

Further, high levels of optimism may be associated with lower HPA axis reactivity and inflammation. For example, Roy et al. (2010) found that higher levels of optimism were linked to lower levels of inflammatory markers such as IL-6, fibrinogen, and homocysteine. Conversely, it may be that pessimism is a vulnerability factor for inflammation. Recall the discussion in Chapter 5 of how inflammation is associated with diseases such as CHD.

Dispositional Constructs Involving Perceptions of Control

A number of dispositional constructs related to health outcomes deal directly with perceptions of control, including Rotter's (1966, 1990) *locus of control*, Kobasa's (1979) *hardiness*, and Antonovsky's (1979, 1987) *sense of coherence (SOC)* construct. According to Rotter's social learning theory, over time we develop generalized expectancies about our actions and the reinforcements that follow them, which are referred to as **locus of control**. When we have an **internal locus of control** (e.g., Alicia) we generally expect that our actions will lead to predictable outcomes and reinforcements. However, when we have an **external locus of control** (e.g., Claudia) we expect that reinforcements and other outcomes will be influenced by outside forces such as luck, fate, coincidence, powerful others, and so forth.

locus of control: general expectancies about the connections between one's actions and the outcomes and reinforcements that follow them.

Rotter's (1966) I-E Scale is typically used to determine if a person has an internal or external locus of control, but many alternative self-report scales also have been developed. For example, the Health Locus of Control Scale (Wallston & Wallston, 1981) was developed to assess the degree of control one expects over one's health.

The locus of control construct has been enormously popular with thousands of studies examining its effects. In general, internal locus of control has been found to be more beneficial than external locus of control when it comes to most stress and health scenarios. For example, the INTERHEART case control study (Rosengren et al., 2004) of 24,767 participants (11,119 of whom had experienced a first MI) from 52 countries that examined psychosocial risk factors for MI, discussed in Chapter 5, concluded that "high locus of control was a significant protective factor." Further, the effect was attenuated but still protective for MIs after statistically adjusting for other health risk variables. Their final calculated population attributable risk (PAR), which is a reflection of the proportion of MI cases attributable to external locus of control if it were a causal factor was 16%.

In another study known as the 1970 British Cohort Study, Gale, Batty, and Deary (2008) assessed locus of control for 11,563 children at age 10 and then evaluated their health outcomes and behaviors at age 30 (7,551 of the original sample) and found that those with an internal locus of control were statistically less likely to report being overweight or obese, less likely to rate their health as fair or poor, and to have less psychological distress even after

◯ INSIGHT EXERCISE **6.1**

If you are curious to know your locus of control, then carefully review the items on the left side and the right side of the table below. Think about which side fits you best—the left or the right?

What Is Your Locus of Control?

Becoming a success is a matter of hard work; luck has little or nothing to do with it.	Getting a good job depends mainly on being in the right place at the right time.
When I make plans, I am almost certain that I can make them work.	It is not always wise to plan too far ahead because many things turn out to be a matter of good or bad fortune anyhow.
What happens to me is my own doing.	Sometimes I feel that I don't have enough control over the direction my life is taking.
Getting people to do the right thing depends upon ability; luck has little or nothing to do with it.	Who gets to be the boss often depends on who was lucky enough to be in the right place first.
People are lonely because they don't try to be friendly.	There's not much use in trying too hard to please people; if they like you, they like you.
Capable people who fail to become leaders have not taken advantage of their opportunities.	Without the right breaks one cannot be an effective leader.
The average citizen can have an influence in governmental decisions.	This world is run by the few people in power, and there is not much the little guy can do about it.

Did you complete the exercise? If you endorsed primarily the left side items then you likely have an internal locus of control, whereas if you believe the right side items fit you best then you probably have an external locus of control. The above items were sampled from Rotter's (1966) I-E Scale.

Source: *Rotter, J.B. (1966), Generalized expectancies for internal versus external control of reinforcement,* Psychological Monographs, *80; 1, No. 609.*

adjusting for other health risk variables. They concluded that "having a stronger sense of control over one's life in childhood seems to be a protective factor for some aspects of health in adult life" (p. 397). Further analyses revealed that if locus of control were causal, external locus of control could account for 10.3% of the overweight, 9.6% of the obese, 13% of those who rated their health fair to poor, and 13.1% of those who were psychologically distressed. Although these were self-report health measures rather than objective measures, they nevertheless reflect a general pattern found in other studies. Locus of control also may play a role in determining the likelihood of starting and maintaining certain health-harming behaviors such as cigarette smoking. For example, Clarke, MacPherson, and Holmes (1982) found that adolescents with internal locus of control were less likely to start smoking, and that among adolescent smokers, those with external locus of control were the ones who stated they were most likely to continue smoking.

Another dispositional construct involving perceptions of control is hardiness. The hardiness construct emerged from stress research as a way of

hardiness: a construct described as a stress-resistant personality that exhibits existential courage through a synergy of the three cognitive elements of control, challenge, and commitment.

describing a *stress-resistant* personality that exhibits existential courage (Maddi, 2006). **Hardiness** is defined as a synergy of three cognitive elements, the three Cs of *control, challenge,* and *commitment* (Kobasa, 1979; Maddi, 2002).

Control (versus powerlessness) is similar to Rotter's internal locus of control concept and refers to confidence in one's ability to cope with difficulties and to have an influence on outcomes.

Challenge (versus security) concerns a sense that stress and change are catalysts for growth and personal development. They are appraised as exciting opportunities and not avoided in favor of easier pathways to comfort or security.

Finally, **commitment** (versus alienation) means to be deeply involved in one's life endeavors and to be true to one's self and values even during periods of high stress. Thus, when persons approach life with existential courage they do not shrink from life's challenges but rather actively engage them in a form of transformational coping that serves to shape the outcome. Hardy individuals also perceive stress and change as less threatening, thus lowering their overall reactivity to stressors. In many ways, the concept of hardiness is similar to the concept of resilience.

Over 25 years of research and more than 1,000 studies have provided mixed evidence for a protective effect of hardiness as a buffer or moderator in the stress-illness link. There are many unresolved issues regarding the construct (see Klag & Bradley, 2004, for a discussion). Let us look at three of these issues.

First, there is some controversy as to whether hardiness is a unitary construct or three separate, somewhat independent, constructs (Carver, 1989). For example, whereas commitment and control have been found to consistently predict health outcomes, challenge has not (Funk, 1992).

Second, negative affectivity and neuroticism are highly negatively correlated with hardiness, suggesting that many of the hardiness-health outcome studies have a serious confound. It may be that high hardiness is a reflection of low neuroticism rather than that hardiness confers an additional protective effect. Most studies have not controlled for neuroticism and those that have often find that hardiness no longer predicts health outcome (Funk & Houston, 1987; Rhodewalt & Zone, 1989) though in a few cases it still does (Maddi & Khoshaba, 1994) (see Maddi, 2002, for a rebuttal of this criticism).

Third, the construct of hardiness was developed primarily through testing men, and many subsequent investigations have exclusively examined men. When women are included in studies of hardiness, the results are typically equivocal or nonsupportive (Benishek & Lopez, 1997; Klag & Bradley, 2004).

The SOC model also concerns dispositional perceptions of control. Recall from Chapter 1 Antonovsky's (1979, 1987) SOC model, which like hardiness is characterized as a *stress resistant* personality style that is comprised of three components. In this case they are *comprehensibility, manageability, and meaningfulness.* Remember that comprehensibility refers to our ability to make cognitive sense of stimuli, manageability to our ability to access internal and external coping resources, and meaningfulness to our capacity to emotionally make sense of environmental demands and see them as worthy of engagement. It is interesting to note that manageability has similarities to Rotter's *locus of control* and Kobasa's hardiness *control* component.

As discussed previously (see Chapter 1), Eriksson and Lindstrom (2005) reviewed over 450 publications of the salutogenic model and concluded that SOC promotes resilience and positive health, including mental health. More recently Surtees, Nicholas, Wainwright, Khaw, and Day (2006) examined mastery, SOC, and mortality from data collected in the prospective EPIC-Norfolk cohort study. They considered SOC to be the most distinctive of all the positive health outcome constructs dealing with personality coping dispositions (e.g., SOC, hardiness, dispositional optimism, and self-efficacy) (Ouellette & DiPlacido, 2001).

The Surtees et al. (2006) study began tracking 20,323 residents (ages 41 to 80 years) of Norfolk, England, after assessing them for sense of mastery (SOM) (similar to Rotter's I-E scale) and SOC. The researchers ascertained at the study's 6-year follow-up that after statistically adjusting for other health risk factors, including biological (e.g., age, sex, disease), behavioral (e.g., cigarette smoking), and psychological (e.g., hostility and neuroticism), that for each standard deviation difference, a higher SOM was associated with a 15% reduction and a higher SOC with a 10% reduction of all-cause mortality. In other words, each standard deviation increase in SOM conferred a 15% reduction in mortality. Likewise each standard deviation increase in SOC conferred a 10% reduction in mortality. A high SOM (but not SOC) appeared to be protective of cardiovascular mortality (17% reduction) and a high SOC (but not SOM) of cancer mortality (11% reduction). Although both constructs were highly correlated with each other, their protective effects against all-cause mortality were independent. The authors suggested that a strong SOC may have direct biological benefits by protecting against physiological reactivity to stressors.

In sum, there is evidence to suggest that high internal locus of control is protective against MI, other negative health outcomes and behaviors, and cardiovascular as well as all-cause mortality. Support for SOC protecting against cancer mortality and all-cause mortality also was found. Though many studies indicate that hardiness buffers stress reactions against illness, the effects observed are mainly specific to men and they may be due to low neuroticism rather than to additional protection that hardiness is alleged to confer.

CHAPTER SUMMARY AND CONCEPT REVIEW

- Models that link personality to stress and health include the biological predisposition model, health-related behavior models, and moderation models.

- Personality refers to an enduring pattern of thoughts, emotions, and behaviors that define an individual and traits refers to the characteristics or structural elements of the personality.

- Eysenck's PEN model of personality consists of the Big Three supertraits of psychoticism, extraversion, and neuroticism.

- Eysenck proposed that introverts have greater cortical arousal than extraverts and this accounts for some of their reserve and social reticence.

- Gray proposed a behavioral approach system (BAS) brain mechanism that is sensitive to reward and a behavioral inhibition system (BIS) that is sensitive to punishment and nonreward.

- Gray's model suggests that extraverts have more positive affect and greater subjective well-being because they have a more dominant BAS, and individuals with high levels of neuroticism have more negative affect and less subjective well-being because they have a more sensitive BIS.

- The Big Five consists of five broad personality dimensions of neuroticism, extraversion, openness, conscientiousness, and agreeableness.

- Of the Big Five, neuroticism is the one that is most closely associated with stress reactivity, higher negative affect, lower positive affect, less subjective well-being, greater use of disengagement coping, a greater chance of developing a clinical or personality disorder, more dissatisfaction in intimate relationships, a greater probability of engaging in problem alcohol use and smoking tobacco, a greater likelihood of involvement in an occupational accident, and perhaps greater mortality (although the findings here are mixed).

- The Type A behavior pattern has generally fallen into disfavor due to failures to replicate promising initial studies.

- Hostility and particular forms of anger expression (e.g., suppressed anger and destructive anger justification) are more robust predictors of coronary heart disease (CHD) than Type A, especially in men, though anxiety may be a better predictor of CHD in women.

- Recently the Type D (distressed) personality has emerged as a predictor for a poor prognosis in patients with heart disease but the construct has met with some skepticism after the Type A disappointments.

- Among the Big Five, conscientiousness has emerged as the broad trait that appears to be the most protective of health and longevity.

- Extraversion rates number one among the Big Five in positive affect and subjective well-being; it also is emerging as positively related to posttraumatic growth.

- Dispositional optimism appears to have a protective effect on health, including protecting against cardiovascular disease in men and women as well as protecting against CHD-related and all-cause mortality in women.

- High internal locus of control appears to be protective against myocardial infarction, other negative health outcomes and behaviors, and cardiovascular as well as all-cause mortality.

- Sense of coherence (SOC) seems to protect against all-cause mortality. In addition, it may protect against cancer mortality.

- The evidence for hardiness as a buffer in the stress-illness link is mixed; the construct and research supporting it are criticized for confounding neuroticism and for failure to find consistent protective effects for women.

CRITICAL THINKING QUESTIONS

1. Why do you think studies have found gender differences in anger-hostility or anxiety as risk factors for CHD? What explains these differences? How can constructive anger expression protect men against CHD? Why do you believe the same protection for constructive anger expression was not found for women in the study discussed in this chapter?

2. How do you account for study findings that the protective effects for optimism and the harmful effects for cynical hostility were both more exaggerated for Black than White women?

3. Which personality factors do you believe leave you more vulnerable to stress? How do they leave you vulnerable? What healthy strategies can you employ to counteract your personality vulnerabilities? Which personality factors do you believe protect you from stress? What ways can you use them for your maximum health and well-being advantage?

4. Why do you think perceptions of control are related to stress and health outcomes? Which theory that includes perceptions of control is your favorite? Why? How does perceived control protect a person against stress and adverse health outcomes?

5. If someone asks you how personality relates to health and longevity, what would you say? What do you consider the three most important findings in this area? Why are these three findings the ones you consider to be the most important?

KEY TERMS AND CONCEPTS

Agreeableness*

Anger

Anger expression

Behavioral approach system (BAS)*

Behavioral inhibition system (BIS)*

Biological predisposition model

Buffer

Challenge

Commitment

Conscientiousness*

Control

Constructive anger expression

Destructive anger justification

Destructive anger rumination

Diagnostic and Statistical Manual (DSM)

Disengagement coping

Dispositions

Engagement coping*

Externalizing disorders

External locus of control

Extraversion*

Eysenck's PEN model*

Facets

Factor analysis

Five Factor Model (FFM)*

Hardiness*

Health-related behavior models

Hostility*

Internalizing disorders

Internal locus of control

Introverts

Locus of control*

Moderation models*

Neurosis

Neurotic cascade

Neuroticism*

Openness*

Personality

Personality disorder

Personality types

Psychosomatic medicine

Psychoticism

Reinforcement sensitivity theory

States

Sixteen Personality Factor (16 PF) Questionnaire

Temperament

The Big Five

The Big Three

Traits*

Type A*

Type B

Type D*

MEDIA RESOURCES

CENGAGE**brain**

Access an interactive eBook, chapter-specific interactive learning tools, including flashcards, quizzes, videos, and more in your Psychology CourseMate, accessed through CengageBrain.com.

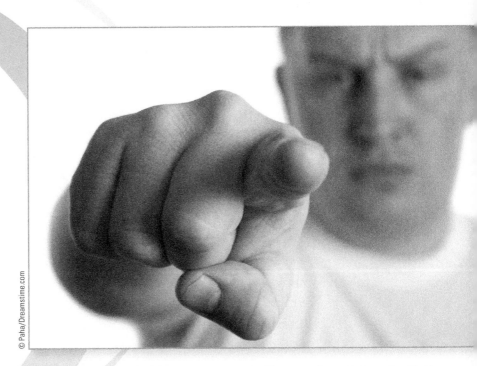

© Paha/Dreamstime.com

Holding on to anger is like grasping a hot coal with the intent of throwing it at someone else; you are the one who gets burned.

~BUDDHA

ANXIETY, ANGER, AND DEPRESSION

Imagine you have a flower garden and ask yourself what it would feel like if you spent a full day prepping your garden and planting your flowers only to find the next morning that half your flowers had been thoroughly excavated by the frisky little neighborhood dog, Skippy. You might get a little annoyed if the next day, after replanting your flowers, you return after your lunch break only to see Skippy digging around in your garden. In fact, after catching Skippy several times with dirty paws as you survey the fresh holes in your garden, you might even get a little hot under the collar.

The next morning after you rise out of bed, you find yourself already pretty irritated as you anticipate the prospect of yet another showdown with Skippy. As you rapidly approach your garden, ready for today's duel, you imagine smoke coming out of your ears. Abruptly, you turn the corner and you spot fresh holes and flowers strewn about. Instantly you are livid. Looking up from the holes and expecting to see Skippy, instead you right away discover a large muscular dog with teeth bared that fixes his eyes on you, growls, and then leans forward in your direction. Uh oh! Now how do you feel? In a blink of an eye, your anger turns to fear.

As you know, anger and fear, the two fight-or-flight emotions, are based on how we mentally appraise the situation. When our appraisals change, our emotions change. Because we can control our appraisals, we can manage our emotions. The idea of controlling our appraisals, the cognitive approach, is one of several broad sets of strategies we will discuss later for managing feelings of anxiety, anger, and depression. The point is that we are not simply passive recipients of our emotions, but rather we unknowingly play an active role in shaping their direction and intensity. Once we understand this connection, we can knowingly learn to manage these emotions as the need arises.

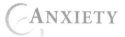

ANXIETY

Mark Twain once remarked, "I am an old man and have known a great many troubles, but most of them never happened." The apprehension and dread of anxiety can feel like trouble even when there is no trouble. Our body reaction is the same to *imagined* trouble (i.e., the saber-toothed tigers of the mind) as to *real* trouble. Our body cannot tell the difference between them even though we can separate the real from the imagined intellectually. What Mark Twain referred to as *troubles*, in this context, we could refer to as anxiety. Anxiety and fear are very similar, but distinctions can be drawn between the two.

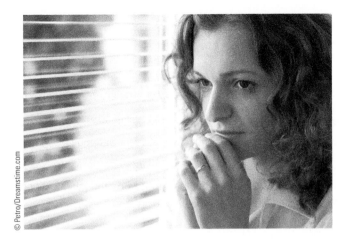

Anxiety is a vague sense of unease about the future.

Before we examine anxiety, let us first look at fear. Generally speaking, **fear** is the emotion we feel when there is concrete danger, such as the feeling of fright you have when suddenly encountering a growling large muscular dog in your flower bed. There is a very real possibility that you could receive some unwanted tooth marks on your leg as that scenario unfolds. So your fear is well founded.

On the other hand, **anxiety** involves more complex and diffuse feelings of uneasiness related to possible impending threats. Anxiety is very future oriented and can capture more abstract threats than fear (e.g., the anxiety of losing face in front of an audience). We often use words like *nervous, apprehensive,* and *uneasy* to capture the anxiety emotions. **Worry** involves mentally recycling concerns—it is the process of repeating our thoughts associated with anxiety.

Besides everyday anxiety, we can feel **existential anxiety,** a form of anxiety associated with *awareness of ultimate concerns* such as death, meaning, freedom, and isolation (Yalom, 1980). These concerns capture the essence of existence and embody the cosmic questions such as "What happens after death?" "What is the meaning of life?" "Why do we exist?" "How much freedom do we really have?" "What is loneliness and why do we experience it?" Certain events such as the death of a loved one, a diagnosis of a serious illness, separation or divorce, difficult choices that have long lasting life consequences (educational, career, or romantic commitments, etc.), traumatic events that evoke a crisis of meaning, midlife or other lifespan transitional passages, and so forth, may trigger existential anxiety.

Both fear and anxiety are related to the *flight* component of the fight-or-flight response. As such, both are natural emotions that generally serve us well to keep us out of danger. For example, the fear we experience when a sudden bolt of lightning strikes close by before a thunderstorm approaches prompts us to seek shelter and thus increases our safety. However, like all good things when overdone, fear and anxiety can present problems. For instance, if we

INSIGHT EXERCISE **7.1**

If you would like, take a few minutes to complete the scale called the "Self-Analysis Questionnaire" to get a reading on your own general level of anxiety. Use the scoring key to see if you are low, midrange, or high in overall anxiety.

Self-Analysis Questionnaire

Read each statement and then mark the appropriate number to indicate how you generally feel. There are no right or wrong answers. Do not spend too much time on any one statement but give the answer which seems to describe how you generally feel.

1. I am a steady person.

Almost Never	Sometimes	Often	Almost Always
4	3	2	1

2. I am satisfied with myself.

Almost Never	Sometimes	Often	Almost Always
4	3	2	1

3. I feel nervous and restless.

Almost Never	Sometimes	Often	Almost Always
1	2	3	4

4. I wish I could be as happy as others seem to be.

Almost Never	Sometimes	Often	Almost Always
1	2	3	4

5. I feel like a failure

Almost Never	Sometimes	Often	Almost Always
1	2	3	4

6. I get in a state of tension and turmoil as I think over my recent concerns and interests.

Almost Never	Sometimes	Often	Almost Always
1	2	3	4

7. I feel secure.

Almost Never	Sometimes	Often	Almost Always
4	3	2	1

8. I have self-confidence.

Almost Never	Sometimes	Often	Almost Always
4	3	2	1

9. I feel inadequate.

Almost Never	Sometimes	Often	Almost Always
1	2	3	4

10. I worry too much over something that does not matter.

Almost Never	Sometimes	Often	AlmostAlways
1	2	3	4

Scoring. Simply add your numbers over the ten questions. Be careful to notice that some of the rows of numbers go up and some go down. The higher your total, the more the trait of anxiety dominates your life. Adult men and women have slightly different scores on average, with women being somewhat more anxious generally.

If you scored **10–11,** your anxiety level is in the lowest 10th percentile.

If you scored **13–14,** your anxiety level is in the lowest 25th percentile.

If you scored **16–17,** your anxiety level is about average.

If you scored **19–20,** your anxiety level is around the 75th percentile.

If you scored **22–24 and you are male,** your anxiety level is around the 90th percentile.

If you scored **24–26 and you are female,** your anxiety level is around the 90th percentile.

If you scored **25 and you are male,** your anxiety level is at the 95th percentile.

If you scored **27 and you are female,** your anxiety level is at the 95th percentile.

SOURCE: *"Self-Analysis Questionnaire" developed by Charles Spielberger in collaboration with G. Jacobs, R. Crane, S. Russell, L. Westberry, L. Barker, E. Johnson, J. Knight, and E. Markes. We have selected the trait anxiety questions from the questionnare, inverting some of the scoring of the negatively worded items for easy self-scoring.*

tremble with fear or anxiety while safely inside our house any time we hear thunder, then these emotions create unnecessary problems for us. If we cognitively process threat-related stimuli such as the thunder in a biased fashion so that our threat assessments are excessive and overused, we can generate anxiety that is debilitating (Ouimet, Gawronski, & Dozois, 2009).

When we experience fear and anxiety with sufficient distress for long enough periods, we can feel suffering or impairment that goes outside the normal boundaries of stress reactions. According to the medical model reflected in the *Diagnostic and Statistical Manual, 4th Edition, Text Revision* ([DSM-IV-TR], American Psychiatric Association, 2000), discussed in Chapter 6, a person can meet the diagnostic criteria for an **anxiety disorder** if other physical causes are ruled out (e.g., hyperthyroidism, adrenal gland tumors, too much caffeine, etc.) and anxiety is excessive and disabling. As you would expect from their suffering or impairment, individuals diagnosed with an anxiety disorder unfortunately have an overall lower quality of life than their healthy counterparts (Olatunji, Cisler, & Tolin, 2007).

Let us briefly look at the primary DSM-IV-TR anxiety disorders: generalized anxiety disorder (GAD), panic disorder, phobic disorders, obsessive-compulsive disorder, and the stress disorder of posttraumatic stress disorder (PTSD). First, be aware that there is a phenomenon known as the *medical student syndrome* where medical students tend to see symptoms in themselves of various diseases they are studying. If you are very conscientious and self-analytical, you may be disposed to see some of the symptoms of these anxiety disorders in yourself. It is possible that you have an anxiety disorder, but then again, you may just be experiencing the medical student syndrome. As you learn more about these disorders it is important to put this information in its proper perspective.

Generalized Anxiety Disorder (GAD)

Mr. Y, a 30-year-old married real estate investment company owner, goes to a local outpatient psychiatric clinic saying that he "is on the verge of a nervous breakdown." He reports that he has always been a "worrier" but not to the extent that his life was affected in any noticeable way. However, over the past year he has been experiencing a "tweaked" feeling of inner agitation and "stays keyed up" most of the time. Mr. Y has frequently complained of stomach upsets and diarrhea over the past 6 months as well as a decreased ability to concentrate at work. (Frances & Ross, 2001, pp. 184–185)

Mr. Y was diagnosed with a **generalized anxiety disorder (GAD)**. Key features of this disorder are his excessive uncontrollable anxiety and worry that had persisted for at least 6 months and that cause him *clinically significant distress or impairment*. As a chronic worrier, Mr. Y's anxiety and worry are out of proportion to events in his environment. People with GAD may experience symptoms such as fatigue, muscle tension, restlessness, irritability, sleep disturbances, or difficulty concentrating. Depression also may be present.

GAD is reported to have a lifetime prevalence of 5.7% (i.e., the percent of people in the general population that will develop the disorder during their lifetime) (Kessler et al., 2005). It is more commonly diagnosed in women than men (American Psychiatric Association, 2000). Gender differences like these are found in many of the anxiety disorders and could be due to multiple causes, the most prominent being that there is greater social approval for females than males to experience and express anxiety-related emotions (McLean & Anderson, 2009). The course of GAD is long term with onset often beginning in childhood or adolescence. Its symptoms, usually exacerbated by stress, generally wax and wane throughout the person's lifespan.

Panic Disorder

A **panic disorder** is characterized by repeated and unexpected panic attacks along with worry and concern about reoccurrence of attacks. **Panic attacks** have a pronounced physiological component that is usually frightening and can cause anxiety about the anxiety (*anxiety sensitivity*). People with a high level of interoceptive sensitivity (i.e., a conscious awareness of internal physiological activity), especially if they are acutely aware of heartbeat activity, are more likely to experience anxiety and anxiety disorders (Domschke, Stevens, Pfleiderer, & Gerlach, 2010). During a first panic attack, it is not uncommon for people to mistakenly believe they are having a heart attack, because symptoms such as a pounding heart, palpitations, rapid heart rate, chest pain, sweating, shortness of breath, numbness, tingling, or dizziness are common to both conditions. Consider the following person's physiological reactions during a panic attack and imagine how easily it could be interpreted as a sign of a heart attack:

> My heart was beating so hard and fast I thought it would jump out and hit my hand. I felt like I couldn't stand up—that my legs wouldn't support me. My hands got icy and my feet stung. There were horrible shooting pains in my forehead. My head felt tight, like someone had pulled the skin down too tight and I wanted to pull it away. . . . I couldn't breathe; I was short of breath. I literally got out of breath and panted like I had run up and down the stairs. I felt like I had run an eight-mile race. I couldn't do anything. I felt all done in; weak, no strength. I couldn't even dial a telephone. . . . (Laughlin, 1967, p. 92)

People may have other fear-related thoughts during a panic attack besides "I'm having a heart attack" including "I'm dying" or "I'm going crazy" or "I'm losing control," all of which may exacerbate the attack. Along with the physiological responses and fear cognitions, the panicked person has an intense feeling of fear. This feeling may lead to a sense of unreality or detachment from oneself. A panic attack usually develops abruptly, peaks within 10 minutes, and then gradually subsides. Panic disorder, more common in women than men, has an age of onset typically occurring in late adolescence or, less commonly, in the mid-30s (American Psychiatric Association, 2000). A credible lifetime prevalence estimate for panic disorder is 4.7% (Kessler et al., 2005).

Phobias

The word *phobia* is Greek for "fear." A person diagnosed with a **phobia** has an unreasonable or excessive fear of a particular object, situation, or activity. The DSM-IV-TR divides phobias into the three broad categories of *agoraphobia, social phobias,* and *specific phobias.* Persons with **agoraphobia** are fearful of being in a public place or outside the home to the extent that it might be difficult for them to leave without embarrassment or to get help should they have a panic attack. Their inhibition about being in such situations could be considered an extreme form of avoidance coping. Examples of fear-provoking situations and events include waiting in a line, being in a crowd, traveling on a bus, crossing a bridge, or leaving their house without a companion. Agoraphobia may be present in people with or without a history of panic disorder. In both cases the fear that drives the avoidance behavior is a dread of having panic-like symptoms in a context of vulnerability. Consider the following person with agoraphobia:

> "I feel tense and fearful much of the time. I don't know what it is. I can't put my finger on it. I am frightened, but don't know what I fear. I keep expecting something bad to happen. I just get all nervous inside. . . . For the past week or so I don't want to get away from the house [which equated for him a refuge and safety]. I fear I might go all to pieces, maybe become hysterical."
>
> The patient continued to discuss this aspect a little further: . . . "I can go into a store [without feeling unduly anxious] but only if my car is parked right close by the store. I fear somehow that something might happen and then I couldn't get back to my car. The farther I get from my car, or from home, the more uneasy I get. The house is like a refuge to me. The farther I get from it, the more uneasy I become. I feel secure in the house. If something happens to me there, something can be done about it." (Laughlin, 1967, p. 107)

Social phobia, as the name suggests, concerns a fear of social activity, specifically the fear of being engaged in a social activity with unfamiliar people that might scrutinize and embarrass them. Persons with social phobias often use avoidance coping so they are not subjected to their feared social activities. Examples of avoided social circumstances include dating, eating in public, writing in front of observing others, public speaking (e.g., giving a speech or presentation), and so forth. They often decline social invitations while keeping secret the real reasons for not accepting. If they do accept these invitations, they generally endure intense anxiety during the event. Social phobias may be generalized or specific to only particular social activities (e.g., eating in public). They typically begin in midadolescence and are generally predated by a history of childhood shyness and social inhibition. A likely lifetime prevalence estimate for social phobia is 12.1% (Kessler et al., 2005).

Specific phobias are intense and exaggerated fears of specific objects or situations other than public places or social contexts covered by the other phobia categories. Examples of common specific phobias include fear of particular animals, storms, or heights; seeing blood or receiving an injection; flying or driving; or fear of choking to name a few. Specific phobia is more common in women than men by a ratio of 2:1 (American Psychiatric Association, 2000). This disorder is considered to be one of the most common of the anxiety disorders (lifetime prevalence estimate is 12.5%; Kessler et al., 2005).

It is important to point out about phobias in general, however, that many people have fears about particular things, events, or situations, especially public speaking. However, such fears generally do not warrant a phobia diagnosis unless they clinically impair a person's ability to function academically, socially, in a job, or in a normal routine. Impairment is one of the hallmarks that distinguishes an anxiety disorder from everyday anxiety.

Obsessive-Compulsive Disorder

A person diagnosed with an **obsessive-compulsive disorder** has recurrent obsessions or compulsions. **Obsessions** refer to *thoughts*, images, or impulses that are intrusive or inappropriate enough to cause a marked elevation of anxiety, whereas **compulsions** refer to *behaviors* or mental acts that are ritualistic and designed to lower anxiety. Common obsessions include anxiety themes concerning contamination, order, doubts, or aggressive or sexual imagery—normal worries about everyday problems do not qualify. Common compulsions include repetitive behaviors, such as hand washing, checking or ordering of objects, or mental acts, such as counting, praying, or silently repeating words. Let us look at Ms. A, a school teacher, who was diagnosed with an obsessive-compulsive disorder, to better understand the symptoms.

> She often spends 3–4 hours a day engaged in checking behaviors. She spends at least an hour going back and forth between her curling iron, the stove, and the front door. After she is finally convinced that everything is as it should be, the thought comes to her that she should check it all again because, if she doesn't, the house may burn down or a burglar may get in. She often retraces her driving path for fear that she has run over someone or something. Report card time is a nightmare for Ms. A because she repetitively checks and rechecks for hours the grades she has recorded. She reports an association between obsessional thoughts about harm coming to her parents and her behaviors. For instance, she feels that she must call her mother every day in the morning and evening, no matter how inconvenient this may be. She says she is obsessed with the thought that if she misses a phone call to check up on her, her mother may have a stroke and die and it will be her fault for failing to call. (Frances & Ross, 2001, pp. 173–174)

Obsessive-compulsive disorder is more likely to begin during the age range of 6 to 15 years for females and from ages 20 to 29 years for males with the disorder being equally common for males and females (total incidence probably less than 2% of the population) (American Psychiatric Association, 2000).

Posttraumatic Stress Disorder (PTSD)

Recall our discussion of PTSD in Chapter 3. PTSD is a reaction to traumatic stressors (death- or injury-related stressors that evoke helplessness, extreme fear, or horror) that results in reexperiencing the traumatic event, avoiding stimuli correlated with the event, experiencing general response numbing, and having persistent increased arousal. Mr. R, a fireman, who was badly burned over a third of his body, was diagnosed with PTSD. After he left the hospital, his symptoms became worse.

> His recurrent nightmares, in which he reexperiences the fire over and over again, have worsened since he has been home, and he is having great difficulty going to sleep—perchance to dream. At the invitation of his co-workers, Mr. R recently visited the fire station with great reluctance. When the fire alarm sounded, he "nearly leapt out of what was left of my skin" and began to tremble and sweat. He left hurriedly, pleading illness. He is very ashamed about having to face his co-workers in his present condition—shaky, sweating, and frightened—instead of his usual brash and fearless self. . . . He feels that he is cracking up: He paces the floor; is afraid to leave the house on his own; and frequently feels dizzy, numb, and detached. (Frances & Ross, 2001, pp. 180)

PTSD has a high frequency of comorbidity (i.e., co-occurrence) with other anxiety disorders, major depressive disorder, and alcohol use disorders—calling some to question whether it is really a distinct syndrome (Rosen & Lilienfeld, 2008). Individuals with PTSD appear to have a greater prevalence of inflammatory-related medical conditions as well as higher levels of inflammatory cytokines (Gill, Saligan, Woods, & Page, 2009). A reasonable estimate of the lifetime prevalence of PTSD reported is 6.8% (Kessler et al., 2005).

Treatments for Anxiety Disorders

This section focuses on the treatments that have the highest level of empirical support for anxiety disorders because it is not within the scope of this text to discuss the vast full range of anxiety treatment approaches. The treatment approaches for anxiety disorders that have the most research support generally fall into three camps: pharmacological (drug therapy), behavioral, and cognitive behavioral. There is substantial evidence for the efficacy of pharmacological treatments for GAD, panic disorder, social phobia, obsessive-compulsive disorder, and PTSD with antidepressants, especially the selective serotonin reuptake inhibitors (SSRIs) being particularly effective when used during initial treatment and later for preventing relapse (Donovan, Glue, Kolluri, & Emir, 2010; Zohar & Westenberg, 2000). SSRIs boost serotonin levels in the brain (an important neurotransmitter of the monoamine family that also includes norepinephrine and dopamine), which then often results in lowered anxiety and depression levels. Prominent SSRIs include Prozac (fluoxetine), Zoloft (sertraline), Paxil (paroxetine), Celexa (citalopram), and Lexapro (escitalopram).

GABA: gamma aminobutyric acid; an inhibitory neurotransmitter that reduces neuronal excitation.

The antianxiety drugs (or anxiolytics), medications that have relaxation and calming effects, are sometimes used to treat anxiety disorders (e.g., to control panic attacks). Most work through the **GABA** (γ-aminobutyric acid) system. GABA is an inhibitory neurotransmitter that reduces neuronal excitation. The primary anxiolytics are in a family of drugs called the benzodiazepines that include Valium (diazepam) and Xanax (alprazolam). Unfortunately, the antianxiety effects of the benzodiazepines are temporary, the drugs can be addictive, and this class of medications is usually accompanied by marked side effects (e.g., drowsiness and, less frequently, memory impairment) (Roy-Byrne & Cowley, 2007). When benzodiazepines are prescribed, it usually is for a short period (e.g., 2 to 4 weeks).

For GAD symptom relief, it should be noted that an alternative nonbenzodiazepine anxiolytic medication called BuSpar (buspirone) is as effective as the benzodiazepines (Roy-Byrne & Cowley, 2007). BuSpar's disadvantage is that it has a delayed benefit (2 to 4 weeks), but its advantage is that it lacks the sedation and addiction drawbacks associated with the benzodiazepines (Roy-Byrne & Cowley, 2007).

Beta blockers such as Inderal (propranolol) are occasionally used to reduce organ system responses to anxiety (Roy-Byrne & Cowley, 2007). These medications block the beta receptor sites on the heart, which reduces the heart's excitatory potential. Thus, heart rate and heart pounding sensations can be reduced during high anxiety performance situations (e.g., giving a speech). For those with a high level of **interoceptive sensitivity**, this class of medications may bring relief in certain situations.

interoceptive sensitivity: having a high conscious awareness of one's internal physiological activity such as one's heartbeat activity.

However, the first line of drug treatment today for most forms of anxiety disorders is the SSRIs because they can be taken daily on a long-term basis with overall better results and fewer complications than other medications. They also reduce any depression symptoms that may accompany anxiety disorders.

exposure therapy: a form of therapy in which the person in treatment systematically confronts the feared event or stimulus in a safe and controlled environment.

The behavioral approach that is most effective in treating anxiety disorders is **exposure therapy**, a form of therapy in which the person in treatment systematically confronts the feared event or stimulus in a safe and controlled environment. Exposure may be through one's imagination (imaginal exposure such as systematic desensitization discussed in Chapter 13), reality (in vivo), or virtual reality. In addition to working with the therapist during sessions, individuals receiving exposure therapy usually engage in homework between sessions (e.g., confronting fearful situations) without the therapist being present to generalize the positive effects outside of the therapeutic setting. The reduction of anxiety or fear symptoms is believed to occur through a classically conditioned process of habituation and extinction. The fear or anxiety response that is linked to the stimulus gradually diminishes over 8 to 12 sessions (a standard length of treatment).

response prevention: refers to the planned practice of inhibiting compulsive behaviors when exposed to a feared event or stimulus.

For obsessive-compulsive disorder, response prevention is added to the exposure therapy. **Response prevention** refers to the practice of the person engaging in planned prevention of compulsive behaviors when he or she is exposed to the feared event or stimulus. Thus, the person with obsessive-compulsive disorder not only undergoes the process of habituation of fear or anxiety through exposure, but when he or she does not act upon the compulsive urge, through using response prevention, the person also learns to recognize that a ritual is not necessary to prevent feared outcomes (e.g., the home will not burn down because the stove was not checked repeatedly).

cognitive-behavioral therapy: a short-term cognitively oriented therapeutic approach that also uses behavioral strategies that is designed to challenge dysfunctional automatic thoughts, assumptions, and beliefs that sustain a particular disorder and to replace them with healthier realistic thinking patterns.

Cognitive-behavioral therapy (one variation is called cognitive restructuring) is a short-term (generally 12 or 16 sessions in versions that use manuals to standardize the process) cognitively oriented therapeutic approach designed to challenge dysfunctional automatic thoughts, assumptions, and beliefs that sustain a particular disorder and to replace them with healthier realistic thinking patterns. Behavioral methods also are integrated into the therapeutic process as needed. For example, Beck, Emery, and Greenberg (1985, p. 63) list the following types of cognitive assumptions associated with GAD and social phobias that are challenged in therapy:

1. "Any strange situation should be regarded as dangerous."
2. "A situation or a person is unsafe until proven to be safe."
3. "It is always best to assume the worst."
4. "My security and safety depend on anticipating and preparing myself at all times for any possible danger."
5. "I cannot entrust my safety to someone else. I have to ensure my own security."
6. "In unfamiliar situations, I must be wary and keep my mouth shut."
7. "My survival depends on my always being competent and strong."
8. "Strangers despise weakness."
9. "They will attack at a sign of weakness."
10. "If I am attacked, it will show that I appeared weak and socially inept."

Such assumptions keep the threat level high in new or social situations and stoke the feelings of anxiety, which in turn can serve as a catalyst for developing and perpetuating an anxiety disorder such as GAD or social phobia.

Meta-analytic studies report that exposure therapy is the most effective treatment for panic disorder when combined "with relaxation training and/ or breathing retraining techniques" (Sanchez-Meca, Rosa-Alcazar, Marin-Martinez, & Gomez-Conesa, 2010, p. 46), for obsessive-compulsive disorder when combined with response prevention (Rosa-Alcazar, Sanchez-Meca, Gomez-Conesa, & Marin-Martinez, 2008), and for specific phobias with in vivo exposure being more effective than imaginal exposure or virtual reality exposure (Wolitzky-Taylor, Horowitz, Powers, & Telch, 2008). In general, meta-analyses also reveal that trauma-focused treatments for PTSD, such as trauma-focused cognitive-behaviorial therapy and eye movement desensitization and reprocessing (a form of treatment that involves reprocessing of traumatic memories at the neurophysiological level leading to the memories being desensitized and restructured) (Shapiro, 2002), are more effective than non-trauma-focused treatments (Ehlers et al., 2010). Meta-analytic studies also report large effect sizes for cognitive-behavioral therapy for the treatment of GAD, panic disorder, social phobia, and PTSD (see Butler, Chapman, Forman, & Beck, 2006, for a review). For social phobia, the addition of exposure to cognitive therapy appears to be a particularly effective treatment approach (Barlow, Allen, & Basden, 2007).

Further, meta-analytic results suggest that emerging new approaches in the area of mindfulness-based therapy (based on principles of present awareness, acceptance, and nonreactivity; see Chapter 14) can have moderate effects in improving anxiety and mood symptoms in persons diagnosed with anxiety disorders (Hofmann, Sawyer, Witt, & Oh, 2010). Mindfulness-based therapy may well be positioned to become the next wave, the "third wave," behind cognitive therapy (the second wave), and behavior therapy (the first wave) (Prochaska & Norcross, 2010, p. 319) in the treatment of these disorders.

Anxiety Management

We all experience anxiety, but for some people the anxiety is severe and chronic enough that getting treatment from a professional is the best way to gain relief. Consulting a physician to rule out any organic causes of anxiety should be the first step for someone with debilitating chronic anxiety. After physical causes are ruled out, the next recommended step would be to consult an appropriate mental health professional for treatment. As discussed earlier, there are many effective treatments for anxiety disorders, especially pharmacological treatments, exposure therapy, and cognitive-behavioral therapy. Just as it makes good sense to seek appropriate treatment for medical conditions, the same applies for psychological conditions.

For the majority of people with everyday anxiety, however, anxiety can be managed without the assistance of medications or a therapist by learning and applying self-management strategies. The idea is generally to keep anxiety levels within an optimal zone during performance tasks (remember the Yerkes-Dodson

Curve discussed in Chapter 1). At other times the goal is simply to keep anxiety from creating too much distress.

There are many different strategies for managing anxiety. Some involve lowering overall diffuse physiological arousal levels, others involve using cognitive approaches, and yet others involve confronting the feared situation directly. Let us look at 10 primary strategies. The idea is to present you with a menu of options—some of which you may already be doing—that you could try out. You could then integrate the strategies that work best for you into your daily living routine.

1. Reduce Use of Stimulants   This commonsense approach has intuitive validity for most people. Reducing or eliminating caffeine or other stimulants can take the edge off anxiety. Some people drink as much as a pot of coffee or several 20-ounce caffeinated soft drinks daily and then wonder why they are feeling stressed and anxious. What they do not recognize is that they are priming their body to be overaroused. Reducing stimulants resets baseline arousal to its normal level so that it takes a lot more stimulation to reach the physiological red zone.

2. Engage in Aerobic Exercise   Engaging in aerobic exercise such as running, biking, or swimming on a regular basis lowers anxiety and depression and elevates mood. Even taking an extended brisk walk can lower anxiety levels. In fact, physical exercise of all types, if done as reasonable workouts, can lower anxiety levels for a number of hours after the exercise. The multiple benefits of and approaches to exercise for health and well-being are discussed in more depth in Chapter 11.

3. Practice Deep Relaxation Exercises   Practicing deep relaxation exercises such as progressive muscle, imagery, or autogenic relaxation twice a day for 20-minute sessions can lower overall anxiety levels. The antidote to anxiety is relaxation. When we feel relaxed we cannot feel anxious. Many people have never really experienced deep natural relaxation until they have practiced one of these exercises and they are amazed at the depth of relaxation and accompanying good feelings they can achieve once they do it. These exercises are described and discussed in more detail in Chapter 13.

4. Meditate   There are many forms of meditation but at least two forms, mantra meditation and mindfulness meditation, have antianxiety benefits when practiced on a regular basis (usually 20 minutes twice a day). There are many benefits to meditation for health, psychological well-being, and managing stress that are discussed in more depth in Chapter 14. Many people consider meditation a good alternative to deep relaxation exercises.

abdominal breathing: also known as diaphragmatic breathing; breathing that involves drawing the first part of the breath into the lower part of the lungs, which results in the abdomen expanding, and then the remaining breath into the upper part of the lungs, which results in the chest expanding.

5. Use Deep Breathing   This exercise often helps with short-term anxiety. Deep abdominal breathing, also known as diaphragmatic breathing, is the preferred method for anxiety reduction. During **abdominal breathing**, the first part of the breath is drawn into the lower part of the lungs, which results in the abdomen expanding. The remaining breath is drawn into the upper part of the lungs, which results in the chest expanding. Several slow abdominal breaths help to lower short-term anxiety. Would you allow yourself a few moments to try it? If so, do Stress Management Exercise 7.1.

STRESS MANAGEMENT EXERCISE **7.1**

Abdominal Breathing

Get into a comfortable sitting position and place your palms on your abdomen. Breathe in through your nose and gently pull the air slowly into your lower lungs. Notice how your hands move outward as your abdomen expands. Now slowly continue to draw more breath to fill out your upper lungs. Notice how your chest expands and your hands move inward as your abdomen contracts. Now hold the breath in your lungs for a count of 3. 1 . . . 2 . . . 3. Now slowly release the air through your nose. Try it again.

Did you try the exercise? How did it feel? You may have been a little self-conscious at first, but this is normal. Did you feel more relaxed afterwards? In the future, you can do this exercise whenever you feel the tension mounting and you have a few moments. Once you learn how to do it, you can go hands free.

6. Accept Anxiety as Natural Accepting that a certain amount of anxiety is normal in many situations helps to undercut the "fear of fear" (e.g., anxiety sensitivity). There are many situations in life that involve some level of social, financial, physical, or other risk. When we encounter these situations, it is normal to feel anxiety. This anxiety helps to prime us to be more vigilant and ready to act. If we try to suppress or deny the anxiety, it only grows. Try not to

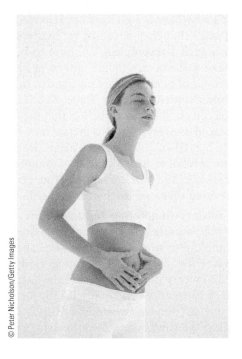

© Peter Nicholson/Getty Images

Hold your palms over your abdomen to learn the process of abdominal breathing.

think of a pink elephant. Try harder. Can you make that pink elephant go away in your mind? Then try harder. The harder we try, the more the pink elephant exerts itself. Why? Because in order not to think of the pink elephant we first have to conjure up an image of a pink elephant. Anxiety works the same way. The more we try to suppress it, the more it exerts itself. So relax and enjoy the ride on the pink elephant, and accept that everyday anxiety is normal.

7. Focus Attention Outward   In performance situations, such as giving a speech to an audience, focusing attention outward can reduce anxiety. People who focus their attention inward, wondering how their performance is coming across, tend to heighten their anxiety with their self-focus. However, individuals who focus on audience members who are reacting positively to their speech tend to feel less self-conscious and thus less anxious when giving their speech. So when you find yourself engaged in self-focus when performing in front of a group, remember to redirect your focus onto another person or even an object at the back of the room and you will find that your mind goes away from self-evaluation thoughts and back to the task at hand.

8. Challenge Anxiety-Generating Belief Systems   Challenge your belief systems such as *need for approval* and *perfectionism*. These beliefs are breeding grounds for worrisome thoughts. Drain the pond of these beliefs and you will not hatch those pesky mosquitoes (i.e., the thoughts) that spring from them. Ask yourself questions such as (1) What evidence supports or refutes this belief? (2) Is this belief rational or logical? (3) What is a more rational belief I can substitute for this irrational belief? Individuals with a high need for approval tend to be anxious when they lack confidence in a new social situation. They make assumptions like "To be rejected is the worst thing in the world," "I can't get others angry at me," and "I have to please others" (Beck et al., 1985, p. 289). Individuals who have a high level of perfectionism tend to be anxious when performing tasks that they have not yet mastered. They carry assumptions such as "I am what I accomplish," "I have to be the best at whatever I do," and "If I make a mistake, I'll fail" (Beck et al., 1985, pp. 289–290). Maintaining high levels of perfectionism puts you at risk for anxiety disorders, eating disorders, and depression (Egan, Wade, & Shafran, 2011). People with these belief systems can challenge their beliefs that they have to be approved of by everyone or succeed at every task. No matter how hard one tries, someone will not like him or her. Also, failure is how people learn how to be successful. Therefore, a certain level of failure should be welcomed as part of the growth and learning experience and not feared. Dysfunctional belief systems and methods for challenging them are discussed further in Chapter 10.

9. Challenge Anxiety-Generating Thoughts   First keep a "Worry Log." The idea is to become a more efficient worrier, condensing a day's worth of worries into a 30-minute session. This is best done at a routine time each day. By concentrating worries into one 30-minute period, most people find that they have less need to worry during the rest of the day. People can easily magnify normal anxiety through worrisome **self-talk** (i.e., the way we mentally talk to ourselves) such as "I'm overwhelmed by this." Once you have identified your worry thoughts, try challenging them by using realistic *anxiety diffuser* self-statements such as, for example, "I have prepared well for this . . . slow down and take it one step at a time." First try them in your worry log. Later, use these realistic challenges mentally in everyday life when you find yourself having worrisome thoughts. See Chapter 10 for more information.

10. Confront Your Fears   As you know from our discussion of the anxiety disorders, one of the most effective ways to overcome fear and anxiety is exposure. Until you put yourself in the feared situation, you are missing your opportunity to desensitize and habituate to it. Avoidance coping only maintains and builds fear and anxiety. Courage is doing what we fear even though we are afraid. If we are not afraid, it is not courage. As the actor John Wayne said, "Courage is being scared to death . . . and saddling up anyway." So exposure is one of the best behavioral strategies you can employ to reduce fear and anxiety. Remember, the idea is to keep fear and anxiety manageable, not to eliminate it. Even some of the most experienced stage actors admit to still having some stage fright.

ANGER

Recall Skippy, the frisky little dog that liked to dig holes in your flower garden? Why would you feel anger when you expect to see Skippy? Why would your anger turn to fear in a flash when you see a much larger and more menacing dog in Skippy's place? As discussed earlier, anger and fear, the two fight-or-flight emotions, are based on how we appraise the situation mentally.

Lazarus (1999, p. 217) explains the *core relational theme* for **anger** as "a demeaning offense against me and mine" with appraisals of "harm to the self and the assignment of blame." Thus, any anger you may have felt toward Skippy was due to your appraisal of having been harmed (i.e., lost work time, possible dead flowers, etc.) by Skippy, the one you blame.

Anger primes us to "fight" or "attack" the offending party (of course we would not attack Skippy, but our anger would prompt us to shoo him out of our garden). Lazarus (1999, p. 217) provides an explanation for why your anger would turn to fear in the following passage—with bracketed comments inserted from the author of this book relevant to Skippy and the flower garden scenario:

> If the attack on the other person [in this case shooing Skippy] who deserves the blame can be accomplished without unreasonable danger [Skippy may be frisky but he is not dangerous], anger is the likely emotion. On the other hand, if we judge that that attack places us at serious risk, anxiety or fright may supersede or accompany anger, especially if the other person [in this case the larger menacing dog] threatens to retaliate [the larger dog had his teeth bared, was growling, and had his eyes fixed on you—a bad sign].

Because Skippy posed a minimal threat to retaliate if you shooed him out of your garden, it was easier to feel anger. However, with the much larger menacing dog, fear was the more adaptive emotion because the anger response could get you in trouble if you tried to shoo the big dog out of your garden.

We can think of anger as being on a continuum from mild anger, considered *irritation* or *annoyance,* to midlevel anger that is usually referred to as being *mad* or *angry,* to high-intensity anger that can be labeled *rage* or *fury.*

Besides Lazurus's definition of anger stemming from a *demeaning offense* or provocation, other reasons for feeling anger may be frustration (being blocked from reaching a goal where aggression fueled by anger may enable removal of the obstacle), competitiveness, or the need to control or dominate. Temporary discomfort factors such as stress, hunger, fatigue, heat, cold, and pain also can elicit angry feelings.

Anger can be a masking or cover emotion for feelings of fear, anxiety, shame, embarrassment, or other emotions that make a person feel vulnerable. Because anger is an empowering emotion, a person who feels powerless might resort to anger to feel in control, to bully, or to intimidate others. *Righteous anger* is an empowering form of anger in which a person expresses indignation, outrage, and moral superiority over another (Lazarus, 1999). This form of anger is sometimes a cover for feelings of vulnerability. For example, a husband who is caught cheating on his wife may resort to righteous anger when she confronts him with the evidence. His anger could take the form of accusations about her "trustworthiness" given that she has "spied" on him. Thus, his shame, humiliation, and lack of trustworthiness are covered by his righteous indignation and finger pointing as he *projects* his own lack of trustworthiness onto his wife.

Anger can be suppressed, inhibited, or directed toward oneself (sometimes referred to as *anger-in*) or it can be outwardly directed (*anger-out*). For example, a student can say, "I'm mad at myself for not doing well on the exam," which is anger-in, or "I'm mad at the professor because I didn't do well on the exam," which is anger-out. As discussed in Chapter 6, anger-in is associated with an increased risk of myocardial infarction (MI) (Dembroski, MacDougall, Williams, Haney, & Blumenthal, 1985). However, certain forms of anger-out, especially *destructive anger justification* also are related to increased coronary heart disease (CHD) risk (Davidson & Mostofsky, 2010). Outward expression of anger is well documented as being related to acute cardiac events (see Chapter 5).

Also, as discussed in Chapter 6, hostility, an attitudinal disposition of cynicism, suspicion, and resentment toward others that may underlie feelings of anger, is a risk factor for CHD (e.g., Chida & Steptoe, 2009). Though the anger-hostility link to CHD has received the most attention, the negative health outcomes of anger-hostility also are linked to hypertension (Rutledge & Hogan, 2002), stroke (Arthur, 2002; Williams, Nieto, Sanford, Couper, & Tyroler, 2002), type 2 diabetes (Golden et al., 2006), and headaches (Materazzo, Cathcart, & Pritchard, 2000; Perozzo et al., 2005). Given these findings, what then is the healthiest approach to the expression of anger?

Supportive evidence for the moderate expression of anger (Eng, Fitzmaurice, Kubzansky, Rimm, & Kawachi, 2003) using *constructive anger expression* through assertively discussing feelings of upset in an attempt to resolve the situation while considering the other person's point of view (Davidson & Mostofsky, 2010) appears to be optimal, at least with respect to minimizing CHD risk. In fact, anger has its benefits in that it can signal a person that there are problems that need to be addressed. It also can energize individuals to take action and to make constructive changes. In relationships, anger can signify that tensions are running high and feelings need to be communicated assertively to lower frictions and address issues.

Although anger can have its benefits, excessive or chronic anger is related to a range of problems and psychological disorders. For example, it is associated with PTSD, depression, substance abuse, and some of the personality disorders (particularly narcissistic, borderline, obsessive-compulsive, antisocial, and paranoid). For instance, feelings of anger may result from a **sense of entitlement** (expecting special rights and privileges) associated with narcissism or from perfectionism often seen in obsessive-compulsiveness when unrealistic expectations are not met. Adolescents who have a conduct disorder, an oppositional defiant disorder, or attention deficit hyperactive disorder may have anger problems as well.

Intermittent explosive disorder (IED) is a psychiatric disorder characterized by episodes of extreme anger and acting out the anger through assaults or the destruction of property. A person with this disorder has "spells" or "attacks" and often feels remorseful afterwards. A recent study found that people diagnosed with IED are at greater risk for developing a number of adverse health conditions such as CHD, stroke, hypertension, diabetes, back or neck pain, headaches, chronic pain, arthritis, and ulcers (McCloskey, Kleabir, Berman, Chen, & Coccaro, 2010). Consider Mr. P, a 46-year-old plumber diagnosed with IED:

> Mr. P's wife reports that their marriage has been reasonably happy despite occasional fights and that there are no grounds for Mr. P's jealousy but says that "if he keeps blowing up like he has been, I will have to leave him." She says that every once in a while Mr. P completely loses control and "becomes a different person." On one occasion, he began breaking up the furniture in the apartment when she got home a little late and he was convinced that she was with another man. On another occasion, he tore up most of her wardrobe because he said she dressed too provocatively. His wife says that it is hopeless for her to try to reason or interfere with Mr. P during these episodes because he goes blindly on with his destructive behavior despite anything she does or says. (Frances & Ross, 2001, p. 262)

Anger can produce a number of harmful effects, especially if it is excessive or inappropriately expressed. One of the most obvious negative features of anger is that it can lead to the destruction of property, such as demonstrated by Mr. P, or even violence. Besides physical aggression, anger also can lead to hurtful verbal aggression in the form of name calling and "hitting below the belt" that can be very destructive to relationships.

Anger can impair a person's ability to function well at work or in interpersonal relationships. Chronically angry people often are seen as "hostile," "hotheads," or "having a chip on their shoulder." People with these characteristics generally are perceived as difficult or unpleasant. Such individuals create transactional dynamics in interpersonal contexts that bring matching anger back on themselves or fearful avoidance behavior in others, which merely compounds their stress.

projection: a defense mechanism in which a person sees in others disowned elements of his or her own personality.

Chronically angry people often lean excessively on the defense mechanism of **projection** and will critically find flaws and weaknesses in others that are really just outward manifestations of disowned elements of their own personality. For example, if Bob has difficulty feeling trust in others, he will see others as untrustworthy and therefore blameworthy rather than acknowledging that he currently has a limited capacity to trust—an issue that he could work on. In other words, chronically angry people are prone to be *externalizers*

TABLE **7.1**　Characteristics of constructive anger versus destructive anger

Characteristics of Healthy, Constructive Anger	Characteristics of Unhealthy, Destructive Anger
1. You express your feelings in a tactful way.	1. You deny your feelings and pout (passive aggression) or lash out and attack the other person (active aggression).
2. You try to see the world through the other person's eyes, even if you disagree.	2. You argue defensively and insist there's no validity in what the other person is saying.
3. You convey a spirit of respect for the other person, even though you may feel quite angry with him or her.	3. You believe the other person is despicable and deserving of punishment. You appear condescending or disrespectful.
4. You do something productive and try to solve the problem.	4. You give up and see yourself as a helpless victim.
5. You try to learn from the situation so you will be wiser in the future.	5. You don't learn anything new. You feel that your view of the situation is absolutely valid.
6. You eventually let go of the anger and feel happy again.	6. Your anger becomes addictive. You won't let go of it.
7. You examine your own behavior to see how you may have contributed to the problem.	7. You blame the other person and see yourself as an innocent victim.
8. You believe that you and the other person both have valid ideas and feelings that deserve to be understood.	8. You insist that you are entirely right and the other person is entirely wrong. You feel convinced that *truth* and *justice* are on your side.
9. Your commitment to the other person increases. Your goal is to feel closer to him or her.	9. You avoid or reject the other person. You write him or her off.
10. You look for a solution where you can both win and nobody has to lose.	10. You feel like you're in a battle or a competition. If one person wins, you feel that the other one will be a loser.

SOURCE: Burns, D. D. (1993). *Ten days to self esteem.* New York: Quill William Morrow.

in that they tend to see their problems as external to themselves. Thus, they are unable to learn and grow from an internal self-examination of these areas of limitations.

Chronic anger also is overstimulating, which makes it difficult to relax or sleep when attempting to take some downtime to recharge. Feelings of anger can disrupt cognitions and make it difficult to think clearly or rationally or to problem solve. In addition, anger can prompt a person to be impulsive and make rash decisions that may be regretted later. Finally, as discussed previously, anger in particular forms and expression can lead to serious unwanted health or psychological consequences. When anger becomes problematic (Table 7.1), anger management strategies can provide effective tools for recognizing anger and applying constructive solution-focused approaches.

Anger Management

Some of the earliest approaches to managing anger were based on catharsis theory. This theory is a logical extension of Freud's *hydraulic model*. According to **catharsis theory,** if anger is not expressed, it builds like steam in a locomotive's steam engine until it explodes. By ventilating anger (i.e., the steam) periodically, the pressure is released and anger is kept manageable. Unfortunately, though therapists in the past encouraged venting and catharsis exercises such as hitting a pillow to release angry feelings, research demonstrates that catharsis theory does not work. Is this a surprise to you? What reasons do you think account for the ineffectiveness of the catharsis strategy?

> **catharsis theory:** a discredited theory of anger management based on the concept that to reduce anger one should ventilate it periodically.

There is a large body of social psychology research showing that catharsis activity is not only ineffective in reducing anger, but it actually *increases* rather than decreases hostility and aggression (see Aronson, Wilson, & Akert, 2010, pp. 374–378, for a discussion). For example, Aronson et al. (2010, p. 375) note that "verbal acts of aggression are followed by further attacks." The reason catharsis does not work is because it hardens thoughts and attitudes that foster blame and derogation of the target of anger. This then leads to self-justification for harboring angry feelings. Such self-justification can lead to acting on the angry feelings in an aggressive way. The unintended effect of catharsis is to add more steam to the steam engine, causing it to overheat and go off the tracks.

An alternative approach to anger management was pioneered by Novaco (1975) who created a multicomponent program called **stress inoculation,** designed to build coping abilities and skills for use in stressful situations. Novaco focused on strategies for managing thoughts that trigger anger when a person is under provocation and on relaxation procedures designed to reduce the arousal component of anger. Following Novaco's lead, empirically based individual and group **anger management** treatments have focused on cognitive approaches, relaxation training, and social skills training to deal with problem anger.

Cognitive approaches involve training in cognitive coping skills through learning to challenge *self-talk* that builds and supports angry feelings like "I don't get mad, I get even" or "I'll show him what a loser he is." They can be replaced with cognitions that diffuse anger such as "My anger reminds me to work toward constructive change" or "I'll try to understand where he is coming from rather than trying to prove I'm right." Relaxation training seeks to reduce the physiological response components of anger using deep relaxation exercises such as progressive muscle relaxation exercises, meditation, imagery, autogenic training, or deep breathing (see Chapters 13 and 14).

It is estimated that between 75% and 80% of anger experiences happen within an interpersonal context (Deffenbacher, Oetting, Huff, Cornell, & Dallager, 1996). Unresolved interpersonal anger may be the result of a person's having insufficient skills to work constructively through differences with others. Social skills training is designed to increase social competency in the areas of listening, assertiveness, negotiation, conflict resolution, and problem solving. The idea is to build social skills so that feelings can be expressed appropriately and tensions and conflicts can be worked through in a constructive fashion.

Through a series of studies, Deffenbacher and his associates determined that cognitive interventions, relaxation training, and social skills training are equally effective in reducing problem anger (both state and trait anger) (Deffenbacher, Oetting, Huff, & Thaites, 1995; Deffenbacher, Story, Stark, Hogg, & Brandon, 1987; Deffenbacher, Thwaites, Wallace, & Oetting, 1994; Hazaleus & Deffenbacher, 1986). Recent studies also have validated the successful use of these approaches on special populations such as, for example, adolescents (Blake & Hamrin, 2007), incarcerated offenders (Walters, 2009), or substance abusers (Fernandez & Scott, 2009).

Just as anxiety is a natural emotion (the flight side of "fight-or-flight"), so is anger (the fight side of "fight-or-flight"). It is only when the frequency, intensity, or expression of anger creates problems for us and others that it needs to be managed. The idea is to own and acknowledge one's anger and not try to suppress or deny it. Once anger is owned, it can be dealt with. Otherwise, a person could have the *pink elephant* problem in which the more anger is suppressed, the more the pink elephant exerts itself. The anger is there, it just is not acknowledged, and, therefore, it finds expression in other ways. For example, underground anger can become manifest in sarcasm, cutting remarks, or passive-aggressive behavior that can be destructive to property and relationships. **Passive-aggressive behavior** is a form of passive resistance to others through procrastination, excuse-making, obstructionism, or poor or destructive performance of tasks where the person engaging in the behavior does not take responsibility for his or her actions or inactions. For example, a teen who reluctantly agrees to a parent's request to wash the family dishes, procrastinates, and then "accidently" breaks a few dishes when finally washing them is engaged in passive-aggressive behavior to avoid having to do the dishes in the future.

It is better to acknowledge anger and then try to reduce its intensity and direct anger-driven behavior toward constructive solutions than it is not to recognize angry feelings. Remember, *constructive anger expression* that involves assertively discussing one's upset while considering the other person's perspective is the most beneficial to one's health and well-being.

As you know from the preceding discussion, there are a number of different effective approaches to managing problem anger. Let us next look at 10 of those that involve arousal reduction, cognitive, behavioral, or social skills strategies. Assertiveness and conflict resolution strategies are very important and are discussed in more depth in Chapter 8. If you experience excessive or problematic anger at times, try some or all of these 10 strategies for reducing anger. Remember, anger is a *choice* based on your appraisal of the situation. Change your appraisals and you will change your emotions.

1. Take Responsibility (a cognitive strategy) As discussed earlier, anger involves assignment of blame. When we blame someone else we are assigning responsibility to that person for the problem. Sometimes we have to swallow our pride and take responsibility for the role we have played in the difficulty. We can ask how we contributed to the problem. Perhaps rather than blaming

passive-aggressive behavior: a form of resistance to others through procrastination, excuse-making, obstructionism, or poor or destructive performance of tasks where the person engaging in the behavior does not take responsibility for his or her actions or inactions.

Skippy for doing what dogs like to do, we could talk to his owner and arrive at a mutual understanding of how Skippy's owner can manage him better. In other words, we can take responsibility for addressing the issue directly with Skippy's owner (something you have probably already considered).

2. Use Humor (a cognitive strategy)   Humor and anger are incompatible. Though Skippy may be annoying, there is something mildly amusing about his frisky persistence to pothole your garden. The ability to find humor and laughter in such situations helps diffuse anger. Humor involves the ability to take a different perspective and to find encouragement in even negative situations. Who knows, maybe you and Skippy could become best of friends.

3. Examine Intentions (a cognitive strategy)   Trying to understand the intentions of the offending party helps us gain perspective on the situation. For example, did Skippy intend to give you a hard time or was Skippy just doing what dogs like to do? For humans, if it was not the intention of the other person to be insulting, offensive, and so on, then perhaps the other person simply needs constructive feedback about how his or her behavior comes across. With constructive feedback, that person may be able to make some positive changes when interacting with you.

4. Use Deep Breathing (an arousal reduction strategy)   The abdominal breathing technique that helps reduce diffuse physiological arousal associated with anxiety also works to reduce anger arousal (refer to the earlier section on anxiety for details). Taking several slow deep abdominal breaths is a good short-term strategy for reducing anger intensity.

5. Practice Deep Relaxation Exercises (an arousal reduction strategy) Practicing deep relaxation exercises such as progressive muscle, imagery, or autogenic relaxation twice a day for 20-minute sessions can lower not only overall anxiety levels, but also anger levels (see Chapter 13). Recall that one of the effective strategies for anger management discussed earlier is relaxation training, which helps to lower overall physiological arousal levels that can add fuel to anger.

6. Take a Time-Out (a behavioral strategy)   If you are angry but an immediate response is not called for (e.g., you receive an offensive e-mail), then take the time to engage in other tasks to buy time and allow your body to calm down. As the body relaxes out of its fight-or-flight response, you will feel less anger. After taking some time to distance yourself psychologically from the problem, you can then address the issue in a more reasoned manner.

7. Challenge Anger-Building Cognitions (a cognitive strategy)   Ask yourself if you are using anger-building thoughts that intensify and perpetuate angry feelings. If so, you may want to substitute thoughts like "I can stay calm and take this point by point" or "Maybe we both have some right ideas" or "I don't need to prove anything" or "My goal is to work toward a constructive solution to the problem." These thoughts keep you focused on keeping arousal levels manageable and on working toward positive outcomes. See Table 7.2 for Novaco's (1975) suggested self-statements for dealing with different stages of provocation.

TABLE **7.2** Examples of Self-Statements for Various Provocation Stages

Novaco's (1975) suggested self-statements used for anger management during different stages of provocation

Preparing for a Provocation:
What is it that I have to do?
I can work out a plan to handle this.
I can manage this situation. I know how to regulate my anger.
If I find myself getting upset, I'll know what to do.
There won't be any need for an argument.
Time for a few deep breaths of relaxation. Feel comfortable, relaxed, and
   at ease.
This could be a testy situation, but I believe in myself.

Confronting the Provocation:
Stay calm. Just continue to relax.
As long as I keep my cool, I'm in control here.
Don't get all bent out of shape; just think of what to do here.
You don't need to prove yourself.
There is no point in getting mad.
I'm not going to let him get to me.
Don't assume the worst or jump to conclusions. Look for the positives.
It's really a shame that this person is acting the way she is.
For a person to be that irritable, he must be awfully unhappy.
If I start to get mad, I'll just be banging my head against the wall. So I
   might as well just relax.
There's no need to doubt myself. What he says doesn't matter.

Coping with Arousal and Agitation:
My muscles are starting to feel tight. Time to relax and slow things down.
Getting upset won't help.
It's just not worth it to get so angry.
I'll let him make a fool of himself.
It's reasonable to get annoyed, but let's keep the lid on.
Time to take a deep breath.
My anger is a signal of what I need to do. Time to talk to myself.
I'm not going to get pushed around, but I'm not going haywire either.
Let's try a cooperative approach. Maybe we are both right.
He'd probably like me to get really angry. Well, I'm going to disappoint him.
I can't expect people to act the way I want them to.

Self-Reward:
It worked!
That wasn't as hard as I thought.
I could have gotten more upset than it was worth.
My ego can sure get me in trouble, but when I watch that ego stuff I'm better off.
I'm doing better at this all the time.
I actually got through that without getting angry.
I guess I've been getting upset for too long when it wasn't even necessary.

SOURCE: Novaco, R. W. (1975). *Anger control: The development and evaluation of an experimental treatment.* Lexington, MA: D.C. Health.

8. Empathize (a cognitive strategy)   Empathy involves trying to understand the other person's perspective (i.e., attempt to walk in the other person's shoes). You may not agree with the other person, but if you can understand where he or she is coming from, it is harder to stay angry. Active listening helps to convey empathy. This form of listening means that you rephrase in your own words what you hear from the other person so that he or she feels heard. Active listeningis illustrated with examples in Chapter 8.

9. Be Assertive (a social skills strategy)   Assertiveness means to be forthright with others while respecting their rights. This contrasts with passivity, which refers to allowing others not to respect our rights or aggressiveness that involves us violating the rights of others. If we feel angry toward another, we can express our concerns or feelings to them in a respectful nonpunitive manner and ask for change. Context is important. For example, within a work context it is probably better to keep expressions of angry feelings out of it, but rather to diffuse tension in the situation by referring to *concerns* such as "I am concerned that I have not heard back from you in a timely manner and as a result I am having difficulty completing my portion of the project. Could you please get back to me in the next 24 hours?" In more intimate relationships, we can label our anger feelings more directly. For example, we could say "I'm feeling irritated when you interrupt me. It makes me think you do not value my point of view. Could you please let me get this off my chest before we discuss it? Then I would love to hear your thoughts."

10. Practice Forgiveness (a cognitive strategy)   Giving the other person the benefit of the doubt and engaging in forgiveness when called for can release you from being tethered to feelings of resentment or desires for retaliation. Recall from Chapter 2 that forgiveness is the act of giving up resentments toward others and letting go of claims for retribution and restitution. Forgiveness can help restore relationships that have been damaged by conflict. It can break people out of endless cycles of revenge and counter-revenge for perceived wrongs. Engaging in forgiveness is associated with lower levels of general physiological and cardiovascular reactivity as well as higher well-being (Bono, McCullough, & Root, 2008; Witvliet, Ludwig, & Vander Laan, 2001).

DEPRESSION

As discussed, when people experience stress they usually have a "fight-or-flight" response with accompanying emotions of anger or anxiety. There is, however, a third negative mood state commonly associated with stress that we have not yet discussed. If people feel helpless or hopeless and overwhelmed by stress, or experience a sense of loss, they also may feel sadness and despair, or experience depressed mood states.

diathesis stress model of depression: stress leads to depression in vulnerable individuals.

In fact, there is substantial evidence for a **diathesis-stress model of depression** (Monroe & Simons, 1991) that stress leads to depression in vulnerable individuals. People who are depressed generally experience more stress including *self-generated stress* than their nondepressed counterparts (Davila, Bradbury, Cohan, & Tochluk, 1997; Hammen, 1991; Holahan, Moos, Holahan, Brennan, & Schutte, 2005). Some feelings of despondency or depression are normal reactions to excessive stress, especially when the stress involves loss. However, at what point does a depressed mood become a problem that needs treatment, in other words, a clinical depression? Consider Nancy's situation described by Seligman, Walker, & Rosenhan (2001):

> Within a two-day period, Nancy received a double blow: she got a C on her Abnormal Psychology midterm, and she also found out that her high school boyfriend had become engaged to someone else. The week that followed was awful. For the first few days, she had trouble getting out of bed to go to class. She burst into tears over dinner one evening and had to leave the table. Missing dinner didn't much matter anyway. She wasn't hungry. Her future looked bleak since she now believed she would never be accepted by any clinical psychology graduate school, and that she would never again find anyone she would love as much. She blamed herself for these failures in the two most important areas of her life. (pp. 249–250)

Nancy responded to the stress of her "double blow" with characteristic sadness, despair, and depressed mood. Is this "normal depression" or "clinical depression"? As Seligman et al. (2001) recount in completing their story, Nancy's mood lifted after a couple of weeks when her instructor gave her and the other students the option of another assignment to substitute for poor grades and her roommate arranged a blind date for her. So in this case, Nancy had a "normal depression" to the stress and losses she encountered. However, if her symptoms had persisted and become more severe, she might then have met the criteria for a diagnosis of a "clinical depression." So as Seligman et al. (2001, p. 250) note, "in many ways, normal depression differs only in degree, not in kind, from the clinical disorder."

What then is a clinical depression? According to the DSM-IV-TR, there are several types of mood episodes, depressive disorders, bipolar disorders, and other mood disorders. Some of these disorders, such as the bipolar disorders, include manic episodes with many features from the other end of the continuum such as inflated self-esteem, grandiosity, talkativeness, need for less sleep, easy distractibility, and greater involvement in risky endeavors. However, for our purposes, we will focus on the most common type of clinical depression referred to as **major depressive disorder** rather than those that involve manic episodes (e.g., bipolar disorder).

major depressive disorder: a mood disorder characterized by experiencing depressed moods or the loss of pleasure that stretch throughout the day almost every day for a least 2 weeks.

A person with a major depressive disorder has at least one major depressive episode that lasts 2 weeks or more "during which there is either depressed mood or the loss of interest or pleasure in nearly all activities" (American Psychiatric Association, 2000). Almost everybody experiences occasional episodes of mild depression or the *blues*. However, a person with a major depressive episode experiences depressed moods that stretch throughout the day almost every day for at least 2 weeks. Besides depressed mood or loss of interest in pleasurable activities, symptoms of this form of clinical depression include most, but not necessarily all, of the following: almost daily insomnia or hypersomnia (sleeping too much), significant weight loss (not due to dieting)

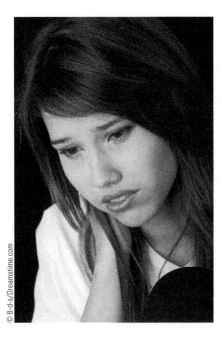

© B-d-s/Dreamstime.com

Depression is more common in females after puberty. Before puberty there are no differences between males and females.

or gain, excessive daily fatigue, feelings of worthlessness or inappropriate guilt, poor concentration, or recurrent suicidal thoughts. As you can see, this is significantly more severe than the *blues*.

Kessler et al. (2005) estimate a lifetime prevalence of 16.6% for major depressive disorder and 20.8% for *all mood disorders*. The average age of onset of major depressive disorder is the mid-20s (American Psychiatric Association, 2000). Female adolescents and adults are twice as likely as their male counterparts to be diagnosed with the disorder (for prepubertal children there are no gender differences in frequency of diagnosis) (Hankin et al., 1998; Weissman & Olfson, 1995).

As discussed in Chapter 5, individuals with severe or chronic medical conditions (e.g., MI) are more likely to experience depression and some of these persons will develop major depression disorder (estimates range from 20% to 25%) (American Psychiatric Association, 2000). Low self-esteem also is a vulnerability factor for depression. As Brown (1998, p. 234) remarks, "low self-esteem puts people at risk for developing depression when a negative life event occurs." Based on assessments of data collected from three longitudinal studies, Orth, Robins, and Meier (2009) concluded that even under low-stress conditions low self-esteem is a vulnerability factor to depression.

Engaging in **ruminative thinking** about one's depression, defined as "a repetitive form of thinking, in which one repeatedly and in an abstract-evaluative way ponders about oneself, and about the possible causes, meaning, and implications of one's sad and depressed feelings" also is a vulnerability factor for prolonging and deepening depressed moods as well as predicting "the maintenance of clinical depression and the onset of new episodes of depression" (Raes, 2010, p. 758).

Clinical depression can be life threatening. Unfortunately, people with major depression are at greater risk for attempting suicide with up to 15% of those diagnosed with the disorder dying as a result of suicide (American Psychiatric Association, 2000).

There are a number of effective pharmacological and psychological treatments for major depressive disorder. An older class of drugs called the **tricyclic antidepressants (TCAs),** which increase brain norepinephrine levels, and another called the **monoamine oxidase inhibitors (MAOIs),** which increase brain serotonin, norepinephrine, and dopamine levels, are now largely supplanted by the newer **selective serotonin reuptake inhibitors (SSRIs).** The SSRIs, which increase brain serotonin levels, are now the first line of effective pharmacological treatment for unipolar depression (Nemeroff & Schatzberg, 2007). First introduced in the late 1980s, the SSRIs are safer because they have less risk for overdose and have fewer side effects (although they can lead to sexual dysfunction) than the TCAs and MAOIs.

Clinical trial studies indicate that an even newer class of drugs, the **serotonin norepinephrine reuptake inhibitors (SNRIs)** that include Effexor XR (venlafaxine XR) and Cymbalta (duloxetine), is as effective as the SSRIs (Nemeroff & Schatzberg, 2007). This new class of medications boosts both serotonin and norepinephrine neurotransmitters in the brain and shows promise in treating individuals who are depressed and who are unresponsive to the SSRIs.

Other alternatives to the SSRIs that are effective for treating unipolar depression include Wellbutrin (bupropion), which increases brain dopamine and norepinephrine levels, and Remeron (mirtazapine), which is a novel antidepressant that affects serotonin and norepinephrine transmission in the brain. Thus, the TCAs, MAOIs, SSRIs, and SNRIs and a few other medications are all effective in treating major depression, though the SSRIs are generally preferred as the first line of treatment due to their longer track record of safety and tolerability. For those who are unresponsive to the SSRIs, physicians or other prescribers may then consider prescribing one of the other effective alternatives.

Meta-analyses and randomized controlled trials demonstrate effectiveness for a number of short-term therapies including behavior therapy (e.g., Lewinsohn, Antonuccio, Steinmetz, & Teri, 1984), interpersonal psychotherapy (e.g., Klerman & Weissman, 1992), and cognitive-behavioral therapy (e.g., Beck, 1967) in treating major depressive disorder (see Craighead, Sheets, Brosse, & Ilardi, 2007, for review). There are several behavioral approaches to treating depression. They have in common, however, the idea of motivating the person who is depressed to be active and engage in more positive (i.e., rewarding) activities. Many people when depressed withdraw and stop engaging in activities they once found pleasurable. As a result, their opportunity for feeling good becomes severely restricted. Because feeling good is an antidote to feeling depressed, the concept is for them to once again get involved in pleasurable activities.

In order to facilitate this process the person who is depressed may require training in recognizing the connections between engaging in positive activities and feeling good by keeping logs and self-monitoring. Training in assertiveness, communication, or other social skill areas such as learning how to reduce depressive behaviors (e.g., complaining, crying, or other behaviors that may keep

selective serotonin reuptake inhibitors (SSRIs): a newer class of antidepressants designed to increase the brain's serotonin levels.

others at arm's length) also may be required to increase the chance that he or she can actively pursue good feelings through social contact (i.e., social rewards).

Interpersonal psychotherapy for depression includes helping persons who are depressed recognize and deal effectively with interpersonal issues that concern their depression. The therapy generally entails around 16 sessions. As Craighead et al. (2007, p. 298) note, "the primary problem areas targeted include unresolved grief, interpersonal disputes, role transitions, and interpersonal deficits (e.g., social isolation)." Thus, as in behavioral social skills training, the social context of the disorder is addressed as a focus of treatment—in this case, the primary focus.

Of all the therapeutic approaches to treating major depression, Beck's (1967) cognitive-behavioral therapy is best known. According to Beck's model (Beck, 1967, 1991; Young, Beck, & Weinberger, 1993), negative thinking patterns are reflected in the *cognitive triad, maladaptive attitudes, automatic thoughts,* and *errors in thinking* that create a vulnerability to depression and sustain it once it takes hold.

The **negative cognitive triad** refers to a tendency among depressed people to view in a negative light (1) the self (e.g., "I am worthless"), (2) the world ("This situation is impossible"), and (3) the future ("I'll never be successful").

Maladaptive attitudes such as "If I do not perform as well as others, it means that I am an inferior human being" or "My value as a person depends greatly on what others think of me" (Beck, Rush, Shaw, & Emery, 1979) are well-springs for **automatic negative thoughts.** Such thoughts are said to be automatic because they seem to happen almost reflexively and without examination or even awareness at times. Thoughts may include "I'm no good," "People don't like me," "I am a failure as a person," "Things will never change," or any one of a myriad of possible streams of unpleasant cognitions.

Errors of thinking refer to cognitive processing styles that are distorted, biased, or illogical. Beck identifies a number of thinking errors including (1) *arbitrary inference* (drawing conclusions without supportive evidence), (2) *selective abstraction* (focusing on a detail that ignores the more important big picture), (3) *overgeneralization* (drawing sweeping conclusions based on limited information), (4) *dichotomous thinking* (thinking in black or white terms rather than shades of gray), (5) *magnification and minimization* (exaggerating small events or trivializing big events), and (6) *personalization* (taking responsibility for events that are not under one's control).

Beck's cognitive-behavioral approach to treating depression involves four phases that typically unfold in less than 20 sessions. In the first phase, behavioral treatment approaches are applied that are designed to encourage participants to become more active. By the second stage, individuals begin the process of learning about and recording their automatic thoughts. The therapist challenges the accuracy of their distorted thoughts and assists them in learning the process of self-challenge. By the third phase, through the assistance of their therapist, individuals learn to identify their negative thinking patterns and biases (i.e., errors of thinking). Finally, in the fourth phase, the therapist helps participants challenge and change maladaptive attitudes that underlie their automatic negative thoughts. In Chapter 10 we will go into more detail about how to challenge any negative automatic thoughts we may have.

negative cognitive triad: a tendency among depressed people in Beck's model of depression to view the self, the world, and the future in a negative light.

automatic negative thoughts: distorted cognitions that occur almost reflexively and sometimes without awareness.

Dealing with Depression

As discussed earlier, everyone has the blues from time to time. Usually, depressed mood states just go away on their own given sufficient time. However, if depressed moods become troublesome or if you suspect you may have a mood disorder, then it is important to see a physician to rule out possible medical causes or to assist you in getting treatment. Let us look at some general strategies for dealing with depression.

1. See Your Physician   There are a number of underlying medical conditions that can cause depression symptoms (e.g., thyroid conditions, diabetes, etc.). By treating these conditions, the depression symptoms usually are alleviated. If one of these conditions is not present, and you have the signs and symptoms of a clinical depression, your physician can assist you with depression medication if indicated or refer you to an appropriate mental health professional for assistance. Do not let feelings of shame or embarrassment prevent you from talking to your physician. In today's world, physicians are accustomed to seeing depression and are ready and available to discuss treatment options with you.

2. Engage in Aerobic Exercise   There is considerable evidence that engaging in aerobic exercise will boost the "feel good" chemicals in your brain and also reduce anxiety that often accompanies depressed moods (see Chapter 11). Being on a regular exercise routine also can be used as a preventive strategy for reducing the likelihood or frequency of future depressed moods. In fact, depressed moods can be motivators to strengthen your desire to also implement other healthy lifestyle strategies such as healthy eating and using stress management.

3. Reduce or Eliminate Alcohol   Alcohol is a central nervous system depressant. Though you may get a temporary mood boost from drinking alcohol, the aftereffects usually will cause you to feel more depressed. Alcohol simply compounds the problem ("Treating Depression Along with Alcohol Dependence," 2010). In addition, the effects of alcohol consumption can lead to disinhibition that in turn can lead to impulse-driven behaviors you may later regret. For example, you may say or do something impulsively that you feel badly about the next day. Thus, feelings of regret, guilt, and self-recrimination are added that only magnify depressed feelings.

4. Get Social   This is counterintuitive because when we feel depressed, we often feel like withdrawing and being alone. However, withdrawal deprives us of a chance to experience social rewards, which can then boost our mood states. Getting active and doing things we enjoy are also counterintuitive because when we feel depressed, we experience less pleasure in activities that we normally find pleasurable. However, as you know from the behavioral treatment research, engaging in pleasurable activities eventually boosts our mood states. The key is to do them even when we do not feel like it.

5. Challenge Negative Thinking   When you are depressed you are likely engaging in distorted thinking. To counteract this tendency, thinking happy thoughts is not an effective strategy. Rather, the cognitive approach that works best is to write down your negative thoughts and ask yourself if the evidence really supports them. Are you engaging in one or more of the six *errors of thinking* discussed earlier? If so, which ones? Identify them to see your pattern.

Replace the written negative thoughts with more realistic ones. Do this written exercise at least twice a day. We all engage in distorted thinking from time to time, so do not be hard on yourself when you do it. Just be aware that it is normal to distort when depressed and you can counter this tendency by replacing distorted thoughts with more realistic ones. If you have suicidal thoughts, share them with someone you can trust and in whom you can confide. This is important. Almost all communities have crisis centers or suicide hotlines listed in their telephone books. The confidential toll-free phone number for the National Suicide Prevention Lifeline is 1-800-273-8255.

POSITIVE MENTAL HEALTH

Much of the information discussed in this chapter is presented through the lens of the DSM framework. However, you should be aware that there are alternative views to the DSM. Although the DSM represents today's predominate view of mental health, it has its drawbacks because it is closely tied to the biomedical *disease* model and what Maddux (2009) refers to as "illness ideology." Maddux (p. 63) contends that although the introduction of the DSM-IV explicitly disavows illness ideology assumptions, "practically every word thereafter is *inconsistent* with this disavowal." He further states that we can easily substitute the word *disease* for *disorder* and have a similar construct system for classification. In fact, the word *psychopathology,* commonly used by mental health clinicians, embodies the blend of *psychology* with *pathology* (i.e., disease).

Maddux (2009) argues that the categories of classification in the DSM are *social constructions* (abstract categories collaboratively agreed upon by those who decide what goes into the DSM) rather than actual diseases that have physical properties. That is not to say that people do not at times feel severely anxious or depressed, but rather to say that even if their symptoms fit into a category designated by the DSM, they do not necessarily have an illness.

Instead of using the illness ideology approach, Maddux suggests using a positive psychology approach such as using *character strengths* to define mental health. He points to the **Values in Action (VIA)** classification system as a good example (Peterson & Park, 2009; Peterson & Seligman, 2004). Character strengths for the VIA system were derived from philosophy, psychology, psychiatry, and youth development as well as virtue catalogs from historical figures (e.g., Benjamin Franklin). Christopher Peterson and Martin Seligman, the originators of the system,discovered 24 strengths for the VIA that they grouped into the six categories of (1) *Wisdom and Knowledge,* (2) *Courage,* (3) *Humanity,* (4) *Justice,* (5) *Temperance,* and (6) *Transcendence.* See Chapter 15 for more information.

Rather than arguing for the replacement of the pathogenic approach (e.g., the DSM) with the salutogenic approach (positive mental states, feelings, and behaviors), Keyes (2009, p. 89) argues for a *"whole states approach"* that incorporates both the "pathogenic and salutogenic paradigms." Hence, he states, mental health is not defined as just the absence of mental illness, but rather the presence of *hedonia* (i.e., happiness) and *positive functioning.*

Keyes (2009) identifies two clusters based on his factor analyses that represent **complete mental health,** one for *hedonia* containing 2 symptom categories

TABLE **7.3** Keyes' complete state model of mental health. To be diagnosed as flourishing a person must score high on at least one hedonic measure and six positive functioning measures.

Categorical Diagnosis of Mental Health (i.e., Flourishing)
Diagnostic criteria Symptom description

Hedonia: requires high level on at least one symptom scale (Symptoms 1 or 2)	
1.	Regularly cheerful, in good spirits, happy, calm and peaceful, satisfied, and full of life (*positive affect past 30 days*)
2.	Feels happy or satisfied with life overall or domains of life (*avowed happiness or avowed life satisfaction*)[a]
Positive functioning: requires high level on six or more symptom scales (Symptoms 3–13)	
3.	Holds positive attitudes toward oneself and past life and concedes and accepts varied aspects of self (*self-acceptance*)
4.	Has positive attitude toward others while acknowledging and accepting people's differences and complexity (*social acceptance*)
5.	Shows insight into own potential, sense of development, and open to new and challenging experiences (*personal growth*)
6.	Believes that people, social groups, and society have potential and can evolve or grow positively (*social actualization*)
7.	Holds goals and beliefs that affirm sense of direction in life and feels that life has a purpose and meaning (*purpose in life*)
8.	Feels that one's life is useful to society and the output of his or her own activities are valued by or valuable to others (*social contribution*)
9.	Exhibits capability to manage complex environment, and can choose or manage and mold environments to suit needs (*environmental mastery*)
10.	Interested in society or social life; feels society and culture are intelligible, somewhat logical, predictable, and meaningful (*social coherence*)
11.	Exhibits self-direction that is often guided by his or her own socially accepted and conventional internal standards and resists unsavory social pressures (*autonomy*)
12.	Has warm, satisfying, trusting personal relationships and is capable of empathy and intimacy (*positive relations with others*)
13.	Has a sense of belonging to a community and derives comfort and support from community (*social integration*)

SOURCE: Keyes, C. L. M. (2005), Mental illness and/or mental health? Investigating axioms of the complete state model of health, *Journal of Consulting and Clinical Psychology*, 73, 539–548. Table 1, p. 541. American Psychological Association.

[a] Life domains may include employment and marriage or close interpersonal relationship (e.g., parenting).

and another for *positive functioning* that has 11 symptom categories (Table 7.3). He states the following:

> To be diagnosed as "flourishing" in life, individuals must exhibit high levels on at least one measure of hedonic well-being and high levels on at least six measures of positive functioning. Individuals who exhibit low levels on a least

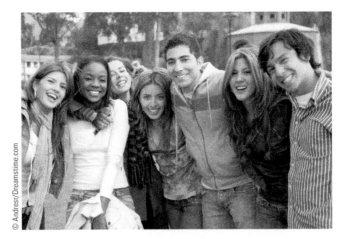

© Andresr/Dreamstime.com

According to Keyes (2005), the MIDUS survey determined that only 17% of the total U.S. population had no mental illness within the last year and were flourishing. What are they doing that enables them to enjoy both good mental health and to flourish?

one measure of hedonic well-being and low levels on a least six measures of positive functioning are diagnosed as "languishing" in life. Languishing in the absence of mental health is synonymous with saying that it is a state of being mentally *un*-healthy. To be languishing is to be in a state of being stuck, stagnant, or empty, and devoid of positive functioning in life. Adults who are "moderately mentally healthy" do not fit the criteria for either flourishing or languishing in life. (Keyes, 2009, p. 90)

In other words, he suggests a continuum from *languishing,* to moderate mental health, to *flourishing.* Further, Keyes contends that this measure of mental health can be used in conjunction with diagnostic measures of mental illness so that each represents information about a person's complete mental health, one pathogenic and the other salutogenic.

To illustrate this approach and his findings, Keyes (2005) reported the following from his analysis of the MacArthur Foundation's 1995 Midlife in the United States (MIDUS) survey results for adults between the ages of 25 and 74: (1) 7% had a mental illness within the last year and were languishing, (2) 14.5% had a mental illness within the last year and had moderate mental health, (3) 1.5% had a mental illness within the last year and were flourishing, (4) 10% had no mental illness within the last year and were languishing, (5) 51% had no mental illness within the last year and had moderate mental health, and (6) only 17% of the total had no mental illness within the last year and were flourishing. Unfortunately, in the United States, according to Keyes' model, only 17% of adults appear to exhibit the highest level of positive mental health.

Alternative approaches to the DSM can give us a window into how to maximize mental health by focusing on our strengths rather than our problem areas. In Chapter 15 we will focus on the concept of positive interventions that naturally stem from the positive mental health approach. Pathogenic models represented by the DSM are useful for describing

positive mental health models: focus on how positive therapy and interventions can maximize flourishing and other optimal positive functioning experiences.

problematic patterns of distress and functioning. A natural and noble goal of these models is to bring relief and reduce suffering for those who are affected. However, **positive mental health models** go beyond this goal to point the way forward toward achieving even more desirable states of thriving or flourishing.

CHAPTER SUMMARY AND CONCEPT REVIEW

- Fear and anxiety are emotional components of the "flight" aspect of the fight-or-flight response.

- Generalized anxiety disorder (GAD) is characterized by excessive uncontrollable anxiety and worry.

- Panic disorder involves repeated and unexpected panic attacks along with worry about reoccurrence of attacks.

- Phobias consist of unreasonable and excessive fears of a particular object, situation, or activity.

- Obsessive-compulsive disorder is characterized by recurrent, intrusive, and inappropriate obsessions manifest as thoughts, images, impulses or compulsions.

- Posttraumatic stress disorder (PTSD) is a reaction to traumatic stressors that includes reexperiencing the traumatic event, avoiding stimuli associated with the event, experiencing general response numbing, and having persistent arousal.

- The first line of drug treatment today for most forms of anxiety disorders is the selective serotonin reuptake inhibitors (SSRIs).

- Effective behavioral approaches to treating anxiety disorders include exposure therapy and response prevention (for obsessive-compulsive disorder).

- Everyday anxiety can be managed using aerobic exercise, deep relaxation, meditation, deep breathing, acceptance of anxiety, focusing attention outward, challenging anxiety beliefs and thoughts, confronting fears, and reducing stimulants.

- Anger represents the emotional component of the "fight" side of the fight-or-flight response.

- Anger relates to assigning blame; being stressed, in pain, or frustrated; masking vulnerability feelings; or needing to feel powerful.

- Moderate expression of anger using constructive anger expression appears to be optimal with respect to minimizing coronary heart disease (CHD) risk.

- Anger can have its benefits in signaling people that problems need to be addressed as well as in energizing them to make constructive changes.

- Intermittent explosive disorder (IED) is characterized by episodes of extreme anger and acting out the anger through assault or property destruction.

- Harmful effects of anger or its expression include verbal and physical aggression; increased interpersonal conflicts; personal insight and growth impairment; inability to relax or sleep; and disruptive thinking, problem solving, and behaviors.

- Novaco's (1975) stress inoculation anger treatment program serves as a basis for anger management treatments that use cognitive approaches, relaxation training, and social skills training.

- Strategies for anger management include taking responsibility, using humor, examining intentions, challenging anger-building cognitions, empathizing, forgiveness, deep breathing, engaging in relaxation exercises, taking a time-out, and being assertive.

- Depression is a third negative mood state commonly associated with stress.

- There is substantial evidence for a diathesis stress model of depression.

- Major depressive disorder is significantly more severe than "the blues."

- The first line of effective pharmacological treatments for depression is the SSRIs.

- Meta-analytic studies demonstrate the effectiveness for behavior therapy, interpersonal psychotherapy, and cognitive-behavioral therapy as psychological treatments for major depressive disorder.

- It is important to see a physician to rule out underlying medical causes that could be generating depression symptoms.

- Engaging in aerobic exercise, reducing or eliminating alcohol, becoming more social, and challenging negative thinking are useful strategies for dealing with depression.

- Maddux (2009) criticizes the DSM for its "illness ideology" focus and its classification system that is based on social constructions.

- Keyes (2009) argues for a "whole states approach" that includes both the pathogenic and salutogenic aspects of mental health.

CRITICAL THINKING QUESTIONS

1. How is anxiety beneficial? How is it detrimental? In what ways is having an anxiety disorder different from experiencing everyday anxiety? How is the approach to managing an anxiety disorder similar or different from managing everyday anxiety?

2. What top three strategies do you believe are most effective for managing any everyday anxiety you may experience? Have you tried these strategies? Did you find them effective? Why did you select these three over the others?

3. How is anger beneficial? How is it detrimental? Why is anger suppression a bad idea? Why is using a catharsis technique a bad idea for dealing with anger?

4. How do you know when anger is a problem that needs to be managed? What are the top three strategies that you could use to manage any problematic anger you may experience? Why do you prefer these three strategies over other ones?

5. Why do you think stress is linked to depression? How can a person create self-generated stress that leads to depressed mood? How do you distinguish between "normal depression" and clinical depression?

6. Why do you think a survey found that the majority of the U.S. population had no mental illness within the last year and had moderate mental health yet did not flourish? What strategies can a person employ to maintain a healthy mental state and at the same time flourish (hint—refer to Chapter 2 for ideas)?

KEY TERMS AND CONCEPTS

Abdominal breathing*

Agoraphobia

Anger

Anger management

Anxiety

Anxiety disorder*

Anxiety sensitivity*

Automatic negative thoughts*

Catharsis theory*

Cognitive-behavioral therapy*

Complete mental health

Compulsions

Diathesis stress model of depression*

Errors of thinking

Existential anxiety

Exposure therapy*

Fear

GABA*

Generalized anxiety disorder (GAD)

Intermittent explosive disorder (IED)

Interpersonal psychotherapy

Interoceptive sensitivity*

Major depressive disorder*

Maladaptive attitudes

Monoamine oxidase inhibitors (MAOIs)

Negative cognitive triad*

Obsessions

Obsessive-compulsive disorder

Panic attacks*

Panic disorder

Passive-aggressive behavior*

Phobia

Positive mental health models*

Projection*

Response prevention*

Ruminative thinking

Selective serotonin reuptake inhibitors (SSRIs)*

Self-talk

Sense of entitlement

Serotonin norepinephrine reuptake inhibitors (SNRIs)

Social phobia

Specific phobias

Stress inoculation

Tricyclic antidepressants (TCAs)

Values in Action (VIA)

Worry

MEDIA RESOURCES

CENGAGE**brain**.com

Access an interactive eBook, chapter-specific interactive learning tools, including flashcards, quizzes, videos, and more in your Psychology CourseMate, accessed through CengageBrain.com.

8

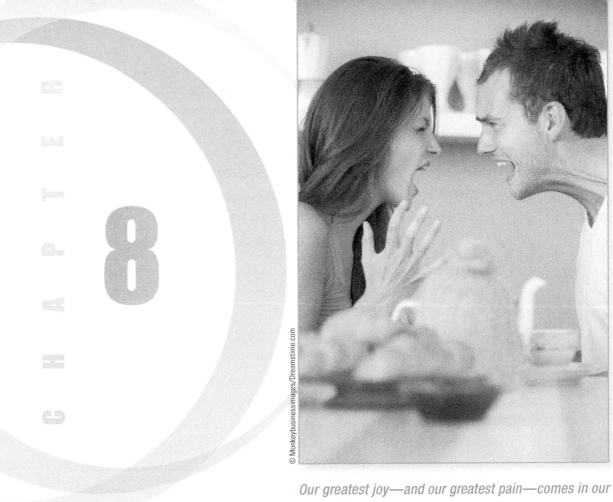

Our greatest joy—and our greatest pain—comes in our relationships with others.

~Stephen R. Covey

© Monkeybusinessimages/Dreamstime.com

INTERPERSONAL STRESS

In Edward Albee's classic play Who's Afraid of Virginia Woolf? the primary characters, George and Martha, are a married couple who engage in round after round of insults, name calling, and verbal abuse. They epitomize what can go wrong in relationships and why relationships, though often joyful, can also be a source of pain and stress. The following dialog from Albee's play (Albee, 1962, p. 152) captures how George and Martha are drawn to each other yet at the same time inflict pain on one another.

George: (*Barely contained anger now*) You can sit there in that chair of yours, you can sit there with the gin running out of your mouth, and you can humiliate me, you can tear me apart . . . ALL NIGHT . . . and that's perfectly all right . . . that's O.K. . . . .

Martha: YOU CAN STAND IT!

George: I CANNOT STAND IT!

Martha: YOU CAN STAND IT!! YOU MARRIED ME FOR IT!!

(A silence)

This picture stands in contrast to Angela's story. Remember Angela from Chapter 2? As a child, Angela was emotionally and physically abused by her mother and endured many hardships as an adult.

"Still, with all that has happened and all the challenges that have come to pass, Angela considers herself to be a very happy person. Her daughter Ella, to whom she is extremely close, brings her endless joy. . . . She has made many friends—indeed, formed a whole community of like-minded people— and they are a pleasure and support to her." (Lyubomirsky, 2007, p. 29)

Thus, in spite of the difficulties relationships may pose, we are social beings who are drawn to the joys and pleasures of our social bonds. Our relationships are a primary source of our overall meaning and happiness in life. The challenge for us then is to figure out how to strengthen social bonds while at the same time lower tensions that are inherent in the bonding process.

There are many types of relationships, including romantic, family, friendships, coworkers, and acquaintances. Although relationships can bring their own stressors, the social networks we develop also can provide us with physical, social, and emotional support that can buffer us against the harmful effects of stress. Our role in developing and maintaining quality relationships influences how we are benefited in return. This is especially true in romantic relationships, where the emotional stakes are higher, and the competing needs and interests of each partner are constantly in play. Thus, there is a dynamic of nurturing oneself, one's partner, and one's relationship that determines the health and success of all three entities. The greatest challenge then is finding the balance point.

Because there are competing needs and interests inherent in any relationship, sustained involved relationships inevitably lead to conflict. How we successfully manage conflict, or at least our part in it, involves a certain way of approaching relationships and the skills that nurture them. Do we want relationships like George and Martha's, or do we want relationships like Angela enjoys? Though the answer is obvious, it is not what we want, but rather how we approach relationships and interpersonal conflict that ultimately determines the results.

INTERPERSONAL CONFLICT

High Drama—Raising Tensions and Creating Distance

One way we can deal with interpersonal conflict is through raising tensions, creating distance, and generally engaging in high drama. If we take this approach, we may be able to win an argument or prevail in a disagreement, but, ultimately, we weaken our relationships. We will succeed in increasing the stress levels of those around us and set up scenarios where the people we care about the most keep their physical or emotional distance. Let us look at some of the primary factors that contribute to creating distance.

Differences   Which is most true, "opposites attract" or "birds of a feather flock together"? There is a considerable body of social psychology research showing that we are most attracted to those who are similar to us in our behaviors, beliefs, attitudes, and worldviews (Berscheid & Reis, 1998; McPherson, Smith-Lovin, & Cook, 2001). Though we may have some opposite traits that add balance to our relationships, if they are too extreme then we are more likely to have diverging needs and goals. These can lead us to sacrifice fulfillment of certain needs and interests, to go it alone, or try to get the other person in the relationship to accommodate our needs.

For example, if Jeff who is an extreme extravert wants to go to a party and his wife Susan who is an extreme introvert wants to stay home and read a good book, they will have to resolve their competing needs. Jeff can stay home and feel unfulfilled, he can try to persuade Susan to sacrifice her needs and come along, or he can go to the party alone. Any of these options can become flash points for potential conflict. However, if both are either introverts or extraverts, they can more easily find common ground to satisfy their mutual needs in these areas.

Power and Control   When differences arise, one high-drama method for dealing with them is to use power and control tactics. Examples include withholding; bullying; or using intimidation, manipulation, or deception. These tactics serve to influence the other person through use of punishment or

negative reciprocity: one person directs a hostile, angry, or accusatory remark toward the other which prompts a negative response in kind from the targeted person, leading to rounds of verbal attacks and counterattacks.

demand-withdraw pattern: a destructive interaction pattern identified by Gottman and Gottman in which demands from one party ultimately lead to withdrawal and stonewalling from the other party.

stonewalling: the fourth step in the demand-withdraw pattern when the withdrawing person withholds attention and puts up a wall that blocks communication and cooperation as a way to punish the demanding person.

through trickery. When a person uses punitive tactics, that person can expect the recipient to experience negative affect. Such feelings may include embarrassment, humiliation, sadness, hurt, anger, anxiety, or depression. Remember George's accusation to Martha that she humiliates him? George clearly feels pain from her punitive tactics. No doubt, Martha feels the same from George's insults (e.g., his comments about the gin running out of her mouth).

The interaction pattern found in George and Martha's relationship is called **negative reciprocity**. One person directs a hostile, an angry, or an accusatory remark toward the other, which in turn prompts a negative response in kind from the targeted person. Each round of verbal exchanges leads to attack and counterattack that escalate tensions and conflict rather than lead to resolution and reduced tension.

Gottman and Gottman (1999) identified another particularly destructive pattern they called the **demand-withdraw pattern** in which one party makes a type of demand on the relationship that leads the other party to withdraw from the interaction rather than attempt to resolve the demand. The demand-withdraw pattern involves four steps: (1) one partner complains or criticizes the other, which prompts (2) the other person to get defensive, (3) to feel contempt toward the person complaining, and (4) then withdraw emotionally or physically. The Gottmans refer to the fourth step as **stonewalling** when the withdrawing person withholds attention and puts up a wall that blocks communication and cooperation as a way to punish the demanding person. Gottman and Gottman (1999) called criticism, defensiveness, contempt, and stonewalling the "Four Horsemen of the Apocalypse" because of their destructive influence on marriages.

Gottman and Levenson (2000) conducted a 14-year longitudinal study that demonstrated that the demand-withdraw pattern of communication is an

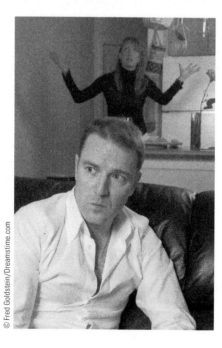

© Fred Goldstein/Dreamstime.com

Stonewalling is a part of the demand-withdraw pattern that predicts divorce.

important factor that predicts later divorce. Other factors include continued relationship dissatisfaction combined with frequent thoughts of dissolving the marriage. Further, negative affect predicts early dissolution of the marriage, and lack of positive affect, later marriage break-ups. Gottman and Levenson (2000) determined that they could use these variables to predict over 90% of the couples who would divorce.

These communication patterns involve the use of power and control tactics and language. In their book entitled *Straight Talk: A New Way to Get Closer to Others by Saying What You Really Mean,* Miller, Wackman, Nunnally, and Saline (1982) characterize two forms of **heavy control communication:** the iron fist and the velvet glove. The iron fist, a form of active *heavy control talk,* uses a sledgehammer to get a point across, whereas the velvet glove, a form of passive heavy control, uses a more indirect approach. Examples of the iron fist include name calling, blaming, accusing, threatening, putting down, ordering, ridiculing, criticizing, taunting, and using sarcasm. Velvet glove communication often involves attempts to manipulate through inducing guilt or sympathy and includes whining, denying, withholding, foot-dragging, playing the martyr, making excuses, and keeping score. Both forms of communication are detrimental to the health of relationships.

Another power and control tactic, game playing, involves the use of deception. Eric Berne's 1964 classic book *Games People Play* chronicles the use of these tactics. There is a hidden agenda with payoffs in game playing that reward the person running the game. The other members are pulled into the drama and unknowingly play their prescribed roles. The mythic **drama triangle** (Karpman, 1968), the most basic prototype for fairy tales and classic stories, is often a game. It involves a persecutor (i.e., villain), victim, and rescuer (i.e., hero) (Figure 8.1). For example, Cinderella (the victim) is persecuted by her wicked stepmother and her stepsisters (the villains) only to be rescued by the handsome prince (the hero).

In real life the drama triangle often involves two people who launch into a dispute and then pull in a third person. This process is called **triangulation** (Bowen, 1978). The third person determines who the persecutor and victim are, and then tries to rescue the victim. For example, young Eric and Lori are

drama triangle: a game played that involves a persecutor, victim, and rescuer.

triangulation: the process whereby two people in dispute pull in a third person.

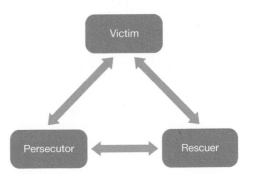

FIGURE **8.1** Drama Triangle

The drama triangle involves a victim, persecutor, and rescuer. Roles often interchange abruptly during the enactment of the drama triangle.

newly married and have a serious argument. Lori (the victim) calls her dad and complains about Eric (the persecutor). Her dad (the rescuer) invites Lori to move back with her parents, which she does.

The curious thing about the drama triangle is that the roles can change abruptly, leaving some of the players feeling dazed and confused. In the example of Eric and Lori, Eric (now the victim) feels violated by Lori's dad (now the persecutor) and pleads with Lori (now the rescuer) for reconciliation. Lori then returns to Eric, leading her dad now to feel like the victim. In short order, Lori's dad has gone from rescuer to persecutor to victim. What is Lori's payoff? She gets attention and social support from her family, she ultimately prevails in her dispute with Eric, and she does not have to take responsibility for any of it. Everyone else feels dazed and confused by what happened.

As you can see, these dramas can play endlessly with the same plot line and alternating players for each role. Although there are clearly cases of true victimization, including, for example, domestic abuse, most everyday disputes are not black and white but really involve shades of gray. We may unconsciously adopt a game role when we feel victimized, judge someone else to be a persecutor, or feel a need to rescue another from a plight. However, these games involve prescribed roles that control our behavior and persons willing to use hidden agendas to receive covert payoffs associated with that control. Thus, they serve to increase rather than decrease stress because they promote high drama and dishonest ways of working through relationship difficulties.

Responsibility   Problem relationships are characterized by blaming, anger, and externalizing responsibility; in other words, it is always the other person's fault. In many ways this externalizing pattern resembles elements of the drama triangle with each party assuming a victim role and seeing the other as the villain, especially during periods of high stress when we have a greater tendency to engage in distorted thinking. As we know, villains deserve to be punished, so we may shift into the hero role to punish the villain.

In his book entitled *The Joy of Conflict Resolution*, Gary Harper (2004) gives an illustration of this process in the classic Popeye cartoons. "The typical plot line of a Popeye cartoon features Popeye taking abuse from the villainous Bluto. Eventually, Popeye reaches the limit of his considerable patience, pops open his can of spinach, and administers Bluto the beating he so justly deserves. And all is well with the world." (p. 5)

Harper cautions that though the hero is perceived as noble and courageous, there is a dark side. The dark side is that the hero can slip into a form of *self-righteousness* in which any action, no matter how aggressive, can be justified as noble as long as the other party is painted as the villain. In the extreme form we can think of how terrorists justify their actions. Terrorists often cast themselves as victims who possess a self-righteous justification for their acts of terror because they cast their targets as villains who deserve punishment. In this way they do not feel responsible for pain and suffering they inflict on others. Likewise, it is a slippery slope for couples to view each other as villains who deserve the punishment they can mete out on one another.

When we assign blame we make what social psychologists call attributions. **Attributions** are causal inferences about why a person engages in a particular

attributions: cognitions people use to explain why a person behaves a certain way.

behavior. We can form internal attributions or external attributions. Similarly, we can make stable attributions or unstable attributions. When we make **internal stable attributions** we attribute the cause of the target person's behavior to personality or traits. **External unstable attributions** refer to temporary situational factors.

Dissatisfied couples tend to attribute each other's negative behaviors to internal stable causes such as "he is a jerk" or "she is a witch." Thus, the target person is regarded as permanently defective or bad in some regard. However, satisfied couples tend to attribute each other's negative behaviors to external unstable factors such as "he's had a bad day" or "she is under a lot of stress" (see Bradbury & Fincham, 1990, for a review). The flip side is also true where positive acts among happy couples are attributed to internal stable causes ("he is a good man" or "she is a caring woman") and in unhappy couples to external unstable causes ("every now and then he can act like a real human being" or "she must have woken up on the right side of the bed this morning, she's actually being nice"). Thus, attributions made by unhappy couples tend to reinforce a view that their partner is a permanent villain, even if that person does good things occasionally, and that their partner is responsible for all the bad things that happen in their relationship. When things go wrong in the relationship, this attributional style considers one side blameless and the other side 100% responsible. No wonder they have difficulty working through their relationship issues.

Low Drama—Lowering Tension and Creating Closeness

Low-drama approaches are designed to reduce tension and conflict, lead to shared problem solving, and result in greater closeness. These approaches value and nurture interpersonal relationships and facilitate personal and relational growth. If you think of an intimate relationship as like a garden, you as the gardener want to add the right amount of light, water, fertilizer, and caring for your garden that will not only sustain it but help it thrive. Too much or too little of these elements can result in stunted growth and sick plants.

Similarities   Because similarities attract, one approach to minimizing conflict and tension is to search for common ground. What areas do you have in common? What are your mutual interests, and in what interests do you diverge? Start with common ground and you have a mutual base to build on. As you explore commonalities, you may find that you are more similar than you think. Acknowledge and recognize these similarities, and it is easier to move toward closeness.

One way to develop shared understandings is to experience authentic empathy for one another. **Empathy** involves putting yourself in the other person's skin and experiencing the world through that person's eyes. It sounds like a hard task, so how do we do it? First, we can look for nonverbal cues. Does the other person look stressed or relaxed? What emotions might that person be feeling? Although there may be cultural differences in the display of emotions, Ekman (1993) and others (Elfenbein & Ambady, 2002) have determined that *facial* displays of the six emotions of anger, fear, disgust, happiness, surprise, and sadness have universal characteristics that are easily decoded regardless of the culture of the observer.

A good primary palette of emotions to start with is the set of emotions of *sad, mad, glad,* and *nervous.* A sad person, like a tired person, will often have a

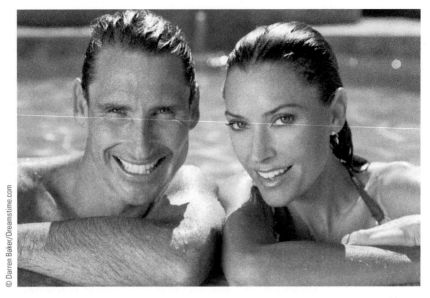

© Darren Baker/Dreamstime.com

Which one has the Duchenne smile? Have you made your choice? If you guessed the man, you are correct. Notice the crinkling around the corners of his eyes that are missing in the woman's smile.

face that looks drawn and a body posture that is more slumped, as if the person is pulling inward to escape from sad news. The person's facial expression may look like a lower intensity version of a crying face. A mad person, with eyes glaring, generally has a more outward focus and a more aggressive posture (e.g., furrowed brow, forward lean, pointed finger, etc.). Anger may be mixed with tension and nervousness as the muscles tighten in response to perceived threat. That person, like the nervous person, is in the "fight-or-flight" mode. Nervousness suggests readiness for flight, so the person may lean away, avoid eye contact, shuffle the feet, fidget, or in some other way indicate a readiness to flee. Finally, glad feelings are associated with higher energy, an uplift of the face and posture, and sparkling eyes. If the person is smiling, it is likely to be a **"Duchenne smile,"** a genuine smile that is characterized by the skin crinkling around the corners of the eyes (i.e., forming crow's feet). Unlike polite smiles, Duchenne smiles are hard to fake because they involve involuntary muscles of the face.

It is important that we communicate our happy feelings to our partner so that he or she can feel gratified, know better what we like, or simply bask in the warm glow of our happiness. **Positive reciprocity** (i.e., expressing how much we like each other's positive qualities and behaviors), the flip side of negative reciprocity, is an important norm for elevating good feelings about one another and the relationship.

A second way to achieve empathy is to use active listening. **Active listening** is a collaborative process of attending to the message being conveyed by the other party and then feeding back an understanding of the message. The feedback forms a loop so that misunderstandings are clarified by each party until the person sending the message feels heard by the listener. As such it is a

Duchenne smile: a genuine smile that is characterized by the skin crinkling around the corners of the eyes.

active listening: a collaborative process of attending the message being conveyed by the communicator and then feeding back an understanding of the message.

two-way process. This contrasts with passive listening, which is a one-way process of one person conveying a message and the other person passively receiving the message. There is no feedback, so the person conveying the message is unsure if he or she is understood by the listener.

At its simplest level active listening involves **paraphrasing** what the other person just said. The paraphrase is often prefaced by statements like "You are telling me that . . . I'm hearing you say that . . . Let me get this straight . . . It sounds like . . . You seem to be saying . . . If I understand you correctly . . . In other words. . . ." If the listener is on target, the talker will give **feedback** and say "that's right" or give some other indication that acknowledges the accuracy of the listener's understanding. However, if the listener is not on target, the person conveying the message may say "I don't think you quite get it" or something to that effect. At that time it is important for the listener to have a nondefensive and nonreactive response and to ask for more information. This process is called **clarifying** and involves a statement like "please tell me more then so I can better understand where you are coming from." With paraphrasing, feedback, and clarifying, it is hoped that the listener can close the loop of understanding between the two parties, bringing them closer together.

Active listening allows both partners to share more deeply in each other's inner worlds. In effect, each partner becomes a mirror for the other. More advanced levels of this form of reflective listening involve identification of feelings and deeper messages that reside beneath the surface messages. Warmth, understanding, and support can be conveyed within a partnership that strengthens social bonds. Conflicts will still occur, but they are now seen through supportive and benign lenses. In this context, conflicts are viewed as challenges that stimulate self-reflection and growth. In fact, a little challenge mixed with a healthy dose of emotional support is the optimal blend for promoting personal growth. Through trial and error we can discover the right mix of light, water, fertilizer, and care that leads to optimal growth of each partner and the relationship.

Constructive Influence   Because each party in a relationship has his or her own needs and interests, it is important to be able to express them in a constructive manner to work out arrangements that are mutually satisfying. We can use constructive influence when we engage in what has been referred to variously as *clean communication, straight talk,* or *assertiveness.* In each of

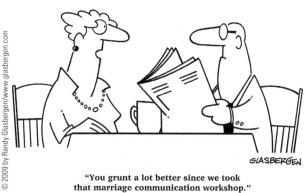

© 2009 by Randy Glasbergen/www.glasbergen.com

**"You grunt a lot better since we took
that marriage communication workshop."**

these methods, there is no iron fist, velvet glove, game playing, or deception, but rather a straightforward expression of one's thoughts, feelings, desires, and observations in a nonjudgmental and respectful way.

In their book entitled *Couple Skills: Making Your Relationship Work,* the authors McKay, Fanning, and Paleg (2006, pp. 57–61) list the "Ten Commandments of Clean Communication." The first six commandments deal with messages they label "pejorative communication." These are the "don'ts." Pejorative messages should be avoided. These include use of heavy control language such as "judgmental words" (i.e., use of zingers that indicate the partner is defective like "you are thoughtless" or "you are childish"); global negative labels (i.e., name calling like "stupid, crazy, evil"); "you" messages that blame or accuse; old history that is brought into the conversation to justify angry feelings; negative comparisons because they are designed to punish and make the partner feel bad; and threats because use of threats is a coercive tactic that involves a potential use of punishment.

The last four commandments are instructive and give us suggestions of what to do. These are the "do's." They are:

- "*Describe* your feelings rather than *attack* with them." This involves use of "I" messages rather than "you" messages. For example, "I feel sad" rather than "You made me cry" or "I am embarrassed" rather than "You embarrassed me." Clean communication involves keeping one's voice at a normal volume rather than overwhelming or flooding the partner with emotion. Each person takes responsibility for his or her feelings when using "I" messages.

- "Keep body language open and receptive." If one's body language is congruent with the message that "we are here to communicate," then communication will flow more freely. Body indicators of openness and receptivity are good eye contact, uncrossed arms, and attentive listening (e.g., leaning slightly forward, nodding, or using active listening).

- "Use whole messages." Whole messages have four parts. It may not always be feasible to use all four parts, but the more parts used, the more information is conveyed in the message and the better the potential for the recipient to understand the communication. The four parts are (1) observations (i.e., neutral statements of fact like "it rained yesterday"); (2) thoughts (i.e., "I" statements about one's personal understandings such as "My idea is . . ." or "I was wondering about . . ." or "The way it seemed to me was . . . ," and so forth); (3) feelings (i.e., "I" statements that identify one's emotions such as, for example, "I feel frustrated" or "I am excited"); and (4) needs, desires, and wants (i.e., "I" statements such as "I want to feel closer to you" or "I need some relief from all this stress," etc.).

- "Use clear messages." Clear messages are not contaminated by subtext or a necessity to read between the lines to understand the intention of the communicator. For example, a "why" question is often a disguised judgment statement. A partner who says "Why are you so messy?" is really making a statement disguised as a question. The statement implies a critical judgment that "You are messy, therefore you are bad—you should clean up after yourself if you want to be good." This is a contaminated message.

McKay et al. (2006, p. 60) present the following as an example of a **whole clear message**: "I notice you're pretty quiet tonight (*observation*). It makes me think you're not interested in me (*thought*), and I feel hurt and a little angry (*feeling*). I'd like for you to talk with me more (*need*)."

Whereas use of whole messages is desirable in close relationships, if you want to return a defective product for a refund or receive compensation from the cleaners for a damaged shirt, you may be more effective using only selected components. These types of scenarios call for simple assertive responses such as "When I brought my shirt in to have it laundered it was new and in fine condition (*observation*). Now as you can see it is badly discolored. I would like to request a reimbursement for the cost of my shirt" (*want*). Though you could also disclose your thoughts or that you are frustrated, disappointed, angry, or upset about the damaged shirt, you have to ask yourself if these disclosures will help or hinder your objective of receiving the reimbursement. Will they raise or lower the potential for dramatic conflict?

Likewise, in work contexts, the use of certain feeling words may up the drama and potential for conflict, so substituting more neutral words may be a better choice. For example, instead of saying to a coworker who has made a costly mistake, "I am *mad* about what has just happened," a worker can say, "I am *concerned* about what just happened." The general rule of assertiveness is to give the **minimally effective response** (Rimm & Masters, 1974) in contexts in which assertion could be met with punishment (e.g., potential blowback from making the assertive statement). If the minimally effective response does not accomplish the objective, then a person can gradually escalate assertive responses if appropriate (e.g., talking next to the supervisor). In other words, what is the least threatening way you can present your position to accomplish your objectives while still upholding your rights and respecting the rights of others? In the workplace, the primary goal is to accomplish particular business objectives rather than to become more transparent to achieve emotional closeness—a goal more appropriate for intimate relationships.

minimally effective response: the least threatening assertive response that can accomplish the objective.

No matter how smoothly communication flows between couples, there will be times when interests will diverge. Remember Jeff and Susan? Jeff, an extravert, wants to go to a party and Susan, an introvert, wants to stay home and read a good book. How do they resolve their differences and still maintain their closeness and function as a partnership? There are a myriad of these types of situations arising in marriages, ranging from the trivial (e.g., whether to attend the party) to the important (e.g., how to best discipline the children). It is at times like these that couples are often unknowingly involved in **negotiations**. The key to successful negotiations is to recognize that it is a normal part of maintaining intimate relationships. When we think of negotiations we often think of two lawyers with briefcases sitting across from each other at a large conference table. However, in everyday life the process consists of a periodic series of ongoing informal exchanges. If each party engages in clean communication; the parties both express their wants, needs, and interests; they maintain a flexible attitude; and they search for similarities and common ground then the chances for them to reach a mutually satisfying outcome are high.

During the first stage of negotiation, each partner can assertively express his or her interests. Both partners can use active listening to process and clarify an understanding of the other's needs. Feedback of understandings helps to convey that each is understood and promotes empathy. Then, in the second stage, the couple will move from discussion of interests to proposals for action. The idea is to present a proposal that best satisfies the needs of both individuals. Proposals can be met with counterproposals that move each closer to their ultimate objectives until they reach a compromise. If, however, an acceptable compromise cannot be reached, then one party can suggest a **time-out** (e.g., "Let's take a break and talk about it later today"), and the subject can be revisited later until a solution is found. Persistence is an important attribute for success in this process. Exiting a disagreement gracefully by taking a time-out, agreeing to disagree, or focusing on the positives are important actions to take to maintain overall harmony in relationships when frustrations run high.

McKay et al. (2006, p. 101) discuss a number of classic compromise solutions. Let us see how four can apply to Jeff and Susan's situation.

1. **"Take Turns"** Susan goes to Jeff's party this week, but Jeff agrees to decline the next party invitation and stay home with Susan for a quiet evening of reading.

2. **"Do Both; Have It All"** Jeff goes to the party and Susan stays at home and reads.

3. **"Trial Period"** Susan agrees to go to the party for one hour, but if she wants to leave after that time they will politely exit.

4. **"Split the Difference"** Half the evening they will attend the party and the other half they will stay home where Susan can read.

Responsibility An important part of using the low-drama approach is to accept responsibility for our thoughts, feelings, and actions. In other words, acknowledge and accept that other people do not control what we think, feel, or do. Likewise, we do not control what other people think, feel, or do. If we are unhappy in a situation only we are responsible for making changes that make us happy, not the other person. We may have a constructive influence on others, but we will never control them. If we change how we approach a problem, perhaps others involved will change in kind, but we cannot expect it. And we certainly cannot expect a partner to make personality changes as a way to resolve conflicts. Ultimately, we are responsible for taking care of our individual needs within the context of maintaining and nurturing our relationships.

Being responsible also means setting limits. When we engage in **limit setting** we are defining what we will agree to or accept from others and what we will not. Limit setting relates to the concept of boundaries. **Boundaries** define your personal space (i.e., the space that defines you as distinct from others). To be assertive means to affirm your right to protect your boundaries from inappropriate intrusions. Though boundaries can refer to physical space, they also refer to psychological space (e.g., privacy).

boundaries:
one's physical and
psychological space.

In its simplest form, protecting one's boundaries means saying "no." For example, if you receive a sales call, you have the right to say, "thank you, but I am not interested." No explanation is required. If the salesperson is persistent and asks for reasons, then you can use the assertive response of the **broken record technique** in which the same statement is simply repeated. "Thank you, but I am not interested." For very persistent callers, after using the broken record technique, a good method is to simply state what you want, what you intend to do, and then exit. "As I've said, I am not interested. Please do not call me again. I am going to hang up now."—click.

In intimate relationships we have the right to be treated with respect and dignity. If we believe we are being mistreated, we have the right to call attention to our feelings and ask that the behavior stop. This is also a form of limit setting. Emotional or physical abuse is never acceptable. Ultimately, if we believe we have exhausted the viable constructive alternatives, we may determine that the best way to set limits is to exit the relationship. Some relationships are toxic and cannot be repaired. If we leave with anger and acrimony, only we can determine whether to finally let go and forgive. Forgiveness does not have to be done in person but may be simply a matter of letting go of past hurts and resentments. Determining when or if to forgive is also a matter of personal responsibility.

STRESS MANAGEMENT EXERCISE **8.1**

Imagine that you are in the following situations. How would you respond using the constructive techniques we have discussed?

■ Your best friend has done poorly on an exam and says, "I studied hard and I still bombed the exam." What would you say to convey empathy?

■ Your romantic partner just said, "We just don't seem to click anymore. Maybe we are just not a good long-term match." Use a whole clear message to convey your thoughts and feelings.

■ You are going out to eat and your friend wants to go to a Chinese restaurant but you are more in the mood for Mexican food. What compromise solution would you propose as part of an informal negotiation?

■ You believe you were treated unfairly by your boss when your boss made a disparaging remark about you in front of your coworkers. You feel embarrassed, hurt, and angry. What minimally effective response could you use to try to prevent this from happening again?

■ You are shopping for a car and the salesperson starts asking you personal questions that you do not feel comfortable answering because you are just browsing, such as how big of a down payment you are prepared to make if you find the right vehicle today. How would you assertively and constructively protect your privacy boundaries and set limits with this salesperson? What would you say if this salesperson persists?

The Stress of Divorce   Of course in marital relationships exiting the relationship may involve divorce—a legal dissolution of the partnership. Up to half of first marriages will result in divorce (Cherlin, 1992) and second marriages have an even greater likelihood of divorce. Some people engage in a serial pattern of marriages with interludes of single life. This new pattern of serial marriages for meeting intimacy needs contrasts with marriage patterns observed in the United States in the latter half of the 19th century when the norm was to have a lifelong marriage; the divorce rate then was very low though steadily rising over the latter half of the century, starting around 5% in 1867 and slowly rising to around 12% by 1900 (Preston & McDonald, 1979).

How stressful is the process of divorce? How difficult is it to adjust to the stress of divorce and its aftermath? To answer these questions we can look at one of the dominant models for explaining the stress of a divorce and its adjustment called the **divorce-stress-adjustment perspective.** As Amato (2000) explains, the stress and adjustment trajectory of a divorce depends on the person, the stressors associated with the divorce, and the moderators or protective factors that serve as shock absorbers for the impact of the divorce. Research indicates that the result of this divorce-stress-adjustment process is that some people show a boost in well-being following a divorce such as a person leaving an abusive partner, others experience a temporary crisis that improves after a transition period until well-being returns to normal levels (the majority), and still others move into a downward spiral from which they never fully recover (Amato, 2000).

Although the divorce experience is usually stressful, it is not always met with painful emotions. For some people, it is met with a feeling of relief. Furthermore, the challenge of dealing with a divorce and its aftermath may stimulate personal growth that ultimately results in higher levels of self-confidence and autonomy—in other words, positive consequences.

The process of divorce is usually initiated by one partner who feels dissatisfaction that later turns into estrangement. That person later experiences a period of mourning upon recognizing that the marriage has no future, which ultimately leads him or her to initiate the divorce—overall more wives than husbands initiate divorce. The other partner (the noninitiator) usually experiences greater stress during the divorce process because that partner has not yet mourned the impending loss nor planned for the dissolution of the marital bond.

Amato (2000) lists the following as stressors or risk factors that make adjustment to divorce more difficult:

- Child custody actions, such as gaining sole custody and responsibility for parenting one's children, or the opposite, losing all custody rights
- Ongoing conflicts with an ex-spouse
- Loss of financial resources that leads to downward economic mobility (more likely to affect women than men, especially custodial mothers)
- Disruption of social and emotional support networks (e.g., in-laws, mutual friends, marital support)

Moderators that serve as protective factors (i.e., shock absorbers) against the stress of the divorce include:

- Individual personal resources such as coping skills, social skills, and self-efficacy (e.g., viewing the divorce as an opportunity for personal growth or to escape a dysfunctional marriage rather than as a personal failing or as a tragedy)
- Interpersonal resources such as building new social support networks (e.g., finding a new partner or meeting new friends)
- Structural resources such as employment, financial resources, community services

Adjustment is better for those who are able to adapt and function well in their new roles following the divorce, who have fewer psychological or health problems, and whose identity and lifestyle are less organized around their former marriage. On the average, most negative affective reactions to divorce such as feelings of anxiety or depression subside within 2 years.

SOCIAL SUPPORT, SOCIAL STRAIN, AND HEALTH

At the beginning of this chapter we visited Angela, who enjoys many positive benefits of her interpersonal relationships, and Edward Albee's characters of George and Martha, who endure a dark, stormy, and stressful relationship. Whereas Angela's social network brings her added resources and an emotional lift, George and Martha's social bond drains their resources and sinks them into a pit of emotional despair. Angela enjoys *social support*, but George and Martha experience *social strain*.

social support: refers to social interactions embedded within a network of social relationships that provide a person with potential access to or receipt of actual or perceived resources from others who are perceived as caring.

Social support refers to social interactions *embedded* within a network of social relationships that provide a person with potential access to or receipt of *actual* or *perceived* resources from others who are perceived as caring (Kaniasty, 2008). According to this construct, we can measure levels of social support from *actual* assistance received that can be objectively verified (e.g., receipt of financial assistance) and from the *perception* of assistance that is subjectively determined (e.g., self-report measures). We also can measure the structural aspect of social support of *embeddedness* through counting the number of meaningful social connections a person has (e.g., marital status, number of friends, etc.). Social support can be physical and tangible (e.g., assistance clearing debris after a hurricane), informational (e.g., reminding an elderly relative to take her medications), or emotional (e.g., being a good listener for a friend who is upset).

social strain: refers to social interactions within a network of social relationships that are a source of stress because they drain resources or provide assistance in an unhelpful manner.

Social strain (Rook, 1990) refers to social interactions within a network of social relationships that are a source of stress because they drain resources or provide assistance in an unhelpful manner. Social strain includes relationships that are characterized by high conflict, hostility, negative emotions, or excessive burdens. George and Martha exhibit a socially strained relationship.

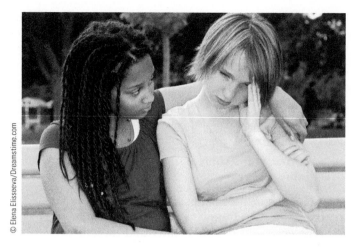

Being emotionally supportive to a friend who is distressed is a form of social support.

Social Support and Health

From Berkman and Syme's groundbreaking 1979 finding showing that Alameda County, California, residents who lacked social support died at higher rates than their high social support counterparts, to the present, researchers have gathered a substantial body of evidence demonstrating that social support is reliably related to better health and increased longevity (for a review, see Graham, Christian, & Kiecolt-Glaser, 2007, and Uchino, 2006). These positive effects are present for measures of actual support, perceived support, and embeddedness.

Ironically, studies conducted measuring *actual* assistance are the most limited and difficult to interpret because they sometimes find that people with the greatest health needs (e.g., disability or illness) receive the most support. In other words, when the health outlook is most dire, the person is most likely to receive actual assistance. This positive correlational finding can lead to the false conclusion that high social support leads to higher rather than lower rates of illness or mortality. In spite of the occasional positive correlation, in general, studies find health benefits from actual support. For example, one study (Herbst-Damm & Kulik, 2005) found that patients who are terminally ill lived 80 days longer when they received *actual* social support from volunteers than those who did not receive support.

In part due to interpretation and practical limitations for studies of *actual* social support, the body of research literature linking *perceived* social support to greater health and well-being is larger, stronger, and more reliable than it is for actual social support. For example, Uchino, Cacioppo, and Kiecolt-Glaser (1996) concluded from their meta-analytic review of studies comprised primarily of measures of perceived social support, that higher support was positively related to overall immune functioning. In addition, a number of studies have found a positive correlation between perceived social support and natural killer (NK) cell activities, cytotoxicity, and numbers (Baron, Cutrona, Hicklin, Russell, & Lubaroff, 1990; Miyazaki et al., 2003).

Studies using quantitative measures of *embeddedness* such as social network size and marital status have also indicated positive health and well-being benefits. Although there have been some contrary findings, in general, the larger the social network size, the better the health outcomes. As Graham et al. (2007, p. 782) note, "the relationship between network size and health outcome rivals that of well-established health risk factors, such as smoking, blood pressure, blood lipids, obesity, and physical activity."

Even having just one person to trust and confide in appears to make a big difference in health status. Marital status seems to be a good indication of that phenomenon, and gender appears to play a role with men showing the strongest benefit from marriage in both disease and mortality statistics (Kiecolt-Glaser & Newton, 2001). By way of illustration of the magnitude and gender differences in the effect, we can look at the mortality statistics for unmarried men and compare them to those of unmarried women. Men who are not married have a 250% greater risk of mortality than married men, and women who are not married have a 50% greater mortality risk than married women (Ross, Mirowsky, & Goldsteen, 1990). Looking at the health benefits of marriage then, we can ask, why do men have 5 times more benefit from marriage than women? Possible reasons are that married women (as compared to married men): (1) do a disproportional amount of housework and childcare (work that can add more stress), (2) are more likely to give than receive spousal informational support (e.g., recommendations, advice, etc.) that shapes good health behavior, and (3) are less likely to depend on their spouse as their only confidant and therefore need him less to meet all their social support needs—the spouse as sole confidant was reported by 15% of wives and 40% of husbands in a study by Harrison, Maguire, and Pitceathly (1995).

How then does social support achieve its beneficial effects? There are two primary models describing how social support promotes health and well-being, the *stress buffer model* and the *direct effect model*. According to the **stress buffer model of social support,** social support *moderates* the effects of stress—that is, it lessens the negative effects of exposure to stressors (i.e., it serves as a shock absorber) (Figure 8.2). This model predicts that social support is beneficial only under stressful conditions (when shock absorbers are most needed). The **direct effect model of social support** suggests that social support has beneficial health and well-being effects independent of the level of stress. In other words, social support is a good tonic that has a positive effect regardless of stress levels (i.e., in high- and low-stress situations) (Figure 8.3).

Empirical support for both models has been reported across a large body of findings. The results depend largely on the ecological context, the type of support, the nature of the stressor, and the outcomes measured. For example, based on his review of the relevant research, Cohen (2004) concludes that the stress buffer model best predicts the effects of *perceived* social support on *health* outcomes in conditions where the need is high. However, Kaniasty (2008) concludes from his review that the direct effect model best predicts *well-being* outcomes. In other words, we are happier and better adjusted when we have social support, and this is true across all levels of stress, including low-stress conditions. However, social support benefits our *health* status only

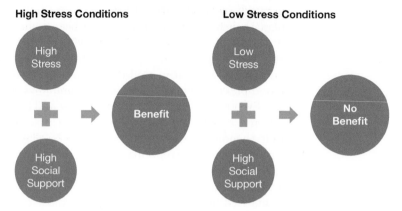

FIGURE **8.2** The stress buffer model of social support suggests that social support moderates the effects of stress so that social support is only beneficial under high-stress conditions.

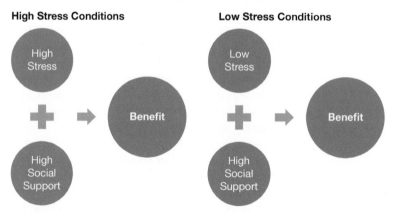

FIGURE **8.3** The direct effect model of social support suggests that social support exerts beneficial effects at all stress levels.

under high-stress conditions. Otherwise (e.g., low-stress conditions), it has no effect.

Through what biological systems does social support have an impact? Uchino (2006) outlines a number of biological pathways through which social support may achieve its positive effects including through the cardiovascular, neuroendocrine, and immune systems. For example, social support may buffer the effects of stress on cardiovascular reactivity. Uchino (2006) notes that higher levels of social support are associated with lower everyday blood pressure levels, less cardiovascular disease, and a slower disease progression for patients who are already suffering from cardiovascular disease. In addition, recent neuroendocrine studies have found that salivary cortisol levels are lower when social support is high (Heinrichs, Baumgartner, Kirschbaum, & Ehlert, 2003; Milagros, King, Ma, & Reed, 2004). The strongest evidence for biological pathways, however, is a positive link between the immune system and social support (see Graham et al., 2007; Uchino et al., 1996). In particular, it seems to dampen the immune system's inflammatory responses to stress. For example, several studies have found that higher social support is associated with lower levels of the cytokine and inflammatory marker interleukin-6 (Costanzo et al., 2005; Friedman et al., 2005, Lutgendorf, Anderson, Sorosky, Buller, & Lubaroff, 2000). As you recall, elevated proinflammatory cytokines such as interleukin-6 are associated with an increased risk of heart disease (see Chapter 5).

Social Strain and Health

What are the health effects of being in a socially strained relationship like George and Martha's, one marked with strife, conflict, and hostility? First, there is considerable evidence that such relationships have a direct negative physiological effect, especially on the cardiovascular system. Kiecolt-Glaser and Newton (2001) reviewed the relevant literature and concluded that (1) marital conflict leads to elevated blood pressure and heart rate, (2) the effects are amplified when conflict is augmented with hostile behaviors, and (3) the effects are more pronounced and prolonged for wives than husbands. Kiecolt-Glaser and Newton (2001) also suggest that the gender discrepancy findings are due to women being more attuned to the emotional quality of the marriage so that wives function as a type of "barometer" for distress in marriages. As a result, when confronted with hostility and conflict from their marital partner, they pay a greater price in the form of cardiovascular reactivity.

Graham et al. (2007) reviewed the research on immunity and social relationships and contend that there is solid evidence reflected in findings of poorer immunological responses, presence of mouth ulcers, or slower wound healing that marital conflict can lead to immune system dysregulation. They also point to a strong body of evidence for immune system dysregulation being associated with the experience of "relationship burden" in the form of long-term caregiving for a loved one, such as a spouse with Alzheimer's disease (see Chapter 4). Therefore, there is considerable evidence that social strain can produce physiological conditions that increase the risk for adverse health.

ADJUSTING TO DIFFERENCES

Alejandro was beaming when he came in to work. His coworker Mark noticed Alejandro's excitement and asked him what it was about. Alejandro told Mark that he was looking forward to his daughter Rosa's Quinceañera. Mark had a blank look on his face. "What is that," he asked? "It's a coming of age celebration for my daughter's fifteenth birthday," Alejandro replied. "Why would you want to do that? Isn't sixteen the age for daughters celebrating these kinds of things? Haven't you ever heard of sweet sixteen?" Mark asked. "Yes, but you don't seem to understand. It's our cultural tradition to celebrate our daughter's fifteenth birthday. We even have a father-daughter dance," Alejandro replied. Mark shrugged his shoulders. "If you say so," he commented and then walked away. Alejandro looked puzzled. His mood deflated as he wondered why his coworker would react in such a dismissive fashion to the news of his daughter's Quinceañera—a celebration that meant so much to him.

The exchange between Alejandro and Mark represents the challenge of adjusting to differences—in this case, different cultural practices. **Cultures** have their own unique values, beliefs, words, and customs, and these are often reflected in art, music, stories, and behaviors that are distinctive. Sometimes a culture is embedded within a surrounding culture or **superculture** (Jones, 1997). When this happens the embedded culture is referred to as a **subculture**. When a person belongs to two cultures, that person is said to be **bicultural**. Alejandro, a Hispanic living in the United States, is bicultural in that he identifies with both a Latino subculture and the superculture. Mark, who is not bicultural, has a difficult time understanding Alejandro's bicultural orientation. Likewise, Alejandro is puzzled by Mark's seeming lack of respect for his subculture.

James Jones (1997, p. 280) remarks in his writings about the unique challenges associated with biculturalism that "one's loyalty, commitment, and identity are challenged by this culturally perceived dualism." For example, members of a subculture may regard another member as disloyal to the culture of origin if that person becomes too closely identified with the superculture (e.g., not being able to speak or understand the native language of one's culture of origin with recent immigrants of the shared subculture). Likewise, members of the dominant culture may regard that same person with suspicion if that person is too closely identified with the subculture (e.g., Mark's dismissive reaction to Alejandro when Alejandro expressed excitement about his daughter's Quinceañera). Jones further notes that "the central challenge of bicultural adaptation is to maintain loyalty and connection to one's culture of origin, while also participating in a personally meaningful way in the broader society" (p. 281).

There are a number of choices for minority group members when dealing with such challenges. LaFromboise, Coleman, and Gerton (1993) outline these choices as (1) *assimilation*—absorption into the dominant culture through severing ties with one's culture of origin, (2) *acculturation*—absorption into the dominant culture while maintaining an identity as a member of the minority culture, (3) *alternation*—modification of cultural behavior to fit the social context in a way similar to the bilingualism model, (4) *multiculturalism*—maintain a distinct identity as a member of two or more cultures, and (5) *fusion*—assimilate but bring a cultural identity that blends with other cultural identities to form a new stronger cohesive whole culture (i.e., melting pot theory).

The adoption of a multicultural identity leads to the formation of an **ethnic identity** that defines the person in part through culture, language, or nation of origin of the subculture. Berk (2007, p. 404) concludes upon reviewing the relevant research for minority adolescent identity development that "a strong, secure ethnic identity is associated with higher self-esteem, optimism, sense of mastery over the environment, and more positive attitudes toward

bicultural: belonging to two cultures.

ethnic identity: defining a person through culture, language, or national origin.

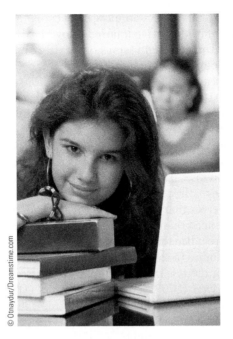

For this Latina, a strong and secure ethnic identity plays a role in coping better with stress and achieving more in school.

one's ethnicity." She further notes that minority adolescents with strong ethnic identities cope with stress better, achieve more in school, and are better adjusted than their counterparts who have weak ethnic identities. Therefore, although maintaining a secure ethnic identity has its drawbacks in that it can emphasize differences, it also has benefits such as promoting positive well-being, adjustment, and achievement.

STRESS AND HEALTH EFFECTS OF RACISM AND DISCRIMINATION

One insidious way that some people deal with racial or ethnic differences is through racism and discrimination. **Racism** is defined as "beliefs, attitudes, institutional arrangements, and acts that tend to denigrate individuals or groups because of phenotypic characteristics or ethnic group affiliation" (Clark, Anderson, Clark, & Williams, 1999, p. 805). **Prejudice** refers to negative *attitudes* and beliefs about a particular group, and **discrimination** to *behaviors* motivated by prejudice that range from social exclusion to aggression (Brondolo, Rieppi, Kelly, & Gerin, 2003). Clark et al. (1999, p. 808) argue that measuring **perceived racism**, "the subjective experience of prejudice or discrimination," is important to understanding the psychological and physiological consequences of the phenomenon. Perceived racism captures the appraisal of exposure to subtle racism, such as microstressors that cannot be adequately measured through objective measures of racism. Though overt racism has declined in recent decades, Harrell (2000, p. 46) notes that

discrimination: behaviors motivated by prejudice that range from social exclusion to aggression.

perceived racism: subjectively experiencing that one is the target of prejudice or discrimination.

microstressors are still quite common, especially for African Americans, examples of which include "being ignored or overlooked while waiting in line, being mistaken for someone who serves others (e.g., maid, bellboy), and being followed or observed while in public."

Most of the research on perceived racism has been conducted with African Americans. Jones (1997, p. 17) makes the case that African Americans are unique among United States minorities in that their history includes "the forced passage from Africa to America; slavery; legally enforced racial segregation and discrimination based on skin color; rigid caste-like category boundaries for racial identification; and persistent lower-class status relative to whites and other immigrant groups." African Americans also have been salient in being in the forefront of many political and judicial battles for civil rights for minorities. As such, Jones observes that prejudice toward Blacks by Whites is more crystallized and pronounced than toward other minorities. This is not to minimize the real effects of prejudice for other minorities, but rather to illustrate why the predominance of studies in the area have focused on African Americans.

Upon reviewing the research on ethnicity and stress of minority groups in the United States, Myers (2009, p. 9) concludes that "African Americans appear to carry the greatest burden of morbidity and mortality from many different illnesses, including heart disease, hypertension, type 2 diabetes, certain types of cancer, adverse birth outcomes and HIV/AIDS." The worst overall health profile among minorities living in the United States, he concludes, is carried by African Americans living in poverty. Racism can play a role as an interpersonal stressor and as a factor that can lead to blocked economic and educational opportunities that can in turn lead to stress related to limited access to resources. Racial stressors also may lead some African Americans to engage in increased health risk behaviors (Guthrie, Young, Williams, Boyd, & Kintner, 2002; Kwate, Valdimarsdottir, Guevarra, & Bovbjerg, 2003), to use less preventive medical services (e.g., mammography and cholesterol screening), and to experience less adequate health care in general (e.g., African American women are 3 times more likely to die in hospitals after hysterectomies than their White counterparts).

One particular focus of researchers examining the racism-health link is racism's association with increased cardiovascular activation. For example, in laboratory studies in which participants are exposed to racist situations, they show elevations in blood pressure and other indicators of increased cardiovascular reactivity (Fang & Myers, 2001; McNeilly et al., 1995). It is unclear, however, the degree to which racism plays a role in the development of hypertension, a disease that inordinately affects African Americans (one-third are hypertensive—Hajjar & Kotchen, 2003). Unlike sickle cell anemia, an inherited disease more common in African Americans, there does not appear to be a hypertension gene that could account for the disease's predominance in African Americans. Therefore, researchers generally suspect that the increased rates of hypertension found in African Americans are related to social phenomena.

Brondolo, Gallo, and Myers (2009) note that recent laboratory and ambulatory (use of portable measuring devices to monitor 24-hour activity) research connects the experience of racism to increased physiological reactivity in the form of increased blood pressure, heart rate, and cortisol—patterns linked to the development of hypertension and other stress-related disorders. Pascoe

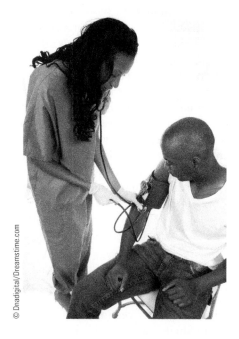

© Dnadigital/Dreamstime.com

What role do social phenomena such as racism and discrimination play in the higher incidence of hypertension found in African Americans?

and Richman (2009) also point to evidence that sustained increases in the activation of the hypothalamic-pituitary-adrenocortical axis increases the allostatic load, which can, over time, lead to the development of variety of health conditions, including cardiovascular disease. Thus, the increase in physiological reactivity and its demand on allostatic load is one likely racism-linked pathway to the development of hypertension. A second proposed pathway is racism-related stress leading to an increased involvement in health risk behaviors (e.g., cigarette use) and less involvement in health beneficial behaviors (e.g., physical exercise). Finally, Woods-Giscombe and Lobel (2008) suggest a third pathway driven by generic stressors such as financial strain that are indirectly linked to race-related discrimination. In their study of African American women, Wood-Giscombe and Lobel (2008, p. 179) found that "generic stress, race-related stress, and gender-related stress made equivalent contributions to African American women's stress and their associations with distress were of similar magnitude." Another study, this one of African American men, found that racism-related stress accounted for 4% to 7% of the psychological distress they experienced (Pieterse & Carter, 2007).

Research in the area of perceived discrimination shows promise in further elucidating the pathophysiology for hypertension and cardiovascular disease as it relates to these phenomena. A recent meta-analysis (Pascoe & Richman, 2009) of 134 samples found that perceived discrimination produces increased stress responses; is associated with engaging in health risk behaviors; and is negatively related to physical health, mental health, and to engaging in health-promoting behaviors.

Additional evidence was presented in a recent study (Richman, Pek, Pascoe, & Bauer, 2010) that asked Black and White participants over a period of 24 hours to wear an ambulatory blood pressure monitor, to complete a measure of perceived discrimination (i.e., interpersonal mistreatment), and to make PalmPilot diary entries that indicated their affective state. The researchers found that regardless of race, participants who reported more perceived discrimination had "steeper nighttime trajectories for systolic and diastolic blood pressure and less nighttime dipping in heart rate over time as compared to those who had reported relatively infrequent discrimination" (Richman et al., 2010, p. 403). In addition, participants with higher levels of perceived discrimination showed greater negative affect and less positive affect after experiencing stress. These results are important because they show a possible mechanism for discrimination leading to hypertension and cardiovascular disease because the cardiovascular nondipping phenomenon is known to increase risk for these diseases.

GENDER DIFFERENCES IN RESPONSE TO STRESS

Are there general differences between men and women in how they respond to stress? According to Shelly Taylor and her colleagues (Taylor, 2006; Taylor et al., 2000), there are. Although Taylor and her associates agree with Cannon's (1932) theory that both males and females have a similar primary *physiological* fight-or-flight response to stress, they disagree that the *behavioral* responses of both genders are the same. They note that much of the early research on stress was done with male rats and humans, and that this influenced early thinking about the process. Indeed, men are behaviorally more likely to fight or flee when threatened; however, they argue that women are more likely to **affiliate**—to seek out others in order to form groups for joint protection. Fight-or-flight behaviors for women, they contend, are not adaptive to survival of the species when women are responsible for carrying a child in pregnancy and later nursing and tending to the child when the child is most vulnerable. They note that it is safer for the protection of her offspring for a pregnant woman or a woman with a child to seek protection in groups than to fight or flee when confronted with a threat (e.g., a predator). Thus, they contend, this behavioral tendency toward affiliation is stronger in females than males.

tend-and-befriend: Taylor's theory that biobehavioral mechanisms influenced by oxytocin influence women toward engaging in affiliative behaviors when under stress.

Taylor and her colleagues further argue that in order for a woman to maximize protection for herself and her offspring when under threat, females have evolved a behavioral mechanism that is biologically driven that prompts them to **tend-and-befriend.** This biobehavioral mechanism is strongly influenced by the hormone oxytocin, which has mild sedative properties and promotes affiliative behavior. **Oxytocin** is a hormone found in high concentrations in nursing women that is believed to facilitate maternal-infant bonding. Thus, this hormonally influenced process leads women under threat to *tend* to their offspring and to *befriend*, that is, to nurture their children and develop, maintain, and use social ties and networks.

oxytocin: a hormone found in high concentrations in nursing women that is believed to facilitate maternal-infant bonding.

There is supportive evidence for the tend-and-befriend theory. For example, Aronson, Wilson, and Akert (2010, p. 462) conclude from their survey of the relevant research that "females are more likely than males to develop intimate friendships, cooperate with others, and focus their attention on social relationships." In general, women also are more prone to seek emotional support from others, especially other women, when under stress (Tamres, Janicki, & Helgeson, 2002).

However, is this emotional support–seeking tendency due to the biobehavioral factors proposed by Taylor and her colleagues or to gender socialization factors that encourage stress-related emotional support seeking in women and discourage it in men? There is scant evidence that gender differences in coping with stress are influenced by differences in oxytocin levels. In addition, after conducting a meta-analysis of gender differences in coping behavior, Tamres et al. (2002, p. 19) concluded that "most of the sex differences in coping were small." Therefore, these small differences could be due to gender socialization differences as likely as biobehavioral factors.

Let us assume for the sake of argument that we discount the gender socialization hypothesis and accept an evolutionary explanation for tend-and-befriend behaviors. Is such an explanation then unique to women? Geary and Flinn (2002) make the case that tending is an important evolutionary mechanism for men as well, because humans are among the few mammals where both genders engage in parenting. They point out that in many mammalian species (e.g., humans, chimpanzees, and dolphins), males are drawn to affiliate and form coalitions to compete for females or to control resources that can be shared with females to help raise offspring, so befriending is an important evolutionary mechanism for males as well. (See Taylor et al. [2002] for a reply to Geary and Flinn's [2002] arguments.) As you are aware from our previous discussion of social support, males also receive important health and well-being benefits from social support. Therefore, whereas gender differences may be present in coping with stress, they are likely small, and tend-and-befriend mechanisms are probably important for men as well, though through different patterns and to a somewhat lesser degree.

CHAPTER SUMMARY AND CONCEPT REVIEW

- In general, people in relationships who have similar interests, beliefs, attitudes, and worldviews have less reason to engage in interpersonal conflict.

- Negative reciprocity and demand-withdraw patterns are interaction styles that are more likely to lead to negative outcomes for relationships.

- The use of heavy control communication is counterproductive to the health of relationships.

- One common game is the drama triangle that involves a persecutor, victim, and rescuer.

- In unhappy relationships one person often blames the other and uses internal stable attributions to justify anger toward the partner when the partner exhibits negative behaviors and external unstable attributions to dismiss positive behaviors as temporary.

- Constructive approaches to resolving interpersonal difficulties involve using strategies that enhance authentic empathy, communicating with whole clear messages, negotiating differences, and accepting responsibility.

- Although the majority of people who go through the divorce process experience a temporary crisis followed by normal adjustment, some experience an immediate boost in well-being, and others, a downward trajectory from which they never fully recover.

- Actual social support, perceived social support, and embeddedness are all positively linked to health and well-being.

- Marriage is positively related to health for both men and women though men appear to enjoy 5 times the benefit of women.

- The weight of evidence seems to support the stress buffer model for perceived social support benefiting health and the direct effect model for social support benefiting well-being.

- Cardiovascular, neuroendocrine, and immune pathways seem to be the systems most positively affected by social support.

- Social strain appears to have a direct negative physiological effect, especially on the cardiovascular system; immune system dysregulation also is a potential by-product.

- Cultural differences can present a challenge for some people.

- A bicultural person belongs to two cultures, usually a subculture and a superculture.

- Adoption of a strong ethnic identity in accordance with the multicultural identity model has benefits in promoting positive well-being, adjustment, and achievement, though it has drawbacks in that it can emphasize differences.

- Laboratory results show that participants exposed to racist situations show more pronounced cardiovascular reactivity including elevation in blood pressure.

- Higher rates of hypertension for African Americans could be due to racism-related increased physiological reactivity that raises allostatic load, increased involvement in health risk behaviors, reduced involvement in health beneficial behaviors, and to greater generic stressors related to financial strain that are indirectly linked to race-related discrimination.

- According to the tend-and-befriend model, women are more likely to seek affiliation in response to threat, which is influenced by the hormone oxytocin.

- There is supportive evidence for the tend-and-befriend model, but gender differences in coping with stress are generally small and may not be related to oxytocin.

CRITICAL THINKING QUESTIONS

1. Why are such a high proportion of the stressors we encounter within the interpersonal domain? How are interpersonal stressors different from other stressors? Why are interpersonal stressors often so concerning compared to stress related to things?

2. Of the interpersonal stressors discussed, which one is most concerning to you that you are currently experiencing? What constructive communication strategies can you use to deal with this interpersonal stressor?

3. How can working through issues of ethnic identity be stressful? In what ways can having a strong ethnic identity be protective against stress for a minority group member? What role do cultural differences play in interpersonal stress? What do you think is the best communication strategy for reducing interpersonal stress related to cultural differences?

4. What elements of perceived racism are probably the most stressful? How can a person who may be a target of perceived racism best cope with it? What communication strategies can that person apply?

5. How important is gender to our understanding stress? What do you believe are some of the primary differences between men and women in the types of stressors they encounter and how they deal with them? How important is the tend-and-befriend model to understanding any patterns of gender differences in response to stress? Explain.

KEY TERMS AND CONCEPTS

Active listening*

Affiliate

Attributions*

Bicultural*

Boundaries*

Broken record technique

Clarifying

Cultures

Demand-withdraw pattern*

Direct effect model of social support

Discrimination*

Divorce-stress-adjustment perspective

Drama triangle*

Duchenne smile*

Empathy

Ethnic identity*

External unstable attribution

Feedback

Heavy control communication

Internal stable attributions

Limit setting

Minimally effective response*

Negative reciprocity*

Negotiations

Oxytocin*

Paraphrasing

Perceived racism*

Positive reciprocity

Prejudice

Racism

Social support*

Social strain*

Stonewalling*

Stress buffer model of social support

Subculture

Superculture

Tend-and-befriend*

Time-out

Triangulation*

Whole clear message

MEDIA RESOURCES

CENGAGE **brain**

Access an interactive eBook, chapter-specific
interactive learning tools, including flashcards,
quizzes, videos, and more in your Psychology
CourseMate, accessed through CengageBrain.com.

© Dpaint/Dreamstime.com

The faster I go, the behinder I get.

~Anonymous

Job Stress

"The customers and my coworkers are contacting me 24/7 through my office phone, my laptop, and my BlackBerry," Lisa complained to her husband. *"I no longer have a personal life. No wonder we don't have quality time together anymore."* What is Lisa's problem? Lisa has a form of job stress known as **technostress** (Brod, 1982, 1988; Small & Vorgan, 2008) where she is asked to adapt to serious and fundamental changes in her job roles that are driven by new technology.

"Your ideas are as stupid and inane as you are for proposing them," Rebecca's supervisor scolded. Rebecca felt the sting of her boss's reprimand. What made it especially hurtful was that her dressing-down was done in front of her coworkers. What is Rebecca's problem? Rebecca feels stress from having a bully boss, an abusive leader.

"I can barely drag myself out of bed each morning to go to work," Kevin confided to his friend. *"I'm physically exhausted and emotionally spent. I've given everything to my job and gotten nothing but grief in return. Lately, I've been snapping at customers. I could get in trouble, maybe even fired, but I don't care anymore."* What is Kevin's problem? Kevin is suffering from burnout due to excessive and prolonged job stress.

technostress: the pressure to adapt to serious and fundamental changes in job roles that are driven by new technology; may also relate to general difficulty adapting to new technology.

Lisa's, Rebecca's, and Kevin's experiences illustrate some of the myriad forms of job stress. What is job stress? In its simplest form, **job stress** is what we experience when the demands of our work exceed our abilities. However, stress at the job is complex and may relate to a lot of different factors including the specific job roles and demands, the employing organization's culture and leadership, interpersonal stressors related to work, whether the training and resources are available when needed to facilitate completing job tasks, the safety and comfort of the physical work environment, work schedules, job and economic security, technology, and the conflict between the demands of work and the desire to maintain a satisfying personal life.

Physiologically, emotionally, cognitively, and behaviorally, job stressors evoke the same fight-or-flight responses as other types of stressors (i.e., the saber-toothed tigers of our minds). As a result, job stress can adversely affect our health and well-being. In addition, it can lead to lost productivity that is costly to an organization staffed with overstressed workers. Job stress can be dealt with at the personal level or systemically within the organization. Overall, the goal for managing job stress is to be able to work in the optimal zone (recall the Yerkes-Dodson Curve from Chapter 1), where performance levels are best, rather than to eliminate work stress altogether.

MODELS OF ORGANIZATIONAL STRESS

Organizational stress, job stress, and work stress are common terms in the area's literature that have overlapping meanings. Organizational stress refers to how the structure and processes of the organization bring about stress, whereas job stress is specific to the roles, tasks, and demands of a specific job within the organization. The following illustrates how these two terms overlap but also differ. When two departments are unable to work collaboratively then it creates organizational stress. This type of organizational stress will have the biggest impact on the worker whose job is most dependent on performing tasks using information from other departments. For example, in this context the engineer at an automobile company who needs the art design from another department to engineer a new car model will experience more job stress than the engineer whose job it is to make a more efficient muffler from designs developed within his or her department. So job stress is affected by organizational stress but at different degrees depending on the nature of the organizational stress and of the jobs most affected within the organization. The term **work stress** is generic and applies to all manner of work-related contexts including the stress of informal work, self-employment, a formal job, or work in an organization.

There are a number of theoretical models of organizational stress, but five of the most popular are the organizational role, the person-environment fit, the job demands-control, the effort-reward imbalance (ERI), and the organizational injustice model. Following is a brief survey of each. We will be revisiting them throughout the chapter.

Organizational Role Stress

Outlined in their 1964 book entitled *Organizational Stress: Studies in Role Conflict and Ambiguity,* Robert Kahn and his associates (Kahn, Wolfe, Quinn, Snoek, & Rosenthal, 1964) established organizational role theory as one of the first major theoretical frameworks specific to the scientific study of stress in the workplace. In their view, stress involves adjustment to work roles. What is a work role? As described by Beehr and Glazer (2005, p. 10), a work "role can be defined as the social character one 'plays' in an organization." Although there are many elements to Kahn and his colleagues' (1964) model of **organizational role stress** known as the role episode model, the most widely studied concepts from their model are *role conflict, role ambiguity,* and *role overload.* Let us look at each.

Role Conflict Two or more role demands are incompatible with each other. For example, being a responsible worker means working overtime to complete your work tasks, but being a responsible parent means going to your child's soccer game instead. This role conflict creates stress.

Role Ambiguity The duties, responsibilities, and performance expectations of the job are not clearly defined by organizational leaders. For example, a new worker in an organization is unsure how much time to devote to report writing and how much to spend improving sagging customer relations. As a result, the new employee experiences stress.

qualitative overload:
a term used within
the role episode model
of organizational
stress, indicating that
the employee does
not have the required
competencies to
complete the tasks.

quantitative overload:
a term used within the
role episode model of
organizational stress
indicating that there are
insufficient resources
to complete the tasks
assigned in the time
provided.

Role Overload   The work load is too great and there are insufficient resources to complete the tasks assigned in the time provided, an experience referred to as **quantitative overload,** or the employee does not have the required competencies to complete the tasks even when there is sufficient time, an experience known as **qualitative overload.**

Have you ever been served a cold meal at a restaurant because the server was too busy waiting on all the other tables to pick up your hot plate when it first came out of the kitchen? If so, perhaps it is because the server was experiencing quantitative overload from being assigned too many tables to get the hot food out on time. Even though the server was competent, it was simply impossible to get all the hot plates out on time with so many tables to serve. However, what if your cold plate was a result of your server having responsibility for a small number of tables but not being able to ever master how to balance the various duties of taking orders, filling tea glasses, and bringing out hot plates on time? That server would have experienced qualitative overload stress from lack of competency to efficiently perform these duties.

Person-Environment Fit Model

**person-environment
(P-E) fit:** a model of
organizational stress
that states that stress
occurs when there is a
poor match between the
worker and the work
environment.

Another model of organizational stress, the **person-environment (P-E) fit** model (Edwards, Caplan, & Harrison, 1998), states that stress occurs when there is a poor fit between the worker and the work environment. Determination of a *misfit* is subjective and occurs when a worker *perceives* that his or her (1) abilities do not match the demands of the organization or (2) needs are not met by the organization—the greater the misfit, the greater the stress. For example, an elementary school teacher who enjoys working with young children is a better fit than one who feels more comfortable working with adults. All things being equal, the teacher who prefers working with children would experience less P-E fit stress than the one who prefers working with adults.

Job Demands-Control (Job-Strain) Model

job demands-control:
a model of organiza-
tional stress that states
that when a worker
experiences high
psychological demands
paired with minimal
control then job strain
occurs.

low decision latitude:
a worker's experience of
having insufficient skills
or authority over one's
job to autonomously
complete the assigned
job tasks.

job strain: the harmful
consequences that result
from exposure to job
stressors.

In the **job demands-control** (also known as job-strain) model (Karasek, 1979), *strain* occurs when a worker experiences high psychological job demands yet has little control over the job (Figure 9.1). This lack of control is known as **low decision latitude,** a condition characterized by having insufficient skills or authority over one's job to complete the job tasks autonomously. According to this model, which medical professionals do you think should have more strain, nurses or physicians? If you guessed nurses then you are correct. Why? Nurses have high psychological demands combined with low decision latitude (low control) (Brown, James, & Mills, 2006) because they have less patient care decision-making authority than physicians. Physicians provide the patient care directives and nurses follow them rather than the other way around.

The term **job strain** is used in this model and other organizational stress contexts to refer to harmful *consequences* that result from exposure to job stressors. There may be emotion-related strains (e.g., frustration, anger, and anxiety), physiological-related strains (e.g., cardiovascular, gastrointestinal, or musculoskeletal problems), and job-related strains (e.g., low motivation, low

	Low Job Demands	High Job Demands
Low Control	Passive Job	High-Strain Job
High Control	Low-Strain Job	Active Job

FIGURE **9.1**   Karasek's Job Demands-Control Model

High demands coupled with low control leads to high job strain.   SOURCE: Cooper, C. L., Dewe, P. J., & O'Driscoll, M. P. (2001), *Organizational stress: A review and critique of theory, research, and applications*, p. 135. Thousand Oaks, CA: Sage. Copyright © 2001 Sage Publications. Reprinted by permission of SAGE Publications.

satisfaction, and absenteeism). According to this model, the less autonomy and control (latitude to make job decisions) one has over one's significant job stressors, the more strain one experiences. A factor like social support from coworkers can serve to moderate or buffer the health consequences of job strain. Likewise, tangible resources like high income can have a protective effect.

Effort-Reward Imbalance (ERI) Model

effort-reward imbalance (ERI) model: a model of organizational stress that states that high-cost low-gain work efforts are stressful.

The **effort-reward imbalance (ERI) model** (Siegrist, 1996) proposes that high-cost, low-gain work efforts are stressful. When we give a lot to our work we expect *reciprocity* in the way of high reward. The reward may be in the form of money, status, or esteem. However, when we experience an imbalance in reciprocity, where high work effort is met with low reward, we experience distress. This loss of control threatens our sense of mastery and self-efficacy over our occupational role status, resulting in further stress such as fear of being laid off or being passed over for promotion.

Organizational Injustice Model

The **organizational injustice model** assumes that stress occurs when the organization's interpersonal transactions, procedures, or outcomes are perceived as unfair (Cropanzano, Goldman, & Benson, 2005). According to this model organizational injustice can occur under a variety of circumstances. For example, organizational injustice occurs when employees are not treated with respect and dignity, if workplace procedures are unethical or inconsistent, or when the organization rewards its employees in ways that are not in proportion to their effort. Therefore, these outcomes are seen as not only unfair but also sources of stress.

STRESS AND OCCUPATIONS

Some occupations and jobs appear to be more stressful than others. Researchers of occupational stress have turned their attention primarily to police, firefighters, social workers, teachers, health care workers, and office and managerial workers because of the stress associated with these occupations. What follows is a brief examination of the stress associated with these occupations. Although this may create a negative impression of these occupations, keep in mind that there also are many positive qualities of these jobs that are not covered due to the limited scope of this section. For example, police, firefighters, social workers, teachers, and health care workers work in noble professions that promote the public good so that we may experience enhanced safety, security, health, well-being, and education. Office and managerial workers perform essential functions for their organizations and businesses so that we may enjoy the goods and services they produce. Therefore, although the focus of this section is on the stress of these professions, this information should not discount their positives. What then are some of the stresses these professions encounter?

Police and firefighters deal with long periods of boredom punctuated by episodes of physical danger. For example, police work involves tedious paper work, red tape, involvement in the court system, and shift work that can each contribute to an officer's overall stress load. Sulsky and Smith (2005, p. 85) remark that "because of the erratic nature of police work, officers often report both work overload (too much to do) and work underload (too little to do)." Police and firefighters have higher rates of alcoholism and divorce than the general population, statistics that may reflect the stress of working in their occupations.

People-oriented service professions such as social workers, teachers, and health care workers generally experience high stress and a greater likelihood of *burnout* (we will discuss burnout in more detail later). Sulsky and Smith (2005, pp. 86–87) note that "social service workers report little positive feedback from their jobs or the public, unsafe work environments, frustration in dealing with bureaucracy and excessive paperwork, a sense of personal responsibility for clients, and work overload. . . . Teachers indicate that excessive paperwork, lack of adequate supplies/facilities, work overload, and lack of positive feedback are salient stressors." Student misbehavior including display of poor attitudes, rudeness, and discipline problems also are stressors indicated by teachers (see Tatar, 2009, for discussion). In the United Kingdom, one study (Jones & Hodgson, 1998) found that teachers reported the second highest rates of depression, anxiety, and work stress among all the occupations surveyed.

The research is sparse in the area of stress of university and college professors but professors also report high stress levels. In a large sample study that surveyed over 1,200 faculty from 80 universities in the United States, the respondents reported that at least 60% of their overall life stress was due to their work stressors (Gmelch, Lovrich, & Wilke, 1984). Although professors may have many *specific* sources of stress such as pressure to publish or to secure funding for research projects, interpersonal conflict stress (see Chapter 8) was found in one study of 124 professors to be their number one *general* stressor (Narayanan, Menon, & Spector, 1999).

Of the medical professionals studied, nurses continue to receive the most research attention. Stressors in the nursing field, especially in the United States, include high-demand, low-control work (low decision latitude), shift work, patient death and dying issues, uncooperative patients or patient family members, and difficulties with physicians and other medical staff (Lambert & Lambert, 2001). Today's chronic worldwide shortage of nurses also often leads to stress due to organizational understaffing issues.

Physicians, too, experience high levels of stress including dealing with difficult patients, death and dying issues, as well as coping with heavy and complex workloads that involve decision-making responsibility that affects the

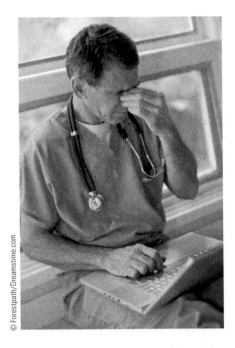

© Forestpath/Dreamstime.com

Nurses experience a high level of stress, but according to Rutledge et al. (2009) physicians reported approximately a 50% average higher emotional stress level than nurses. If nurses have lower decision latitude than physicians, why would physicians score significantly higher on emotional stress? What other model could better explain these findings?

health and longevity of their patients. A recent study (Rutledge et al., 2009) of 185 physicians and 119 nurses working in teaching hospitals asked participants to carry handheld computers so they could record their stress levels when randomly prompted throughout each work day during the study's 1-week time span. The study found that physicians reported approximately a 50% average higher emotional stress level than nurses. These results run contrary to what the job demands-control model predicts that we discussed earlier. Recall that the model predicts that nurses would have more stress because they have lower decision latitude than physicians. The authors of the study did not test the job demands-control model so they did not address this issue and the reasons for these findings are not established. Perhaps related to this excess stress, the rate of divorce, suicide, and abuse of prescription drugs among physicians is higher than in the general population (Council on Scientific Affairs, 1987; O'Connor & Spickard, 1997; Sotile & Sotile, 1996).

Surprising to some, clerical and secretarial work are highly stressful occupations. In fact, results from the seminal prospective Framingham Heart Study indicated that coronary heart disease rates were nearly twice as high among women clerical workers as homemakers (Haynes & Feinleib, 1980). Compared to academic and sales work, clerical work rates the highest in work overload and perceived lack of control (Narayanan et al., 1999).

Although managers have greater job control than many occupational groups, they also report high levels of stress. Upon reviewing the relevant literature, Sulsky and Smith (2005, p. 90) concluded that "some important stressors for managers are work overload, conflict and ambiguity in defining the managerial role, and difficult work relationships." Managers who have difficulty coping with these stressors are more likely to report higher levels of anxiety, depression, and alcohol consumption.

WORK STRESS AND HEALTH

Work stress, like any form of stress, may affect one's health and well-being. Researchers in the area have focused primarily on models of work stress that are used to predict cardiovascular disease. Three models in particular seem to have predictive value. The one most often cited and tested is the job demands-control (also known as job-strain) model (Karasek, 1979) discussed earlier. However, the previously discussed ERI model and the organizational injustice model also are important models establishing a link between work stress and adverse health.

Kivimaki et al. (2006) conducted a meta-analysis of 14 prospective cohort studies involving a total of 83,014 employees that examined the association between work stress (as measured by the job-strain, ERI, or organizational injustice model) and coronary heart disease (CHD). The authors of the study determined that work stress confers an additional 50% excess CHD risk. After adjusting for other potential CHD risk variables, Kivimaki et al. (2006) estimated that workers who experience high job strain (high demand and low control) have a 1.16 risk ratio, high efforts and low reward (ERI model) a 1.58 risk ratio, and organizational injustice a 1.62 risk ratio. They also noted that some individual studies found no CHD risk for job strain, and that such examples of inconsistent evidence could be due to methodological issues such as how frequently job strain was assessed. All the studies that found no CHD risk only assessed job strain once rather than over multiple points in time.

The INTERHEART study first discussed in Chapter 5 examined 5,426 workers across 52 countries who had experienced a first myocardial infarction (MI) and matched them to controls of the same age, gender, and site. Results indicated that workers who experienced several periods of stress had risk adjusted odds of an MI of 1.38, but those who had *permanent* stress at work were more than twice as likely to experience an MI as their matched controls (adjusted odds ratio of 2.14) (Rosengren et al., 2004).

Another large-scale investigation, the Whitehall II study, examined 10,308 London-based civil servants (white-collar office workers) over multiple phases spanning from 1985–1988 (phase 1) to 2002–2004 (phase 7). Using a measure of job strain (demands-control model), they determined that among 37- to 49-year-old participants by phase 2, "there was a clear dose-response association between greater reports of work stress and higher risks of incident CHD events" (Chandola et al., 2008, p. 642). In other words, the more work stress the workers experienced, the greater the likelihood they would have an MI. Their average adjusted risk ratio was 1.68. The investigators also found evidence of a higher morning rise in cortisol among workers with higher work stress. In addition, they were able to determine that negative health behaviors such as poor diet and low physical activity and the metabolic syndrome (see Chapter 5) explained about one-third of the risk of work stress on CHD.

One study (Wang et al., 2007) found that women hospitalized after an acute coronary event with high job strain at baseline experienced coronary artery diameter *narrowing* of 5.2% at a 3-year follow-up—suggesting that work stress accelerated their coronary artery disease progression. Yet women in the group who had no significant marital or work stress at baseline had coronary artery diameter *widening* of 7.1% at that same follow-up—suggesting an improvement.

Another study by Gallo, Bogart, Vranceanu, and Walt (2004) determined that women who had both a lower status occupation and high job stress had higher ambulatory systolic blood pressure, an autonomic nervous system reaction that likely puts them at greater risk for cardiovascular disease.

Thus, there appears to be abundant evidence that certain types of work stress contribute to the development of cardiovascular risk including MI. The causal mechanisms are not yet clearly known, though stress-related negative health behaviors, the metabolic syndrome, autonomic nervous system, and neuroendocrine factors likely play a role. Although models of work stress help us understand their role in the development of heart disease and MI, they are not the whole story.

Shift Work and Other Work Schedules

Another important area of investigation that reveals a link between work and negative health consequences is work schedule—specifically shift work, night work, and long-hour work schedules. Think of a time when you traveled by air across time zones, perhaps during a red-eye flight. What did your body feel like afterwards? Were you alert and full of energy or did you feel drowsy and sluggish? How about a time when you may have stayed up most of the night cramming for an exam? Were you at your best the next day? Chances are that if you had any of these experiences, it impaired your concentration and overall ability to function well the next day. The reason for your feeling "jet lag" or lack of concentration after pulling an all-nighter is because it disturbed your *circadian rhythm*. **Circadian rhythm** refers to our 24-hour biological cycle linked to the light-dark cycle that regulates our internal physiological processes such as, for example, core body temperature, hormone levels, blood pressure, heart rate, and so forth. When this is disturbed, it disrupts our concentration and ability to perform work tasks well.

circadian rhythm: the 24-hour biological cycle linked to the light-dark cycle that regulates one's internal physiological processes.

Working nights means we are working at times when our circadian rhythm is at low ebb, like a car in idle. According to our biological programming, this is a problem because it creates a mismatch—our biological engine idles during work time and cranks up during sleep time. Because we are fighting our natural rhythms, we tend to have disturbances in both our wake (e.g., fatigue, drowsiness) and sleep phases (e.g., insomnia, sleep disruptions) of the circadian cycle.

shift work: a type of work schedule that involves large periods of work outside the normal daylight hours.

Shift work, a type of work schedule that 20% to 25% of workers follow, "refers to any regular employment outside the 7 a.m.–6 p.m. interval" (Sulsky & Smith, 2005, p. 100). It may include rotating shifts in which workers are on a system that changes shifts periodically (e.g., from a morning shift to an evening shift) or on an unchanging permanent shift (e.g., always a night shift). Documented adverse effects of shift work include chronic fatigue, loss of sleep, declines in memory and cognitive functioning, family and social life disruptions, and detrimental health conditions (Bourdouxhe et al., 1999; Rouch, Wild, Ansiau, & Marquie, 2005).

What are some of the detrimental health conditions associated with shift work? The most prevalent health problems found are those related to the gastrointestinal (GI) system. For example, Costa (1996, p. 10) noted that shift workers often complain about digestive disorders such as "disturbances of appetite, irregularity of the bowel movements with prevalent constipation, dyspepsia, heartburn, abdominal pains, grumbling and flatulence." More serious conditions such as chronic gastritis and peptic ulcers also are more prevalent. One reason suggested for the increased prevalence of GI problems among shift workers is that they have less access to healthy and nutritional foods during the night shift. However, current evidence does not support this hypothesis. Therefore, GI vulnerability of shift workers is more likely due to other factors such as sleep deficits or circadian rhythm disruptions (Vener, Szabo, & Moore, 1989).

Shift work also seems to increase risk for cardiovascular disease. Boggild and Knutsson (1999) reviewed 17 relevant studies and estimated that shift workers have a 40% increased risk for cardiovascular disease than their day worker counterparts. For example, Kawachi et al. (1995) in the Nurses' Health prospective study of 79,109 female nurses found that long-term rotating shift work (i.e., 6 or more years) as compared to never working shifts conferred a 1.51 adjusted elevated risk of CHD. That is, nurses who worked long-term rotating shifts were one and a half times more likely to develop CHD.

Working long hour schedules also is associated with negative effects, including adverse health effects (Van der Hulst, 2003). Although the research is sparse in the area, working long hours (more than 60 hours a week) as well as lack of sleep may be associated with an increased risk for experiencing an MI (Liu & Tanaka, 2002). In Japan, the phenomenon of working long hours leading to an early death is common enough that the Japanese have a word to describe it. The word *karoshi* literally means "death from overwork." Such long hour schedules may be detrimental to health because they lead to "increased fatigue, reduced motivation, prolonged exposure to work stressors, and the use of poor lifestyle habits such as smoking, lack of exercise, and inadequate diet" (Totterdell, 2005, p. 41). Therefore, both shift work and working long hours positively correlate with increased cardiovascular risk.

A few large-scale prospective studies indicate that shift work and night work also increase the risk of breast cancer and colorectal cancer. For example, the Nurse's Health Study followed 78,562 women nurses for 10 years, and those who worked 30 or more years on the night shift showed a relative risk for breast cancer of 1.36 (Schernhammer et al., 2001). Likewise, a similar number of nurses from the Nurse's Health Study were tracked for the same period and the women who worked for 15 years or more were found to have a 1.35 relative risk of developing colorectal cancer (Schernhammer et al., 2003).

Why did these night workers have an increased risk of cancer? Although the exact mechanisms are not known, the most popular hypothesis relates to the hormone melatonin. The **pineal gland,** a tiny gland shaped like a pine cone (hence the name *pine*al) in the center of the brain, releases melatonin during the dark phase and inhibits its release during the light phase of the light-dark circadian cycle. **Melatonin** lowers our body temperature and causes drowsiness, which helps us sleep at night. The hormone typically reaches its peak

melatonin: a hormone released by the pineal gland that lowers one's body temperature and causes drowsiness.

concentration in the middle of the night. However, environmental lighting, such as the lighting in a hospital during the night, inhibits melatonin production.

Melatonin has an inhibiting effect on the production of estrogen and on the growth and proliferation of cancer cells. Therefore, suppression of melatonin through exposure to light during the nighttime peak concentration periods likely results in an overall reduced level of blood melatonin levels. The reduced levels of melatonin weaken its ability to suppress estrogen, which then has an indirect effect on breast cancer risk. Estrogen is known to directly stimulate hormone-sensitive tumors in the breast. Further, a reduction in melatonin levels directly limits the amount of anticarcinogenic protection this hormone can provide. Schernhammer et al. (2003) note that some studies indicate that patients with colorectal cancer have lower levels of melatonin, supporting the contention that suppressed melatonin may be a mechanism explaining the increased colorectal cancer risk for night workers. In addition, the direct anticarcinogenic effect of melatonin applies to other cancer types as well, such as breast cancer.

In a review of the literature on the relationship between shift work and cancer, Costa, Haus, and Stevens (2010) note that sleep deprivation among shift workers may lead to immune suppression, which also may contribute to increased risk for cancer. Further, disruption of the circadian clock genes that regulate cell cycles can lead to uncontrolled cellular growth, a condition associated with tumor growth. They suggest that, although there is supportive evidence for the connection between shift work and cancer, more work needs to be done before we can more accurately assess the complex factors that may contribute to shift workers' increased cancer risk.

WHAT IS BURNOUT?

Remember at the beginning of this chapter Kevin confided to his friend that he was physically exhausted and emotionally spent? Kevin suffers from burnout. Have you ever experienced burnout? If so, how did you know you were burned out? What do you think caused your burnout? If you are like most people, you have an intuitive understanding of burnout. You recognize when you feel burned out. You probably see it as caused by work, school, or caregiving stress. You know that it feels like emotional depletion—that your emotional reserves are exhausted. It negatively affects your motivation and ability satisfactorily to complete your work in a timely fashion or provide your service (e.g., caregiving) with a positive outlook.

Most of us have at one time or another experienced some burnout, and as a result we have an experiential understanding of the phenomenon. Nevertheless, surprisingly, researchers still struggle with reaching a consensus on a precise definition. Arie Shirom (2011, p. 223), one of the leading researchers in the area, defines **burnout** "as an affective reaction to ongoing stress whose core content is the gradual depletion over time of individuals' intrinsic energetic resources, including the components of *emotional exhaustion, physical fatigue,* and *cognitive weariness.*" Notice that the key words are *affective, ongoing stress, gradual depletion, energy, emotional exhaustion, physical fatigue,* and *cognitive*

burnout: emotional exhaustion and depletion due to ongoing stress with corollary physical and mental fatigue.

INSIGHT EXERCISE **9.1**

If you would like to determine your burnout level, then take the short version of Malach-Pines (2005) Burnout Measure.

Burnout Measure: Short Version

Please use the following scale to answer the question: When you think about your work overall, how often do you feel the following?

1	2	3	4	5	6	7
never	almost never	rarely	sometimes	often	very often	always

Tired _____

Disappointed with people _____

Hopeless _____

Trapped _____

Helpless _____

Depressed _____

Physically weak/Sickly _____

Worthless/Like a failure _____

Difficulties sleeping _____

"I've had it" _____

In order to calculate your burnout score add your responses to the 10 items and divide by 10 _____.

Now that you have taken the measure and determined your overall burnout score, what does it mean? According to Malach-Pines (2005), if you scored between 0 and 2.4 you have little or no burnout. A score of 2.5 to 3.4 indicates that you are at risk for burnout. Unfortunately, a score of 3.5 or higher means that you are burned out with high burnout being in the 4.5 to 5.4 range and very high burnout in the 5.5 or higher range. If you are burned out you may want to use some of the strategies discussed in this chapter for dealing with burnout or consult a counselor for more assistance.

How well do you think this measure captures the concept of burnout as you may have experienced it? The concept of burnout measured by this instrument is slightly different than the three-component burnout constructs presented by Arie Shirom or Christina Maslach that are discussed elsewhere in this section. Notice also that the Malach-Pines measure directly taps depression, which suggests that the author of this scale believes there is some overlap between burnout and depression. The issue of how much overlap there is between burnout and depression is an important question that is discussed later in this section. In spite of its differences from the other constructs of burnout, this quick snapshot instrument gives you a good overall indication of your general level of burnout.

SOURCE: *Based on Malach-Pines, A. (2005), The Burnout Measure, Short Version,* International Journal of Stress Management, *12, 78–88. Appendix, p. 88.*

TABLE **9.1**   The Top Three Themes Associated with Vigor

Shraga and Shirom (2009) interviewed participants to determine what themes they associated with vigor. Quotes of the participants indicate their personal experiences with vigor.

Theme	Quote
Meaningful interactions	"This [vigorous] feeling doesn't necessarily have to do with my job's conditions. It is often more related to people: a warm connection, a good one, an interaction can create this feeling." "When people around me are nice, when they express to me their appreciation for something I did." "Behaviors of true friendship, friends that come to support you when it is needed."
Challenge	"About a week ago, my boss gave me a special project, something quite complex. I did it, and I did it well although it was complicated. It made me feel very satisfied and I felt vigorous. . . ." "A few days ago a man came to see me. He had some very unclear symptoms and I sent him to take some tests, based on my diagnosis. The test results showed that I was right on the mark, although his situation was very unique. This challenge of solving an unusual problem, giving a correct diagnosis [creates this feeling of vigor]." "I had a creative idea on how to solve a major problem we had been having for a long time." "Interest in the work, just this week a new project came in and I learnt a new subject, something mentally intriguing."
Success	"It happened when I was working on a project, which turned out to have a very successful result. I felt I had received very positive feedback . . . from the result of the work itself. This made me feel emotional energy and had a physical effect as well." "Feeling vigorous comes from success, like when I built this program that worked properly and everyone was happy with it." "When I get the end-product and see that the investment was worthwhile."

SOURCE: Shraga, O., & Shirom, A. (2009), The construct validity of vigor and its antecedents: A qualitative study, *Human Relations*, 62; 2, 271–291. Copyright © 2009 Sage Publications. Reprinted by permission of SAGE Publications.

vigor: represents the positive pole on a burnout continuum in Shirom's model of burnout characterized by emotional, physical, and cognitive vibrancy.

weariness. So according to Shirom, burnout is a long-term process mediated by our emotional reactions to stress that saps our emotional, physical, and mental energy reserves. According to his model, a worker with opposite characteristics will have **vigor,** a positive psychological state characterized by *emotional energy, physical strength,* and *cognitive liveliness* (Shraga & Shirom, 2009). Workplace meaningful interactions, challenge, and success are the top three activities positively related to vigor (Shraga & Shirom, 2009) (Table 9.1). Could promoting workplace vigor then be a good antidote to burnout?

Christina Maslach (1998), the pioneer researcher in the area most closely associated with the measurement and conceptualization of burnout, presents a similar though slightly different definition and model of burnout. Maslach's (1998, p. 68) initial interest in the phenomenon was spurred by a general recognition that many workers in the helping professions (e.g. therapists, human service providers, educators, health care professionals) experience stress from their "ongoing and intense level of personal, emotional contact." She notes that the term *burnout* emerged from everyday language and not from scholarly theory. Therefore, she attempted to determine what the term represented through developing a self-report instrument that captured the phenomenon as understood by the general population. Her original instrument, the Maslach Burnout Inventory (MBI) (Maslach & Jackson, 1986), focused on the people-oriented occupations. Later versions were applied to other occupational categories as well.

Based on Maslach's understanding of the concept from her test development research, she presents a three-dimensional model of burnout. The dimensions are *emotional exhaustion, cynicism*, and *reduced efficacy*. Let us look at each.

1. Emotional Exhaustion   A person feels emotionally depleted, drained, and lacking in emotional resources. Two of the major reasons for this exhaustion are work overload or work-related interpersonal conflicts. Although the evidence does not support a negative relationship between the whole construct of burnout and work performance, it does support the specific dimension of emotional exhaustion as being related to declines in work performance (Taris, 2006). This dimension represents the *individual stress* component of burnout.

2. Cynicism   Originally referred to as *depersonalization,* this dimension refers to disillusionment, a loss of idealism, negativity, detachment, hostility, and lack of concern. Cynicism represents a way to protect oneself against the overload of emotional exhaustion—to create a buffer of detachment. This dimension represents the *interpersonal* component of burnout.

3. Reduced Efficacy   This dimension is characterized by feelings of diminished self-efficacy, personal competency, and productivity. These feelings arise from a self-assessment of one's inadequacy to help others or to be an effective worker. Counter to what one would expect the evidence does not support the idea that reduced efficacy due to burnout leads to objective work performance declines (Taris, 2006). This dimension embodies the *self-evaluation* component of burnout.

Maslach (1998) regards burnout as residing on one end of a continuum with *engagement* anchoring the other end. **Engagement** represents the positive polarity of her three dimensions and "consists of a state of high *energy* (rather than exhaustion), strong *involvement* (rather than cynicism), and a sense of *efficacy* (rather than a reduced sense of accomplishment)" (Maslach, 1998, p. 73). Burnout can be prevented by focusing on ways to reduce its risk or by focusing on how to strengthen engagement. According to Maslach, work settings that foster the three components of engagement, that is, energy, involvement, and efficacy, are more likely to promote employee well-being and productivity.

engagement: represents in Maslach's model of burnout the positive polarity of her three dimensions characterized by high energy, involvement, and sense of efficacy.

As you may notice, burnout has some qualities such as fatigue and loss of energy that are similar to depression. You might wonder if burnout is just depression under a different name or a distinctly different phenomenon. If so, you are in good company because researchers ask the same question. Let us look at their evidence to gain some clarity about the concept of burnout. First, we can see that burnout is conceptually different than depression because it is usually associated with work environments as compared to depression, which generalizes across many situations. Second, upon closer inspection, note that there is more complexity in the clinical syndrome of depression than burnout because depression includes a wide range of symptoms not typically associated with burnout such as suicidal ideation, ahedonia (lack of pleasure), and significant weight loss (not due to dieting) or gain to name a few. Last, the research indicates that although burnout and clinical depression are moderately correlated, sharing around 26% of their variance, they also are distinct constructs with *cynicism* and *reduced efficacy* only weakly overlapping with depression (see Shirom, 2011, for discussion).

Upon reaching advanced stages of burnout, persons may ultimately develop symptoms of depression if their general coping strategies fail, but advanced burnout states do not necessarily lead to depression. Instead, advanced burnout could lead to a hardening of one's cynical detached perspective toward clients or customers, that is, to the development of a *dehumanizing* outlook toward them. Such a hardened outlook could coexist with depression or stand alone as a symptom independent of depression (Shirom, 2011).

BURNOUT AND HEALTH

Are there adverse health consequences associated with burnout? Melamed et al. (2006a) reviewed the empirical evidence primarily from longitudinal studies but also from some case control studies (cross-sectional) using measures of vital exhaustion (Kop, Hamulyak, Pernot, & Appels, 1998) and burnout using the Shirom-Melamed Burnout Measure (SMBM) (Toker, Shirom, Shapira, Berliner, & Melamed, 2005). The **vital exhaustion** concept relates to burnout and involves a low-energy state, sleep disturbances, extreme fatigue, irritability, and feelings of demoralization, whereas the SMBM measures Shirom's (2011, p. 223) burnout construct of "emotional exhaustion, physical fatigue, and cognitive weariness" discussed earlier. Both seem to tap into the physiological dimensions of burnout.

In general, Melamed et al. (2006a) determined that after adjusting for traditional cardiovascular risk factors, workers with high levels of vital exhaustion had a two- to threefold increased risk of experiencing future CHD, of having a fatal MI, or of experiencing sudden cardiac death. Burnout also is associated with a relative risk of a CHD and an MI of the same magnitude as vital exhaustion. These researchers caution that the measures of vital exhaustion and the SMBM overlap somewhat with measures of depression (e.g., fatigue, loss of energy), and as a result, there is the possibility that these measures tap into depression. Because depression also is a risk factor for heart disease (see Chapter 5), future researchers will need to include measures of depression in their studies to tease out its effects from those of burnout before they can get a more valid assessment of the independent effects of burnout on health.

Ahola, Vaananen, Koskinen, Kouvonen, and Shirom (2010) recently conducted a 10-year prospective study of 7,396 Finnish forest industry employees using the Maslach Burnout Inventory–General Survey and found that after making adjustments for traditional risk factors, the emotional exhaustion measure of the inventory statistically predicted all-cause mortality for younger employees. They determined that the most common causes of death among the burned-out workers were alcohol use related, coronary artery disease, suicide, accidents, lung cancer in men, and breast cancer in women. Ahola et al. (2010) suggest that some of these causes may be related to burnout's overlap with depression and some to traditional mechanisms for developing coronary diseases. For instance, suicide deaths more likely relate to depression rather than burnout. However, the coronary artery disease deaths found are likely related to mechanisms that link specifically to burnout, though we cannot entirely rule out the role of possible depression. For example, Melamed et al. (2006a, p. 206) presented evidence that vital exhaustion and burnout are related to coronary risk factors such as "the metabolic syndrome, dysregulation of the hypothalamic-pituitary-adrenal axis along with sympathetic nervous system activation, sleep disturbances, systemic inflammation, impaired immunity functions, blood coagulation and fibrinolysis, and poor health behaviors" (see Chapter 5).

Besides burnout's role in the development of cardiovascular disease, it also predicts the development of type 2 diabetes. In a prospective study of 677 apparently healthy workers followed for 3 to 5 years, Melamed and his associates (Melamed, Shirom, Toker, & Shapira, 2006b) determined that burnout at baseline increased the risk of developing type 2 diabetes by almost twofold even after adjusting for other relevant risk factors. In addition, Melamed (2009) discovered in his prospective study of 650 workers who were healthy at baseline that their initial burnout levels predicted their risk of developing neck, shoulder, or low back pain at the study's 3- to 5-year follow-up. He found a 1.67 increased risk after adjusting for possible confounding variables. Therefore, it appears that burnout is not only a risk for heart disease, but also for other health conditions such as type 2 diabetes and musculoskeletal pain.

BURNOUT PREVENTION AND TREATMENT

Although there is voluminous research on the phenomenon of burnout, there is surprisingly little empirical evidence documenting how to prevent and treat it. Sulsky and Smith (2005) reviewed several organizational strategies for reducing burnout that include (1) hiring additional employees to reduce individual employee work overload—though realistically, they acknowledge, this is usually not feasible; (2) instituting job orientations and realistic job preview programs for new employees to prevent burnout by dispelling any initial unrealistic perceptions, that is, over-idealizations, that new employees may have about the job; (3) giving employees realistic and timely job performance feedback to prevent any false perceptions of low self-efficacy; (4) arranging for the use of worker social support groups; and (5) using workplace group cognitive restructuring intervention programs (cognitive-behavioral approaches; see Chapter 10) to reduce burnout. Each of these strategies should work in theory though, to date, most have not been empirically tested. There is, however, some empirical support for the use of cognitive restructuring interventions. The researchers van Dierendonck, Schaufeli, and Buunk (1998) found that cognitive restructuring training that focused on workers looking at their situation differently; examining their expectations, goals, and plans; as well as learning relaxation skills reduced emotional exhaustion, but not the other two components of burnout represented by Malach's model (i.e., cynicism and reduced efficacy).

Smith and Moss (2009) write about the importance of *self-care* to prevent burnout and impairment of psychologists. Their recommendations are applicable to other helping professionals and many other occupational groups as well.

As the name implies, **self-care** means that each individual takes responsibility for using strategies that prevent or minimize burnout and other forms of professional impairment. Some of these approaches are broad and designed to enhance one's emotional well-being such as staying self-aware (e.g., monitoring burnout tendencies), using humor, sharing quality time with friends and family, setting limits and boundaries, engaging in wellness behaviors (exercise, good diet, regular sleep), enjoying leisure activities including taking vacations, and practicing one's spiritual beliefs. Their other approaches focus on occupational strategies such as staying current and informed to maintain or increase professional competencies (e.g., attending professional development workshops), consulting with other professionals on a regular basis (including perhaps a mentor), exercising greater control over one's work environment when appropriate, and maintaining a healthy balance between work and personal life.

WORKPLACE HARASSMENT AND DISCRIMINATION

workplace discrimination: hostile behaviors directed toward workers by other employees because of the target persons' identity group characteristics.

sexual harassment: the engagement in gender-based insulting or hostile behaviors, sexual coercion, or the application of unwanted attention or pressure of a sexual nature not tied to job outcomes by one worker to another worker.

Besides the models of workplace stress discussed earlier, workplace harassment and discrimination also are important stressors. **Workplace harassment** refers to hostile behaviors directed toward workers by other employees because of the target persons' identity group characteristics such as age, gender, national origin, race, religion, disabilities, or sexual orientation. **Workplace discrimination** refers to workers receiving adverse employment opportunities because of their identity group's characteristics.

Most of the stress research in the area of workplace harassment has been conducted on **sexual harassment.** Gender-based harassment may include one or more of the following: (1) insulting or hostile behaviors targeting gender, (2) unwanted attention or pressure of a sexual nature that is not tied to job outcomes applied by one worker to another worker, or (3) **sexual coercion,** a form of pressure for sexual involvement tied to job outcomes (e.g., sex for promotion). In their review of the research in the area, Rospenda and Richman (2005) estimate that at least 50% of women will likely experience workplace sexual harassment in their lifetime and 15% of men have been sexually harassed. They further estimate that 40% of racial and ethnic minorities will experience worker discrimination during their lifetime. African Americans will experience an even higher percentage. Research documenting the percentage of harassment and discrimination based on other characteristics (e.g., age, disability, sexual orientation, religion) is minimal and hard to quantify accurately, although there is plenty of anecdotal evidence documenting older age, younger age, disability, and sexual orientation workplace harassment and discrimination.

Rospenda and Richman (2005) note that research points to women who are single, younger, and less educated as the demographic group most likely to be sexually harassed. Besides these demographic factors, other factors that are associated with higher levels of sexual harassment include organizational tolerance of this behavior (e.g., lax policies and enforcement), work contexts where men significantly outnumber women, or contexts where women are working in traditionally "male" occupations (e.g., construction, law enforcement, engineering).

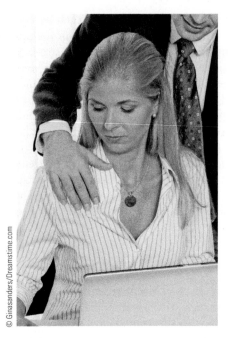

© Ginasanders/Dreamstime.com

Sexual harassment at work is a cause of job stress. At least 50% of women will likely experience workplace sexual harassment in their lifetime. Men may also be sexually harassed. What would you do if you were being sexually harassed at work?

Sexual harassment stress is associated with a greater likelihood of job turnover, use of sick leave, and loss of work productivity (United States Merit Systems Protection Board [USMSPB], 1995). Rospenda and Richman (2005) also note that anxiety, distress, and depression are common adverse reactions to workplace harassment and discrimination. On average, individuals who experience sexual harassment report higher levels of alcohol consumption including alcohol abuse (Richman et al., 1999). In addition, anecdotal evidence suggests that sexual harassment, like other forms of stress, is associated with an increase in physical symptoms such as headaches, insomnia, fatigue, GI disturbances, and teeth grinding among others (Gutek & Koss, 1993). Likewise, racial discrimination is linked to physical symptoms such as greater cardiovascular reactivity (see Chapter 8).

An employee who is experiencing harassment or discrimination has several options available. One strategy is to use the minimally effective response discussed in Chapter 8. Use of the minimally effective response involves setting limits by starting with a minimal level of assertion that can accomplish the objective and escalate in measured steps from there if necessary. For example, a simple matter of fact statement that "I am feeling uncomfortable with X (e.g., your hand on my shoulder)" may be sufficient to cause the offending party to stop, especially if the person is unaware that the behavior is inappropriate. If that minimal response is ineffective, escalating levels of assertiveness may include the following with "1" being the minimum response and "4" the maximum in this example: (1) "as I said, I am feeling uncomfortable with X" stated in a more emphatic manner; (2) "I am feeling uncomfortable and I would like for you to stop (or remove your hand)"; (3) "please stop (or remove your hand), this is unacceptable"; and (4) "if you continue (or do not remove your hand) I will inform your supervisor." Informing a supervisor or a Human Resources representative is always an option if the offensive behavior pattern persists. Keeping a detailed log of interactions with the offending party also is a good idea. In the United States, federal laws enforced by the Equal Employment Opportunity Commission (EEOC) protect against workplace discriminatory harassment based on age, gender, national origin, race, religion, or disabilities.

From an organizational perspective the most effective intervention against harassment and discrimination is a strong and consistently enforced organizational policy. Although there is less research documenting the effectiveness of training programs aimed at both fostering empathy toward victims and changing attitudes and beliefs of potential perpetrators, such programs also may decrease the incidence of harassment and discrimination within the organization.

TIME MANAGEMENT

"Now here you see, it takes all the running you can do, to keep in the same place. If you want to get somewhere else, you must run at least twice as fast as that," explained the Red Queen to Alice in Lewis Carroll's *Through the Looking Glass* (Carroll, 2004, p. 175). Sometimes no matter how fast we work, it is not fast enough to complete our tasks in a timely fashion. The stress of work overload can affect us at our place of employment, home, school, or other areas of everyday life. We can lighten work overload by limit setting (e.g., saying "no" to more requests) when feasible, negotiating a more realistic workload, or changing jobs, but often it is a matter of time management. **Time management** refers to using our time efficiently to accomplish our goals. Effective use of time is a good stress management tool because it reduces the feeling of pressure when we have a backlog of unfinished work or impending deadlines. It improves our productivity and frees time for leisure activities like hobbies, exercise, recreation, and socializing that recharges us and reduces stress.

Before we examine how to manage our time better, let us first look at how we waste it. Five major time wasters are lack of goals, too many goals, procrastination, perfectionism, and boundary intrusions.

1. Lack of Goals   People who do not set goals waste valuable time because they do not know where they are headed. They are like hikers lost in a forest with no compass or sense of direction. Most of their time is spent wandering aimlessly covering the same ground without ever finding their way out. Some individuals suffer from "paralysis of analysis." They often will ruminate endlessly about which goal to pursue and believe there is never sufficient information to make a commitment. Fear of making the wrong decision or too much stress also can create indecisiveness about which goals to pursue.

2. Too Many Goals   These people have too many irons in the fire because they have too many goals and become quickly overloaded. They may experience concentration difficulties or physical fatigue as the worries and pressures of unfinished tasks mount from their tendency to spread themselves thin.

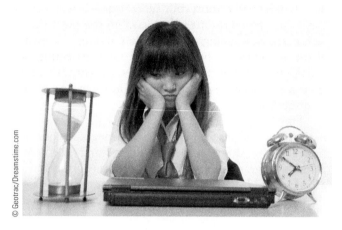

© Geotrac/Dreamstime.com

The stress of time mismanagement

3. Procrastination Individuals who procrastinate view certain tasks as aversive and try to avoid them as long as possible. As a result, they squander valuable time until their deadline is about to approach and then rush to complete the task at the last minute. Some enjoy the thrill of their brinkmanship, the adrenalin rush of living on the edge. Others simply are unable to self-motivate until the anxiety of their impending deadline becomes intolerable. In both cases, they increase the risk of receiving negative consequences if they do not complete their project on time (e.g., a grade penalty for a student's late paper).

Procrastinators may avoid dealing with unwanted or unpleasant tasks by using distraction, daydreaming, wishful thinking, or other methods to kill time so that there is insufficient time left to work on the avoided task. They then can rationalize that they will do the task tomorrow. At the workplace these individuals are often on the prowl for other coworkers to chat with to run out the clock. Procrastinators do better if they nibble on their project a little at a time from the start rather than gorge on it at the last minute, that is, break the big project down into smaller, bite-sized chunks for easier management.

4. Perfectionism Perfectionists often become immersed in trivial detail and lose sight of the big picture. They lack a sense of proportionality and have difficulty calibrating their time to match the importance level of the task. As such, they waste a great deal of time on minor tasks instead of allocating their time proportionally to ensure that major tasks receive the lion's share of their time. They also may engage in endless cycles of repetitive checking and rechecking of their work product in pursuit of perfection. Often perfectionists will avoid working on tasks that they do not feel supremely competent to work on, which leaves the task unattended. In addition, they may be difficult work partners because they sometimes get angry at themselves and others who do not live up to their unrealistic standards and may consequently slow down the progress of their collaborative work projects.

5. Work Interruptions Interruptions, whether they are phone calls or drop-ins, can consume a lot of your time. Some complex projects require a warm-up period before you can build the momentum you need to work steadily toward completion (e.g., creative writing). Once the momentum is interrupted, the project comes to a screeching halt. So these projects in particular need blocks of uninterrupted time to ensure timely completion.

TIME MANAGEMENT STRATEGIES

Linden (2005, p. 97) notes that whereas time management solutions and strategies are very popular in stress management programs and manuals, there is "not a single published, controlled trial of the effect of time management on any hard, stress-related index." Most accounts of time management effectiveness are anecdotal. He further remarks that "given that time management programs have a clearly described set of steps, concrete learnable skills, and a convincing rationale, one would expect positive outcomes, which makes the lack of research all the more striking" (Linden, 2005, p. 97). There is, however, some limited research that demonstrates time management training results in enhanced perception of the control of time, greater job satisfaction, and less job-related somatic tension (see Claessens, van Eerde, & Rutte, 2007, for review). So the concept and strategies of time management are very rational and logical for managing stress, and there is some evidence for their effectiveness, but unfortunately there is generally a lack of hard empirical validation. With that understanding in mind, let's look at seven popular time management strategies.

1. Keep a Daily Time Log The idea is to record information about how you use your time. This raises your awareness of particular times or situations where you are wasting time or could be working in a way that uses time more efficiently.

2. Establish Goals and Prioritize Use a "To-Do List." On the list record all the tasks that you need to do. Large or complex tasks should be broken down into smaller tasks that are also listed. Then prioritize your tasks using an A, B, C goal system. "A" goals are top priority goals (e.g., paying the rent) that have important positive or negative consequences associated with their completion. "B" goals are important, though second to "A" goals (e.g., mowing the lawn). Finally, "C" goals are given the lowest priority (e.g., reorganizing a storage closet). Goals can be reprioritized later if needed so that a "B" priority goal can be upgraded to an "A" goal or downgraded to a "C" goal (e.g., the grass is now tall enough to warrant upgrading the "mowing the lawn" goal to an "A" level). "C" goals that are not completed in 1 month are deleted from the list. This is a rolling list so task items that are completed are deleted and new tasks are added as they arise. Use the Pareto principle to determine how to allocate your time (see the Pareto principle next).

Pareto principle: the principle that only 20% of one's goals contain 80% of the total value; therefore, good time management involves spending most of one's time on the most important 20% of one's goals.

3. Follow the Pareto Principle The Pareto principle states that only 20% of your goals contain 80% of the total value. Therefore, you will wisely use your time by focusing most of it on the 20% with the most value, the "A" priority goals, because the other 80% of your goals contain only 20% of the total value. In other words, spend most of your time on your most important goals because they will reap a disproportionately greater amount of reward.

4. Prune and Weed   File or throw away paper when it crosses your desk rather than letting it pile up. Archive or delete already-read e-mail messages that are filling your inbox. The idea is to process paper or electronic information once rather than repeatedly, unless it is important and needs to be retrieved later. Set limits so that optional tasks are not added to your "To-Do" list when you are experiencing work overload.

5. Set Boundaries to Manage Your Physical Work Space and Technostress   Closing your office door sends an implicit message that you are busy and not to be interrupted unless it is important. Reply to e-mails, text, or phone messages at scheduled times each day rather than throughout the day (e.g., once in the morning and once in the late afternoon). Turn off your cell phone during periods when you are working on a task and wish not to be interrupted. Take time out from focusing on digital media to prevent digital overload (Small & Vorgan, 2008). Manage or limit *digital fog* (digital mental haze), *data smog* (digital overload), *screen sucking* (online addiction), *frazzing* (frantic but ineffective multitasking), and *technostress* to prevent *techno-brain burnout* (Walsh, 2011).

6. Delegate when Feasible and Appropriate   Delegating lower priority tasks enables you to focus more of your time and energy on "A" priority tasks. Many who are reluctant to delegate are perfectionists who believe that if they do not do it themselves, it will not be done correctly. They want to micromanage every detail of the project and do not have the confidence in others to complete the task according to others' styles. In order to change, they need to let go of some of that "need to control" in exchange for getting additional time to pursue their most important goals.

7. Schedule Relaxation Time   Scheduling relaxation time to recharge your batteries seems counterintuitive to some (e.g., Type A personalities). However, the idea is to work more efficiently rather than to just work harder. Charlesworth and Nathan (1985) tell a story about a young man who wanted a job as a lumberjack. The boss tried him out for a week but noticed that although the young man was strong, he chopped down fewer trees each day, starting with 10 trees on Monday and by Friday the aspiring lumberjack was struggling to fell even one tree.

> "Sir," he said, "I'm working harder and harder, but I'm afraid I'm a disappointment to you. I have yet to fell one tree today." "Why do you do so little?" the boss asked. "I'm really trying, Sir," was the response. "Have you taken the time to sharpen your ax, boy?" The boy answered, "No, sir, I really haven't had time because I have been so busy working." The lesson: work sharper, not harder. (p. 230)

STRESS MANAGEMENT EXERCISE 9.1

Managing Time Stress

Would you like to become a better time manager? Have you ever tracked how you use your time? You might be surprised to learn what your time wasters are. Do you ever experience any technostress? If so, you may benefit from determining how much time you spend using digital media including social networking, texting, and online gaming? Keep a log for 48 hours of normal activity. Although it is tempting, you are encouraged not to alter your regular patterns just because you are keeping a log. After all, this exercise is for your benefit. Once you determine where you are using your time inefficiently, develop an action plan for better time management. Refer to the seven time management strategies discussed in this chapter for guidance. Next implement your plan. Try it for a week and see how well it works. If it works well, you may want to continue the plan. If it does not, try making some modifications and develop a new plan for implementation. Remember to "work sharper, not harder" if you want to manage your time stress.

JOB-RELATED WELL-BEING

Let us assume that you work in a job where you manage your job stress well. That is a good start. Now, given that stress is not an issue, does it follow that you must be happy in your job? As you know from previous chapters, even if you eliminated any negative feelings you may have about your job because you were managing your job stress efficiently, at best you would move into a neutral state unless you added positive feelings. So in order to experience happiness and well-being at work, you would need not only to manage your stress well, but also to add positive thoughts and feelings. Subtraction of stress will only get you so far. Addition of positive thoughts and feelings is also required for job satisfaction. Thus, two reasonable goals for obtaining job satisfaction are to manage job stress well *and* strive for job-related well-being.

As discussed in Chapter 2, one way to experience well-being is to be "in the zone," to experience *flow*. Recall that flow refers to "the experience of complete absorption in the present moment" (Nakamura & Csikszentmihalyi, 2009, p. 195). We are most likely to experience flow when we work on tasks that challenge us while at the same time we feel some sense of mastery over them. If we are overwhelmed by tasks we are likely to feel anxiety (a stress emotion), but if we are not sufficiently challenged by them we feel boredom, which is not a pleasant state either. In addition, according to **self-determination theory** (Deci & Ryan, 1985; Ryan & Deci, 2000), when we are intrinsically motivated (i.e., the joy of doing it) to move toward *realistic* goals (i.e., the experience of *competence*) we choose (i.e., the experience of *autonomy*), we have a better chance of experiencing well-being. When the goals are associated with positive relationship qualities (i.e., the experience of *relatedness*) like affiliation, community, and self-acceptance rather than purely self-centered goals like financial success, we are even more likely to experience well-being. Further, when we make good progress toward our goals, we experience enhanced well-being. In sum, a job is more

self-determination theory: when one is intrinsically motivated to move toward realistic goals one chooses, one has a better chance of experiencing well-being.

likely to foster well-being if it supports our ability to experience flow, pursue intrinsically motivating goals that we have some say in choosing, develop and maintain positive connections with other employees when working on our goals, and experience a good rate of forward progress toward achieving our goals.

This also is a good start, but not a complete picture because the ingredients that go into high job satisfaction are varied and complex. Peter Warr (2005, p. 555) presented a framework of 10 major elements of the job environment that determine well-being at work. As you will see, some of these overlap with the previous constructs discussed.

1. "Opportunity for Personal Control" This includes aspects of previously discussed self-determination theory such as autonomy, freedom of choice, and the ability to make decisions about how to conduct one's work.

2. "Opportunity for Skill Use" The ability to use one's skills and talents in the job relates to the experience of competence, also an important need according to self-determination theory.

3. "Externally Generated Goals" Goals presented by others (e.g., organizational leaders) should be reasonable so that we do not experience quantitative or qualitative job overload. They should be communicated clearly to avoid creating role conflicts. And there should be sufficient resources to accommodate the job demands if we are to experience good job satisfaction.

4. "Variety" Varying routines and changing the nature of work tasks help to prevent boredom. This also introduces new challenges that can foster the development of new skills and promote the experience of flow as long as the new challenges do not exceed our capacities.

5. "Environmental Clarity" Timely and accurate feedback about worker performance and communication about the consequences of satisfactory and unsatisfactory work behavior help to reduce ambiguity. Clarity about the future security of the job reduces uncertainty.

6. "Availability of Money" Salary and overall income play a role in overall job satisfaction. Workers tend to use a **social comparison** process of comparing their pay with other workers' pay in the same job category. If they believe their pay is less than others' pay with similar experience working the same job, they are more likely to be dissatisfied (Clark & Oswald, 1996).

7. "Physical Security" If a worker feels endangered because of unsafe working conditions, then it goes without saying that he or she is more likely to be dissatisfied. Environmental physical stressors such as excessive heat or noise also can reduce satisfaction. A comfortable, safe, and ergonomically healthy work environment is optimal.

8. "Supportive Supervision" Effective leadership and supportive management can create work environments that are more positive and conducive to employees satisfactorily fulfilling work goals.

9. "Opportunity for Interpersonal Contact" The opportunity to have satisfactory social relationships at work is important because coworkers provide many of the social rewards (e.g., validation, social support) that come with the job. However, if there is frequent interpersonal conflict, then social rewards are diminished and employees are less likely to be satisfied.

10. "Valued Social Position"   Having a job that has meaning to the worker is important. The job's status or the prestige of the occupation also can play a role in job satisfaction.

WORK STRESS ORGANIZATIONAL INTERVENTIONS

Given the pervasiveness of work stress, organizations often ask what they can do to assist their employees to cope better with organizational stressors. Organizational work stress interventions aim at the employee directly or the organization itself and may be either preventive or recovery oriented. These differences reflect levels of interventions known as *primary, secondary*, and *tertiary prevention* (Table 9.2).

Primary prevention strategies attempt to minimize the source of stress and to promote a supportive organizational culture. **Stress audits** are used to identify problem areas. They involve all employees in a department or an organization completing self-report questionnaires. Then resources are directed to these areas to make positive changes such as changing personnel policies, "improving communication systems, redesigning jobs, or allowing more decision making and autonomy at lower levels" (Cooper, Dewe, & O'Driscoll, 2011, p. 338). Hurrell (2005) reviewed the relevant literature for primary prevention strategies involving what he calls *socio-technical interventions*, such

TABLE **9.2**   Primary, secondary, and tertiary workplace stress management interventions.

Primary Interventions
Scope: Preventative—Reduce the number and/or internsity of stressors *Target:* Alter work environments, technologies, or organizational structures *Underlying assumption:* Most effective approach to stress management is to remove stressors *Examples:* Job redesign; role restructuring; organizational restructuring
Secondary Interventions
Scope: Preventative/reactive—Modify individuals' responses to stressors *Target:* Individual *Underlying assumption:* May not be able to remove/reduce stressors, so best to focus on individuals' reactions to these stressors *Examples:* Stress management training; communication and information sharing; "wellness" programs
Tertiary Interventions
Scope: Treatment—Minimize the damaging consequences of stressors by helping individuals cope more effectively with these consequences *Target:* Individual *Underlying assumption:* Focus is on "treatment" of problems once they have occurred *Examples:* Employee assistance programs; counseling

SOURCE: Cooper, C. L., Dewe, P. J., & O'Driscoll, M. P. (2001), *Organizational stress: A review and critique of theory, research, and applications*, p. 189, Thousand Oaks, CA: Sage. Copyright © 2001 Sage Publications. Reprinted by permission of SAGE Publications.

as modifying workloads (reducing work overload), changing work schedules, and improving work processes (e.g., better participation in decision making), and concluded that there is generally good evidence for their effectiveness in reducing objective measures of stress (e.g., blood pressure, sick days taken).

Secondary prevention involves teaching stress management skills. This educational approach is usually multimodal and includes training in relaxation, time management, assertiveness, lifestyle management, or any one of a host of traditional stress management skills. These skills usually are taught to groups of employees at the work site. Cartwright and Cooper (2005) examined the literature in the area and lamented that there is a shortage of good methodologically sound research evaluating the organizational and individual impact of these programs. They concluded that "there is considerable evidence to suggest that any measured benefits decay rapidly over time and are rarely maintained beyond 6 months posttraining" (Cartwright & Cooper, 2005, p. 617).

Tertiary prevention deals with employees who need rehabilitation and recovery assistance because they have developed mental or physical health conditions related to stress. An example of this approach is an Employee Assistance Program (EAP), a program that provides "counseling, information, and/or referral to appropriate internal or external counseling treatment and support services for troubled employees" (Cooper et al., 2011, p. 339). EAPs are usually a component of the organization's Human Resources Department as an employer-funded benefit. The actual service, however, is typically delivered by health, counseling, and wellness professionals through another organization that has a contract with the host organization. Distressed employees can receive immediate attention by being referred to their company's EAP. Cooper et al. (2011, p. 346) concluded from their examination of the research in the area that employees report high levels of satisfaction with EAPs, but that given the practical and methodological limitations (e.g., confidentiality for employees using the service, difficulty conducting longitudinal research) of the limited evaluation research of EAPs, "it is simply not possible to draw general conclusions about the effectiveness of these interventions."

A POSITIVE PSYCHOLOGY APPROACH

Nelson and Simmons (2011) present a holistic model of stress that applies theory and research of positive psychology to the study of work stress. The unique aspect of their as yet untested model is that they promote the idea that organizations should focus on generating employee *eustress* along with preventing *distress*. They see factors found in Antonovsky's (1979, 1987) sense of coherence (SOC) model such as *meaningfulness* and *manageability* as well as other positive psychology factors such as *hope, positive affect, satisfaction, commitment,* and *vigor* as indicators of eustress. If employees learn to savor eustress experiences alongside learning how to cope with distress, then they will more likely achieve success in managing their work stress than if they simply focus on managing distress. Examples of generating eustress include managers establishing meaningful goals to generate hope, sharing more information to increase worker satisfaction, and redesigning jobs to enhance features that workers find positive and engaging. See Figure 9.2 for their complete model.

Stressors
- Role demands
  - Role conflict
  - Role ambiguity
  - Work-home
- Interpersonal demands
  - Diversity
  - Leadership
  - Team pressures
  - Trust
  - Status
- Physical demands
  - Temperature
  - Indoor climate
  - Air quality
  - Illumination
  - Noise
  - Office design
- Workplace policies
  - Promotion
  - Discrimination
  - Benefits
  - Downsizing
- Job conditions
  - Routine jobs
  - Work overload
  - Job security
  - Wages
  - Sexual harassment
  - Skill discretion

Savoring

Eustress
- Hope
- Positive Affect
- Vigor
- Meaningfulness
- Manageability
- Satisfaction
- Commitment

Individual differences
- Optimism
- Hardiness
- Locus of Control
- Self-Reliance
- Sense of Coherence

Distress
- Anger/Hostility
- Job Alienation
- Frustration
- Negative Affect
- Burnout
- Anxiety

Coping

Outcomes
- Physical Health
- Mental Health
- Work Performance
- Spouse's Health
- Marital Quality
- Quality of Care for Children
- Quality of Friendships
- Community Involvement

FIGURE **9.2**   Nelson and Simmons's (2011) Holistic Model of Stress   SOURCE: Nelson, D. L., & Simmons, B. L. (2011), Savoring eustress while coping with distress: The holistic model of stress in J. C. Quick & L. E. Tetrick (Eds.), *Handbook of Occupational Health Psychology*, 2nd ed., pp. 55–74. Washington, DC: American Psychological Association.

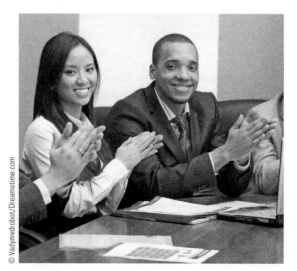

© Vadymvdrobot/Dreamstime.com

According to Nelson and Simmons's (2011) holistic model, organizations should not just focus on preventing employee distress but also on promoting employee eustress.

- One form of organizational stress is organizational role stress and includes role conflict, role ambiguity, and role overload such as quantitative overload and qualitative overload.

- The person-environment (P-E) fit model of organizational stress sees a perceived misfit between a worker's characteristics and those of the work environment as a source of stress.

- The job demands-control (also known as job-strain) model states that stress results from a worker experiencing high psychological job demands with little job control.

- The effort-reward imbalance (ERI) model suggests that high-cost, low-gain work efforts are stressful.

- The organizational injustice model assumes that perceived unfairness with outcomes, procedures, and interpersonal transactions in the organization are stressful.

- The research suggests that certain occupations and jobs are stressful, including the work of police officers, firefighters, social workers, teachers, nurses, physicians, clerical workers, and managers.

- Adverse cardiovascular health effects from work strain, ERI, and organizational injustice stress are reported in a number of prospective studies of initially healthy participants.

- Shift work predicts higher rates of gastrointestinal (GI) problems, coronary heart disease (CHD), breast cancer, and colorectal cancer.

- Working long hour schedules is associated with an increased risk of myocardial infarction (MI).

- Burnout involves the gradual depletion of personal energy such as emotional reserves or resources.

- Studies indicate that burnout and the overlapping concept of vital exhaustion are related to adverse cardiovascular health conditions.

- Other adverse health conditions associated with burnout include the development of type 2 diabetes and musculoskeletal pain.

- Workplace harassment and discrimination lead to stress.

- Racial discrimination is associated with greater cardiovascular reactivity.

- Being the target of sexual harassment increases the likelihood of being less productive at work, experiencing adverse physical or mental health symptoms, using sick leave, abusing alcohol, or leaving the job.

- According to self-determination theory, well-being will result when we are working toward realistic goals that we have chosen because we are intrinsically motivated to pursue them.

- A work environment framework that supports well-being includes the opportunity to experience autonomy, competency, work variety, environmental clarity, money, physical security, effective and supportive leadership, satisfactory relationships with coworkers, reasonable external goals, and a job with meaning or status.

- Time can be wasted through lack of goals, too many goals, procrastination, perfectionism, and boundary intrusions.

- Time management strategies include keeping a daily time log, establishing goals and prioritizing, following the Pareto principle, pruning and weeding, setting boundaries, delegating, and scheduling relaxation time.

- Organizational work stress interventions include primary, secondary, or tertiary prevention strategies.

- Nelson and Simmons (2011) present a holistic model of stress that promotes the idea that organizations should focus on generating employee eustress along with preventing distress.

CRITICAL THINKING QUESTIONS

1. Which of the five models of organizational stress best applies to your current job or to your role as a student? In what ways does it apply? What are the most effective strategies you can use for dealing with this type of stress?

2. How are vigor and engagement similar and different? What are the top three strategies you can use to prevent burnout at school or work? How can you increase your vigor and engagement in school or work?

3. When you procrastinate on school or work assignments, what are the primary reasons? What are the top three strategies you can employ to prevent procrastination?

4. Of Peter Warr's (2010) 10 major elements of the job environment that determine well-being at work, what are the top three that most determine your well-being? Why did you select these three? Explain each.

5. In what ways can employers reduce employee distress? How can they best promote employee eustress?

KEY TERMS AND CONCEPTS

Burnout*	Emotional exhaustion	Low decision latitude*	Organizational stress
Circadian rhythm*	Engagement*	Melatonin*	Pareto principle*
Cynicism	Job demands-control*	Organizational injustice model	Person-environment (P-E) fit*
Effort-reward imbalance (ERI) model*	Job strain*		
	Job stress	Organizational role stress	Pineal gland

Primary prevention	Role overload	Sexual harassment*	Time management
Qualitative overload*	Secondary prevention	Shift work*	Vigor*
Quantitative overload*	Self-care	Social comparison	Vital exhaustion
Reduced efficacy	Self-determination	Stress audits	Workplace discrimination*
Role ambiguity	theory*	Technostress*	Workplace harassment
Role conflict	Sexual coercion	Tertiary prevention	Work stress

MEDIA RESOURCES

CENGAGE **brain**

Access an interactive eBook, chapter-specific
interactive learning tools, including flashcards,
quizzes, videos, and more in your Psychology
CourseMate, accessed through CengageBrain.com.

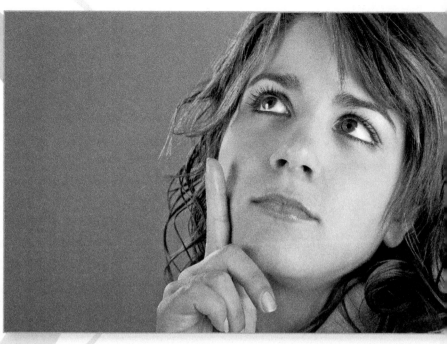

It's not what you think you are—but what you think,
you are.

~UNKNOWN

CHAPTER 10

COGNITIVE AND BEHAVIORAL APPROACHES

We can go through our daily lives coping with a myriad of stressors—from small hassles like a shoelace that snaps with no time left to major life events that seismically shake and fracture the very ground we stand on. Consider the following account from a mother interviewed by Keesee, Currier, and Neimeyer (2008, p. 1157). "My son's murder was a bizarre, random event that occurred on Christmas eve morning as he left a diner after having breakfast. He was accosted by a carjacker who had burglarized a nearby service station and who took his car and shot him at point-blank range. My son died all alone, without ever having an opportunity to see his family. I have never been able to make any sense of this event. The fact that one can make no sense of it makes the death very difficult to bear."

This was a mother's account 8 years after her 34-year-old son's senseless death as she still struggles to cope. How would any of us cope with such a painful and heartbreaking loss? The loss of one's child is especially dreadful because it violates the natural order of things that death takes parents long before their children. To cope, a parent may try to make sense of the loss, sense-making; or extract some threads of meaning from the loss, meaning-making; or use any one of a number of different cognitive and behavioral strategies.

T his chapter takes a closer look at these strategies and examines how we use them to cope with stress, including traumatic stress, and explores which strategies are most effective.

GENERAL TYPES OF COPING STRATEGIES

Recall from Chapter 1 that **coping** refers to the effective use of resources and strategies to deal with internal or external demands (Coyne & Holroyd, 1982). Another definition of coping is "the efforts we take to manage situations we have appraised as being potentially harmful or stressful" (Kleinke, 2007, pp. 290–291). Folkman and Moskowitz (2004) note that the field of coping came into its own during the decades of the 70s and 80s spurred by the 1966 publication of Richard Lazarus's book entitled *Psychological Stress and the Coping Process*. At the time, Lazarus's cognitive-behavioral approach to understanding coping processes was novel compared to the more orthodox approaches that employed Freudian defense mechanisms to explain similar phenomena.

TABLE **10.1**   An example of a coping strategy for each of the four major coping categories

Problem-Focused Coping	Emotion-Focused Coping	Support-Seeking Coping	Meaning-Making Coping
"I made a plan of action and followed it."	"I got busy with other things that helped me feel better."	"I tried to get emotional support from friends or relatives."	"I looked for something good in what was happening."

Since those early days, researchers have made great strides in understanding the predominant coping strategies people use. What did they discover? According to Folkman and Moskowitz (2004), coping strategies divide into four major categories: problem focused, emotion focused, support seeking, and meaning making. See Table 10.1 for an example of each.

One of the first theoretical groupings of coping strategies, suggested by Folkman and Lazarus (1980), splits coping strategies into the two broad-based categories of problem-focused coping and emotion-focused coping. **Problem-focused coping** involves dealing with the perceived cause of the distress (i.e., the problem), whereas **emotion-focused coping** entails managing the distress caused by the problem (i.e., the negative emotions).

To illustrate the differences between the two, you are invited to complete Insight Exercise 10.1.

The **goodness of fit hypothesis** (Folkman, 1984) suggests that coping is most effective when there is a good fit between the coping strategy and the amount of control you can exert over the stressor. In situations in which you can exert a high level of control over the stressor, then problem-focused strategies are the best fit; however, when you can exert little or no control over the stressor, then emotion-focused strategies are the best fit. In other words, if you can make the problem go away by solving it, then your best coping strategy is to tackle the problem. However, if you cannot make the problem go away, then your best coping strategy is to manage your emotional reactions to the stressor rather than trying to solve an insolvable problem.

Although there is substantial support for the goodness of fit hypothesis in coping, Folkman and Moskowitz (2004) conclude after examining the relevant studies that the empirical evidence for its validity is not always consistent. In many cases the fit hypothesis is supported, but in other cases there are inconsistencies. For example, women who experienced a failed in vitro fertilization attempt—an outcome that is largely uncontrollable—who used emotion-approach coping adjusted better than those who used problem-focused coping in one study (Terry & Hynes, 1998), supporting the goodness of fit hypothesis. Yet, when women in this same study used an escapist strategy, a form of emotion-focused avoidance coping, they showed poor adjustment even though there was a good fit between their perception of low controllability and their coping strategy. In another study (Macrodimitris & Endler, 2001), people with type 2 diabetes who used active problem-focused coping to manage their controllable health condition showed less depression. However, contrary to the goodness of fit hypothesis, their use of problem-focused coping was not related

problem-focused coping: dealing with the perceived cause of the distress.

emotion-focused coping: managing the distress caused by the problem.

INSIGHT EXERCISE **10.1**

First, think of your most stressful encounter in the last month. Have you thought of it? Now indicate which of the coping responses on the checklist you used to deal with the stressor.

What Is Your Coping Strategy?

Coping Responses Checklist

1	Made a plan of action and followed it.
2	Tried to see the positive side of the situation.
3	Took things a day at a time, one step at a time.
4	Got busy with other things that helped me feel better.
5	Tried not to act too hastily or follow my first hunch.
6	Got away from things for a while.
7	Knew what had to be done and tried harder to make things work.
8	Made a promise to myself that things would be different next time.
9	Bargained or compromised to get something positive from the situation.
10	Exercised more to reduce tension.

The checklist above, adapted from Billings and Moos (1984), categorizes items as either problem-focused coping or emotion-focused coping. Did you find that you endorsed mostly odd numbers or even numbers? If you endorsed mostly odd numbers, then your predominant approach to coping with the stressor was problem focused, but if you endorsed mainly even numbers then your primary approach was emotion focused. Perhaps you used a combination of both.

The next question you might ask yourself is how effective were your coping strategies. How much control did you have over the stressor? One idea, known as the goodness of fit hypothesis discussed elsewhere in this section, suggests that if you have control over the stressor then problem-focused coping strategies are best, but if you have no control over the stressor then emotion-focused strategies are best. Did your results match the goodness of fit hypothesis?

to perceptions of control. On the other hand, their employment of emotion-focused coping when combined with low perceptions of control was associated with better psychological adjustment, supporting the goodness of fit hypothesis.

Billings and Moos (1981) divided coping into three categories: *active cognitive* such as planning, which uses mentally oriented problem-focused coping; *active behavioral* such as trying harder, which employs action-oriented, problem-focused coping; and *avoidance coping*, which is a form of emotion-focused coping that may involve using cognitive or behavioral strategies. See Table 10.2 for examples of how these coping strategies would divide if separated into four categories. Note, however, that Billings and Moos (1981)

TABLE **10.2**   Examples of cognitive and behavioral coping strategies for problem-focused coping and emotion-focused avoidance coping. Note that Billings and Moos (1981) lumped together cognitive and behavioral avoidance coping into one category called simply avoidance coping but divided problem-focused coping into active cognitive and active behavioral coping strategies.

	Problem-Focused Coping	Emotion-Focused Avoidance Coping
Cognitive	"I made a plan of action."	"I refused to believe that it happened."
Behavioral	"I took additional action to try to get rid of the problem."	"I tried to reduce tension by eating more."

lumped together cognitive and behavioral avoidance coping into one category called, simply, avoidance coping.

Avoidance coping items include "kept my feelings to myself," "avoided being with people in general," "refused to believe that it happened," and "tried to reduce tension by eating more" (Holahan & Moos, 1987, p. 949). In general avoidance coping is effective as a strategy for dealing with minor or transient irritations such as those that may soon go away on their own. However, for serious or chronic problems, avoidance coping only brings temporary relief from distress. It is not an effective long-term strategy. At best avoidance coping amounts to sweeping problems under the rug. What happens to the rug after repeated sweepings? The rug becomes lumpy and difficult to walk on, reminding us that the problems, though hidden, are still there and getting bigger. In addition, avoidance coping interferes with our ability to experience personal growth from negative experiences or feedback. How can people learn from their difficulties if they do not even acknowledge them or attempt to deal with them? Kleinke (2007, p. 305) concluded after reviewing the relevant research that "unsuccessful copers respond to life challenges with denial and avoidance. They either withdraw from problems or react impulsively without taking the time and effort to seek the best solution."

Sometimes *distancing* as a strategy of avoidance coping (e.g., "I went on as if nothing had happened") can be adaptive, but other forms of avoidance coping such as *escape-avoidance* (e.g., "I wish that the situation would go away or somehow be over with") are generally maladaptive (Folkman & Lazarus, 1988a). For example, if you are waiting at home for results of a biopsy test to see if you have cancer, putting aside worrisome thoughts for that day can be beneficial for temporarily managing your fear and anxiety, but wishing the problem would go away is not. Likewise, if you are later informed that the results of the test are positive, going into denial and using a strategy of refusing to believe the results can be disastrous long term even though this strategy can temporarily alleviate anxiety.

Besides problem-focused coping and emotion-focused coping, factor analytic studies suggest that *support seeking* is another important independent coping strategy (Amirkhan, 1990). Examples of support seeking include "confided your fears and worries to a friend or relative," "sought reassurance from those who know you best," and "went to a friend for advice on how to change the situation" (Amirkhan, 1990, p. 1070). Recall the importance of social support for health and well-being discussed in Chapter 8.

Although problem-focused coping, emotion-focused coping, and social support-seeking coping categories are important for cataloging the broad strategies of how people deal with stress, by the decade of the 90s, researchers had determined that without considering the use of meaning-based coping, these three categories were not sufficient. A fourth general category of coping proposed by Park and Folkman (1997) draws on how people use cognitive strategies to derive meaning from stressful situations. This fourth category, known as **meaning-making coping**, is coping that uses our values, beliefs, and goals to shape meaning in stressful situations that are generally not conducive to the use of problem-focused coping such as long-term caregiving for a loved one with dementia or loss of a loved one.

According to Park and Folkman's (1997) meaning-making coping model, the meaning of an event is appraised through attributions, primary appraisals, and secondary appraisals. See Figure 10.1 for an illustration of the process.

meaning-making coping: to use one's values, beliefs, and goals to shape meaning in stressful situations that are generally not conducive to the use of problem-focused coping.

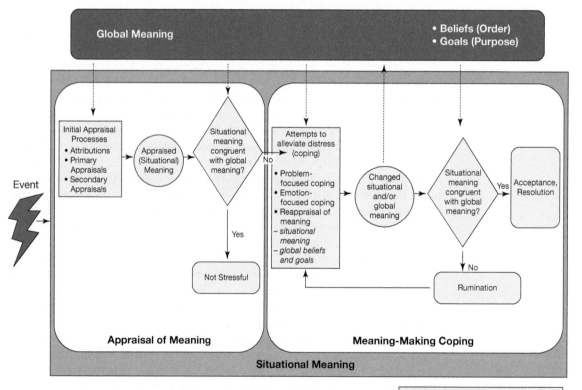

FIGURE **10.1** Park and Folkman's (1997) model of meaning-making coping SOURCE: Park, C. L., & Folkman, S. (1997), Meaning in the context of stress and coping, *Review of General Psychology, 1,* 115–144. Reproduced with permission via Copyright Clearance Center.

When situational meaning is incongruent with global meaning, the event is considered stressful. What is global meaning? **Global meaning** is a product of our system of core values, beliefs, and goals that we use to interpret our experiences of the world. **Global beliefs** cover broad areas "such as fairness, justice, luck, control, predictability, coherence, benevolence, and personal vulnerability"; and **global goals** cover "ideals, states, or objects that people work toward being or achieving or maintaining, such as relationships, work, wealth, knowledge, and achievement" (Park, 2008, p. 972).

Recall in the beginning of this chapter the anguish of a mother whose son was inexplicably murdered. Although we can only respectfully guess her beliefs and goals, the traumatic event likely led to a discrepancy between her global beliefs such as "people are benevolent and the world is coherent" and her situational experience of "my son was murdered in a senseless act." Further, her likely global goals of wanting good health for her family and close family relationships were violated by her son's sudden and tragic loss of life. This is the type of seismic event that creates distress often associated with meaning-making coping. She may have used other forms of coping such as emotion focused or support seeking to reduce her distress, but ultimately she was faced with how to resolve the discrepancy between her global and situational frameworks for meaning.

In order to restore shaken or lost meaning, changes need to be made to either the situational meaning or the global meaning, or both, to bring them into alignment with each other. Meaning making includes the use of cognitive restructuring (reworking existing assumptions and beliefs and replacing them with new ones) to fit the specific situational event meaning into the wider global meaning framework (i.e., assimilation) or to change the wider global meaning framework to conform to the specific situational event meaning (i.e., accommodation). This process produces *cognitive products* known as ***meanings made***. Failure to resolve these discrepancies leads to poor adjustment and ruminative attempts to come to terms with the event. Good adjustment occurs when the meaning-making process leads to congruency between situational and global meaning that in turn leads to acceptance or resolution.

For example, perhaps the bereaved mother could make some meaning out of her son's death through thinking that it brought the surviving family members closer together—if indeed it did—which would be congruent with her global goals (i.e., assimilation) of wanting to be emotionally close to her family. Alternatively she could change her global beliefs that the world is coherent and see the world as a lot more random and dangerous than she previously believed (i.e., accommodation), changing her worldview to fit the situation. Perhaps in doing so she might believe that she now has more personal strength and wisdom that come with acceptance of events she cannot control. The **assimilation** process of adding new information (i.e., the situational meaning) to an already existing schema or cognitive framework (i.e., her global meaning) is more common than the **accommodation** process of changing the larger organizing schema (i.e., her global meaning) to fit the smaller one (i.e., the situational meaning).

Candace Lightner, the 1980 founder of Mothers Against Drunk Driving (MADD), used meaning-making coping to cope with the death of her 13-year-old daughter, Cari, who was killed by a drunk driver while walking in a bicycle lane in their suburban neighborhood. The offender was a 47-year-old man who had three previous drunk driver convictions. The police officer informed Candace that the offender would likely serve no prison or jail time even though the man who killed her daughter was out on bail for a previous drunk driving offense, a hit and run. Candace soon met Cindi Lamb, whose 5-year-old daughter, Laura, became quadriplegic when a swerving drunk driver traveling 70 mph crashed into their car on a highway. Together they founded MADD to strengthen the laws against drunk driving and support its victims. The MADD website honors Cari Lightner and Laura Lamb. For Cari "it was her life, and her death, that became a rallying cry to end the tragedy of drunk driving" (MADD, 2010).

MEASUREMENT OF COPING STRATEGIES

Measures of coping often use retrospective self-reports in the form of checklists similar to the one you were invited to complete in Insight Exercise 10.1. Respondents are generally asked about the coping strategies they used to manage a stressful event that occurred within a certain period, such as the last month. Alternatively they are asked to check the coping strategies they would use if they experienced hypothetical stressful encounters presented to them in vignettes.

The 50-item Ways of Coping Scale that measures eight types of coping was one of the first checklist coping inventories (Folkman & Lazarus, 1980, 1988b). This inventory measures coping strategies labeled confrontive coping, distancing, self-controlling, seeking social support, accepting responsibility, escape-avoidance, planful problem solving, and positive reappraisal. Other popular coping inventories are the Coping Inventory for Stressful Situations (Endler & Parker, 1990), the Coping Strategy Indicator (Amirkhan, 1990), and the Coping Response Inventory (Moos, 1993).

Retrospective coping inventories suffer from the same issues discussed in Chapter 4 regarding inventories that ask for recall of stressful life events. That is, people often have difficulty remembering events accurately and may have memory distortions or biases when answering. Some researchers have attempted to get around this problem by using momentary accounts of coping such as asking about the most stressful experience the research participant had that day or during another proximal interval, commonly 48 hours.

One study (Stone et al., 1998) that compared reports of retrospective coping with those of momentary coping found that the retrospective approach underreported cognitive coping strategies and overreported behavioral coping strategies relative to the information collected using momentary coping data. Which then is most accurate, the retrospective or the momentary reports? That is not entirely clear because even the study's researchers noted that participants making momentary reports may also forget or omit information. For example, because the participants had to report information repeatedly, they may have thought that they had already reported particular coping strategies that they in fact had not reported. Further, they may have focused on more concrete well-defined stress-related problems in their momentary reports rather than larger, more abstract problems that become more apparent across longer time spans. Thus, the momentary reports may not be as sensitive a measure for collecting information on how people cope with more abstract stress-related problems as retrospective checklists.

Some researchers use narrative approaches in which participants identify a stressor and then give an account of how they coped with the stressor. The content of the narratives are then analyzed to determine the types of coping strategies used. An advantage of this approach is that it can uncover novel coping strategies that are not included on a checklist. However, the narrative approach, too, has its shortcomings. For example, unlike checklists that prompt one's memory about different coping strategies, narratives have no prompts and so coping strategies that are used may be forgotten. Folkman and Moskowitz (2004, p. 751) conclude, "there is no gold standard for the measurement of coping. . . . The measurement of coping is probably as much art as it is science. The art comes in selecting the approach that is most appropriate and useful to the researcher's question."

SPECIFIC TYPES OF COPING STRATEGIES

As discussed earlier, there are at least four general types of coping strategies and a number of different coping inventories. These coping inventories provide a finer-grained analysis of coping styles than can be obtained by simply measuring the four general approaches. They also are useful in spelling out how to conceptualize specific coping strategies. Each inventory lists different variations of specific coping strategies based on the authors' understanding of the coping process. A good illustration of specific coping strategies is represented by the Coping Orientations to Problems Experienced (COPE) Scale created by Charles Carver and his colleagues (Carver, Scheier, & Weintraub, 1989), an instrument that measures 14 coping styles. The styles are listed next along with a sample item for each. Imagine also the following scenario. Andrea lives in a dorm and needs to study for her upcoming exam. Unfortunately for her, other students, including her roommate, often visit with each other and have a good time in her dorm room while she is studying. How does she cope? An example is given next of each coping method that Andrea might use, some adaptive and some maladaptive. Which coping strategies would you use?

- **Active coping**—taking measures to remove or lessen the problem. "I take additional action to try to get rid of the problem." Andrea asks her roommate and her roommate's friends if they would not mind going to one of the other dorm rooms to visit because she has to study. When they leave she puts a "do not disturb sign" on her door.

- **Planning**—thinking about and deciding on future actions for dealing with the problem. "I make a plan of action." Andrea plans her day so that she can study in her dorm room at times when her roommate is attending classes.

- **Suppression of competing activities**—intentionally setting aside other projects to focus on the problem. "I put aside other activities in order to concentrate on this." Andrea turns off her television, cell phone, and other related electronic devices so she can concentrate on studying.

- **Restraint coping**—deliberately waiting until the time is right to act. "I hold off doing anything about it until the situation permits." Andrea does her errands during the early part of the day when she is most distracted and then studies later in the day when things are quiet and she is least likely to be interrupted.

- **Seeking social support for instrumental reasons**—seeking information, assistance, or advice from others. "I try to get advice from someone about what to do." Andrea forms a study group and studies for her exam with the group.

- **Seeking social support for emotional reasons**—seeking sympathy or understanding from others. "I try to get emotional support from friends or relatives." Andrea calls her boyfriend and shares with him her concerns about the distractions she faces and her worries about her upcoming exam.

- **Positive reinterpretation and growth**—reframing or reappraising the stressor in a more positive or benign light. "I look for something good in what is happening." Andrea comes to view her exam and dealing with study distractions as practice for later career-and-relationship challenges because they help her grow intellectually and emotionally.

- **Acceptance**—acknowledging the reality of the stressor or that it cannot be changed. "I learn to live with it." Andrea accepts that there is nothing she can do about her roommate and all the distractions and tries to study in spite of the difficulties.

- **Turning to religion**—finding comfort in religion or religious practices. "I seek God's help." Andrea prays that God will help her find the strength and courage she needs to persevere in her studies in spite of the many distractions she faces.

- **Focus on and venting emotions**—expressing feelings. "I let my feelings out." Andrea vents her feelings of frustration to a friend about how difficult it is to study when she has to live with a roommate who is frequently inconsiderate.

- **Denial**—not believing the stressor is real or acting as though it is not real. "I refuse to believe that it has happened." Andrea sees she has an upcoming exam listed on her class syllabus, but thinks that it must be a typo because the timing of the exam does not seem quite right to her, especially because she had already planned to go out with her boyfriend around that time.

- **Behavioral disengagement**—reducing efforts to act on the stressor. "I give up the attempt to get what I want." Andrea decides that studying is not worth the trouble, so she chats with her roommate and friends instead of studying.

- **Mental disengagement**—using tactics such as distraction to take one's mind off the stressor. "I go to movies or watch TV, to think about it less." Andrea decides to watch her favorite show on television to take her mind off her worries rather than study for her exam.

- **Alcohol-drug disengagement**—using substances to avoid thinking about the stressor. "I drink alcohol or take drugs in order to think about it less." Andrea sneaks a bottle of rum into her dorm room and starts drinking rum and Coke to deal with the stress of her upcoming exam.

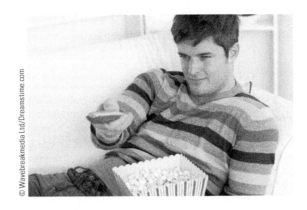

Watching television to deal with stress uses mental disengagement as a coping strategy.

Factor analyses of 11 dimensions of the COPE Scale reveals that these specific styles of coping tend to group into the four general factors discussed previously of problem-focused/active (i.e., active coping, planning, restraint), emotion-focused/avoidance (e.g., denial, mental disengagement, alcohol-drug disengagement), social support coping (e.g., seeking social support for instrumental reasons, seeking social support for emotional reasons), and meaning-making coping/positive cognitive restructuring (e.g., positive reinterpretation and growth, acceptance) (Zautra, Sheets, & Sandler, 1996).

Another way to conceptualize the different specific coping strategies is to think of them as intersecting along two dimensions: problem focused versus emotion focused and approach versus avoidance coping (Table 10.3). **Approach coping** involves using strategies to reduce or eliminate the stressor or its effects (e.g., distress). **Avoidance coping** in this context refers to disengaging from the stressor or its effects. For example, problem-focused approach coping involves planning, whereas problem-focused avoidance coping involves behavioral disengagement. Emotion-focused approach coping involves cognitive restructuring, whereas emotion-focused avoidance coping involves denial. Nes and Segerstrom (2006) determined in their meta-analytic review of 50 studies with a total of 11,629 participants that dispositional optimism was positively related to approach strategies ($r = .17$) and negatively associated with avoidance strategies ($r = -.21$). As you recall from Chapter 6, dispositional optimism is associated with a number of positive health and well-being benefits. The authors of the meta-analytic review suggest that approach coping strategies could likely serve as meditational mechanisms for the positive adjustment findings generally found in research studies of optimism.

One form of coping that stands out in the COPE and some other coping scales as somewhat different from the others is "turning to religion." When asked, many people report that they turn to their religious beliefs or practices to cope with stress. The COPE has four items that are examples of religious-based coping: (1) "I seek God's help," (2) "I put my trust in God," (3) "I try to find comfort in my religion," and (4) "I pray more than usual." Other measures have none or even fewer religious-based coping items. For example, the Ways of Coping Scale has one item. As discussed in Chapter 2, there is a growing body of evidence suggesting that engaging in religious or spiritual activity confers

approach coping: using strategies to reduce or eliminate the stressor or its effects.

avoidance coping: disengaging from the stressor or its effects.

© Wavebreakmedia Ltd/Dreamstime.com

TABLE **10.3**   Examples of coping strategies that intersect along the two dimensions of approach coping versus avoidance coping and problem-focused coping versus emotion-focused coping.

	Problem-Focused Coping	Emotion-Focused Coping
Approach Coping	Planning Seeking instrumental support Task-oriented coping Active coping Confrontive coping	Cognitive restructuring Seeking emotional support Turning to religion Acceptance Positive reinterpretation
Avoidance Coping	Problem avoidance Behavioral disengagement	Denial Distancing Mental disengagement Wishful thinking Social withdrawal

SOURCE: Nes, L. S., & Segerstrom, S. C. (2006), Dispositional optimism and coping: A meta-analytic review, *Personality and Social Psychology Review*, 10, 3, 235–251. Copyright © 2006 by Sage Publications. Reprinted by permission of SAGE Publications.

positive health and well-being effects. The health and well-being benefit findings could be due to a number of factors including social support, meaning-making, and religious-based coping. Such findings have spurred a growing interest in studying religious-based coping.

Researchers studying religious-based coping note that it is important to distinguish this specific subset of religiosity from general religiosity. Why? **Religious-based coping** refers to the use of religious methods to reduce stress, whereas general religiosity does not necessarily have that aim. Psychologist and pioneer religiosity/spirituality researcher Kenneth Pargament and his colleagues (Pargament, Smith, Koenig, & Perez, 1998, p. 710) argue that religious-based coping adds a unique component to the study of coping and thus "religious coping cannot be 'reduced' to nonreligious forms of coping."

religious-based coping: the use of religious methods such as prayer to reduce stress.

In spite of this assertion, Park (2005) emphasizes the overlap between religious-based coping and meaning-making coping. Park (2005, p. 721) concluded from her cross-sectional study of 169 bereaved college students that "religion was related to meaning-making coping, as reflected in positive reappraisal coping, and to adjustment in terms of subjective well-being and stress-related growth. Further, the association of religion with these adjustment outcomes was mediated by positive reappraisal coping." In other words, religion seemed to produce its positive subjective well-being and stress-related growth effects primarily through engendering a type of meaning-making coping called positive reappraisal coping. Figure 10.2 demonstrates through a path analysis the higher strength of the pathway between religion and subjective well-being when the effects of meaning-making coping as a mediator are included in the process. Along with meaning-making coping, other traditional general types of coping such as seeking social support and emotion-focused coping may overlap with religious-based coping methods also.

Pargament, Koenig, and Perez (2000) created the RCOPE to measure a wider range of religious coping strategies than traditional measures. They found through the RCOPE, after controlling for demographic and global religious variables, that religious coping contributed unique variance to adjustment. Better

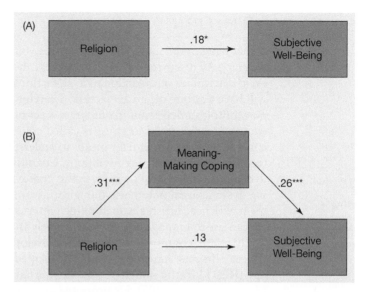

FIGURE **10.2** Park's (2005) study indicates in the first path analysis (A) that religion significantly (indicated by the asterisk) predicts subjective well-being. However, the second path analysis (B) shows that meaning-making coping mediates the effect. Notice the high significant (indicated by the double asterisks) path coefficients indicating that religion predicts meaning-making coping and meaning-making coping predicts subjective well-being. When meaning-making coping is taken into account in path analysis B, the direct path between religion and subjective well-being is no longer significant.   SOURCE: Park, C. L. (2005), Religion as a meaning-making framework in coping with life stress, *Journal of Social Issues, 61*, 4, 707–729. Copyright © 2005 Blackwell Publishing. Reproduced by permission of Blackwell Publishing.

adjustment was associated with certain forms of religious coping such as positive reappraisals, forgiveness, and support, and poorer adjustment with other forms such as spiritual discontent and reappraisals of a punishing God.

Particular forms of religious-based coping may be associated with adverse health outcomes and reduced longevity. In a 2-year longitudinal study of elderly patients who were medically ill, Pargament, Koenig, Tarakeshwar, and Hahn (2001) were the first to find that particular forms of religious-based coping predicted early mortality. Using a brief form of the RCOPE, these researchers determined that coping items that reflected religious struggle such as "Wondered whether God had abandoned me" and "Questioned God's love for me" predicted up to a 10% increased risk of early mortality even after controlling for other relevant variables. Thus, in terms of coping with their illnesses, such forms of religious-based coping may be indicative of a poor prognosis and early mortality.

In general then, which coping strategies discussed are the most effective overall for managing stress? Although approach coping seems to be the most successful and avoidance coping the least successful, there appears to be no best strategy for every situation. The key is *flexibility* and the ability to use a wide range of coping strategies to fit the specific context or situation. As Kleinke (2007, p. 305) concludes after reviewing the coping literature, "people who cope most successfully are those who are equipped with a battery of coping strategies and who are flexible in adapting their responses to the situation."

COGNITIVE RESTRUCTURING

cognitive primacy: the idea that cognitions influence how one responds to stress.

cognitive restructuring: a technique used in cognitive-behavioral therapy of challenging dysfunctional automatic thoughts, assumptions, and beliefs and replacing them with healthier realistic thinking patterns.

rational-emotive behavior therapy (REBT): a cognitive therapy developed by Ellis that involves active disputation of irrational beliefs.

catastrophize: to cognitively maximize the perceived negative consequences of an event.

Is that bang in the night you hear outside your bedroom window a cat or a cat burglar? As discussed in earlier chapters, how we appraise and interpret an event determines our reaction to it. If we think the worst and *catastrophize,* we will have a strong negative reaction. Therefore, our cognitive filters play an important role in determining our stress reactions. The idea that cognitions influence how we respond to stress is called **cognitive primacy.** To understand the concept of cognitive primacy means to understand that we can change our stress reactions by changing our cognitions. **Cognitive restructuring,** a technique used in cognitive-behavioral therapy, in this context refers to the process of challenging dysfunctional automatic thoughts, assumptions, and beliefs and replacing them with healthier realistic thinking patterns. One of the most important tools we can use to manage our stress effectively is cognitive restructuring.

Modern cognitive therapy was developed primarily by two theorists, Albert Ellis and Aaron Beck. Ellis developed **rational-emotive behavior therapy (REBT)** in the mid-1950s as an alternative to traditional psychoanalysis (Ellis & Dryden, 2007). He proposed an ABC model whereby "A," an **activating event** such as receiving a poor exam grade, is interpreted through "B," one's **beliefs,** leading to emotional and behavioral **consequences,** "C." If "B" is irrational, then a student who receives a poor exam grade is likely to have an exaggerated emotional response to "A" such as depression, shame, anger, or anxiety that is out of proportion to the event. In other words, the student will **catastrophize** and see the event as having catastrophic meaning. In order to engage in cognitive restructuring, the student will need to **dispute** the irrational beliefs that led to "C." Therefore, we can add "D" (i.e., dispute) to the process, now making it an ABCD model.

Examples of irrational beliefs that would need to be disputed include a high need for perfection or approval. Such beliefs have two main characteristics. They (a) are absolutistic and (b) generate attributions that are overgeneral and unrealistic. The absolutistic quality of the belief is signaled by use of words such as *must, should, have to,* and *need to.* For example, with perfectionism, a student can think "I have to be perfect in all that I undertake. If I am not, I am worthless, a failure, and will never amount to anything." The first sentence represents the absolutistic nature of the belief, and the last sentence the unrealistic overgeneralization. REBT therapists use techniques such as debating, bibliotherapy (therapists providing reading material to clients that provide additional support for treatment), social skills training, and role playing to assist the client in challenging irrational beliefs.

self-talk: the silent internal dialogue people have with themselves.

We can self-challenge our irrational beliefs through asking ourselves questions such as (1) What evidence supports or refutes this belief? (2) Is this belief rational or logical? (3) What is a more rational belief that I can substitute for this irrational belief? For example, a perfectionist can use **self-talk,** the silent internal dialogue we have with ourselves, to say "I would like to have done well on the exam, but even though I didn't do well, I am still a worthwhile person who in the past did well on other exams and will do well in the future." In this way, the absolutistic language of *have to* is substituted with more flexible language such as *I would like to* and the consequences are not seen as a reflection of self-worth or future catastrophes.

Beck (1967) independently created his system of cognitive psychotherapy based on his research and clinical practice with depression. He later widened his focus to include treatment of other areas such as anxiety, substance abuse, personality disorders, and marital problems. As discussed in Chapter 7, Beck's cognitive therapy focuses on challenging *maladaptive attitudes* (e.g., "If I do not perform as well as others, it means that I am an inferior human being") that serve as well-springs for *automatic negative thoughts* (e.g., "I'm no good," "People don't like me," "I am a failure as a person," "Things will never change").

These automatic negative thoughts tend to follow particular dysfunctional patterns that produce systematic *errors of thinking,* in other words, cognitive processing styles that are distorted, biased, or illogical. As discussed in Chapter 7, such errors include (1) *arbitrary inference* through drawing conclusions without supportive evidence, (2) *selective abstraction* through focusing on a detail that ignores the more important big picture, (3) *overgeneralization* through drawing sweeping conclusions based on limited information, (4) *dichotomous thinking* through thinking in black or white terms rather than shades of gray, (5) *magnification and minimization* through exaggerating small events or trivializing big events, and (6) *personalization* through taking responsibility for events that are not under one's control.

Using Beck's approach to cognitive restructuring we can ask basic questions such as (1) What evidence supports this thought? (2) What is another way of thinking about it? (3) If the negative thought were true, what would be its implications? In addition, using the **triple column method** as a daily exercise we can challenge and replace stressful automatic negative thoughts. David Burns (1993, p. 52) illustrates how to employ this method through using his "Daily Mood Log" that has a left-hand column heading of "Negative Thoughts," a middle column heading of "Distortions," and a right-hand column heading of "Positive Thoughts." Following is Burns's (1993, p. 50) list, which provides a detailed breakdown of distorted thinking categories to use in his exercise.

triple column method: a daily exercise used for cognitive restructuring designed to identify, challenge, and replace automatic negative thoughts.

- **All-or-nothing thinking**—dichotomous thinking or black-and-white thinking. "I am either a winner or a loser. There are no shades of gray."
- **Overgeneralization**—taking a specific example and seeing it as global. "It never ends. I got bad news today, but then again, my life is nothing but bad news."
- **Mental filter**—focusing only on bad qualities or events. "I don't fly on planes because they crash too often."
- **Discounting the positives**—overlooking one's positive qualities. "Yes, I have done well in college, but I'm really not that smart."
- **Jumping to conclusions**—engaging in *mind reading,* that is, assuming others are thinking badly of you; or *fortune telling,* that is, predicting negative outcomes. "I know she thinks I'm not in her league and will probably laugh at me when I ask her out on a date."

- **Magnification or minimization**—exaggerating or downplaying the importance of something. "My stomach hurts. It must be appendicitis." "Yes I smoke, but I'll outlive all you nonsmokers."
- **Emotional reasoning**—confusing feelings for facts. For instance, feeling like one is incompetent is seen as evidence that one is incompetent. "How do I know I'm incompetent? Because I feel incompetent, that's how."
- **"Should" statements**—absolutistic statements. "I should be more outgoing. I'm too shy."
- **Labeling**—using negative labels about oneself or others rather than describing the event. "If I wasn't such a weak person, I would have stood up to her."
- **Blame**—internalizing or externalizing responsibility inappropriately. This thinking style involves blaming others for outcomes you are responsible for or blaming yourself for outcomes you had no control over. "If I had gotten more hits, we would have won the game." "If you had gotten more hits, we would have won the game."

The first step in using the triple column method is to write down all your negative or stressful thoughts in the first column. Next, identify any distortions in your thoughts and write them down in the second column. See Figure 10.3

DAILY MOOD LOG

Negative Thoughts Write down the thoughts that make you upset.	Distortions Use the Distorted Thinking chart.	Positive Thoughts Substitute other thoughts that are more positive and realistic.
1. I'm a born loser.	1. all-or-nothing thinking, overgeneralization, mental filter, discounting the positives, magnification, emotional reasoning, "should" statements, labeling, blame.	1.
2. I'll never get another job.	2.	2.
3. I'm letting my family down.	3.	3.

FIGURE **10.3**   Example Using Burns's Daily Mood Log

This log shows how one can begin to use the Triple Column Method.   Source: Burns, D. D. (1993), *Ten days to self-esteem*, p. 50, New York: Quill William Morrow.

STRESS MANAGEMENT EXERCISE **10.1**

Employing the Triple Column Method

Would you like to try the triple column method? If so, take out a sheet of paper and make three columns using the headings of "Negative Thoughts," "Distortions," and "Positive Thoughts." Next write down all the negative thoughts you can think of that currently stress you. Do not censor yourself, but rather let them spill out onto the paper. You can tear up the paper when you are through so that no one can read your private thoughts.

Next, start with your first thought and determine the types of distortions it represents. Write these down. Write as many as are applicable. Move now to the third column. Think of an alternative thought that captures the idea more realistically, and write it down. For example, if your thought is "I am a born loser," a more realistic positive thought is "I have had some setbacks, but so has everyone else. I've had successes in the past and will continue to have them in the future."

When recording your positive thoughts ask yourself the following questions. Does the positive thought "put the lie to the negative thought"? Does the evidence support your alternative thought? If so, it is a good one. If not, keep working on it until it meets these criteria.

Now go through and challenge each negative thought using the same process. When you finish the process, ask yourself how you now feel. Do you feel an uplift, like a burden has been removed? Are you less stressed? If so, how do you know? Perhaps you feel less stress emotions like anxiety, anger, or depression. If you do, then you are in good company because this simple exercise often alleviates negative feelings for those who use it. If you find this exercise effective, you can continue to use it on a daily basis as a way to reduce ongoing stress and experience more positive feelings.

for an example of how to start the first two columns. Last, in the third column, write substitution thoughts that are more realistic than the stressful thoughts. The third column thoughts are not Pollyannaish or rose-colored glasses thoughts, but rather thoughts that you have evidence to support. Thus, the realistic thoughts should be *affirming, valid, realistic*, and "put the lie to the negative thought" (Burns, 1993, p. 53).

STRESS INOCULATION TRAINING

stress inoculation training (SIT): Meichenbaum's cognitive-behavior modification training program designed to prepare individuals for stressful future encounters or treat current excess stress.

Donald Meichenbaum (1985, 1996) developed **stress inoculation training (SIT)** as a cognitive-behavior modification training program to prepare individuals for stressful future encounters or to treat current excess stress. The inoculation concept is based on the principle of fortifying individuals with coping skills (i.e., inoculating them) so that when they encounter anticipated stressful events they will be prepared. SIT uses a combination of cognitive and behavioral skill-building approaches such as educating, raising self-awareness (i.e., self-monitoring), cognitive restructuring, problem solving, relaxation training, and rehearsing. It consists of three phases: the (1) "conceptual

TABLE **10.4** Examples of self-statements used in stress inoculation training for dealing with pain

Preparing for the Painful Stressor
What is it you have to do?
You can develop a plan to deal with it.
Just think about what you have to do.
Just think about what you can do about it.
Don't worry; worrying won't help anything.
You have lots of different strategies you can call upon.

Confronting and Handling the Pain
You can meet the challenge.
One step at a time; you can handle the situation.
Just relax, breathe deeply, and use one of the strategies.
Don't think about the pain, just what you have to do.
This tenseness can be an ally, a cue to cope.
Relax. You're in control; take a slow deep breath. Ah. Good.
This anxiety is what the trainer said you might feel.
That's right; it's the reminder to use your coping skills.

Coping with Feelings at Critical Moments
When pain comes just pause; keep focusing on what you have to do.
What is it you have to do?
Don't try to eliminate the pain totally; just keep it under control.
Just remember, there are different strategies; they'll help you stay in control.
When the pain mounts you can switch to a different strategy; you're in control.

Reinforcing Self-Statements
Good, you did it.
You handled it pretty well.
You knew you could do it!
Wait until you tell the trainer about which procedures worked best.

SOURCE: Meichenbaum, D. (1977), *Cognitive behavior modification: An integrative approach.* New York: Plenum Publishers. Used by permission.

educational phase," (2) "skills acquisition and skills consolidation phase," and (3) "application and follow-through phase" (Meichenbaum, 2007, p. 501).

In the conceptual educational phase the goal is to help clients understand their stress-related problems through collecting information and then presenting the information to them in a collaborative manner that engenders hope. The second phase emphasizes the development of coping skills for dealing with target stressors. These may include use of coping self-statements (Table 10.4), anger management, cognitive restructuring, relaxation, assertiveness training, problem solving, use of social support, emotion-focused coping to deal with uncontrollable stressors, and so forth. Last, the application and follow-through phase involves practice applying these skills during increasing levels of stress. Role playing, modeling, and exposure to real-life stress situations are used as well as techniques to prevent relapse such as learning to identify and rehearse for high-risk situations.

Meichenbaum (2007) notes that since SIT's inception in the mid-1970s (Michenbaum, 1977), the training program has a history of successful use with medical patients (e.g., dealing with pain or preparing for medical procedures such as surgery), psychological or emotional difficulties (e.g., posttraumatic stress disorder [PTSD], anxiety, anger), performance anxiety (e.g., public speaking, athletic competitions, dating), professional groups (e.g., nurses, teachers, probation officers), and people going through stressful life transitions (e.g., unemployment, reentering college, relocating to another country). The typical length of SIT is 8 to 15 sessions over a 3- to 12-month period with some booster sessions at follow-up.

LEARNED OPTIMISM

Seligman (1991) suggests that people can learn to be optimistic just as they can learn to be helpless. As you are aware, optimism is associated with many positive coping strategies, health, and well-being benefits. People who realize **learned optimism** are able to cultivate positive expectations when they see connections between their efforts and outcomes. In order to do this, they must challenge pessimistic causal attributional explanatory styles (Abramson, Seligman, & Teasdale, 1978). **Causal attributions** are cognitions that address the "Why?" question. For example, we may ask ourselves "why did the bad event happen?"

People tend to use the three dimensions of **attributions** of *stable/unstable, global/specific,* and *internal/external* to answer the "Why?" question. A man could think "I asked her out on a date and she said no because" (a) "I am defective" or (b) "I am not her type." If he thought "a," then he is making a stable, global, internal attribution that his condition is permanent (i.e., stable), that it will likely affect him with anyone he asks out on a date (i.e., global), and that he is the cause of her rejection (i.e., internal). What will he think and feel before asking another woman out for a date? Odds are that his pessimistic explanatory style will lead him to feel anxiety and to expect another rejection.

If, on the other hand, he thought "b" (i.e., "I am not her type"), then he is making an unstable, specific, external attribution that his condition is temporary (i.e., unstable), that it applies only to the woman he just asked out for a date (i.e., specific), and that the outcome was due to her tastes (i.e., external). Now what would he think before asking another woman out on a date? As you probably determined, in this case he is using an optimistic explanatory style and is less likely to expect rejection or to feel as anxious when asking another woman out for a date.

Schulman (1999) explains that optimism can be learned through using cognitive training techniques such as the ABCD disputation method advocated by Albert Ellis (Ellis & Dryden, 2007). In addition, Seligman, Reivich, Jaycox, and Gillham (1995) developed a 12-week program called the Penn Optimism Program to assist children who are at risk for depression to learn optimistic thinking through changing their attributional explanatory styles.

attributional retraining (AR): programs designed to change attributional explanatory styles to cultivate learned optimism or a greater sense of personal control over outcomes.

A related approach, known as **attributional retraining (AR)**, has been used successfully for more than two decades to improve college students' academic achievement. The AR approach encourages students to use attributions of control (as opposed to attributions of no control) after poor academic performances. Studies indicate that AR generally leads to modest improvements in academic performance (Perry, Hechter, Menec, & Weinberg, 1993; Perry, Stupnisky, Hall, Chipperfield, & Weiner, 2010).

ADDITIONAL COPING STRATEGIES

There are a number of other strategies for coping with stress including expressive writing, self-forgiveness, humor, pets, and music. A brief discussion of each follows. Other strategies such as physical exercise, nutrition, and relaxation exercises are covered in depth in subsequent chapters.

Expressive Writing

Do you know anyone who keeps a journal? If so, have you ever wondered why they go through all the trouble to write down their personal thoughts and feelings on a regular basis—especially if no one else reads these self-disclosures? What are they getting out of it that keeps them going back to their journal? Is there something therapeutic about journaling? Since the early days of Freudian psychoanalysis, many psychotherapists warned that it is harmful to our psychological and physical health to "hold it all inside." Could it be, especially with people who have experienced trauma, that pouring it out on *paper* is beneficial? To answer this question, James Pennebaker designed a writing exercise known as **expressive writing** that asks participants to write their thoughts and feelings about their most upsetting or traumatic experiences.

expressive writing: a therapeutic writing exercise in which participants are asked to write their thoughts and feelings about their most upsetting and traumatic experiences.

In one of his seminal studies, Pennebaker and his colleagues (Pennebaker, Keicolt-Glaser, & Glaser, 1988) asked participants to engage in expressive writing while control participants wrote about trivial or mundane matters. Each group followed their exercises for 4 consecutive days. What did they find? As predicted, the expressive writing group when compared to the control group reported less distress at a 3-month follow-up, used the health center less often during the course of the study, and showed immune system benefits reflected in greater T-lymphocyte responses. Indeed, there did appear to be therapeutic benefits to journaling.

Since those early beginnings, over 200 studies have been conducted to determine the benefits of expressive writing. Most, but not all, found overall positive effects. A recent meta-analytic review (Frattaroli, 2006) determined that expressive writing has a very modest positive effect size of $r = .075$ for mental and physical health. Do such studies indicate that to achieve benefits you must write about upsetting experiences or trauma like the participants in Pennebaker and his associates' (1988) seminal study did for 4 consecutive days? And what theory best explains these benefits when they occur?

After reviewing the empirical results of the last two decades of expressive writing studies, Smyth and Pennebaker (2008) conclude that (1) people do not need to write about trauma or negative experiences to reap benefits of expressive writing because writing about positive experiences also leads to gains of a similar magnitude, (2) several days of writing are not necessary because benefits can accrue when writing within 1 day, and (3) there does not seem to be one theoretical process that best explains why expressive writing works—in many ways it is still a mystery.

Since the early days of research in the area, the emergence of the Internet and social networking sites like MySpace and Facebook opened new venues for expressive writing (Smyth & Pennebaker, 2008). Given the immense popularity of social networking sites, especially among younger generations, there may be a major paradigm shift underway in predominant ways to express one's thoughts and feelings through writing—in this case, writing to strengthen social bonds. Could the therapeutic benefits of expressive writing account for some of the attraction of social networking sites? What do you think?

Self-Forgiveness

Have you ever considered self-forgiveness to be a coping response? Recall the health and well-being benefits of forgiveness discussed in Chapter 2 indicating that elevated forgiveness levels are often later followed by higher levels of psychological well-being; that forgiving imagery can lead to less cardiovascular reactivity; and that forgiving personalities are less likely to exhibit hostility, anger, depression, and anxiety? Given these findings, then does not it make sense to direct compassion and forgiveness toward oneself as a coping response? If you answered "yes," then you might be surprised to know that "self-forgiveness has been largely neglected by psychological researchers" (Hall & Fincham, 2008, p. 174).

Self-forgiveness refers to the constructive process of letting go of a desire to punish, retaliate, or act destructively toward oneself due to one's perceived transgressions. It does not absolve a person from taking responsibility for objective acts of wrongdoing. Taking responsibility may involve making a commitment to never again commit the offensive acts or to make reparations to persons who have been harmed by such acts (Fisher & Exline, 2006; Hall & Fincham, 2005).

The small body of research literature on the practice suggests that self-forgiveness is more likely to occur when the transgressing person (a) feels less guilt about the transgression, (b) engages in more conciliatory behavior toward the victim, and (c) perceives the victim as more forgiving (Hall & Fincham, 2008).

In the health area, sometimes receiving a cancer diagnosis leads to self-blame. For example, smokers with lung cancer sometimes blame themselves for their past smoking behavior that they see as having caused their cancer. In cases such as tobacco smoking, self-blame can lead to positive health behaviors such as quitting smoking. However, in general, self-blame is associated with greater distress and a poorer adjustment to cancer (see Friedman et al., 2007, for discussion). Breast cancer survivors also may blame themselves for bringing about their cancer, yet the cause of their breast cancer is usually unknown. A recent study indicates that women being treated for breast cancer who engaged in self-blame reported greater mood disturbance and a lower quality of life than their counterparts who did not self-blame (Friedman et al., 2007). A self-forgiving attitude among women undergoing breast cancer treatment is associated with "less mood disturbance and a better quality of life" (Romero et al., 2006, p. 29).

Humor

The sign on the plumber's truck reads *A Flush Beats a Full House*. What possessed the plumber to evoke images of plumbing problems in this way? Perhaps the plumber thought that humor can take some of the stress out of our plumbing calamities. Humor reframes problems in ways that create positive affect,

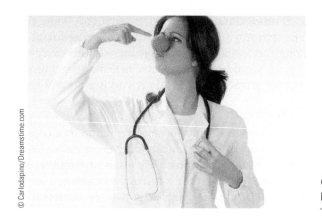

© Carlodapino/Dreamstime.com

Can we laugh ourselves
back to health?

emotional distance, and a new perspective. As a result, the stress feels lighter
and the problem less serious.

Humor as a coping strategy received significant attention from health researchers after Norman Cousins wrote his now famous 1976 book called
Anatomy of an Illness. In the book Cousins described his strategy of taking
high doses of vitamins and watching humorous television and movie clips such
as *Candid Camera* and the Marx Brothers to facilitate the remission of his
rare and painful rheumatoid disease called *ankylosing spondylitis.* Cousins
(1978) later presented his case to physicians and others in the health field
through his article published in the prestigious *New England Journal of
Medicine.* Since that time, the use of laughter and humor as a strategy to combat illness has become popular folklore. After several decades of research in
the area, what does the evidence now tell us?

Martin (2002, p. 219) concludes from his review of the relevant research
that "despite the popularity of the idea that humor and laughter have significant health benefits, the current empirical evidence is generally weak and inconclusive." Most of the research involves laboratory studies where participants
are exposed to comedy conditions. These studies usually suffer from methodological problems such as poor controls and small sample sizes. Actual laughter is rarely measured. When it is, there is no attempt to discern whether the
laughter is real or feigned. Opposite of the commonly held belief that laughter
lowers blood pressure, Martin (2002, p. 218) concludes that "experimental
studies indicate that laughter is actually associated with short-term increases
in blood pressure and heart rate, but no longer-term effects."

coping humor: using
humor to cope with
stress.

More positive results are found for using **coping humor,** a strategy of
using humor to cope with stress. For example, Kuiper, Grimshaw, Leite, and
Kirsh (2004) demonstrated that coping humor is linked to higher levels of self-
esteem, perceived competency, and positive affect as well as less anxiety,
depression, and negative affect. Further, they demonstrated that some sense-
of-humor styles are associated with positive psychological well-being such
as affiliative humor (e.g., "I laugh and joke a lot with my friends) and
self-enhancing humor (e.g. "Even when I'm by myself, I am amused by the ab-
surdities in life"), whereas others are associated with negative psychological

well-being such as self-defeating humor (e.g., "I often get carried away in putting myself down if it makes my family and friends laugh") and belabored humor (e.g., "I react in an exaggerated way to mildly humorous comments") (Kuiper et al., 2004, p. 147). Their ironic conclusion is listed in the title of their article that reads "Humor Is Not Always the Best Medicine" (p. 135).

Pets

Do you have a dog, cat, bird, or another pet friend waiting for you when you come home from school, work, or other activities? If so, do you feel happy anticipating the greeting from your furry or feathery friend upon your return? Do you feel a sense of well-being when bonding with your pet? You may have heard that interacting with your pets can lead to positive physiological effects, but is this popular belief supported by the research? Let us look at the answer to that question.

Overall, there are very few studies assessing the physiological benefits of **human-animal interaction.** Some of the results are inconsistent. However, there are two conclusions we can generally draw from the research (Virues-Ortega & Buela-Casal, 2006). First, longitudinal studies suggest that human-animal interaction through pet ownership can result in lower blood pressure and heart rate. Second, interacting with pets can buffer autonomic reactivity to acute stress. The primary mechanism for these effects seems to be a special kind of social support. Pets give **nonevaluative social support.** That is, when our pets give their social support we do not in any way feel criticized or judged by them.

Recent research indicates that human oxytocin hormone may play a role in the bonding process for women with their pet dogs but not for men and their dogs. Recall from Chapter 8 Shelly Taylor's (2006) tend-and-befriend model that oxytocin, a hormone found in high concentrations in nursing women that is believed to facilitate maternal-infant bonding, has calming properties. Oxytocin may play a role in social bonding, the affiliative process, and stress relief. Miller et al. (2009) found that women who engaged in 25 minutes of interaction with their pet dog immediately after returning home from work showed elevated serum oxytocin levels compared to a control condition where these same women spent the identical amount of time reading a neutral book without their dog present. The effect was not found for men.

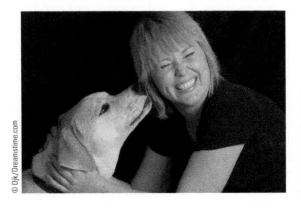

Women who engaged in 25 minutes of human-animal interaction with their pet dog immediately after returning home from work showed elevated serum oxytocin levels.

© Djk/Dreamstime.com

This intriguing study suggests an additional mechanism that explains the physiological benefits of human-animal interaction, at least for women dog owners. Perhaps oxytocin combined with nonevaluative social support plays a role in stress relief for such women when interacting with their dogs.

Music

If "music has charms to sooth a savage breast, to soften rocks, or bend a knotted oak" as William Congreve wrote in his 1697 play *The Mourning Bride,* then surely it also can help us manage stress (Congreve, 1967, p. 326). **Music** has been used throughout the ages for enjoyment and mood regulation (Conrad, 2010). Some forms of music are more relaxing than others, and, as we know, all of us have our own tastes. For example, some find Gregorian chants or New Age music relaxing and others not. Can listening to music lead to positive health effects?

Let us look at the fascinating results of a study (Charnetski, Brennan, & Harrison, 1998) of college students who listened for 30 minutes to a "smooth jazz" tape, a tone/click stimulus, a radio music broadcast that included commercials, or no sound (i.e., silence). Saliva samples were collected before and after their listening experience to determine immunoglobulin A (IgA) levels. The results indicated that IgA levels increased but only in the condition where participants listened to smooth jazz music. What was it about listening to music that caused their enhanced immune system responsiveness? The cause is unknown, but the study's authors speculate that it could be due to increased relaxation, positive affect, direct physiological influences such as the music's increasing their parasympathetic activity, or to music's directly affecting neuronal discharge rates.

A more recent randomized study (Conrad et al., 2007) of 10 patients who were critically ill found that when researchers played the slow movements of Mozart's piano sonatas the patients showed physiological responses indicating stress reduction. What were these physiological responses? Patients who received the music intervention compared to controls had lower blood pressure, heart rate, and plasma concentrations of epinephrine and the proinflammatory cytokine interleukin-6 as well as increased plasma concentrations of growth hormone. The patients who received music intervention also required less sedative drugs to achieve the level of sedation induced in control patients. This study is limited by its small sample size but is intriguing nevertheless. Based on the study's results, the authors suggest that music relaxes the sympathetic-adrenal-medulla system (SAM) and the hypothalamic-pituitary-adrenal axis (HPA), which then positively mediates immune system responses.

The limited research on the beneficial physiological effects of music is still in its infancy and only some types of music appear to produce beneficial effects. However, as Conrad (2010, p. 1981) notes, "music may well be a potentially powerful tool for improving clinical outcomes with little known risk when applied appropriately and judiciously. Whether music in medicine will grow to be widely accepted as an adjunctive therapy will depend on a better understanding of its role through clinical and scientific experimentation."

CHAPTER SUMMARY AND CONCEPT REVIEW

- Problem-focused coping refers to dealing with the perceived cause of distress, whereas emotion-focused coping involves managing distress caused by the problem.

- Active strategies involve problem-focused approaches and avoidance strategies use emotion-focused approaches.

- Avoidance coping may be an effective strategy for dealing with minor or transient irritations, but for serious or chronic problems it is not very successful.

- Support-seeking coping involves seeking informational or emotional support from others.

- Meaning-making coping is coping that uses our values, beliefs, and goals to shape meaning in stressful situations that are generally not conducive to the use of problem-focused coping.

- Retrospective coping inventories, momentary reports, and narrative accounts are methods used to measure coping styles.

- Dispositional optimism is positively related to approach coping strategies and negatively associated with avoidance coping strategies.

- In general, approach coping is more successful than avoidance coping.

- Religious-based coping has some features that overlap with meaning-making coping.

- Cognitive restructuring is a strategy for challenging dysfunctional thoughts, assumptions, and beliefs and replacing them with healthier realistic thinking patterns.

- Rational-emotive behavior therapy (REBT) is based on the ABC model of an activating event being interpreted through one's beliefs, which in turn leads to emotional or behavioral consequences.

- Beck's (1967) cognitive psychotherapy approach is similar to REBT, but it focuses on challenging maladaptive attitudes and automatic negative thoughts rather than irrational beliefs.

- The triple column method is an exercise for challenging dysfunctional thoughts by writing down stressful thoughts in the first column, identifying and labeling the type of distortions they represent in the second column, and writing down more realistic substitution thoughts in the third column.

- Stress inoculation training (SIT) is a cognitive-behavior modification training program that includes education, self-monitoring, cognitive restructuring, problem solving, relaxation training, and rehearsal.

- Optimism can be learned through cognitive training techniques such as the ABCD disputation method or through changing attributional explanatory styles.

- Expressive writing has a very modest positive effect on mental and physical health.

- Self-forgiveness refers to the constructive process of letting go of a desire to punish, retaliate, or act destructively toward oneself due to one's perceived transgressions.

- The evidence suggesting that humor and laughter confer health benefits is weak at best but there is support for the psychological benefits of coping humor.

- Research on pet ownership suggests that human-animal interaction can result in lower blood pressure and heart rate as well as buffer autonomic reactivity to acute stress.

- Some research indicates that music can lead to enhanced immune system responsiveness and reductions in stress hormones and proinflammatory cytokines.

CRITICAL THINKING QUESTIONS

1. Why do you think that dispositional optimists are more inclined to use approach coping and disinclined to use avoidance coping strategies? In what ways could this pattern of coping account for the positive health and well-being benefits associated with dispositional optimism?

2. Do you believe that religious-based coping represents a distinct form of coping that is different from problem-focused coping, emotion-focused coping, social support-seeking coping, and meaning-making coping? How is religious-based coping similar to or different from other forms of coping, especially meaning-making coping?

3. Do you share with others your personal thoughts and feelings on any of the social networking sites? If so, do you experience any therapeutic benefits such as positive feelings from your self-expressions? How do you explain any benefits you may experience from your self-expressions?

4. Have you experienced the calming effects of having a pet greet you at the end of the day? What do you believe accounts for these calming effects? Are some types of pets such as dogs more calming than others? If so, why do you think that is?

5. What do you think accounts for the beneficial health effects of music? What type of music do you believe is most effective for helping you unwind from stress? Do you think certain types of music (e.g., classical) would be equally effective in reducing the effects of stress for anyone who listens, or does the music have to be specific to the taste of the listener to be effective? Explain.

KEY TERMS AND CONCEPTS

Accommodation

Activating event

Approach coping*

Assimilation

Attributional
retraining (AR)*

Attributions

Avoidance coping*

Beliefs

Catastrophize*

Causal attribution

Cognitive primacy*

Cognitive restructuring*

Consequences

Coping

Coping humor*

Dispute

Emotion-focused coping*

Expressive writing*

Global beliefs

Global goals

Global meaning

Goodness of fit
hypothesis

Human-animal
interaction

Learned optimism

Meaning-making
coping*

Meanings made

Music

Nonevaluative social
support

Problem-focused coping*

Rational-emotive behavior
therapy (REBT)*

Religious-based coping*

Self-forgiveness

Self-talk*

Stress inoculation
training (SIT)*

Triple column method*

MEDIA RESOURCES

CENGAGE**brain**.com

Access an interactive eBook, chapter-specific
interactive learning tools, including flashcards,
quizzes, videos, and more in your Psychology
CourseMate, accessed through CengageBrain.com.

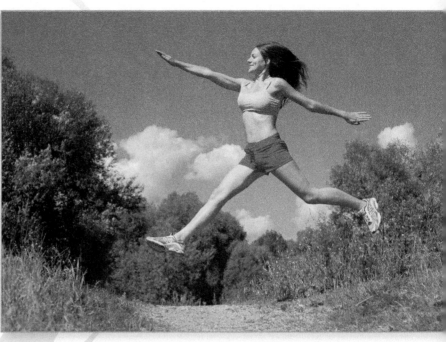

It is exercise alone that supports the spirits, and keeps the mind in vigor.

~CICERO

CHAPTER 11

PHYSICAL ACTIVITY AND EXERCISE

Imagine if you will that you are talking to a college student friend named Erica. Your conversation eventually comes around to, of all things, brands of toothpaste. Out of the blue, Erica announces to you that she doesn't really care about brands of toothpaste because she no longer brushes her teeth. Taken aback, you ask her why? "Well, tooth brushing is boring, it takes too much time, toothpaste gets expensive, and I have better things to do. Besides, I brushed my teeth for many years and got tired of it," she proudly proclaims. What would you think?

Perhaps you would think that tooth brushing as part of a daily routine is a small price to pay to keep your teeth healthy. That just because Erica brushed her teeth for many years doesn't mean she can stop now if she wants to maintain healthy teeth. You might think that maybe she better make tooth brushing a higher priority in her life if she wants to prevent cavities and gum disease and keep her teeth in the future.

Fast-forward now 30 years. You see Erica for the first time since your conversation with her in college all that many years ago. She gives you a big smile. What do you see? Is it a pretty picture?

You might now be wondering what Erica's dental hygiene practice has to do with physical exercise. After all, this is a chapter on physical activity and exercise. Then again, you may have already figured it out.

Remember the joy of running, jumping, and playing when you were a child? If we abandon the regular physical activity we enjoyed so much as children, over the years we prematurely invite diseases of aging—and like Erica's smile, it's not a pretty picture. Maintaining our overall physical health requires ongoing physical activity. Like brushing our teeth on a regular basis, building and maintaining a lifetime habit of regular physical activity is a vital part of choosing a healthy lifestyle. In addition, it is a powerful stress management tool.

According to the U.S. National Center for Health Statistics (Pleis, Lucas, & Ward, 2009), only 33% of adult Americans engage in regular leisure-time physical activity. Whereas another 31% of adults at least engage in *some* leisure-time physical activity, the remaining 36% are considered *inactive*. It is as though a new variety of *Homo sapiens* has emerged, the *sedentarians*. How then did so many people in the industrialized world get to

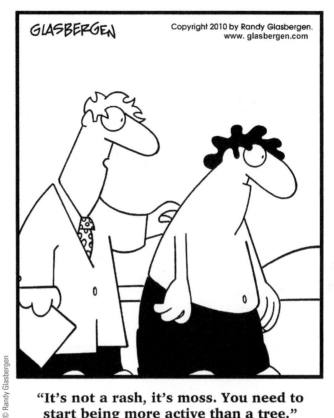

"It's not a rash, it's moss. You need to
start being more active than a tree."

be so sedentary? We have bodies made for movement and physical activity, and yet we generally live lifestyles of inactivity and comfort. Sedentary lifestyles contribute to many of the "diseases of comfort" (Mitchell, Church, & Zucker, 2008, p. 234) such as cardiovascular disease and type 2 diabetes that are so prevalent today.

How are sedentarians different from their active prehistoric ancestors? Actually, their body structures are the same, but their activity levels are vastly different. Whereas prehistoric humans were constantly on the move physically searching for food, fleeing from predators, or fighting physical threats in order to survive, sedentarians are mostly stationary, often spending vast amounts of time standing in place or anchored to their desks at work and then ensconced in their living room sofas or easy chairs at home. Mental movement is the sedentarian's primary exercise. When stressed, sedentarians mentally fight or flee the saber-toothed tigers of their minds while their adrenaline-charged bodies sit idle.

What can we do to reverse this historically recent trend toward sedentarianism? Is the goal to transform sedentarians into marathoners? No, the goal is much more reasonable—to simply encourage sedentarians to once again become *activarians*—to rouse their active vibrant selves (Mitchell et al., 2008). In fact, today's modest recommendations from the U.S. Department of Health and Human Services' (2011) physical activity guidelines for Americans are that we engage weekly in a minimum of 150 minutes of moderate-intensity aerobic activity or 75 minutes of vigorous activity spread throughout the week. The agency also recommends some strength training exercises twice a week (Tables 11.1 and 11.2). The American College of Sports Medicine (ACSM) and the American Heart Association (AHA) have similar guidelines to engage in moderate-intensity aerobic exercise for a minimum of 30 minutes

TABLE **11.1**   Benefits of weekly moderate-intensity aerobic physical activity

Levels of Physical Activity	Range of Moderate-Intensity Minutes a Week	Summary of Overall Health Benefits	Comment
Inactive	No activity beyond baseline	None	Being inactive is unhealthy.
Low	Activity beyond baseline but fewer than 150 minutes a week	Some	Low levels of activity are clearly preferable to an inactive lifestyle.
Medium	150 minutes to 300 minutes a week	Substantial	Activity at the high end of this range has additional and more extensive health benefits than activity at the low end.
High	More than 300 minutes a week	Additional	Current science does not allow researchers to identify an upper limit of activity above which there are no additional health benefits.

SOURCE: U.S. Department of Health & Human Services (2008). Physical activity guidelines for Americans. Retrieved from http://www.health.gov/paguidelines.

TABLE **11.2**   The U.S. Department of Health and Human Services' current physical activity guidelines for adult Americans

Key Guidelines for Adults
• All adults should avoid inactivity. Some physical activity is better than none, and adults who participate in any amount of physical activity gain some health benefits.
• For substantial health benefits, adults should do at least 150 minutes (2 hours and 30 minutes) a week of moderate-intensity, or 75 minutes (1 hour and 15 minutes) a week of vigorous-intensity aerobic physical acitvity, or an equivalent combination of moderate- and vigorous-intensity aerobic activity. Aerobic activity should be performed in episodes of at least 10 minutes, and preferably, it should be spread throughout the week.
• For additional and more extensive health benefits, adults should increase their aerobic physical activity to 300 minutes (5 hours) a week of moderate-intensity, or 150 minutes a week of vigorous-intensity aerobic physical activity, or an equivalent combination of moderate- and vigorous-intensity activity. Additional health benefits are gained by engaging in physical activity beyond this amount.
• Adults should also do muscle-strengthening activities that are moderate or high intensity and involve all major muscle groups on 2 or more days a week, as these activities provide additional health benefits.

SOURCE: U.S. Department of Health & Human Services (2008). Physical activity guidelines for Americans. Retrieved from http://www.health.gov/paguidelines.

TABLE **11.3**   Moderate- and vigorous-intensity aerobic physical activity examples

Moderate Intensity
• Walking briskly (3 miles per hour or faster, but not race-walking)
• Water aerobics
• Bicycling slower than 10 miles per hour
• Tennis (doubles)
• Ballroom dancing
• General gardening

Vigorous Intensity
• Racewalking, jogging, or running
• Swimming laps
• Tennis (singles)
• Aerobic dancing
• Bicycling 10 miles per hour or faster
• Jumping rope
• Heavy gardening (continuous digging or hoeing, with heart rate increases)
• Hiking uphill or with a heavy backpack

SOURCE: U.S. Department of Health & Human Services (2008). Physical activity guidelines for Americans. Retrieved from http://www.health.gov/paguidelines.

(up to 60 minutes) per day for 5 days a week or vigorously intense aerobic exercise for 20 to 30 minutes per day for a total of 75 to 150 minutes per week as well as twice a week of resistance training (i.e., strength training, weight lifting) (Chodzko-Zajko et al., 2009). These are very reasonable recommendations and can be done by even the most stationary sedentarians.

moderate-intensity activity: bodily movement such as brisk walking that produces a sustained heart rate of around 60% of one's maximum capacity.

vigorous activity: bodily movement such as running that produces a sustained heart rate of at least 70% of one's maximum capacity.

Moderate-intensity activities include brisk walking, water aerobics, and doubles tennis to name a few. How do we know if we are engaging in moderate-intensity activity? We know when we are able to talk during the activity but cannot sing. As we further intensify our activity levels, we know that we have entered the **vigorous activity** zone when we can speak only a few words at a time before we need to pause our words to catch our breath. Examples of vigorous activities include aerobic dance, swimming laps, and running or race walking. See Table 11.3 for examples of moderate and vigorous activities.

For some people even 150 minutes of moderate-intensity activity, usually divided into five 30-minute sessions, seems like too much time. However, there is hope even for these individuals to spring into action as well. A recent randomized control study (Church, Earnest, Skinner, & Blair, 2007) published in the prestigious *Journal of the American Medical Association* revealed significant dose-dependent fitness improvements for previously sedentary individuals for even as low as 75 minutes per week of moderate-intensity activity; this amounts to just 15 minutes a day, 5 days a week. Within reason more is better, but the point is that even low doses of regular physical activity can have a meaningful impact on our health.

INSIGHT EXERCISE **11.1**

Are you a sedentarian or an activarian? If you are an activarian, congratulations; you are receiving the many benefits exercise gives you. If you are a sedentarian and you want to transform back into your active, vibrant activarian self, it is probably easier than you think. First it is a matter of looking at your obstacles to starting an exercise program. Which of the following apply to you?

What Are My Exercise Barriers?

1	I don't know how to start an exercise program.
2	I do not have a good place or facility to exercise in.
3	Exercise is too expensive.
4	Exercise takes too much time.
5	I don't have the energy to exercise.
6	It is unsafe to exercise.
7	I am overweight and do not look good in exercise clothing.
8	My friends are sedentarians and they wouldn't like it if I started exercising.
9	I have too many other responsibilities that get in the way of exercising.
10	I have health problems that prevent me from exercising.
11	My smoking gets in the way of exercising.
12	I don't have the confidence to exercise.

After reading the rest of this chapter and talking to one of your activarian friends, brainstorm some ideas for overcoming these barriers. You will find many suggestions and ideas throughout this chapter. Collect and generate as many ideas as possible and then try out a few that seem most reasonable. Once you have addressed the barriers, you are ready to move from contemplating exercise to actually doing it.

MEANING OF PHYSICAL ACTIVITY, EXERCISE, AND FITNESS

physical activity: health-enhancing bodily movement.

physical exercise: planned physical activity designed to exert one's body for health and fitness benefits.

Before we discuss the positive benefits of physical activity, let us define some terms. What do you think the differences are among physical activity, exercise, and fitness? They are overlapping concepts, but they also are different in some respects. Physical activity refers to your bodily movement. Typing on a keyboard, lifting weights, or making the bed are all examples of physical activity. However, for the purpose of this discussion, **physical activity** will mean "bodily movement that enhances health" (U.S. Health and Human Services, 2008, p. 3). **Physical exercise** is planned physical activity designed to exert your body for health or fitness benefits. Of the examples listed previously, only one is physical exercise. Which one? Of course, only weight lifting is physical exercise.

In order to understand the term *physical fitness,* we have to answer the question *fit for what*? In other words, what are we trying to achieve? Are we trying to play a sport, run long distances, lift heavy objects, stretch into different yoga positions, or accomplish some other goal that involves physical activity? In order to accomplish one of these goals, we must develop or maintain various elements of **physical fitness** such as "cardiorespiratory function, relative leanness, muscular strength, muscular endurance, and flexibility" (Howley & Franks, 2007, p. 17). However, which components of physical fitness we target depends on our goal. If we want to stretch into different yoga positions, then flexibility is one of our most important fitness components to develop. Muscular strength is obviously important for weight lifting.

However, if our goal is to strengthen our heart and lower our risk of cardiovascular disease and premature death, then cardiorespiratory fitness is the element of fitness we need to focus on. **Cardiorespiratory fitness,** otherwise known as aerobic fitness, refers to the ability of the body's heart, blood vessels, and lungs to supply oxygen-rich blood to the muscles during sustained physical activity. **Aerobic** means "with air" (i.e., oxygen) and contrasts with **anaerobic,** which indicates "without air." Whereas jogging is a form of aerobic exercise because you can continue to oxygenate your body while you jog, sprinting is a form of anaerobic exercise because at some point during your sprint your bodily systems can no longer sustain their oxygen supplies to maintain energy demands. This lack of oxygen will soon stop your sprint to allow you to catch your breath so you can restore your body's oxygen deficit. Cardiorespiratory fitness can be measured directly using a treadmill test and recording peak absolute oxygen consumption. Like all forms of fitness, it is a product of the **FITT principle,** that is, frequency, intensity, time, and type of physical activity.

Prior to the 1968 publication of physician Kenneth Cooper's book *Aerobics,* the medical community viewed regular physical exercise as a luxury rather than a necessity. However, Cooper was a strong advocate for jogging and aerobic exercise and was one of the catalysts for the jogging craze that followed the publication of his book. His idea was to push our levels of speed and endurance. He inspired walkers to jog and joggers to run faster and longer (Mitchell et al., 2008). By the 1990s, however, the spirit of the times began to change when increasing evidence pointed to important health benefits from more modest activity goals. The U.S. National Institutes of Health (NIH) Consensus Development Panel reviewed the new body of fitness evidence and recommended a minimum of 30 minutes of moderate-intensity physical activity most, if not every day, of the week (NIH, 1996). Today, the U.S. government's health standard of 150 minutes of moderate-intensity exercise a week discussed earlier is closely aligned with this NIH panel recommendation.

Throughout this chapter, then, as we discuss the health and psychological benefits of physical activity and exercise, the emphasis will be on aerobic fitness because this is the component of fitness that has the largest body of supportive research. However, it should be noted that there is a growing body of evidence demonstrating that strength training (also known as resistance training) provides important benefits as well, including lessening the signs and

cardiorespiratory fitness: also known as aerobic fitness; refers to the ability of the body's heart, blood vessels, and lungs to supply oxygen-rich blood to the muscles during sustained physical activity.

aerobic: with air/oxygen.

FITT principle: fitness is a product of frequency, intensity, time, and type of physical activity.

symptoms of diabetes, osteoporosis, arthritis, back pain, obesity, and depression (Centers for Disease Control and Prevention, 2011e). The benefits of strength training also is mentioned, but less frequently, throughout this chapter. One of the psychological benefits of physical activity and aerobic fitness is the ability to combat the adverse effects of stress. However, as we will soon discuss, there are many other psychological and physical benefits as well.

BENEFITS OF AEROBIC ACTIVITY AND EXERCISE

If there ever was a lifestyle panacea for health and well-being, physical activity and exercise probably comes the closest. Granted, it has its drawbacks, including time commitment, effort, and risk of physical injury. However, its range of benefits is probably the most sweeping of all positive lifestyle endeavors we could choose. Benefits of initiating and maintaining ongoing aerobic fitness include the following:

- Strengthens the heart and cardiovascular system
- Reduces risk of cardiovascular disease
- Reduces body fat, risk of the metabolic syndrome and of developing type 2 diabetes
- Reduces risk of cancer
- Boosts the immune system
- Combats bone mass loss due to aging and osteoporosis
- Increases life expectancy
- Buffers stress
- Reduces anxiety
- Reduces depression
- Enhances psychological well-being
- Improves sleep
- Improves cognitive performance
- Builds self-confidence, self-esteem, and self-efficacy

Let us next look at evidence for some of these benefits, grouping them together into two broad but overlapping categories of, first, health and, second, well-being.

HEALTH BENEFITS OF PHYSICAL ACTIVITY

Early studies laid the groundwork for establishing a connection between health benefits and physical activity. For example, a seminal study in the 1950s by Jeremy Morris and his colleagues (Morris, Heady, Raffle, Roberts, & Parks, 1953) was the first to document a relationship between levels of physical activity and incidence of coronary heart disease (CHD). Their study demonstrated that the physically active conductors on London's celebrated double-decker buses had a lower incidence of heart disease than their more sedentary bus-driving coworkers.

A decade later, Harold Kahn (1963) observed that U.S. letter carriers who walked their routes had lower CHD death rates than their postal counterparts who worked in sedentary clerical positions. Even more revealing was evidence he observed that when the active letter carriers switched to sedentary postal clerical jobs, within the span of a little over 5 years their CHD death rates grew to match those of their peers who had spent their entire postal careers as clerks.

In the next decade, Ralph Paffenbarger and his associates also published landmark studies (Paffenbarger, Gima, Laughlin, & Black, 1971; Paffenbarger, Laughlin, Gima, & Black, 1970) on the topic where they reported that the San Francisco longshoremen whose jobs involved high levels of activity (e.g., cargo handling) had lower CHD rates than their counterparts whose jobs entailed more sedentary work. Later in the decade Paffenbarger's research group (Paffenbarger, Wing, & Hyde, 1978) determined that Harvard University alumni who expended higher levels of energy each week had a lower risk of fatal and nonfatal heart attacks than their peers who expended lower levels of energy.

osteoporosis: a skeletal
disease involving loss of
bone density.

In the ensuing years, more research was conducted that uncovered physical activity protection and sedentary risk for a number of diseases including stroke; hypertension; certain cancers; metabolic syndrome; type 2 diabetes; and **osteoporosis,** a skeletal disease involving loss of bone density. In addition, more prospective studies with tighter controls were conducted that presented even stronger evidence of a link between exercise and reduced risk of early death and heart disease.

After five decades of research on physical activity and health, the evidence is now incontrovertible that regular physical exercise reduces the risk of early mortality, cardiovascular disease, stroke, hypertension, breast and colon cancer, and type 2 diabetes; there also is important indirect evidence supporting the use of weight-bearing exercise to protect against bone loss due to osteoporosis (Warburton, Charlesworth, Ivey, Nettlefold, & Bredin, 2010, p. 212). Governmental agencies (e.g., U.S. Department of Health and Human Services, 2011; Public Health Agency of Canada, 2011) and assessments from recent reviews (Bassuk & Manson, 2010; Warburton et al., 2010), including a position stand from the ACSM (Chodzko-Zajko et al., 2009), support these conclusions. For example, Warburton and his colleagues (Warburton et al., 2010) conducted a sweeping review of the research on the effects of exercise on early mortality and disease prevention by first identifying all the studies on the topic that met their inclusion criteria going back to the 1950s. One inclusion criterion for their review was that the study must have used at least three levels of exercise. They needed this information to determine any dose-response relationships. Most of the studies that satisfied their inclusion criteria were prospective cohort investigations. Next they critically examined the methodology and evidence of the body of research they culled. The reviewers then graded the level and quality of the research evidence according to the following scale: Level 1 indicates the highest-quality evidence and level 4 the lowest; grade A merits the strongest and grade C the weakest recommendation for action.

TABLE **11.4** Summary of findings from Warburton et al. (2010) for the effects of physical exercise/fitness on seven primary health outcomes

Type of Health Risk	Number of Studies That Met Inclusion Criteria	Quality of Research	Average Percentage Reduction from Physical Activity/ Fitness	Minimum Recommended Dosage of Moderate Activity	Dose-Response Relationship?
All-Cause Mortality	70	Level 2 A	31%	30 minutes most days of the week.	Yes
Cardiovascular Disease	49	Level 2 A	33%	30 minutes most days of the week. Even 1 hour of brisk walking per week confers benefits.	Yes
Stroke	25	Level 3 A	31%	30 minutes most days of the week. Brisk walking effective.	Yes
Hypertension	12	Level 3 A	32%	30 minutes most days of the week.	Yes
Breast and Colon Cancer	76	Level 2 A	30%	30 to 60 minutes most days of the week.	Yes
Type 2 Diabetes	20	Level 2 A	42%	30 minutes most days of the week.	Yes
Osteoporosis	2	Level 3 A	Reduces risk but further research is required to determine the percentage reduction	30 minutes most days of the week. Must be load-bearing exercise.	Yes

What did they conclude? As indicated in Table 11.4, all categories received the strongest recommendation to use exercise as a preventive strategy; the empirical level of evidence was strongest for exercise reducing the risk of all-cause mortality, cardiovascular disease, breast and colon cancer, and type 2 diabetes though strong evidence also was found for stroke (both ischemic and hemorrhagic) and the prevention of hypertension. The evidence was indirect for using physical activity to minimize the risk of osteoporosis due to only a small number of studies meeting the authors' methodological criteria.

The use of exercise as a strategy to reduce each type of risk appears to confer benefits according to a dose-response relationship. It is not a linear relationship, but rather one in which sedentary individuals who start an exercise program

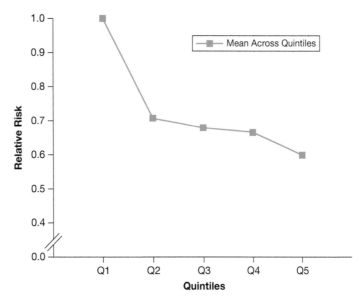

FIGURE **11.1**   Physical activity dose-response curve for all-cause mortality reported by Warburton et al. (2010). Notice that the most dramatic drop in risk occurs when moving from the bottom level of physical activity (sedentary level represented by the first quintile) to the next highest level (represented by the second quintile).   SOURCE: Based on Warburton et al. (2010).

show the most dramatic changes in risk reductions as they go from sedentary to minimally active; gains in dosage build from there with diminishing returns as a person's activity level reaches the maximum on the continuum. In general, each category of risk follows a pattern similar to that observed for all-cause mortality seen in Figure 11.1.

Based on their review and examination of the dose-response benefits, Warburton and his associates (2010) concurred with other authorities, including the Canadian government, that a minimum of 30 minutes most days of the week of moderate-intensity activity is generally advisable for an optimal risk reduction, and up to 60 minutes is even better. For example, the Canadian government's physical activity public health message is that "Every little bit counts, but more is even better—everyone can do it!" (Public Health Agency of Canada, 2011, p. 2). In addition, Warburton and his colleagues (2010) note that in some cases, such as reducing cardiovascular disease risk, even 1 hour of brisk walking per week confers benefits.

Aerobic exercise is the type of exercise with the largest body of supportive evidence for reducing cardiovascular disease risk. However, some studies document CHD prevention benefits for resistance exercise as well. For example, one study (Tanasecu et al., 2002) found that men who lifted weights for a minimum of 30 minutes each week in the study later exhibited a 23% reduced risk of developing CHD than those who did not weight train. The exercise-related risk reduction benefit for cardiovascular disease is similar in magnitude for men and women and appears to be the same across ethnicities (Bassuk & Manson, 2010; Warburton et al., 2010).

Possible mechanisms for reducing CHD through exercise are the reduction of body fat (especially in the midregion where it is most dangerous), blood pressure, and inflammation, along with the control of insulin sensitivity, blood sugar levels, and blood lipid levels (Bassuk & Manson, 2005). A single 30-minute bout of moderate-intensity aerobic exercise can reduce blood pressure (Hamer, Taylor, & Steptoe, 2006). Physical activity also raises high-density lipoproteins (HDL) (the "good" cholesterol) (Ferguson et al., 1998). As a result, the ratio of good cholesterol to total cholesterol becomes more favorable, a risk reduction result that may not be evident by just examining the total cholesterol. The ratio of HDL to total cholesterol is a far more important health risk indicator than total cholesterol by itself.

Reviews of the evidence of physical activity and cancer prevention from epidemiological studies reveal that exercise is associated with an average 20% to 30% reduction in risk of cancers of the breast and a 30% to 40% of the colon (Lee, 2003); each hour of weekly physical activity is associated with a 6% lower risk of breast cancer (Monninkhof et al., 2007). There is some evidence that ongoing physical activity may reduce breast cancer risk through promoting an increase in apoptosis (cellular death) of tumor cells and through reducing circulating estrogen levels; changes in estrogen metabolism can result in a decrease in breast epithelial cell proliferation (Coyle, 2008). However, more research is needed to determine the exact mechanisms responsible for exercise-related breast cancer prevention.

Mechanisms explaining the beneficial effects of exercise on colon cancer have been rarely tested, but the primary hypotheses include accelerating transit of food through the colon, reducing bile acid secretion, improving immune function, reducing serum cholesterol, and changing insulin and prostaglandin levels (Quadrilatero & Hoffman-Goetz, 2003). Recall from Chapter 4 that exercise can boost the immune system when done in moderation (Nieman, Henson, Austin, & Brown, 2005; Roger, Colbert, Greiner, Perkins, & Hursting, 2008). However, too much exercise such as running marathons and engaging in long-distance endurance athletic events can actually temporarily weaken immune system responsiveness, leading to higher illness rates (Anglem, Lucas, Rose, & Cotter, 2008; Nieman, 1995).

Exercise is especially important as a prevention strategy for those at high risk of developing type 2 diabetes, such as individuals with metabolic syndrome (see Chapter 5). Recently, the ACSM and the American Diabetes Association (2010, p. 2282) issued a joint position statement in which they concluded that "high-quality studies establishing the importance of exercise and fitness to diabetes were lacking until recently, but it is now well established that participation in regular PA [physical activity] improves blood glucose control and can prevent or delay T2DM [type 2 diabetes], along with positively affecting lipids, blood pressure, cardiovascular events, mortality, and quality of life."

Based on research from the Nurses' Health Study, Hu and his colleagues (2001) estimated that 87% of new cases of type 2 diabetes in women could be prevented through maintaining a healthy diet, normal weight, and regular exercise. For those who already have type 2 diabetes, aerobic exercise yields

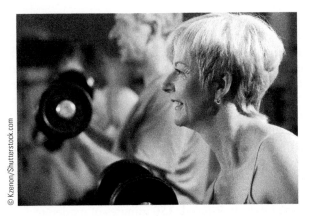

Weight training can reduce the risk of coronary heart disease, diabetes, and osteoporosis.

weight-bearing exercise: a form of exercise like walking and weight lifting in which the muscles work against the full effect of gravity.

visceral fat: the internal fat that pads the liver and abdominal organs.

benefits in controlling blood sugar, but adding resistance training alongside a weekly aerobic routine is even more effective (Sigal et al., 2007).

There is compelling evidence that engaging in **weight-bearing exercise** (muscles work against the full effect of gravity) such as walking, running, and resistance training benefits bone health, but there is only limited research on how this form of exercise can reduce the actual incidence of osteoporosis (Warburton et al., 2010). Note that swimming is not considered a weight-bearing exercise and so is not helpful in preventing osteoporosis. Evidence for the bone health benefits of weight-bearing exercise includes documentation of an inverse relationship between physical activity and the incidence of bone fractures in postmenopausal women and in other populations, including men (Feskanich, Willett, & Colditz, 2002; Kujala, Kaprio, Kannus, Sarna, & Koskenvuo, 2000). One of the few studies that examined the effect of exercise on incidence of osteoporosis found a dose-response relationship for women age 20 or older (Robitaille et al., 2008).

Physical activity seems to be especially effective in reducing the more dangerous type of fat known as **visceral fat** (Kay & Fiatarone Singh, 2006), the internal fat that pads the liver and abdominal organs. Visceral fat contrasts with the more common **subcutaneous fat** that is found just beneath the skin—the type of fat that can be removed during liposuction. Excess visceral fat as measured through use of imaging techniques is an independent risk factor for all-cause mortality (Kuk et al., 2006). It also is a stronger risk factor for heart attacks (as indicated by waist size) than body mass index (Yusuf et al., 2005). In addition, it is linked to colorectal cancer (Otake et al., 2005), breast cancer (Schapira et al., 1994), metabolic syndrome, and an increased circulation of proinflammatory cytokines such as TNF-α and IL-6 (Kyrou, Chrousos, & Tsigos, 2006).

As the medical director of the world-renowned fitness research center, the Cooper Clinic, Mitchell and his colleagues note, "If you were to take samples of subcutaneous and interior fat tissue, place them in separate laboratory dishes, and drip some stimulating chemicals onto them, the interior fat would respond with six times more harmful secretions, such as inflammatory molecules, than the subcutaneous tissue" (Mitchell et al., 2008, p. 29).

Thus, whereas excess fat and obesity pose a health risk, visceral fat is the most dangerous. A person can reduce visceral fat through exercise without changing his or her overall **body mass index (BMI)** (Kay & Fiatarone Singh, 2006). Note that BMI is a measure of the size of the body based on height and weight that is often used to estimate body fat. However, it is not always the most accurate proxy for body fat because a person can weigh more because of excess muscle rather than fat. For example, when Arnold Schwarzenegger was body building, he would have been considered overweight according to the BMI metric, yet his percentage of body fat was actually very low. Thus, exercise can be protective of health even when it is not noticeably apparent through BMI due to its ability to reduce visceral fat.

Although exercise is an important component of weight control, unless caloric intake is reduced, 150 minutes of moderate aerobic activity per week is generally not sufficient to lose weight. Based on examining the relevant body of evidence, the Institute of Medicine (Trumbo, Schlicker, Yates, & Poos, 2002) recommends 60 minutes per day of moderate-intensity activity (e.g., 3 to 4 miles per hour of walking or jogging) to prevent weight gain. And the ACSM (Donnelly et al., 2009) recommends over 250 minutes per week of moderate-intensity exercise to achieve clinically significant weight loss. It is important to point out that in general people who are overweight will benefit as much from regular physical activity as people who are normal weight because weight and exercise exert relatively independent influences on health (U.S. Department of Health and Human Services, 2008).

The ACSM also notes that resistance training does not facilitate weight loss, but that it does reduce health risk by increasing muscle mass and reducing fat mass. Thus, more fat is lost but more muscle mass is gained, resulting in a stronger and healthier person who may experience no net weight loss. In addition, because even during rest muscle burns far more calories than fat, strength training can produce as much as a 15% greater metabolic rate, making it easier to lose weight on dietary weight loss plans (Centers for Disease Control and Prevention, 2011e).

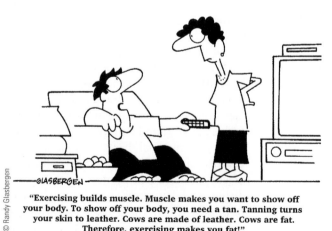

© Randy Glasbergen

"Exercising builds muscle. Muscle makes you want to show off your body. To show off your body, you need a tan. Tanning turns your skin to leather. Cows are made of leather. Cows are fat. Therefore, exercising makes you fat!"

WELL-BEING BENEFITS OF PHYSICAL ACTIVITY

In general the body of research conducted over the last two decades indicates that the immediate effects of exercise include lessening negative mood states and magnifying positive mood. For example, a study (Hansen, Stevens, & Coast, 2001) designed to test how much exercise is needed before a person feels better found improvements in mood after only 10 minutes of moderate-intensity aerobic exercise. Reductions in anxiety state generally occur after a bout of moderate to intense aerobic exercise with the immediate relaxation benefits typically extending for at least several hours (Raglin, 1997). Longer-term exercise protocols as well as direct measures of fitness also show more sustained benefits, such as overall reduced negative affect often coupled with enhanced well-being. The effects are not sustained, however, if an exercise program is discontinued.

Studies examining the effects of exercise on negative affect and mood have examined clinical and nonclinical populations. To date, exercise-related depression studies are more numerous than exercise-related anxiety studies. Researchers also have studied the effects of exercise on positive well-being as determined by measures of quality of life and psychological or emotional well-being.

Although testing the effects of exercise on psychological states seems like an easy process, investigators early on learned that they confronted a host of questions and methodological issues. For example, large-scale population epidemiological studies indicate that one of the risk factors for developing depressive symptoms is a sedentary lifestyle (Farmer et al., 1988). However, does this mean that the reverse is true—that physical activity protects against depression? We will look at evidence that can provide some answers to this question later.

Because symptoms of depression often include fatigue and withdrawal tendencies, when researchers find a negative correlation between physical activity and depression, does it mean that depression contributes to inactivity or that inactivity contributes to depression? Are cheerful people more likely to exercise, which perhaps contributes to a false perception that exercise creates good feelings? What do you think? These are the types of questions investigators had to address by using appropriate research methodology, some forms of which we will examine soon.

Other issues concern **expectancy effects.** If participants in an exercise group are given more attention than subjects in other conditions, such as a wait list control condition (i.e., placement on a waiting list for treatment), then will the exercisers show elevations in mood because of their positive expectations and the attention they receive from staff or because of the effects of exercise itself? How can we best differentiate exercise effects from expectancy effects?

Even comparing exercise to an effective antidepressant medication can be problematic because differences between an effective medication and an equally effective exercise protocol are not expected to be statistically significant. Without a control group for expectancy factors we cannot rule out the expectancy effect's contribution to the outcome for either treatment group. Therefore, we need an adequate prospective design with good experimental controls to determine the efficacy of exercise on these psychological states and conditions.

These studies are less common because using more complex and tightly controlled research designs is more costly and labor intensive for researchers.

In spite of these methodological issues and constraints, investigators have made substantial headway in establishing the efficacy of physical exercise as a tool for reducing anxiety and depression and for boosting psychological well-being. Although early studies were fraught with methodological problems, over the years investigators began employing tighter experimental controls through using randomized controlled trials, considered a gold standard for establishing efficacy of clinical treatments. These "trials" are studies in which participants are randomly assigned to groups where the intervention being tested (e.g., exercise) is compared to one or more control groups that receive an already established treatment, a placebo, or no intervention.

For example, some of the exercise intervention studies include comparison groups that use treatments such as certain types of medication (e.g., Zoloft) or psychotherapy (e.g., cognitive therapy) that have well-established efficacy. In addition, studies may use placebo controls such as a group that engages in stretching rather aerobic exercise or that receives placebo pills. **Placebo pills** are inert pills that control for expectancy effects because participants believe these pills may contain active medicinal ingredients. Along with a growing body of studies using higher quality research methodology, the research literature now also contains a number of meta-analyses that point to the psychological benefits of exercise.

For example, a recent meta-analytic review (Wipfli, Rethorst, & Landers, 2008) of 49 randomized controlled studies examining primarily nonclinical populations reported a moderate to large effect size of -0.48 for anxiety reduction in exercise groups (94% of which were aerobic exercise groups) compared to no-treatment control groups. Only three studies included in the meta-analysis focused on clinical groups. The effect size detected for these clinical groups was -0.52, an effect comparable to the overall effect size in magnitude. The investigators also found that exercise was slightly better than other commonly used treatments for anxiety, such as stress management education or relaxation/meditation, but not more effective than cognitive-behavioral therapy or drug treatment. The effect sizes reported in this meta-analysis are impressive, especially given that the analysis included only randomized controlled trials.

The following randomized controlled study illustrates the use of exercise as an intervention for anxiety in a clinical population. In this study by Broocks et al. (1998), participants diagnosed with severe panic disorder were randomly assigned to a 10-week aerobic exercise group, a group that received an antidepressant medication (clomipramine), or a group that received a placebo pill to control for expectancy effects. The results indicated that exercise was more effective than a placebo but less effective than the antidepressant medication.

Studies evaluating the effects of exercise training on depression find even larger effect sizes than those for anxiety. For example, a meta-analytic review that included only studies identified by the study authors as randomized controlled trials found an impressive average effect size of -1.1, which was over a 1 standard deviation difference in lower depression scores for exercisers compared to no-treatment control nonexercisers (Lawlor & Hopker, 2001).

The authors of the meta-analytic study noted that the effect size was similar to that of cognitive-behavior therapy, but did caution that though the studies they included in their meta-analysis were the best quality they could find, they believed that the included studies did not control adequately for expectancy effects.

A later prospective randomized controlled trial did include an important control for expectancy effects (Blumenthal et al., 2007). Participants diagnosed with major depressive disorder were randomly assigned to one of four groups where they were given a 4-month protocol of (1) exercising at home, (2) exercising in a group, (3) taking a daily dose of the antidepressant medication sertraline (Zoloft), or (4) taking a placebo pill. What did the researchers find? They reported that the exercise effect (home and group) was comparable in magnitude to the effect of the antidepressant medication, and each condition was more effective than the placebo (Blumenthal et al., 2007).

Does engaging in physical activity have a protective effect against later development of depression? Although there are some mixed findings, when examining the studies with better methodology, it appears that it does. For example, using a large-scale community sample from the Alameda County Study, epidemiologists (Strawbridge, Deleger, Roberts, & Kaplan, 2002) were able to determine that physical activity was protective against developing later depression both through cross-sectional and longitudinal analyses even after controlling for potentially confounding variables.

Insomnia and depression often are comorbid (see Chapter 7), suggesting that any antidepressant effects of exercise may also indirectly benefit sleep quality and duration. A meta-analytic review by Kubitz, Landers, Petruzzello, and Han (1996) presented evidence that both acute and long-term regular exercise improve sleep duration and increase the amount of slow wave sleep (also known as deep sleep). The authors noted that "fit individuals not only fell asleep faster, but also slept somewhat deeper and longer (with less awake time) than unfit individuals" (Kubitz et al., 1996, p. 285). Further, a recent study by Reid et al. (2010) found that aerobic exercise leads to improvements in self-reported quality and duration of sleep for individuals with insomnia while reducing their depression. Is, then, improved sleep quality merely a by-product of lessened depression, or is the improvement independent of the antidepression effect? What do you think? After controlling for the effects of depression, the investigators determined that exercise had an independent beneficial effect on sleep, suggesting that exercise may have a direct rather than indirect positive influence mediated only through lessening depression symptoms.

How about positive well-being? What do the research studies reveal about the effects of exercise on positive well-being measures? A meta-analytic study (Netz, Wu, Becker, & Tenenbaum, 2005) of exercise interventions in advanced-age participants without clinical disorders found that the effect size for psychological well-being was 3 times greater than for control groups; aerobic exercise was the type and moderate-intensity activity was the activity level that were the most beneficial. The study's authors noted that physical activity had a significant effect on self-efficacy and that well-being was linked to indicators of cardiovascular fitness.

Is there a dose effect for exercise and depression as well as for well-being? Investigators (Galper, Trivedi, Barlow, Dunn, & Kampert, 2006) found an inverted graded dose relationship between cardiorespiratory fitness as measured by a treadmill test and measures on a depression scale in 5,451 men and 1,277 women as well as a positive graded dose response between cardiorespiratory fitness and a self-report measure of emotional well-being. In other words, they determined that the greater the cardiorespiratory fitness, the lower the depression and the higher the emotional well-being. The peak beneficial dose was 11 to 19 miles of walking, jogging, or running per week. Strengths of the study included its use of large samples and objective measures of fitness. A weakness of the study is that it was cross-sectional rather than prospective. As a result, the investigators could not establish cause-effect relationships.

However, a randomized controlled trial (Dunn, Trivedi, Kampert, Clark, & Chambliss, 2005) of participants with mild to moderate depressive disorder who were randomly assigned to different levels of aerobic exercise groups or to an exercise placebo control group (a stretching and flexibility protocol) for a 12-week period did find greater reductions in depression scores for the high-energy expenditure group (i.e., public health dose of 17.5 kcal/kg/week) than the lower-energy expenditure group (i.e., low dose of 7 kcal/kg/week) or the control group; there were no differences between the control group and the low-dose group, suggesting that a minimal threshold level of activity is needed to produce an antidepressant effect.

Putting the findings of these two studies together, it does appear as though exercisers must maintain a minimum threshold of activity to see beneficial effects. Beyond that minimum level exercise appears to generally lead to dose-dependent benefits until it reaches a peak beyond which there are no additional significant benefits. The optimal doses are generally in range with the recommendations from the U.S. Department of Health and Human Services' (2011) physical guidelines for Americans of a minimum of 150 minutes a week of moderate-intensity exercise spread out over most days of the week.

Both anxiety and depression are positively correlated with stress (see Chapter 7), and as discussed previously, there is evidence that both are reduced by exercise. Further, anxiety is the emotion associated with the flight component of the fight-or-flight response. Because the fight-or-flight's neuroendocrine response to stress is designed to prepare us for physical action, then should not physical activity be a natural way to reduce the physiological consequences of stress? There appears to be some support for this idea. For example, a meta-analytic review by Hamer et al. (2006) found that 30 minutes or more of moderate-intensity exercise lessened blood pressure responses to laboratory-induced stressors. Higher fitness levels also are associated with less proinflammatory cytokine responses to mental stressors (Hamer & Steptoe, 2007). Therefore, physical exercise does seem to buffer the effects of stress.

What mechanisms explain the positive psychological benefits of exercise such as reducing anxiety and depression and boosting well-being? Although the mechanisms are not empirically established, hypotheses fall into two camps: physiological and psychological. Physiological hypotheses mainly center on (1) facilitating synaptic transmission of brain monoamines

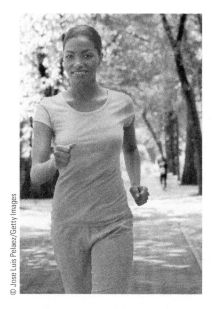

Aerobic exercise such as brisk walking reduces anxiety, depression, insomnia, and other effects of stress while boosting well-being.

© Jose Luis Pelaez/Getty Images

or (2) boosting brain endorphin levels. The **monoamines** are the "feel good" neurotransmitters present in the brain such as serotonin, norepinephrine, and dopamine. If exercise facilitates monoamine action in the brain, then it should produce antidepressant effects just as antidepressant medications boost mood states (see Chapter 7). There is some suggestive evidence that serotonin metabolism increases after exercise due to an increase in the brain's supply of serotonin's precursor molecules (aan het Rot, Collins, & Fitterling, 2009; Chaouloff, 1997; Ransford, 1982), but more research is needed to confirm the monoamine hypothesis.

Endorphins are the body's natural opiates. They reduce pain sensations and create feelings of euphoria. Although endorphins are usually elevated in the bloodstream during intense exercise (up to a fivefold increase) (Farrell, Gates, Maksud, & Morgan, 1982), there is continued controversy as to whether they are responsible for exercise-related mood enhancement (Dishman & O'Connor, 2009). Part of the controversy stems from studies that show that blocking the action of endogenous opioids (i.e., endorphins) with the drug naloxone does not always block the "runner's high" that is sometimes associated with intense exercise. **Runner's high** is a phenomenon in which a runner experiences euphoria precipitated by the act of running. The mechanism generally hypothesized to account for the phenomenon is that running increases brain endorphin activity, which produces the "high." Any supportive evidence from blood plasma studies is indirect at best for establishing a link between endorphins and mood enhancement because these studies do not measure brain endorphin activity directly and it is unknown if even limited amounts of circulating endorphins can cross the blood-brain barrier during exercise. In addition, surveys indicate that many runners do not report experiencing euphoria during or after exercise; instead they are most likely to report feeling relaxed and least likely to report feeling euphoric (Dishman & O'Connor, 2009).

Nevertheless, a recent study by Boecker and his colleagues (2008) using brain imaging (positron emission tomography) of 10 experienced distance runners who were selected for the study because they had reported experiencing runner's high previously is the first to present direct evidence that brain opioid changes after exercise are linked to mood elevation. These researchers recorded brain images before and after exercise and determined that the amount of endogenous opioids released in the frontolimbic areas of the brain was linked to the degree of euphoria reported. This study is an important first step toward establishing a direct causal mechanism for exercise boosting mood states, but the results do not necessarily generalize to all aerobic exercisers because experiencing runner's high during or after exercise is not the norm. In addition, the sample size of the study was small, and the duration of exercise was longer than average (2 hours of continuous exercise), further limiting generalization to a typical exerciser.

The main *psychological* hypotheses for exercise boosting mood states are that it (1) increases self-efficacy or self-esteem or (2) facilitates social interaction. A number of studies find that gaining a sense of mastery over challenging activities such as exercise can lead to increases in self-efficacy, self-confidence, or self-esteem (Butki, Rudolph, & Jacobsen, 2001; Ensel & Lin, 2004; Netz et al., 2005). However, exercise-related increases in self-efficacy are not always correlated with decreases in negative affect as would be expected from this hypothesis. For example, Butki et al. (2001) found that after a bout of exercise, participants' self-efficacy scores increased and their anxiety scores decreased, but there was no significant correlation between self-efficacy and anxiety. Therefore, self-efficacy increases could not account for anxiety decreases.

The social interaction hypothesis states that physical activity is often done with others and that social support and social rewards play a role in exercise-related mood enhancement. However, this hypothesis does not take into account the fact that exercise is often a solitary activity that is not always done in groups or with partners. If social interaction is a primary explanatory mechanism, then people who exercise in groups should have higher mood benefits than those who exercise at home alone. There is contradictory evidence for this hypothesis. For example, Blumenthal et al. (2007) found no significant differences in reduced depression scores for participants who were randomly assigned to a home exercise group when compared to those in a group exercise condition; both groups, however, showed benefits over placebo controls.

To summarize, it appears that there is substantial evidence for the efficacy of physical exercise as a strategy to reduce anxiety and depression, even in clinical populations, with the effect being greater for depression than anxiety. Exercise also seems to counteract insomnia and buffers the physiological effects of stress. Further, there is evidence that regular exercise boosts psychological well-being. Optimal mood-enhancing dosage levels of exercise appear to be in the range of the U.S. Department of Health and Human Services' (2011) recommendation of a minimum of 150 minutes of moderate-intensity aerobic activity spread out over the week. Although there are a number of hypothetical mechanisms explaining these beneficial effects, each has only limited empirical support.

Last, a slightly different but also important well-being benefit of physical activity is its effect on cognitive performance. Meta-analyses reveal a positive relationship between cardiovascular fitness and cognitive performance in older adults (Angevaren, Aufdemkampe, Verhaar, Aleman, & Vanhees, 2008; Colcombe & Kramer, 2003). For example, Colcombe and Kramer (2003, p. 128) found that "fitness training increased performance 0.5 SD [standard deviations] on average, regardless of the type of cognitive task, the training method, or participants' characteristics."

In a review of the relevant empirical literature, McAuley, Kramer, and Colcombe (2004, p. 216) noted that "although fitness effects were observed across a wide variety of tasks and cognitive processes, the effects were largest for those tasks that involved executive control (i.e., planning, scheduling, working memory, interference control, and task coordination) processes." **Executive control** tasks are associated with memory and higher cortical functions.

Similarly, a recent meta-analytic study by Smith et al. (2010) found that aerobic exercise was associated with improvements in cognitive processing speed, attention, executive control, and memory. Such findings are supported by brain studies that demonstrate less cortical brain tissue loss (Colcombe et al., 2003) and greater hippocampus volume (Erikson et al., 2009) in aerobically fit older adults. Also, physical activity during midlife may protect against developing dementia (e.g., Alzheimer's disease) in late adulthood (Andel et al., 2008).

Do the cognitive benefits of exercise also extend to young adults? In a recent study by Aberg et al. (2009) using a massive database of over one million Swedish men born between 1950 and 1976 who enlisted in the military, investigators were able to determine that increases in cardiovascular fitness between the ages of 15 and 18 positively predicted, after controlling for potential confounding variables, how well these young men would perform on intelligence tests at age 18. Improved aerobic fitness led to higher intelligence scores. In addition, muscle strength was not linked to cognitive performance, suggesting that the effects were specifically due to cardiovascular fitness rather than other fitness factors.

The authors speculate that, based on animal studies, aerobic exercise increases circulating levels of certain brain-enhancing biochemicals that cross the blood-brain barrier. These biochemicals have a complementary effect on regions of the brain such as the hippocampus. This effect is especially beneficial to adolescents and young adults because during that period of development their brains have greater plasticity than in later years.

executive control: cognitive tasks associated with memory and higher cortical functions such as working memory, planning, and scheduling.

BEGINNING AN EXERCISE PROGRAM

If you are not fit and you want to begin a physical activity program, the **Physical Activity Readiness Questionnaire (PAR-Q)** (Public Health Agency of Canada, 2011, p. 26) is a good screening tool to determine if you are ready for physical activity (Figure 11.2). The PAR-Q asks seven questions about any experiences you may have had such as a loss of consciousness, a heart condition, chest pain, dizziness, bone or joint problems, medications, or any other reason to suggest the need to talk to a physician before starting an exercise program.

The PhysicaL Activity Readiness Questionnaire (PAR-Q)

Becoming more active is <u>very safe</u> for most people, but if you're in doubt, please complete the questionnaire below.

Some people should check with their doctor before they start becoming much more physically active. Start by answering the seven questions below. If you are between the ages of 15 and 69, the PAR-Q will tell you if you should check with your doctor before you start. If you are over 69 years of age, and are not used to being very active, definitely check with your doctor first.

YES	NO	
☐	☐	1. Has your doctor ever said that you have a heart condition and that you should only do physical activity recommended by a doctor?
☐	☐	2. Do you feel pain in your chest when you do physical activity?
☐	☐	3. In the past month, have you had chest pain when you were not doing physical activity?
☐	☐	4. Do you lose your balance because of dizziness or do you ever lose consciousness?
☐	☐	5. Do you have a bone or joint problem that could be made worse by a change in your physical activity?
☐	☐	6. Is your doctor currently prescribing drugs (for example, water pills) for your blood pressure or heart condition?
☐	☐	7. Do you know of any other reason why you should not do physical activity?

<u>If you answered YES</u> to one or more questions, talk with your doctor before you start becoming much more physically active.

<u>If you answered NO</u> to all questions, you can be reasonably sure that you can start becoming more physically active right now. Be sure to start slowly and progress gradually – this is the safest and easiest way to go.

Delay becoming much more active if:

- You are not feeling well because of a temporary illness such as a cold or a fever – wait until you feel better; or
- You are or may be pregnant – talk to your doctor before you start becoming much more active.

Note: If your health changes so that you then answer YES to any of the above questions, ask for advice from your fitness or health professional.

FIGURE **11.2** Physical Activity Readiness Questionnaire (PAR-Q)

The PAR-Q is a useful screening tool to determine readiness to begin physical activity.
SOURCE: Public Health Agency of Canada (2011). Canada's handbook for physical activity guide to healthy active living. Retrieved from http://www.phac-aspc.gc.ca/hp-ps/hl-mvs/pag-gap/pdf/handbook-eng.pdf.

In general, the ACSM (2005) identifies high-risk individuals for physical activity as those with a known history or symptoms of cardiovascular, pulmonary (i.e., lung), or metabolic disease (e.g., diabetes). Moderate-risk individuals are men over the age of 45 or women over the age of 55. Moderate- and high-risk individuals should obtain a physician's consent before engaging in a *vigorous*-intensity exercise program, but according to the ACSM standards, moderate-risk individuals can feel comfortable engaging in *moderate*-intensity exercise without a physician's consent. They further suggest that men who are 45 years of age or younger and women 55 years or younger who have no symptoms of these diseases are considered low risk and can engage in vigorous-intensity exercise without a physician's consent.

One of the best ways to increase physical activity is through walking because walking does not require special facilities or expensive equipment. Walking can be done indoors (e.g., shopping malls) or out and is the most popular form of activity among those who meet the U.S. government's recommended exercise goals (Lee & Buchner, 2008).

Brisk walking is a good way to achieve moderate-intensity exercise. Moderate-intensity exercise is defined in several ways (Table 11.5). One way to tell if you are in the moderate-intensity zone is to determine your target heart rate using a standard formula. The formula is based on your age, a maximum heart rate of 220, and the goal of reaching 60% of your maximum:

- (220 minus age) times (.60)
- For a 30-year-old it would be $(220 - 30) \times (.60) = 114$ beats per minute

TABLE **11.5**   Indicators of moderate- and vigorous-intensity activity

Moderate-Intensity Activity	Vigorous-Intensity Activity
Can talk but cannot sing	Need to pause our words to catch our breath
Walking 3 to 4 miles per hour	Walking or jogging faster than 5 miles per hour
60% of maximum heart rate	At least 70% of maximum heart rate
60% of VO_2R*	At least 70% of VO_2R
RPE** between 12 and 13	RPE between 14 and 16
Expending 3.0 to 5.9 METs***	Expending greater than 6 METs

© Cengage Learning 2013.

*VO_2R is oxygen uptake reserve, an indicator of the maximum amount of oxygen a person can consume during physical activity.

**RPE is the Rating of Perceived Exertion (Borg, 1988) using a 6 to 20 scale. A person gives a subjective self-rating of his or her intensity level using the following scale: 6 indicates no exertion; 9, very light; 11, light; 13, somewhat hard; 15, hard; 17, very hard; and 20, maximal.

***METs refer to metabolic equivalents. One MET is equivalent to the amount of energy expended when sitting quietly. Brisk walking is equivalent to about 4 METs.

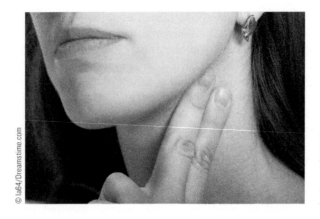

An easy way to measure your heart rate is to feel your carotid artery, which is the artery that runs vertically along the neck.

This formula is used very commonly, though it can over- or underestimate a given person's target heart rate (Whaley, Kaminsky, Dwyer, Getchell, & Norton, 1992). Nevertheless, it is a handy guide to use without necessitating precise treadmill testing. Given its imprecision, however, it is best to use it as an approximation rather than an absolute standard.

An easy way to measure your heart rate is to feel your carotid artery, which is the artery that runs vertically along your neck. You can feel it by placing two fingers a couple of inches below your jaw line close to your windpipe. Do this on only one side of your neck. Do not press too hard because this can activate a reflex that reduces your heart rate, and keep your thumb off your neck to get the best measure. For a quick calculation, count the beats for 6 seconds and add a zero to the end. For very sedentary individuals it is best to start at 50% of maximum heart rate for the first few weeks and then gradually build intensity to the 60% level.

Before starting a walking program it is helpful to have a comfortable pair of walking shoes and loose-fitting clothing. Investment in a good pair of walking shoes is the most important clothing purchase you can make for walking because wearing these shoes adds cushioning and support to protect your feet and act as shock absorbers for the rest of your body. Another helpful tool is a pedometer. A **pedometer** is an inexpensive measuring device that can be clipped to your waist to count your steps and distance traveled by foot.

pedometer: a measuring device that can be clipped to a person's waist that counts the person's steps and distance traveled by foot.

If you are just beginning a walking program, it is best to start modestly rather than overdoing it because too much too soon can actually discourage continued participation—especially if it results in soreness or injury. Start out at a slower pace initially to get your body warmed up before increasing your pace. Always give yourself a cooldown period at the end of the activity where, like your warm-up, you once again slow down the pace, but this time to cool down. You can measure your distance with the pedometer and should have the ultimate goal of completing around 2 miles during your 30-minute walk. See more on how to begin a brisk walking program later in this section.

An alternative to a brisk walking program is to use a step counter to simply count the total number of steps you take each day. The goal is to eventually reach 10,000 steps per day because this goal is roughly equivalent in steps to 30 minutes of moderate-intensity activity taken most days of the week (Manson,

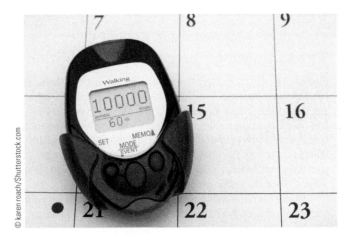

A pedometer or step counter is a good tool for counting 10,000 steps each day when walking for a healthy heart.

Skerrett, Greenland, & VanItallie, 2004; Wilde, Sidman, & Corbin, 2001). Investigators (Hultquist, Albright, & Thompson, 2005) provided empirical support for this goal by showing that sedentary women asked to walk 10,000 steps per day over a 4-week interval walked more on average at 10,159 steps than their 30-minute-per-day brisk-walking counterparts, who walked 8,270 steps each day. Every step is important toward maintaining health and preventing disease.

Sedentary individuals may average as little as 2,000 to 3,000 steps per day (Mitchell et al., 2008). This contrasts with members of the Old Order Amish representing the other end of the continuum, whose men were recorded averaging over 18,000 steps per day and women over 14,000 steps (Bassett, Schneider, & Huntington, 2004). They live their lives principally farming while eschewing modern conveniences such as automobiles or electrical appliances. As such, they live a very active lifestyle from dawn to dusk, rarely sitting except to eat a meal, and consequently have a very low prevalence of obesity (Bassett et al., 2004). It is interesting to note, however, that they maintain low rates of obesity in spite of a high caloric "pre-World War II rural diet" of "meat, potatoes, gravy, eggs, vegetables, bread, pies, and cakes" (Bassett et al., 2004, p. 84). In many ways, the Old Order Amish are living active lifestyles similar to our not-so-distant agrarian ancestors who had low obesity rates. So setting a goal of 10,000 steps is a good realistic challenge to turn around a sedentary lifestyle without creating too much hardship such as forsaking modern conveniences like the Old Order Amish.

To begin the program, log a baseline level of 3 full days of steps, putting a pedometer or step counter on first thing in the morning and not taking it off (except to shower) until going to bed at night. Next divide the figure by 3 to determine your average number of steps per day. Then, during subsequent weeks add 500 more daily steps each week to this baseline until you reach the 10,000 steps per day level (Mitchell et al., 2008).

STRESS MANAGEMENT EXERCISE **11.1**

Stress Busting Through Step Counting

One of the best motivators for increasing your activity level is an inexpensive step counter or pedometer. Step counters only count steps, whereas pedometers count steps and also miles. Either will do fine for this exercise. Purchase a step counter and follow the program outlined in this chapter for getting a baseline. Record your stress level at the end of the day using a 10-point scale with 1 indicating that you hardly feel any stress and 10 that you feel overwhelming stress. After determining your steps and stress level baselines, begin the program of adding 500 steps each week to your daily step count.

At the end of each day, chart your data and record your progress. After the first week answer the following questions. As you increased your number of steps did you notice any changes in your stress levels? As you increased your step count did you become more relaxed? Did you experience more good feelings and a greater sense of well-being?

Continue this exercise each week until you reach the 10,000 steps per day goal. Once you reach that goal you will have good insight into how well the step program helps with your stress and well-being. Continue on with your new program or switch to another form of exercise if that suits you better. Enjoy your activity journey!

To get more steps into the day take the stairs rather than the elevator when feasible, park in lots where you have to walk a greater distance to your destination, and take a walk during your lunch break (Manson et al., 2004). Keep in mind that even doing yard work, gardening, or household chores can add steps. If you are anchored to a desk working on a computer, take the time to get up and walk around your work area periodically to get your blood flowing and add more steps into your day.

Now let us go back to the details of starting a brisk-walking program. What is the best way for beginners to go about building a brisk-walking routine that meets or exceeds the 150-minute-per-week U.S. government recommendation? The following is based on the medical director of the Cooper Clinic and his associates' recommendations for a 5-day-a-week physical activity routine (Mitchell et al., 2008).

- To begin a brisk-walking program, during the first week start by walking approximately 1.5 miles in around 20 minutes.
- Then by the second week build to 2 miles in around 30 minutes.
- If you want to build to around 4 miles in 60 minutes, do so gradually over the course of 10 weeks.

Note that it is not within the scope of this chapter to cover all the different types of exercise activities. However, it is important to briefly mention resistance exercise and flexibility activities. The U.S. Department of Health and Human Services (2011) recommends doing muscle strengthening (i.e., resistance) exercises twice or more a week that involve all the body's major muscles. (See Faigenbaum & McInnis, 2007, for more information on starting a resistance training program.) Health professionals may also recommend supplementing routine aerobic exercise and resistance training with activity that increases flexibility and balance. Hatha yoga, Quigong, Tai chi (a form of Quigong), and Pilates are taught at many community fitness and wellness centers; each focuses on improving muscular flexibility, balance control, and muscular strength (see La Forge, 2007, for more information).

MAINTAINING AN EXERCISE PROGRAM

Starting an exercise program is the easy part. The difficult part is maintaining a good exercise routine. Unfortunately, the initial enthusiasm over starting a new project can wane over the first several months, which can lead to declining motivation to continue. As a result, drop-out rates are high. Missed sessions due to inclement weather, injuries, busy schedules, or other issues can lead to relapses and temporary periods of inactivity. Worse, relapses can lead to the experience of the *abstinence violation effect,* an effect first studied in people who experienced relapses when trying to stop smoking or abusing drugs or alcohol (Marlatt & Gordon, 1985). The **abstinence violation effect** is a process whereby a person experiences a relapse back to a previous habit or lifestyle and then uses all-or-nothing thinking to justify abandonment of the newly adopted lifestyle. For example, a person might use the following self-talk: "I haven't exercised now for the past week. I've failed. This isn't working. So I might as well give up trying to exercise."

What then are the keys to maintaining an exercise program?

- **Avoid overdoing exercise.** Some people think that if moderate intensity is good then high intensity is better. Driven Type A individuals may want to engage in competitions to push themselves to higher levels of fitness. Although competitions can be fun, we are more likely to suffer an injury if we unnecessarily push ourselves too hard and too fast into high-intensity exercise. Once we have an injury, it can prevent or discourage us from continued participation in later physical activity. Think of physical activity as an ongoing healthy lifestyle endeavor. You want to keep your body as injury-free as possible to go the distance rather than sprinting toward possible injury to meet a competitive goal.

- **Challenge negative thinking.** If you have thoughts that discourage you, challenge your negative thinking with positive self-talk using the cognitive restructuring techniques you learned in Chapter 10. Be your own nurturing and positive coach. For example, Buckworth (2007, p. 234) lists the following common negative thoughts and positive challenges: "I'm fatter than everyone in the class" challenged with "Everyone has to start somewhere. Other people have worked long and hard to get where they are"; "I've tried to stay with exercise and each time I failed" challenged with "Every time I begin a new exercise program, I get closer to sticking with it for good"; and "It's just

abstinence violation effect: a process whereby a person experiences a temporary relapse back to a previous habit or lifestyle and then uses all-or-nothing thinking to justify abandonment of the newly adopted habit or lifestyle.

impossible to find time to exercise with my schedule" challenged with "I can take a little time for myself to exercise every day because I deserve it. I'm the one in control."

- **Look for intrinsic rewards.** Select a type of exercise that is the most fun for you so that intrinsic rewards are built into the activity. Recognize that during the initial stages of maintaining a new exercise program, your primary motivation will be fueled by your determination and enthusiasm. An emotion such as enthusiasm is great to get you going, but it tends to wear off as the novelty of the new endeavor fades. In addition, there will be other competing interests for your time and energy as well as periods of discouragement or boredom. Therefore, look for the other immediate benefits to sustain your motivation, such as your increased self-esteem or self-efficacy, reduced stress, anxiety or depression, and the boost you get in overall good feelings. Remind yourself of how good you feel after a bout of exercise compared to how you felt before exercise. If you are motivated by extrinsic rewards, then give yourself a tangible reward each time you pass particular exercise milestones. It could be something small like a star you post on a chart or bigger like tickets to the big game or a new article of clothing to fit your more toned body. Remember also, if you are walking, jogging, or running, use your pedometer to log your activity levels. Checking the steps walked or miles traveled after exercise on your pedometer is a rewarding experience.

- **Maintain a regular routine.** It is best if physical activity is built into your schedule so you do not even have to think consciously about it, like tooth brushing. If you have a morning exercise routine, then follow the same time schedule each morning. Make it as easy on yourself as possible even if it means putting your workout shoes and clothes beside your bed at night. Do not skip exercise just because you do not feel like it. Do you skip brushing your teeth because you do not feel like it? Why not? Because you probably do not want to be like Erica, introduced at the beginning of the chapter. Instead, like most people you want to take care of your health and well-being.

- **Find a workout partner.** Evidence (Trost, Owen, Bauman, Sallis, & Brown, 2002) indicates that we are more likely to maintain an exercise program if we have someone else to work out with. Workout partners can encourage and give each other social support during times when motivation wanes. Interesting conversations between partners during exercise routines also can make time seem to pass more rapidly, like reading a good book or watching a good movie. See Table 11.6 for a more complete though not exhaustive listing of positive predictors as well as negative predictors and barriers to maintaining regular physical activity.

- **Avoid the abstinence violation effect.** Recognize that it is normal to have lapses. For example, if you are ill, you should not be exercising. Likewise, if you have an injury that needs to heal, do not stress the

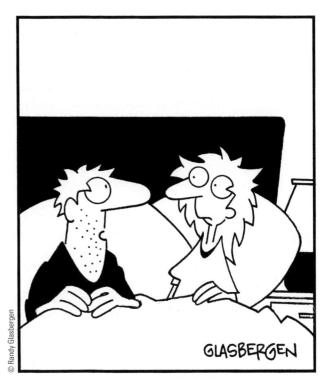

"I was going to get up early to go running, but my toes voted against me 10 to 1."

TABLE **11.6**   Positive predictors and negative predictors/barriers to maintaining regular physical exercise

Positive Predictors	Negative Predictors and Barriers
Normal weight	Overweight or obese
History of physical activity	No history of physical activity
High self-efficacy for physical activity	Low self-efficacy for physical activity
Time for exercise/good time management	No time for exercise/poor time management
Perception of having sufficient strength and energy for exercise	Perception of having insufficient strength and lack of energy for exercise
No tobacco smoking	Tobacco smoking
Social support for exercise	No social support for exercise
Good physical environment for physical activity (safe, good facilities, pleasant environment)	Poor physical environment for physical activity (unsafe, poor facilities, unpleasant environment)
Not self-conscious about appearance	Self-conscious about appearance (female)

SOURCE: Based on Eyler et al. (1999).

relapse prevention:
the process of identi-
fying high-risk relapse
situations and then
avoiding the risks, mak-
ing alternative plans, or
planning how to best
deal with these risks if
encountered.

injury further through exercising. It is smart to think long term and give the injury a chance to heal fully before resuming exercise. Any lapse is just a temporary condition that can be followed by resuming exercise as soon as feasible. In addition, practice **relapse prevention** by identifying high-risk situations such as travel, extra work, events that involve drinking or eating too much, and upcoming inclement weather. Avoid these risk situations when feasible or make alternative plans to maintain exercise when confronted with a high-risk situation. For example, if possible, exercise indoors when the weather is not conducive to outdoor physical activity. If you do slip, have a plan ready for how you will get back into your exercise routine.

EUSTRESS, FLOW, AND PHYSICAL ACTIVITY

As a final thought, recall from Chapter 1 that eustress is a positive form of stress. It is a type of stress that is challenging, satisfying, and even enjoyable. Remember also from Chapter 2 the concept of flow, a feeling of being "in the zone" when you are immersed in an activity that feels intrinsically rewarding. Engaging in sports and other physical activities is sometimes associated with flow. For example, Russell (2001, p. 83) found that "college athletes appear to have similar experiences of flow states, regardless of gender or sport type." Although flow does not always occur during physical activity, there are times when you may lose yourself in the activity, experience an altered sense of time, and a greater sense of control. It is at this time that you are experiencing flow. Researchers (Schuler & Brunner, 2009) have found that flow increases motivation among marathon runners to continue running in the future because they experience flow as a reward of the activity. Could it then be that one additional stress management and well-being benefit of physical activity is that it can produce flow? Thus, in this context physical activity can be seen as an example of eustress, a positive stress that we find both challenging and rewarding.

CHAPTER SUMMARY AND CONCEPT REVIEW

- A number of governmental agencies as well as the American College of Sports Medicine (ACSM) recommend a minimum of regular moderate-intensity aerobic exercise and some resistance training.

- Physical activity, physical exercise, and physical fitness are different but overlapping concepts.

- There are different types of fitness, but developing and maintaining cardiorespiratory fitness is the primary physical activity goal for preventing health risk, enhancing psychological well-being, and increasing longevity; adding strength training also plays an important role.

- The evidence is strong for the health benefits of physical exercise, with the highest level of empirical support found for regular physical exercise reducing the risk for all-cause mortality, cardiovascular disease, breast and colon cancer, and type 2 diabetes, followed by the next level of compelling evidence for stroke and hypertension prevention, and then indirect evidence for it minimizing the risk of osteoporosis.

- Health benefits of regular physical exercise follow a nonlinear dose-response relationship with the most dramatic gains in risk reduction observed for sedentary individuals when they first begin a program of physical activity.

- Physical activity seems to be especially effective in controlling visceral fat, a type of fat that is more dangerous than the more common subcutaneous fat.

- Controlling for expectancy effects and using good quality prospective research methods such as randomized controlled trials are critical toward establishing the efficacy of physical exercise as an intervention for anxiety and depression.

- Evidence indicates that regular aerobic activity has a moderate to large effect size for anxiety-state reduction and an even larger effect size for reducing mild to moderate symptoms of depression; the effect seems to be dose dependent but requires a minimum threshold to have an effect.

- Engaging in regular aerobic exercise appears to have a protective effect against later development of depression.

- Evidence supports the idea that regular aerobic activity reduces insomnia, buffers the physiological effects of stress, improves cognitive performance, and increases psychological well-being.

- The potential mechanisms that explain the psychological benefits of exercise are not empirically established, but there is some support for both physiological and psychological explanations.

- Before beginning an exercise routine, it is important to assess your physical activity risk level to determine if you should obtain a physician's consent.

- Walking programs using a pedometer to establish a 2-mile, 30-minute walk or 10,000 steps per day routine are some of the best ways to meet the general recommendations for regular physical activity.

- Resistance training and routines that increase flexibility and balance also are activities that can develop other components of fitness.

- Maintaining a regular exercise program involves ongoing lifestyle planning and effectively dealing with relapses.

- Physical activity may involve the experience of flow leading to eustress.

CRITICAL THINKING QUESTIONS

1. How do lack of physical activity and depression contribute to each other? Why would engaging in regular physical activity have a protective effect against later developing depression?

2. Why do you think the mood-boosting effects of exercise can occur within 10 minutes of ongoing physical activity, but the anxiety reduction effects generally occur after exercise?

3. What is it about engaging in regular physical activity that makes it an effective strategy for managing stress? In your opinion, how does it rank with other stress management strategies? What properties give it a low, medium, or high ranking compared to other strategies?

4. How much physical activity do you get on a daily basis? If you currently have a low level of physical activity, what strategies can you employ to boost your activity levels? What is your most important first step toward implementing these strategies?

5. Are people who experience flow during exercise experiencing eustress? If so, why? If not, why not? What other factors besides flow can lead a person to experience physical activity as a form of eustress?

KEY TERMS AND CONCEPTS

Abstinence violation effect*

Aerobic*

Aerobic fitness

Anaerobic

Body mass index (BMI)

Cardiorespiratory fitness*

Endorphins

Executive control*

Expectancy effects

FITT principle*

Moderate-intensity activity*

Monoamines

Osteoporosis*

Pedometer*

Physical activity*

Physical Activity Readiness Questionnaire (PAR-Q)

Physical exercise*

Physical fitness

Placebo pills

Relapse prevention*

Runner's high

Subcutaneous fat

Vigorous activity*

Visceral fat*

Weight-bearing exercise*

MEDIA RESOURCES

CENGAGE **brain**.com

Access an interactive eBook, chapter-specific interactive learning tools, including flashcards, quizzes, videos, and more in your Psychology CourseMate, accessed through CengageBrain.com.

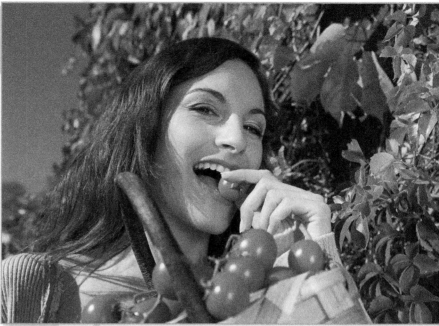

© Image Source/Jupiter Images

It's difficult to think anything but pleasant thoughts while eating a homegrown tomato.

~LEWIS GRIZZARD

NUTRITION

Are you more like Jeremy or Melinda? When you are under stress, do you eat more or less? Perhaps stress does not affect how much you eat. If so, you are unique because the majority of people have eating patterns that change when under stress. For example, one study (Willenbring, Levine, & Morely, 1986) found that 48% of participants reported that like Melinda, they ate less when under stress, 44% were similar to Jeremy and ate more, and 8% reported no stress-related changes in their eating patterns.

Another study (Macht, Haupt, & Ellgring, 2005) specifically looked at the effects of an impending exam (3 to 4 days earlier) on eating, using a field design with a control group. Students were given beepers and randomly beeped 10 times during their normal waking hours to remind them to record their stress levels, the amount they had just eaten since they were last beeped, and their reasons for eating. Compared to the participants who did not have an impending exam, the students in the exam anticipation group reported more stress and more of a tendency to use eating to distract them from tension or negative emotions (e.g., fear) they experienced when anticipating their upcoming exams. College student stress also predicts the **night-eating syndrome,** a type of problematic eating often leading to weight gain in which a person eats very little in the morning but overeats at night (Wichianson, Bughi, Unger, Spruijt-Metz, & Nguyen-Rodriguez, 2009).

There also is evidence that when we do overeat in response to stress, we are more likely to eat unhealthy foods. For example, using a daily diary and a series of questionnaires, researchers (O'Connor, Jones, Ferguson, Conner, & McMillan, 2008) were able to determine that when participants in their natural settings experienced greater daily hassles, they ate more high-fat and sugar snacks and cut down on their main meals and vegetables. Laboratory studies (e.g., Oliver, Wardle, & Gibson, 2000) also demonstrate that stress, at least for emotional eaters, is associated with eating foods high in fat and sugar. These studies illustrate how stress can indirectly affect health through its influence on eating patterns. As discussed in Chapter 5, there is evidence that eating a diet high in fruits and vegetables and low in saturated fat decreases the risk of cardiovascular disease and perhaps even cancer. Therefore, this type of stress eating works against our own best health interests.

There are a number of proposed psychological or biological mechanisms that explain stress-motivated eating. Perhaps you have thought of some of them? Many of these suggest that eating helps a person regulate negative mood. Individuals who attempt to regulate their negative affect through eating are referred to as **emotional eaters.** These individuals can be identified using the Emotional Eating Scale, a scale that measures a person's tendency to cope with anxiety, anger, or depression through eating (Arnow, Kenardy, & Agras, 1995).

How does eating regulate negative affect? Three primary psychological mechanisms proposed are that eating (1) distracts a person from self-awareness and negative feelings similar to the process of how a good movie or book takes our mind off our troubles and transports us emotionally to a different place, (2) boosts positive feelings because we often experience eating as pleasurable, or (3) creates a sensation of bodily relaxation. Recall in the exam stress study (Macht et al., 2005) that the investigators found evidence for distraction as the principal mechanism. However, the other two mechanisms are also plausible for other scenarios. Can you think of a stressful situation in which you ate primarily to boost positive feelings or to feel more relaxed?

A potential physiological mechanism for mood alteration includes *self-medicating* through eating foods that boost serotonin levels (recall from Chapter 7 that serotonin is one of the "feel good" neurotransmitters). Many of the foods that boost serotonin are called *comfort foods.* For example, carbohydrate-rich foods like high-fat sugar snacks that are low in protein can minimize increases in cortisol and negative mood elevations in response to stress, presumably through boosting brain tryptophan levels, a precursor to serotonin (Markus et al., 1998). Individuals who are high-cortisol stress reactors are more likely to exhibit emotional eating in response to daily hassle stress than low-cortisol stress reactors, suggesting that cortisol may play a role in triggering the emotional eating process (Newman, O'Connor, & Conner, 2007).

restraint eaters: individuals who normally limit their food intake to maintain or lose weight.

Besides emotional eaters, individuals who normally limit their food intake to maintain or lose weight, known as **restraint eaters,** also are more likely to show increased eating when under stress (O'Connor et al., 2008; Wallis & Hetherington, 2004). Why are restraint eaters more likely to eat during stress? The motivation is unclear but may relate to a greater preoccupation with food related to having to restrain oneself when wanting to eat particular foods. Stress may impair a person's ability to inhibit eating when that person is thinking or obsessing about these "forbidden" foods.

FOOD AND NUTRIENTS

In order to better understand how food plays a role in our health and well-being, we need to first take a closer look at the different categories of food and their nutrients. As we know, food is animal or plant material that we ingest to provide energy and nourishment. The ingredients in food that provide energy or that sustain our cells and tissues are called **nutrients.** Nutrients divide into macronutrients and micronutrients. The **macronutrients** are the big nutrients, those that we consume in large quantities to fulfill our energy requirements, whereas the **micronutrients** are the essential substances we need in very small quantities like the vitamins and minerals. Macronutrients further divide into the three categories of carbohydrates, protein, and fat.

phytochemicals: bioactive compounds found in plants that are not essential nutrients for sustaining life.

Phytochemicals represent another category of substances found in food. The term *phytochemical* (*phyto* is Greek for "plant") means compounds found in plants that are bioactive but are not essential nutrients for sustaining life. Later, when we discuss the concept of food as medicine, we will focus on beneficial phytochemicals. Another substance found in the plants we eat is fiber. Although technically a carbohydrate, **fiber** is different from starchy carbohydrates because it consists of the plant's indigestible cellulose components. For the purpose of this chapter, fiber is treated as a separate food component rather than as a carbohydrate. Fiber is beneficial to our health but provides no life-sustaining energy. Last, of course, we need sufficient water to maintain life. So water is a nutrient category by itself. In sum, we need our macronutrients, micronutrients, and water to sustain life. Our health can benefit from nonnutrient plant substances such as fiber and phytochemicals as well.

Let us now take a closer look at types of foods, starting with the macronutrient called carbohydrates. The carbohydrates divide into the simple and complex. **Simple carbohydrates** include sugars like those found in honey, milk, fruit, and table sugar that consist of single or double glucose units, whereas **complex carbohydrates** are long-chain glucose molecules that we call starches. Glucose is one of the body's primary fuels. Did you know that our brains are fueled almost exclusively by glucose rather than proteins or fats? Glucose also is an important source of fuel for our skeletal muscles. Most healthy eating plans recommend that the highest percentage of the macronutrients we eat consist of carbohydrates.

The Institute of Medicine is an independent nonprofit organization established through the U.S. National Academy of Sciences to provide advice to the nation regarding health issues. According to the Institute of Medicine's Food and Nutrition Board's (2002) most current guidelines for a healthy balance of macronutrients, we should consume 45% to 65% of our total macronutrients from carbohydrates, 10% to 35% from protein, and 20% to 35% from fats (Figure 12.1).

simple carbohydrates: macronutrient sugars that consist of single or double glucose units.

complex carbohydrates: also known as starches; consist of macronutrient long-chain glucose molecules.

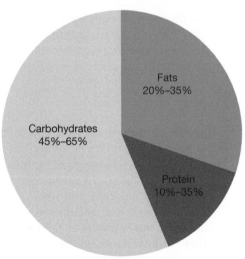

FIGURE **12.1** The Institute of Medicine's Food and Nutrition Board's (2002) most current guidelines for a healthy balance of macronutrients   SOURCE: The Institute of Medicine's Food and Nutrition Board, 2002.

With the exception of fructose (fruit sugar, also found in honey), simple carbohydrates are rapidly absorbed into the bloodstream unless they are eaten in their natural plant form (Brand-Miller, 2003). Fiber slows down the absorption of sugar and allows for a more gradual dose to enter the bloodstream. When fiber is removed through processing, then the processed carbohydrates cause spikes in blood sugar levels when eaten and are said to be foods with a **high-glycemic index/load.** These foods also cause strong insulin responses due to their glucose-spiking tendencies. **Insulin** is the hormone secreted by the pancreas used to transport glucose to the body's cells where the sugar molecules are burned as fuel or converted into **glycogen** (a compound also known as animal starch that is a molecule consisting of long chains of glucose) and stored in the liver and muscles. Excess glucose is then converted into fat and stored in adipose (fat) tissue (Guyton & Hall, 2006). Along with the majority of simple sugars, carbohydrates that have most of their fiber removed such as bleached refined flours generally have a higher glycemic index. These include, for example, white bread and crackers. Many cereals, potatoes, and varieties of rice such as white rice also are high-glycemic index foods, whereas dairy, whole grains, fruits, vegetables, and legumes (e.g., peas, beans, lentils) are low-glycemic index foods (Foster-Powell, Holt, & Brand-Miller, 2002).

Why does the glycemic index matter when choosing food? Low-glycemic foods are preferred in many healthy eating plans because they tend to be more nutrient dense than high-glycemic foods like chips, pretzels, and doughnuts, which are generally stripped of their natural micronutrients or other beneficial substances like fiber during processing. **Nutrient density** refers to the quantity of nutrients packed into the calories consumed. Highly processed foods may contain **empty calories,** a term that indicates that the calories consumed have very little nutritional value. If we load up on empty calories, we have little room left for nutritional calories and can potentially become nutritionally deficient over time even though we are consuming adequate calories.

There also may be health-protective reasons to consider eating low- rather than high-glycemic foods. For example, evidence gathered primarily through observational epidemiological studies indicates that low-glycemic index foods facilitate feelings of fullness and fight obesity, improve insulin sensitivity, lower triglycerides, increase high-density lipoprotein (HDL) levels as well as lower the risk of type 2 diabetes, cardiovascular disease, and colon and breast cancer (Brand-Miller, 2003). However, even though low-glycemic foods may have health benefits, the issue of whether they should be recommended in diet plans for disease prevention is controversial. For example, the American Diabetes Association (ADA) (2004), a group that should be most concerned with this issue, does not emphasize using the glycemic index in making food decisions, but instead advises individuals to consider total carbohydrates as opposed to particular types of carbohydrates when choosing dietary plans. Though the current evidence is suggestive, more research is needed, specifically high-quality experimental research such as randomized controlled trials, before we can determine more definitively if eating low-glycemic index foods can prevent chronic diseases such as heart disease, type 2 diabetes, and cancer.

high-glycemic index/ load: foods that spike blood sugar levels.

glycogen: also known as animal starch; a long-chain glucose molecule stored in the body's liver and muscles.

empty calories: the food consumed has calories but very little nutritional value.

As discussed previously, fiber is the indigestible component of carbohydrates. The human digestive system cannot break down this nonstarch polysaccharide to use its contents for fuel or nutrients. If we ate nothing but fiber, we could fill our stomachs but still starve. As a result, fiber was once thought useless, as waste to be removed through processing, which led to the production of food products almost devoid of fiber like white bread. We now know that fiber has value. In fact, it has a number of health benefits due to its ability to lower circulating low-density lipoprotein (LDL) levels through binding cholesterol and carrying it out of the body through the gastrointestinal (GI) tract before the LDL can reach the bloodstream. It reduces demands on the insulin system by slowing down the release of glucose from foods eaten, and it prevents constipation by stimulating the movement of food through the GI tract at a steady pace. Although the evidence is inconclusive regarding whether eating a high-fiber diet prevents colon cancer (Institute of Medicine, 2002), it is strong regarding fiber's benefits in promoting cardiovascular health and preventing metabolic syndrome (see Chapter 5). For example, one study (Rimm et al., 1996) found that total fiber intake was associated with a 40% reduction in coronary heart disease. Many other studies established similar benefits (Pereira et al., 2004).

Cereal fiber, a type of fiber found in whole grains, seems especially effective in preventing heart disease as well as metabolic syndrome (Brown, Rosner, Willett, & Sacks, 1999; McKeown, Meigs, Liu, Wilson, & Jacques, 2002). The Food and Nutrition Board of the Institute of Medicine (2002) recommends that men 50 years and younger consume 38 grams of total fiber each day and women in the same age category, 25 grams. Older individuals need less—for men, 30 grams, and for women, 21 grams. Foods high in fiber include whole fruits, nuts, seeds, and grains as well as legumes, oatmeal, and many vegetables. The U.S. Department of Agriculture (USDA) and U.S. Department of Health and Human Services' (USDHHS) *Dietary Guidelines for Americans, 2010* (2010) recommend that Americans get at least half of their grain consumption through whole grains.

In addition to carbohydrate, protein is another important food nutrient. **Protein,** a macronutrient that consists of building blocks called **amino acids,** is used as raw material to build and repair the structures of almost every part of our body. Proteins we eat are broken down into their amino acid components and then reassembled into body structures such as hair, muscle, and collagen. Our blood cells employ these amino acids and assembled proteins to carry oxygen in the form of hemoglobin, antibodies to fight diseases, enzymes to catalyze biochemical processes, and hormones to act as chemical messengers. Proteins also can fuel the body, but the body prefers to use stored carbohydrates or fats first because amino acids from proteins undergo more steps to convert into glucose in a process, known as *gluconeogenesis,* or into fatty acids through *ketogenesis* before their energy can be liberated (Guyton & Hall, 2006).

The body loses about 20 to 30 grams of protein each day through a process known as remodeling or "obligatory degradation of protein" and must, therefore, replace it through foods ingested (Guyton & Hall, 2006, p. 857). In order to prevent an overall loss of protein from the body, we need to consume a minimum of at least 20 to 30 grams of protein daily from food. Overall, this is a small amount of our total caloric intake, but we should consume more than this to be safe. The Institute of Medicine (2002) suggests that we consume a minimum of 10% of our average daily calories in protein or at least 8 grams per 20 pounds of body weight (e.g., 64 grams for a 160-pound person). It recommends a maximum of 35% protein for our total caloric intake.

essential amino acids: amino acids needed by the body that must come from dietary sources because the body cannot synthesize them.

There are a total of 20 amino acids from protein that the human body needs, but almost half of these, the **essential amino acids,** must come from dietary sources because the body cannot synthesize them. Proteins are found in both animal sources such as meat, fish, poultry, eggs, and dairy products as well as foods from plant sources such as vegetables, beans, nuts, seeds, and grains. Although all animal sources of protein contain the total essential amino acids and are, therefore, known as **complete proteins,** individual foods from different plant sources may be lacking one or more of them. Hence, most plant proteins are known as **incomplete proteins.** An exception is soy, a legume that is often used by vegetarians for its protein content because it is a plant source that has all the essential amino acids. Generally, a good combination of foods that contain plant protein such as nuts, seeds, grains, legumes, and vegetables will provide all the amino acids the body needs. As a legume, beans are an excellent source of protein that additionally contain beneficial zinc, potassium, and fiber. Vegans (i.e., individuals who eat no animal sources of food) need to be careful that they consume the right combination of plant-based foods (e.g., beans and rice combined) to ensure that they receive all their essential amino acids.

complete proteins: proteins that contain all the essential amino acids.

Whether amino acids come from animal or plant sources makes little difference from a nutritional standpoint. From a health standpoint, amino acids from plant sources often are accompanied by fiber, carbohydrates, phytochemicals, and, generally, healthy fats, whereas amino acids from animal sources are usually accompanied by unhealthy fats like saturated fat (a major exception is seafood). Therefore, plant-based protein often has some health advantages over animal-based protein. Why is fat so often an issue when it comes to developing healthy eating plans? Before we answer that question, let us first look at what fat is.

The third macronutrient, **fat,** consists of fatty acids and their related organic compounds. As noted earlier, the Institute of Medicine (2002) suggests that fat constitute 25% to 35% of our total dietary intake. We can identify fat in food we eat because it has a slick, oily, creamy, or greasy texture. As unappetizing as these descriptors may sound, we like fat because it tastes good. Low-fat foods can taste bland unless other ingredients, usually sugar, are added to compensate for their lack of flavor. The body uses fat in many ways including through its cell membranes, in building hormones, as a form of insulation, and for energy storage. Alongside glucose, fat is an important source of energy. **Triglycerides** are the fatty acid form of fat generally stored in fat cells and later burned for energy.

Some people avoid high-fat foods because of concerns about health risks and weight gain, but fat is actually very beneficial if eaten in the right form and quantity. However, all fats are not created equal in terms of their health benefits and risks. Conversely, all fats, whether from animals or plants, saturated or unsaturated, are equal in their high caloric content. The following list shows the caloric content per gram of the macronutrients:

- Fat = 9 calories per gram
- Carbohydrate = 4 calories per gram
- Protein = 4 calories per gram

Due to the higher caloric content of fat, more than double that of carbohydrate or protein, one successful weight loss strategy often employed is to reduce our total fat consumption. This strategy is an indirect way of managing our calorie intake because weight loss is ultimately a function of calories-in and calories-out. In other words, it is a function of burning more calories than we consume. Weight loss strategies are discussed in more detail later in this chapter. For now, let us explore different types of fat and their health benefits or risks.

saturated fats: a form of fat that is solid at room temperature and is found primarily in animal sources such as meat and dairy.

- **Saturated fats**—This form of fat is solid at room temperature and is found primarily in animal sources such as meat and dairy. It also is found in some plant sources such as cocoa butter, coconut, and some tropical oils. According to the American Heart Association (AHA) (2011a), saturated fat raises levels of LDL (the bad cholesterol), which increases our risk of heart disease. Therefore, the AHA advises that we limit this form of fat to no more than 7% of our total daily calories. Another reason to limit saturated fat—the American Cancer Society (2011b) cautions—is that consuming too much red meat (a source of saturated fats) may increase the risk of some cancers such as colon and prostate cancer. Note that excessive consumption of processed meats such as sausage and bacon is also associated with an increased risk of colon cancer.

trans-fats: generally vegetable oils that have been chemically modified to make them solid through a process called partial hydrogenation.

- **Trans-fats**—These fats are generally vegetable oils that have been chemically modified to make them solid through a process called *partial hydrogenation*. Some stick margarines and shortening consist of trans-fats. This type of fat also is found in many processed snack foods, pastries and other bakery items, as well as deep-fried foods. Trans-fats may create an even greater risk of heart disease than saturated fats through their ability to elevate circulating LDL levels (Institute of Medicine, 2002). For this reason, the American Heart Association (2011a) recommends that we consume no more than 1% of our total calories from trans-fats. In other words, avoid them whenever possible.

- **Cholesterol**—The body manufactures this sterol compound and uses it as a component of our cell membranes or in steroidal hormones such as the corticosteroids. Our body makes all we need and, therefore, does not require it in food. In fact, the Institute of Medicine (2002, p. 5) lists cholesterol along with saturated fats and trans-fats as "not required at any level in the diet." Cholesterol is present in meat and eggs. Contrary to what was once believed, we now know that the relationship between cholesterol consumed and blood cholesterol levels is weak and mainly a concern for people with heart disease or high LDL levels. The American Heart Association (2011a) recommends that we limit cholesterol to less than 300 mg per day. For people with coronary heart disease or high LDL levels, the AHA recommends consuming less than 200 mg per day. As a reference point, one egg contains around 200 mg, so an egg a day is within the guidelines for most people. The yolk contains the cholesterol, so removing the yolk and eating just the egg whites can provide an animal source of protein without the cholesterol.

monounsaturated fats: plant-based fatty acids that have one double-carbon bond that are liquid at room temperature.

- **Monounsaturated fats**—These plant-based fatty acids, liquid at room temperature, are considered healthy fats because they reduce circulating LDL and total cholesterol levels, raise HDL, and reduce the risk of heart disease (Institute of Medicine, 2002; Mensink, Zock, Kester, & Katan, 2003). Olive oil; peanut oil; nuts like almonds, pecans, and hazelnuts; seeds such as sesame seeds and pumpkin seeds; and avocados are good sources of monounsaturated fats.

polyunsaturated fats: fatty acids found in plant-based foods and fish with more than one double-carbon bond that are liquid at room temperature.

- **Polyunsaturated fats**—These healthy fats are found in plant-based foods and also found in fish. Foods that are good sources of polyunsaturated fats include soybean, sunflower, corn, and flaxseed oils as well as fatty marine fish and walnuts. On the whole, these foods have the same beneficial properties for the cardiovascular system as monounsaturated fats. They can lower LDL and total cholesterol, raise HDL, and protect against heart disease.

Two important types of long-chain polyunsaturated fats that the body requires from food because it cannot manufacture them are the **essential fatty acids** called omega-3 fatty acids and omega-6 fatty acids. **Omega-3 fatty acids** have received significant recent attention for their cardiovascular benefits. Indeed, evidence suggests that omega-3 fatty acids have anticlotting effects; are protective against heart disease; and reduce heart rate, blood pressure, cardiac arrhythmias (i.e., abnormal heart rhythms), and the risk of sudden cardiac death (Leaf, 2007). In addition, there is evidence that they exert anti-inflammatory effects through, for example, suppressing proinflammatory cytokines such as tumor necrosis factor-α, interleukin 1β, and interleukin-6 (Simopoulos, 2006). Because inflammation appears to promote chronic diseases like cardiovascular disease, omega-3 fatty acids may play a protective role through their anti-inflammatory properties.

omega-3 fatty acids: long-chain polyunsaturated essential fatty acids found primarily in fatty marine fish and some plant sources known for their cardiovascular and anti-inflammatory benefits.

Omega-6 fatty acids are prevalent in most Western diets because they are found in high percentages in many refined vegetable oils used in processed foods such as safflower, soybean, sunflower, cotton seed, and corn oil. Some contend (Simopoulos, 2006) that omega-6 fatty acids are proinflammatory and, therefore, should not be overconsumed unless balanced with an equal consumption of omega-3. Olive oil, a monounsaturated fat, is considered the gold standard for a low omega-6 fatty acid plant oil.

In the Western world there have been dramatic changes during the last 100 years in the characteristics of our food supply and in our eating habits. On average we now consume a lopsided ratio of omega-6 over omega-3 fatty acids. How large is the imbalance? Astoundingly, we consume 16 times more omega-6 than omega-3, yet some experts argue that our human evolutionary history, along with studies of mammals in nature, suggest that we should be consuming a 1:1 ratio for good health (Simopoulos, 2006). Others (Sacks, 2011) counter that recent evidence indicates this ratio is not relevant when considering health and that omega-6 like omega-3 is also effective in reducing inflammation, lowering LDL, and protecting against heart disease (Mozaffarian et al., 2005; Willett, 2007). Therefore, they argue that there is no need to be concerned about the omega ratio as long as we consume enough of both essential fatty acids to meet the body's requirements. After all, they contend, if both are good fats, then combining the good with the good in any ratio is healthy.

Regardless of where one stands on the issue, if we are eating a typical Western diet we likely get a sufficient supply of omega-6 but may not get enough omega-3. Therefore, it is probably a good idea to eat more walnuts, ground flax seeds, and wild-caught fatty marine fish such as salmon, sardines, and herring because these foods are high in omega-3 that the body needs but cannot manufacture. As discussed in Chapter 4, the vegetarian sources of omega-3 fatty acids contain alpha-linolenic acid (ALA) and do not contain the more important marine sources of eicosapentaenoic acid (EPA) and docosahexanoic acid (DHA) found in fish oils. It appears, however, that our body does convert a limited amount of ALA into EPA and DHA, but the rest is burned as fuel. Fortunately, ALA also has cardiovascular protective effects but it is unknown if it exerts these effects indirectly through converting to EPA and DHA or through taking direct beneficial action on the cardiovascular system (Sacks, 2011). Leafy vegetables like spinach and kale as well as animal fat from grass-fed animals also may contain ALA. It seems that grass contains ALA and animals that eat grass then store ALA in their fat.

Consuming 8 ounces of seafood per week including the lower mercury content fish such as salmon, herring, sardines, trout, Atlantic and Pacific mackerel, anchovies, and Pacific oysters will provide an average of 250 mg per day of EPA and DHA, an amount associated with reduced risk of cardiac-related death (USDA & USDHHS, 2010). Fish oil supplements provide an effective alternative for those who want their marine omega-3s but are unable to include enough fish in their diet. Likewise, for those still concerned about possible mercury contaminants from eating fish, especially large marine fish like tuna, fish oil supplements offer a viable EPA/DHA substitute if the supplements have been molecularly distilled to remove any contaminants—a process that is now common and typically indicated on the label.

Last, let us look at the micronutrients, the vitamins and minerals found in dietary sources. **Vitamins** are essential organic substances (from life-forms), and **minerals** are inorganic elements the body needs in minute amounts to support growth, to maintain bodily tissues, and to metabolize food. Just as a car engine even with a tank of gas cannot run without spark plugs, we cannot burn our carbohydrate, fat, or protein fuel without vitamins and minerals. The body can manufacture some vitamins such as D vitamins made during sun exposure to the skin, but most vitamins and all minerals need to be obtained from dietary or supplement sources. When we do not consume or make the vitamins our body requires, we develop metabolic deficits that have adverse health consequences. For example, a long-term lack of vitamin C can result in scurvy, a condition in which wounds fail to heal, the connective tissues of the body weaken, and blood vessels hemorrhage due to the inability of the body to make sufficient collagen (Guyton & Hall, 2006). Long ship voyages of 20 to 30 weeks without fresh fruits or vegetables during the 15th through 18th centuries often resulted in sailors developing scurvy until British navy physician James Lind determined in the mid-1700s that citrus juice could prevent the disease (National Institutes of Health [NIH] State-of-the-Science Panel, 2006). Unfortunately, his recommendation to the Royal Navy that limes could protect British sailors from scurvy was not implemented until almost 40 years later (American Dietetic Association, 2009). Finally it became so common for British sailors to sail with supplies of lime juice to prevent scurvy that they developed the nickname "limeys." We now know that the vital protective ingredient in citrus juice is ascorbic acid, otherwise known as vitamin C.

Vitamins are stored in all cells in the body to some extent as well as in the liver. Vitamins A, D, E, and K, the four fat-soluble vitamins, are stored for longer periods than the water-soluble ones, vitamin C and the B-complex vitamins (i.e., thiamine, riboflavin, niacin, B_6, folate, B_{12}, biotin, and pantothenic acid). For example, vitamin A is stored in the liver for 5 to 10 months but most of the B-complex vitamins are lost within a few days (Guyton & Hall, 2006). For this reason, daily intake of vitamins through food or other sources, especially the water-soluble ones, is recommended.

Ideally, we should be able to get our vitamins and minerals through a balanced diet, but as Bruce Ames and his colleagues (Ames, McCann, Stampfer, & Willet, 2007, p. 522) argue, "we are far from achieving this goal, especially among the poor." They also note that particular populations may need to take vitamin supplements even if they are eating an ideal diet. For example, vitamin B_{12} deficiencies may develop in older people due to age-related declines in their ability to efficiently absorb this vital micronutrient—in its crystalline form found in supplements it is more readily absorbed than from foods. Vitamin D_3, manufactured from the skin's exposure to ultraviolet rays, is less efficiently generated with age and is diminished in dark-skinned individuals. The USDA and USDHSS's Dietary Guidelines for Americans (2010) also note that Americans consume too little calcium, vitamin D, and potassium. Thus, it may be prudent to take a daily multivitamin/mineral supplement as insurance, preferably one with "USP" (United States Pharmacopeia) on the label. The USP designation indicates that the supplement meets independent testing quality criteria. Today more than half of Americans take vitamin supplements (NIH State-of-the-Science Panel, 2006). Although there is substantial evidence documenting that we need vitamins and minerals in our food or in supplements to prevent clinical deficiency disorders, is there any reason to take vitamin and mineral supplements for other reasons, such as to prevent chronic diseases like coronary heart disease and cancer?

An NIH-sponsored State-of-the-Science Panel (2006) of independent medical professionals sought to address this question by looking only at evidence from randomized controlled trials (intervention-based studies). Thus, they excluded large-scale epidemiological observational studies, resulting in a conservative approach that unfortunately could miss important evidence. As a result, they found few rigorous studies in their review that support a recommendation one way or the other to take supplements; most studies found no beneficial health effects.

The NIH State-of-the-Science Panel (2006, p. 367) did highlight the positive health effects of a few single and double vitamin/mineral component supplements when they concluded that "on the basis of single studies and analysis of secondary outcomes, there is a suggestion that selenium may reduce the risk for prostate, lung, and colorectal cancer; that vitamin E may decrease cardiovascular deaths in women and prostate cancer incidence in male smokers; and that vitamin A paired with zinc may decrease the risk for noncardia stomach cancer in rural China." Further, they noted that postmenopausal women who take calcium in combination with vitamin D can reduce bone fracture risk and increase their bone mineral density. They also strongly advised against smokers taking high-dose β-carotene supplements because two large-scale studies found increased lung cancer incidence and mortality in smokers who took these supplements.

What about the question of whether multivitamins could prevent chronic diseases? What did the panel conclude? The panel was not able to make a determination primarily because of the presence of confounding variables in the studies they reviewed. For example, "fortified" foods (i.e., foods that have vitamins and minerals added) are commonly eaten in regular diets, making it difficult to separate health benefits due to multisupplements from those due to food fortification. In addition, even the best controlled studies do not isolate the specific effects of the individual components of the multisupplements taken by participants. Thus, any health benefits found may only be due to one or two components of the multisupplement, meaning that the remaining components may be superfluous. The panel concluded that "the present evidence is insufficient to recommend for or against the use of MVMs [multivitamin/multiminerals] by the American public to prevent chronic disease" (NIH State-of-the-Science Panel, 2006, p. 370). Given the low risk of harm from taking a daily multivitamin/mineral supplement at recommended doses, and the panel's conservative approach for determining what evidence they examined, it is probably a wise precaution to take these supplements as insurance in spite of the panel's lack of recommendation (Ames et al., 2007).

Last, the USDA and USDHHS note in their Dietary Guidelines for Americans (2010), that Americans consume far too much of one mineral, sodium (Figure 12.2), usually in the form of salt in processed foods rather than through table salt. They recommend taking in no more than 2,300 milligrams (mg) and less than 1,500 mg for "persons who are 51 and older and those of any age who are African American or have hypertension, diabetes, or chronic kidney disease." Why? Limiting sodium is recommended because as the guidelines caution, "a strong body of evidence in adults documents that as sodium intake decreases, so does blood pressure. Moderate evidence in children also has been documented that as sodium intake decreases, so does blood pressure" (USDA & USDHHS, 2010, p. 21). Higher chronic blood pressure increases the risk of cardiovascular disease and kidney disease. One of the best ways to reduce sodium intake is to eat less processed foods and more fresh foods.

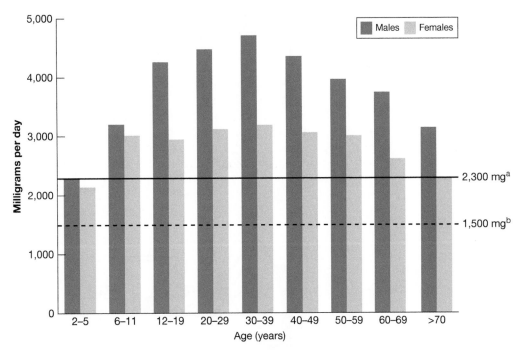

FIGURE **12.2** Average Sodium Intake of Americans by Age and Gender

As can be seen, Americans in almost every age category consume far too much sodium.

SOURCE: U.S. Department of Agriculture and U.S. Department of Health and Human Services (USDA & HHS). (2010). *Dietary Guidelines for Americans, 2010* (7th ed.). Washington, DC: U.S. Government Printing Office.

FOOD AS MEDICINE

The U.S. Department of Health and Human Services (2000) *Healthy People 2010* began the first decade of the 21st century with the public health initiative of achieving a goal that at least 75% of Americans would eat 2 to 4 servings of fruit and 50% consume 3 to 5 servings of vegetables per day by the end of the decade. How did Americans do? Unfortunately, by the later part of the decade only 16.4% of the population met the fruit consumption goal and 29.4% met the vegetable consumption goal (Wright, Hirsch, & Wang, 2009). This is unfortunate because as the USDA/USDHHS's Dietary Guidelines for Americans (2010, p. 35) report, fruits and vegetables contain many beneficial ingredients that are generally "underconsumed in the United States, including folate, magnesium, potassium, dietary fiber, and vitamins A, C, and K." In addition the guidelines point out that "moderate evidence indicates that intake of at least $2^{1}/_{2}$ cups of vegetables and fruits per day is associated with a reduced risk of cardiovascular disease, including heart attack and stroke. Some vegetables and fruits may be protective against certain types of cancer."

Besides the beneficial fiber, vitamins, and minerals fruits and vegetables contain, they also contain bioactive substances known as phytochemicals. These phytochemicals, like many pharmaceuticals derived from plants, may

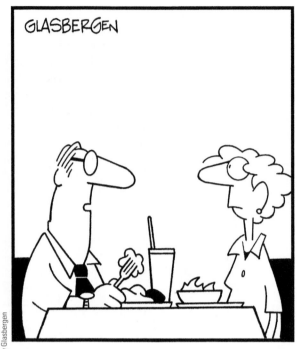

© Randy Glasbergen

**"My doctor told me to eat 5 fruits and vegetables
every day. Today I had 3 raisins and 2 peas."**

functional foods: foods
that have added health
benefits beyond their nu-
tritional value.

have health benefits. For example, did you know that the bioactive ingredient in
aspirin, salicylic acid, was originally derived from the bark of the willow tree?

Certain foods contain more beneficial properties than others. These foods
are known as functional foods. Choosing to consume more *functional foods*
over conventional foods is based on the idea that functional foods have added

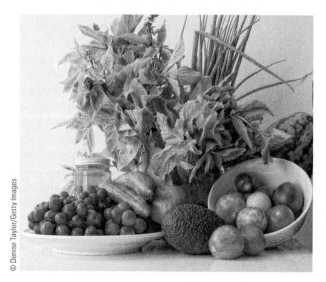

© Denise Taylor/Getty Images

Fruits and vegetables
contain phytochemicals
that are protective
against cardiovascular
disease and perhaps
certain types of cancer.

health benefits beyond their nutritional value. Although the United States through its regulatory agency, the Food and Drug Administration (FDA), does not officially recognize the category of *functional foods*, this categorical label is recognized in Canada, Europe, and Japan (see American Dietetic Association, 2009, for discussion). The concept of food as medicine is not novel. In fact, the founder of medicine, Hippocrates, advised over 2,500 years ago to "let food be thy medicine and medicine thy food."

Although the FDA does not recognize a separate broad category of food called functional foods, it does allow qualified health claims (i.e., claims of health benefits) for specific whole foods and supplements. The FDA rates the scientific evidence for each food, allowing stronger claims to be made when the evidence is stronger. There must be significant scientific agreement to support a claim before the FDA will authorize its use on food labels or for marketing. For example, to reduce the risk of cardiovascular disease, the FDA reports that moderate scientific evidence supports consuming omega-3 fatty acids found in fish and supplements; moderate evidence also supports eating hazelnuts, peanuts, pecans, almonds, pistachios, walnuts, and some pine nuts; low levels of support exist for olive oil; and the lowest level of support is documented for corn oil. Other examples of FDA rulings include its permission for marketers to use statements indicating that low–saturated fat and low-cholesterol diets that include sufficient servings of whole oats or soy proteins "may reduce the risk of heart disease" and that selenium supplements and antioxidant vitamins may reduce the risk of certain cancers (American Dietetic Association, 2009, p. 739). The last reference to antioxidants is important because there is considerable burgeoning research interest in determining the health benefits of antioxidants. What exactly are antioxidants and how are they beneficial to our health?

antioxidants: chemicals found in particular vitamins, minerals, and phytochemicals that reduce oxidative stress.

oxidative stress: the adverse effects of oxygen free radicals on cells.

Antioxidants are chemicals found in particular vitamins, minerals, and phytochemicals that reduce oxidative stress (Table 12.1). **Oxidative stress** refers to the adverse effects of oxygen free radicals on our cells primarily from by-products of normal cellular metabolism. Our cells have their own natural antioxidants in the form of, for example, superoxide dismutase (SOD) that neutralizes most free radicals, but as we age there is indirect evidence that our cellular defenses against oxidative stress begin to slip, exposing us to greater oxidative stress damage and vulnerability to the diseases of aging such as cancer and heart disease (Knight, 2000). In theory when free radicals damage cells, they may also contribute to potential anomalies of the cell or its DNA that increase the chance of normal cells prematurely aging or mutating into cancer cells.

To illustrate oxidative stress, think of what happens to an old car over the years once it is consigned to a junkyard. After decades of sitting in the junkyard, it is covered with rust. Rust is the by-product of the car's metal structure oxidizing. Sometimes we can even see rust holes on the rusting car's body where the oxidation has literally eaten through the metal. Our body's cells also can suffer from oxidation damage if they are not sufficiently protected. They need their own version of rust-proofing to minimize the damage. Likewise, if you cut an apple in half and set it out for a few hours you will notice that the open halves turn brown. Why? The more vulnerable cells of the interior of the apple are exposed to oxidative stress once they are no longer protected by the apple's outer covering. However, if you squeeze lemon juice

TABLE **12.1**   Examples of Antioxidant Vitamins and Minerals

Vitamins	Daily Reference Intakes*	Antioxidant Activity	Sources
Vitamin A	300–900 µg/d	Protects cells from free radicals	Liver, dairy products, fish
Vitamin C	15–90 mg/d	Protects cells from free radicals	Bell peppers, citrus fruits
Vitamin E	6–15 mg/d	Protects cells from free radicals, helps with immune function and DNA repair	Oils, fortified cereals, sunflower seeds, mixed nuts
Selenium	20–55 µg/d	Helps prevent cellular damage from free radicals	Brazil nuts, meats, tuna, plant foods

SOURCE: Chart adapted from Food and Nutrition Board Institute of Medicine DRI reports and National Institutes of Health Office of Dietary Supplements

*DRIs provided are a range for Americans ages 2–70.

onto the freshly cut apple halves, a few hours later the open halves will still be white. Why? The lemon juice contains vitamin C, which acts as an antioxidant and protects the cells in the apple from prematurely oxidizing.

Plants also need to protect themselves from oxidation stress and often do so with brightly colored green, blue, orange, yellow, and red antioxidant pigments in their leaves, fruit, and other structural components. In addition, because plants cannot flee from their predators they have to produce biochemical defenses against insects, fungi, bacteria, and herbivores. These biochemical defenses are often the phytochemicals that give some vegetables a strong sulfur smell (e.g., onions) or a slightly bitter or astringent taste that cause many of us to turn up our noses at a plate full of vegetables. Our taste buds for bitter provide an early warning against swallowing toxic substances because many of the most toxic plant species have an alkaline bitter taste. As Beliveau and Gingras (2007) suggest, over the course of evolution, humans learned to overcome a natural aversion to many of the nontoxic varieties of plants that have less appealing taste or smell characteristics as we expanded our dietary repertoire to include eating more plant species for our survival. As a result, many of the phytochemicals that protect these plants may also protect us in various ways when we eat them, including probably as yet undiscovered ways.

It is an oversimplification to think that phytochemicals are beneficial just for their antioxidant properties because these bioactive chemicals may act in other health-protective ways as well. A look at Table 12.2 shows the most commonly recognized phytochemicals and their known properties. For example, the flavonoids, a member of the largest group of over 4,000 currently identified compounds called **polyphenols,** are often brightly colored and include berries, red grapes, apples, citrus, green tea, cinnamon, and cocoa. We

polyphenols: antioxidant phytochemicals consisting of over 4,000 currently identified compounds.

TABLE **12.2** Beneficial components of foods

Examples of Functional Components*		
Class/Components	Source*	Potential Benefit
Carotenoids		
Beta-carotene	carrots, various fruits	neutralizes free radicals, which may damage cells; bolsters cellular antioxidant defenses
Lutein, Zeaxanthin	kale, collards, spinach, corn, eggs, citrus	may contribute to maintenance of healthy vision
Lycopene	tomatoes and processed tomato products	may contribute to maintenance of prostate health
Flavonoids		
Anthocyanidins	berries, cherries, red grapes	bolster cellular antioxidant defenses; may contribute to maintenance of brain function
Flavanols—Catechins, Epicatechins, Procyanidins	tea, cocoa, chocolate, apples, grapes	may contribute to maintenance of heart health
Flavanones	citrus foods	neutralize free radicals, which may damage cells; bolster cellular antioxidant defenses
Flavonols	onions, apples, tea, broccoli	neutralize free radicals, which may damage cells; bolster cellular antioxidant defenses
Proanthocyanidins	cranberries, cocoa, apples, strawberries, grapes, wine, peanuts, cinnamon	may contribute to maintenance of urinary tract health and heart health
Isothiocyanates		
Sulforaphane	cauliflower, broccoli, Brussels sprouts, cabbage, kale, horseradish	may enhance detoxification of undesirable compounds and bolster cellular antioxidant defenses
Phenols		
Caffeic acid, Ferulic acid	apples, pears, citrus fruits, some vegetables	may bolster cellular antioxidant defenses; may contribute to maintenance of healthy vision and heart health

(continued)

TABLE **12.2** *(continued)*

Examples of Functional Components*		
Class/Components	Source*	Potential Benefit
Sulfides/Thiols		
Diallyl sulfide, Allyl methyl trisulfide	garlic, onions, leeks, scallions	may enhance detoxification of undesirable compounds; may contribute to maintenance of heart health and healthy immune function
Dithiolthiones	cruciferous vegetables—broccoli, cabbage, bok choy, collards	contribute to maintenance of healthy immune function
Whole Grains		
Whole grains	cereal grains	may reduce risk of coronary heart disease and cancer; may contribute to reduced risk of diabetes

Source: Chart adapted from International Food Information Council Foundation: Media Guide on Food Safety and Nutrition: 2004–2006.

*Not a representation of all sources

can identify the sulfides/thiols by their smell, a result of their higher sulfur content and include onions, garlic, and the cruciferous vegetables like broccoli and cabbage. Certain fruits, vegetables, spices, and teas may have anti-inflammatory and detoxification effects alongside their antioxidant properties, which also could account for their beneficial health effects. Is the answer then to Hippocrates' advice to "let food be thy medicine and medicine thy food" to eat more fruits and vegetables? Let us look briefly at some of the evidence for consuming more fruits and vegetables to protect against cardiovascular disease and cancer.

Recall the largest of its kind international INTERHEART case-control study (Yusuf et al., 2004) discussed in Chapter 5 comparing 15,152 cases of acute myocardial infarction (MI) with 14,820 controls, which found a 30% reduction in MI risk associated with consuming fruits and vegetables every day. A recent meta-analytic review (He, Nowson, Lucas, & MacGregor, 2007) that included only prospective cohort studies found a 17% reduction in coronary heart disease (CHD) risk associated with increasing fruit and vegetable consumption to 5 servings per day from less than 3 servings. The authors speculate that the beneficial CHD risk effects could be due to the fruits' and vegetables' micronutrients, fiber, and antioxidants because antioxidants can reduce atherosclerosis.

Some expert reviewers (Vainio & Weiderpass, 2006, p. 111) of the epidemiological studies of fruits and vegetables for cancer prevention found that "there is limited evidence for a cancer-preventive effect of fruits and vegetables for cancer of the mouth and pharynx, esophagus, stomach, colon-rectum, larynx, lung, ovary (vegetables only), bladder (fruit only), and kidneys." The reviewers also estimated that as many as 5% to 12% of cancers could be prevented if people with low fruit and vegetable intake would consume more of these foods. A more current review (Key, 2011) is, however, somewhat more skeptical of the evidence, acknowledging that epidemiological studies have found moderately reduced risk for cancers of the upper GI tract but noting that there may be some confounds from smoking and alcohol use in these studies. The author concludes that "no protective effects have been firmly established" (Key, 2011, p. 6). Nevertheless, the FDA (2011) finds the evidence strong enough to allow the following health claims to be made: "Low fat diets rich in fruits and vegetables (foods that are low in fat and may contain dietary fiber, vitamin A, and vitamin C) may reduce the risk of some types of cancer, a disease associated with many factors."

Clearly, more research is needed to establish stronger evidence for the link between eating more fruits and vegetables and reducing cancer risk. However, consuming more targeted fruits and vegetables may be an even more effective anticancer strategy. Although not an inclusive list, fruits and vegetables that are under investigation for potential anticancer effects include tomatoes; green tea; garlic; onions; soy; the spice turmeric; grapes; berries such as strawberries, raspberries, and blueberries; citrus; and cruciferous vegetables such as cabbage, broccoli, kale, and Brussels sprouts (Beliveau & Gingras, 2007). It is no coincidence then that the Dietary Guidelines for Americans 2010 (USDA & USDHHS, 2010, p. 32) recommends eating a variety of vegetables and especially more "dark-green and red and orange vegetables and beans and peas."

What general eating pattern then seems to be most healthy? There are three healthy eating patterns that have received the most research attention, the **DASH (dietary approaches to stop hypertension)**, Mediterranean-style, and vegetarian patterns. According to the Dietary Guidelines for Americans 2010 (USDA & USDHHS, 2010, p. 73), the DASH plan "emphasizes vegetables, fruits, and low-fat milk and milk products; includes whole grains, poultry, seafood, and nuts; and is lower in sodium, red and processed meats, sweets, and sugar-containing beverages than typical intakes in the United States." The **Mediterranean-style eating pattern** "emphasizes vegetables, fruits and nuts, olive oil, and grains (often whole grains). Only small amounts of meats and full-fat milk and milk products are usually included. It has a high monounsaturated to saturated fatty acid intake ratio and often includes wine with meals." Fish also is usually an important component. Vegetarian eating plans vary. **Lacto-ovo vegetarians** include milk and eggs in their primarily plant-based diet and **vegans** do not consume any food from animal sources. As the Dietary Guidelines for Americans 2010 (USDA & USDHHS, 2010) notes, the predominance of research shows reduced cardiovascular disease risk for all three eating patterns along with less cardiovascular disease incidence for the Mediterranean-style pattern, lower blood pressure for DASH and the vegetarian patterns, and a lower overall mortality rate for the Mediterranean-style and vegetarian eating patterns.

COFFEE, TEA, CAFFEINE, AND STRESS

The two most popular beverages in the world excluding water are coffee and tea, but do they increase or decrease stress? Given that both of these beverages contain caffeine, and caffeine is a stimulant, what are their effects on our overall health? Perhaps you are a regular consumer of one or both of these beverages and are curious to know the answers to these questions. What does the evidence suggest?

In order to make the beverage we call **tea,** leaves from the plant *Camellia sinensis* are gathered and then processed into black, green, or Oolong tea. About 78% of the world's consumption of tea is black tea, 20% green tea, and only 2% Oolong tea (Butt & Sultan, 2009). Black tea is the standard tea consumed in most Western countries and is fully fermented, whereas **green tea,** a tea developed from fresh tea leaves that are steamed or dried in a way that minimizes oxidation and therefore preserves the green pigment, is more popular in Asian countries. Oolong tea is semifermented and is most popular in certain regions of China.

The composition of green tea is about 30% polyphenols and black tea, 5%, with another 25% of black tea consisting of oxidized phenolic compounds (Chacko, Thambi, Kuttan, & Nishigaki, 2010). The primary polyphenols found in green tea are flavonols, otherwise known as **catechins,** that include epigallocatechin-3-gallate (EGCG), epigallocatchin, epicatechin, and epicatechin-3-gallate. **EGCG** constitutes 67% of the total polyphenols of green tea and is the phytochemical that likely accounts for most of its presumed beneficial health properties (Fassina et al., 2004). Because the catechins of green tea are not oxidized, they retain their antioxidant properties and can reduce oxidative stress more effectively than black tea, making green tea the preferred beverage of the two for health-protective effects. Both green tea and black tea also have a number of other bioactive compounds, including caffeine and the amino acid theanine, which is discussed later (see Chacko et al., 2010). There is limited but not established evidence from animal and human studies that the catechins in green tea reduce cardiovascular risk and defend against cancer (Butt & Sultan, 2009; Chacko et al., 2010; Hirano et al., 2002). Cancer prevention mechanisms found in various studies indicate that the polyphenols in green tea may promote apoptosis (programmed suicide of aberrant cells); inhibit tumor growth, metastasis (proliferation), and angiogenesis (the ability of the tumor to feed itself through growing blood vessels); and stimulate cytotoxic T cells to take action against microtumors (Butt & Sultan, 2009; Fassina et al., 2004).

Like green tea, coffee contains several phenolic antioxidants. These compounds may increase "the resistance of LDL to oxidative modification" and prevent atherosclerosis because the oxidation of LDL likely plays a key role in plaque formation (Natella, Nardini, Belelli, & Scaccini, 2007, p. 604). In addition, the anti-inflammatory properties of the antioxidants present in coffee may be responsible for the results of the prospective Iowa Women's Health Study (Andersen, Jacobs, Carlsen, & Blomhoff, 2006) that found, after controlling for other relevant variables, lower death rates from cardiovascular disease and other inflammatory diseases such as diabetes, liver cirrhosis, and Parkinson's disease in coffee drinkers than non-coffee drinkers. A recent meta-analytic review (Yu, Bao, Zou, & Dong, 2011, p. 1) of epidemiological evidence suggests that coffee consumption has protective effects against some types of cancers—"an increase in consumption of 1 cup of coffee per day was associated with a 3% reduced risk of cancer." The nascent human research examining the health-protective effects of green tea and coffee are promising, though more prospective randomized controlled studies are needed to firmly establish these benefits.

What about the effects of stress? What role can tea or coffee play in amplifying or reducing stress effects? One caveat for an individual who is under stress is to consider caffeine's stimulant effects on the nervous system. **Caffeine** has the ability to stimulate our body's neurons by lowering their threshold for excitability (Guyton & Hall, 2006). As a result, caffeine activates the sympathetic-adrenal-medulla axis (SAM) and the hypothalamic-pituitary-adrenal axis (HPA), causing elevations in serum catecholamines and cortisol as well as mild increases in blood pressure, especially under stressful conditions, and the cortisol effects are only partially lessened by developing a caffeine tolerance through daily caffeine intake (Lovallo et al., 2005). High doses of caffeine are commonly associated with anxiety reactions, especially in individuals with anxiety disorders, whereas moderate doses are associated with reduced depressive symptoms and improved alertness, attention, and cognitive performance (Lara, 2010).

The Mayo Clinic staff (2011) suggests that 500 to 600 mg per day of caffeine is a good cutoff point for avoiding caffeine's unwanted effects. Generic brewed coffee has the most caffeine at 95 to 200 milligrams per 8 ounces, followed by black tea at 40 to 120 mg per 8 oz, and then green tea at around 35 mg per 8 oz—note also that an equivalent 8 oz amount of a soft drink like Coca-Cola Classic is 23 mg (although individual container sizes are generally larger) and an energy drink like Red Bull (8.3 oz in a container) is 76 mg (Mayo Clinic, 2011). So caffeine is more likely to be an issue with coffee drinkers and strong black tea drinkers (unless the beverage is in a decaffeinated form) than green tea consumers. Therefore, to avoid magnifying the effects of stress, the number of cups of these beverages should be monitored and limited so as not to exceed 600 mg per day of caffeine.

Interestingly, if tea has caffeine that excites the body's nervous system, why is it often associated with rituals of relaxation? Andrew Steptoe and his colleagues (Steptoe et al., 2007) sought the answer to this question using a randomized double-blind study with participants either assigned to a 6-week active tea group (the equivalent of 4 cups of black tea per day) or a placebo group. Both groups received their beverage in a form that disguised its sensory properties through addition of fruit flavoring and caramel coloring. Further, the placebo group's beverage was modified so that it contained an equal amount of caffeine to that found in the black tea group. After 6 weeks of consuming their respective beverage, participants were given stressful behavioral challenges. Both groups showed similar substantial increases in cardiovascular responses and ratings of subjective stress to the behavioral challenges. However, afterwards the active tea group showed faster recovery from these

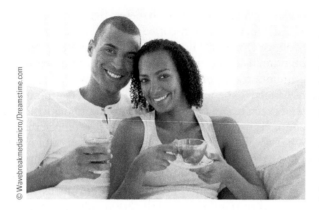

Tea's EGCG has sedative effects and its amino acid theanine increases brain wave patterns associated with relaxation. In addition green tea appears to have properties that provide some protection against cardiovascular disease and perhaps some types of cancer.

stressors in the form of lower cortisol, subjective stress, and platelet activation than was found in the placebo group.

In attempting to explain their findings, the authors noted that EGCG has sedative effects and the amino acid theanine increases brain alpha wave activity, a brain wave pattern often associated with relaxation. They speculated that the more rapid stress recovery for the active tea group to the stress challenge was likely due to the psychopharmacological properties of some of these polyphenols and other non-caffeine-related bioactive ingredients found in tea. Thus, it appears that consuming tea may offer some additional benefits in the way of stress recovery beyond whatever health-protective effects it may have.

STRESS MANAGEMENT EXERCISE **12.1**

Caffeine and Stress

How much caffeine do you consume on a daily basis? In this exercise you are encouraged to keep a stress log and record your caffeine consumption. Three times a day (morning, afternoon, and evening) record your stress levels on a 10-point scale with 1 indicating that you hardly feel any stress and 10 that you feel overwhelming stress. In addition, record the time of day and your caffeine consumption. For example, you would record "1 p.m., drank a 20 ounce cola" if that is what you did. At the end of the week look for patterns connecting your caffeine consumption and your stress levels. If you see a connection, begin to taper off the caffeine during the next week. Tapering off high levels of caffeine can help to reduce any withdrawal effects (i.e., headaches).

After tapering, continue to record your stress levels and caffeine consumption. Do you notice a reduction in stress levels? If so, you may want to eliminate or drastically reduce your caffeine consumption (perhaps switch to green tea or its decaffeinated version) to help you better manage stress. This simple strategy can make a big difference in reducing your overall stress levels.

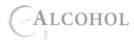ALCOHOL

Like tea and coffee, alcoholic beverages such beer, wine, and distilled liquors are popular beverages in many countries, including the United States where approximately 50% of U.S. adults drink alcohol on a regular basis and another 14% do so infrequently (USDA & USDHHS, 2010). Whereas moderate alcohol consumption is associated with a number of health benefits including reduced CHD risk and increased longevity, excessive drinking is linked to many health problems including numerous types of morbidity (i.e., diseases) as well as early mortality. Moderate drinking of alcohol is defined as "1 drink per day for women and up to 2 drinks per day for men" (USDA & USDHHS, 2010, p. 31). One drink of alcohol is generally defined as 12 ounces of beer, 5 ounces wine, or 1.5 ounces of liquor (USDA & USDHHS, 2010). Alcohol is calorie dense at 7 calories per gram and is considered empty calories because it has no micronutrients.

As a drug, **alcohol** is a central nervous system depressant with relaxation effects on the body that is often used by those who drink it to unwind, relax, or reduce the effects of stress. It also may be used to elevate mood, increase self-confidence in social situations, loosen inhibitions, or relieve boredom. As is well known, alcohol has addictive properties and can create dependency and withdrawal symptoms if abused. Excessive drinking has many health risks, including "cirrhosis of the liver, hypertension, stroke, type 2 diabetes, cancer of the upper gastrointestinal tract and colon, injury, and violence" (USDA & USDHHS, 2010). Due to its ability to impair judgment and reaction time, alcohol is the primary cause of motor vehicle accidents in the United States (MedlinePlus, 2011).

Moderate consumption of alcohol has anti-inflammatory effects but heavy consumption elevates proinflammatory cytokines (Goral, Karavitis, & Kovacs, 2008). The evidence is strong that moderate alcohol consumption lowers the risk of cardiovascular disease and all-cause mortality (USDA & USDHHS, 2010). Numerous studies (Di Castelnuovo, Rotondo, Iacoviello, Donati, & Gaetano, 2002) report a J-shaped curve with the lowest risk of mortality occurring at moderate levels of alcohol use (the bottom of the J) followed by slightly higher mortality associated with abstinence (the beginning of the J) and then a sharply elevating mortality rate with heavy alcohol consumption (the stem of the J). The lowered risk of cardiovascular disease at moderate doses may be in part due to alcohol's low-dose ability to reduce inflammation (Romeo et al., 2007), raise HDL, and counteract blood-clotting tendencies (American Heart Association, 2011b). For women, even one drink a day can slightly elevate the risk of breast cancer, so women who are already at higher breast cancer risk due to family history or other factors should not drink alcohol (American Cancer Society, 2011).

You have probably heard about the health benefits of drinking red wine. Is moderate drinking of wine superior to drinking other alcoholic beverages for health? What does the evidence suggest? Numerous studies have focused specifically on the health benefits of moderate consumption of red wine. Wine first began to receive attention when researchers noticed that the French eat a diet rich in saturated fats like Americans yet have significantly fewer heart attacks. The main difference between their eating patterns is that the French have a higher level of wine consumption. This phenomenon became known as the "French paradox" (Renaud & Lorgeril, 1992). Does wine then confer an added health benefit over other alcoholic beverages?

Some studies have found evidence supporting the hypothesis that moderate consumption of wine reduces the risk of cardiovascular disease to a greater extent than other alcoholic beverages such as beer (Di Castelnuovo et al., 2002). Such differences may be due to the polyphenols found in wine, which are especially high in red wine given that its red color is due to the skin of the grapes being used in the fermentation process where these compounds are especially concentrated. Along with the polyphenols, the plant hormone **resveratrol,** a vasodilator and antioxidant found in high concentrations in red wine, is believed to play a health-protective role by some experts (Saleem & Basha, 2010). Therefore, **red wine,** in particular, is believed by some to have health advantages over other types of alcoholic beverages, including white wine.

Many other experts are not convinced that red wine confers any additional cardiovascular protection over other alcoholic beverages (Lin, Kelsberg, & Safranek, 2010). For example, the American Heart Association (2011b) contends that other lifestyle variable confounds in epidemiological studies, including whether participants eat more fruits and vegetables or exercise more could account for the advantage that red wine drinkers have in cardiovascular risk over drinkers of beer or spirits. They also note that getting more polyphenols can be accomplished by eating more fruits and vegetables, that raising HDL can be done through exercise, and that reduction of blood clotting can be achieved through taking a daily low-dose aspirin. Therefore, they contend, there is no compelling reason for abstinent individuals to begin consuming red wine.

In addition, other experts (Harvard Heart Letter, 2010) note that the studies done to date with resveratrol almost exclusively use cell cultures or nonhuman subjects such as yeast, fruit flies, roundworms, and mice yet no human studies to date have examined the long-term health and longevity benefits of the compound. Therefore, they remain skeptical of any resveratrol health claims.

TOBACCO USE

Tobacco leaves can be used in a smokeless form such as snuff and chewing tobacco or by burning them and inhaling their smoke through puffing on cigarettes, cigars, or pipes. It is well known that tobacco use is the single greatest cause of preventable death, yet 21% of American adults continue to smoke cigarettes (Centers for Disease Control and Prevention [CDC], 2011c). Fortunately, the long-term trend is positive with the number of American adult smokers now half that of the mid-1960s.

Men are more likely to smoke than women, and adults with less education are more likely to smoke than adults with higher education levels (Paharia, 2008). According to the U.S. Centers for Disease Control and Prevention's publication called "Tobacco Use: Targeting the Nation's Leading Killer: At a

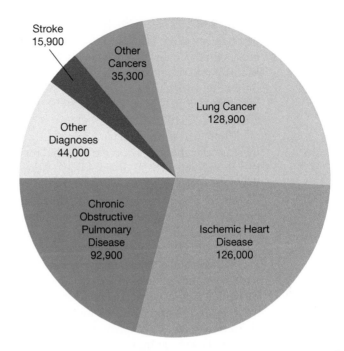

Stroke
15,900

Other
Cancers
35,300

Other
Diagnoses
44,000

Lung Cancer
128,900

Chronic
Obstructive
Pulmonary
Disease
92,900

Ischemic Heart
Disease
126,000

FIGURE **12.3**   Cause and number of deaths attributable to cigarette smoking in the United States

SOURCE: Centers for Disease Control and Prevention (CDC) (2010b). Tobacco use: Targeting the nation's
leading killer: At a glance 2010. Retrieved from http://www.cdc.gov/chronicdisease/resources/
publications/aag/osh_text.htm

Glance 2010," cigarette smoking accounts for 443,000 deaths in the United
States each year from a variety of causes including lung and other cancers,
ischemic heart disease, chronic obstructive pulmonary disease, stroke, and a
number of other diseases (Figure 12.3). The publication also cautions that secondhand smoke causes heart disease and lung disease in adult nonsmokers
and contributes to medical problems for children such as acute respiratory infections, sudden infant death syndrome, and asthma attacks. Further, smokeless tobacco, cigars, and pipes are not harmless to their users because they
contribute to oral, lung, esophageal, and larynx cancers.

Nicotine found in tobacco is an addictive drug that affects the "feel good"
neurotransmitters in the brain such as norepinephrine, serotonin, and dopamine
while also increasing heart rate and blood pressure (Paharia, 2008). Activation
of the dopaminergic pathway's reward systems in the brain may account for
nicotine's highly addictive properties. Most smokers are aware of the health
consequences of smoking, and 70% report they would like to quit. However, less
than 5% who make an attempt on their own stay permanently quit after a single
attempt with the majority of those wanting to quit going through a long-term
process of intervals of smoking cessation followed by relapses (Perkins, 2010).

How does smoking relate to stress? Do people smoke in an attempt to regulate their stress? Smokers will report that they smoke more when they experience negative affect due to stress, and studies confirm this belief (Perkins,

2010). Smokers seem to be trying to regulate their negative mood states through smoking. However, does this self-regulation strategy work? Although most smokers believe that their smoking-to-relieve-stress behavior is effective, according to recent research designed to test this hypothesis, it is not; smoking only relieves negative affect caused by nicotine withdrawal and not negative affect caused by stress (Perkins, 2010; Perkins, Karelitz, Conklin, Sayette, & Giedgowd, 2010).

There are several pharmacologically based smoking cessation tools that increase the chance of success by relieving withdrawal symptoms or reducing the pleasurable effects of smoking. These include the use of one of the three FDA-approved medications for smoking cessation of (1) nicotine replacement therapy delivered in the form of gum, lozenge, or a patch; (2) taking bupropion (Zyban), which is an antidepressant medication that inhibits the reuptake of dopamine and norepinephrine; or (3) use of a more recently approved medication called varenicline (Chantix).

Although not an exhaustive list, behavioral strategies that are most effective for smoking cessation are varied and include the following: self-monitoring through keeping a log of cigarettes smoked to identify emotional and behavioral triggers; using fading of nicotine through slowly reducing the number of cigarettes smoked per day until quit day; employing self-regulation strategies such as chewing gum, taking a walk, or doing relaxation exercises; and receiving monetary rewards for abstinence. Other strategies include addressing weight gain concerns; participating in cognitive-behavioral therapy; using relapse prevention strategies through identifying relapse triggers and planning for high-risk situations; and employing acceptance-focused strategies that focus on learning how to accept smoking urges, negative moods, and other unpleasant experiences associated with quitting rather than trying to change them (Bricker, 2010; Paharia, 2008; Perkins, 2010).

Obesity and Weight Loss

body mass index (BMI): an estimate of body fat based on a formula that uses height and weight.

obese: having a body mass index of 30 or above.

In the United States and many parts of the developed world the growing number of overweight and obese individuals is at epidemic proportions (Berghofer et al., 2008; USDA & USDHHS, 2010). The National Task Force on the Prevention and Treatment of Obesity (2000) defines **overweight** as a **body mass index (BMI)** of 25 to 29.9 and **obese** as 30 or above. BMI can be computed using the formula weight (pounds) divided by height (inches) squared multiplied by 703. However, it is much simpler to use a BMI calculator like the one on the National Heart Lung and Blood Institute's (2011) website at http://www.nhlbisupport.com/bmi/bminojs.htm or to use a BMI table (Table 12.3). With the standard BMI cutoff for obesity of 30, we can see that an average height woman at 5'4" and man at 5'10" would weigh 174 pounds and 209 pounds, respectively, to be considered obese. Using this standard, according to the CDC (2011f), 34% of Americans age 20 or over are obese and another 34% are overweight. This compares to the late 1970s when only 15% of adult Americans were obese (USDA & USDHHS, 2010). The prevalence of obesity is

TABLE **12.3** Body Mass Index (BMI) Table

Height (inches)	Normal						Overweight					Obese										Extreme Obesity															
BMI	19	20	21	22	23	24	25	26	27	28	29	30	31	32	33	34	35	36	37	38	39	40	41	42	43	44	45	46	47	48	49	50	51	52	53	54
	Body Weight (pounds)																																			
58	91	96	100	105	110	115	119	124	129	134	138	143	148	153	158	162	167	172	177	181	186	191	196	201	205	210	215	220	224	229	234	239	244	248	253	258
59	94	99	104	109	114	119	124	128	133	138	143	148	153	158	163	168	173	178	183	188	193	198	203	208	212	217	222	227	232	237	242	247	252	257	262	267
60	97	102	107	112	118	123	128	133	138	143	148	153	158	163	168	174	179	184	189	194	199	204	209	215	220	225	230	235	240	245	250	255	261	266	271	276
61	100	106	111	116	122	127	132	137	143	148	153	158	164	169	175	180	185	190	195	201	206	211	217	222	227	232	238	243	248	254	259	264	269	275	280	285
62	104	109	115	120	126	131	136	142	147	153	158	164	169	175	180	186	191	196	202	207	213	218	224	229	235	240	246	251	256	262	267	273	278	284	289	295
63	107	113	118	124	130	135	141	146	152	158	163	169	175	180	186	191	197	203	208	214	220	225	231	237	242	248	254	259	265	270	278	282	287	293	299	304
64	110	116	122	128	134	140	145	151	157	163	169	174	180	186	192	197	204	209	215	221	227	232	238	244	250	256	262	267	273	279	285	291	296	302	308	314
65	114	120	126	132	138	144	150	156	162	168	174	180	186	192	198	204	210	216	222	228	234	240	246	252	258	264	270	276	282	288	294	300	306	312	318	324
66	118	124	130	136	142	148	155	161	167	173	179	186	192	198	204	210	216	223	229	235	241	247	253	260	266	272	278	284	291	297	303	309	315	322	328	334
67	121	127	134	140	146	153	159	166	172	178	185	191	198	204	211	217	223	230	236	242	249	255	261	268	274	280	287	293	299	306	312	319	325	331	338	344
68	125	131	138	144	151	158	164	171	177	184	190	197	203	210	216	223	230	236	243	249	256	262	269	276	282	289	295	302	308	315	322	328	335	341	348	354
69	128	135	142	149	155	162	169	176	182	189	196	203	209	216	223	230	236	243	250	257	263	270	277	284	291	297	304	311	318	324	331	338	345	351	358	365
70	132	139	146	153	160	167	174	181	188	195	202	209	216	222	229	236	243	250	257	264	271	278	285	292	299	306	313	320	327	334	341	348	355	362	369	376
71	136	143	150	157	165	172	179	186	193	200	208	215	222	229	236	243	250	257	265	272	279	286	293	301	308	315	322	329	338	343	351	358	365	372	379	386
72	140	147	154	162	169	177	184	191	199	206	213	221	228	235	242	250	258	265	272	279	287	294	302	309	316	324	331	338	346	353	361	368	375	383	390	397
73	144	151	159	166	174	182	189	197	204	212	219	227	235	242	250	257	265	272	280	288	295	302	310	318	325	333	340	348	355	363	371	378	386	393	401	408
74	148	155	163	171	179	186	194	202	210	218	225	233	241	249	256	264	272	280	287	295	303	311	319	326	334	342	350	358	365	373	381	389	396	404	412	420
75	152	160	168	176	184	192	200	208	216	224	232	240	248	256	264	272	279	287	295	303	311	319	327	335	343	351	359	367	375	383	391	399	407	415	423	431
76	156	164	172	180	189	197	205	213	221	230	238	246	254	263	271	279	287	295	304	312	320	328	336	344	353	361	369	377	385	394	402	410	418	426	435	443

SOURCE: Adapted from *Clinical Guidelines on the Identification, Evaluation, and Treatment of Overweight and Obesity in Adults: The Evidence Report.*

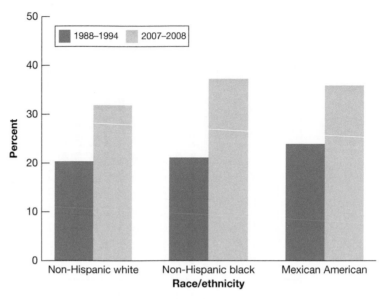

FIGURE **12.4**   Obesity prevalence for non-Hispanic White, non-Hispanic Black, and Mexican American men in the United States   SOURCE: Ogden, C., & Carroll, M. D. (2010). National Health and Nutritional Examination Survey (NHANES). Prevalence of overweight, obesity, and extreme obesity among adults: United States, trends 1976–1980 through 2007–2008. Retrieved from http://www.cdc.gov/NCHS/data/hestat/obesity_adult_07_08/obesity_adult_07_08.pdf.

even higher for African Americans and Mexican Americans, especially among women (Figures 12.4 and 12.5). Doing the math, it is easy to see that according to the BMI, greater than two-thirds of the U.S. population is either overweight or obese. Of course, as we know from Chapter 11, the BMI is not a perfect metric for determining body fat because a lean individual with a high proportion of muscle (e.g., a professional athlete or body builder) could be considered overweight by this standard because muscle weighs more than fat. A more precise measure of obesity is based on determining percent body fat. When using instruments that estimate body fat, a normal weight woman has 25% body fat and a normal weight man, 15% to 18%, but an obese woman has at least 35% body fat and an obese man, 25% (Faulconbridge & Wadden, 2010).

As you are well aware, obesity is a serious health concern. Why is obesity such a concern? The health consequences of obesity include a higher risk of hypertension, heart disease, stroke, colon cancer, breast cancer, type 2 diabetes, arthritis, gallbladder disease, sleep apnea, depression, and early mortality (CDC, 2011d; Paharia & Kase, 2008). For example, obesity is associated with a 10-fold increase in risk for developing type 2 diabetes (Paharia & Kase, 2008). The excess fat carried in obesity is proinflammatory and may contribute to many of the chronic diseases associated with obesity (Guest, Gao, O'Connor, & Freund, 2007).

How do people gain weight and become obese? Weight gain is a matter of **calorie imbalance,** that is, consuming more calories than one expends. The

calorie imbalance: consuming more calories than one expends or vice versa.

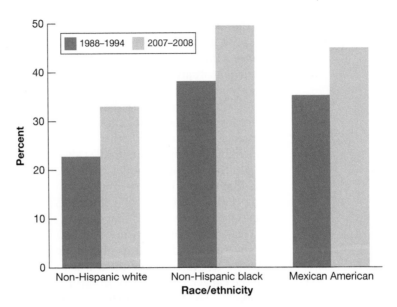

FIGURE **12.5** Obesity prevalence for non-Hispanic White, non-Hispanic Black, and Mexican American women in the United States   SOURCE: Ogden, C., & Carroll, M. D. (2010). National Health and Nutritional Examination Survey (NHANES). Prevalence of overweight, obesity, and extreme obesity among adults: United States, trends 1976–1980 through 2007–2008. Retrieved from http://www.cdc.gov/NCHS/data/hestat/obesity_adult_07_08/obesity_adult_07_08.pdf.

excess calories are stored as fat. Obesity results when the calorie imbalance leads to an ongoing long-term accumulation of fat deposits. Some people are more prone to develop obesity than others. Why? There are several models that attempt to explain individual differences in tendencies toward obesity including the weight set point model, the genetics model, and the positive incentive model.

The **weight set point model** (Stallone & Stunkard, 1991) proposes that weight is determined by a set point that acts as an internal regulator similar to a thermostat. When fat stores decrease below the set point, physiological mechanisms activate to bring the fat stores back to set point. People with higher set points then have a greater tendency to put on excess weight and ultimately become obese. There is some evidence for this model from indications that when **leptin,** an adipose tissue hunger hormone, falls along with fat stores, it signals the hypothalamus to induce hunger (Erlanson-Albertsson, 2005). Thus, leptin may be one of the mechanisms that supports the weight set point.

Why would some people have higher set points predisposing them toward obesity? Genetics may be the answer. For example, studies including examination of twins reared apart suggest a high heritability component of BMI and weight (Schousboe et al., 2004; Stunkard, Harris, Pedersen, & McClean, 1990). Evolution may play a role in this process because the gene pool has a greater chance of surviving when there is a broad range of genetic variation to match a myriad of environmental conditions. Evolutionary theory would suggest then that it is adaptive to genetically predispose some members of the human gene pool to retain more fat stores so that these individuals would survive famines while others perish. However, during periods of abundance, such as the current situation in the developed world, the opposite is true in that having a genetic tendency toward obesity is harmful to survival.

Although the weight set point and **genetics models of obesity** can explain tendencies toward weight gain for select individuals, they do not explain why the majority of people and other mammals will overeat and ultimately become overweight when appealing food is always available for ongoing consumption. The **positive incentive model** challenges the set point idea and instead proposes that motivation to eat is primarily driven by the anticipated pleasure of eating (Pinel, Assanand, & Lehman, 2000). This explains our desire to eat sweet, fatty, or salty foods that in nature would signal dense calorie foods that we would binge on to ensure our survival through the next famine. These foods were more difficult to obtain for our distant ancestors so we are programmed to overconsume them when they are available. Thus, most people have the capacity for obesity in this model, not just people with high weight set points. The point is driven home by the statistic that two-thirds of Americans are currently overweight or obese in part because of the cheap availability of a wide variety of appealing foods including fast foods.

Does stress play a role in developing obesity? There are some indications that it can be a contributing factor. For example, family stress is a risk factor for childhood obesity (Koch, Sepa, & Ludvigsson, 2008). In adults, stress increases cortisol levels that in turn have an impact on rapid weight gain that contributes to the development of stress-related obesity (Vicennati, Pasqui, Cavazza, Pagotto, & Pasquali, 2009). High cortisol can increase eating, change fat metabolism, and affect the action of hormones like insulin and leptin, resulting in greater fat stores, especially visceral fat (Vicennati et al., 2009).

If we have lost our caloric balance, how then do we get it back? Ultimately, no matter what the dietary plan, it is always a matter of calories-in and calories-out. We gain 1 pound of fat for every 3,500 excess calories we consume. Therefore, a reasonable goal for weight loss is to change the caloric balance so that we are running a deficit of 500 calories per day. This would result in 1 pound per week of fat (not water weight) lost. Over the course of a year that would equal a weight loss of 52 pounds. Using a Dietary Guidelines 2010 table (Table 12.4), we can determine our normal caloric needs and then reduce from there.

Behavioral strategies for weight loss all involve this principle of calorie reduction. Popular choices for calorie reduction include low-fat eating, low-carbohydrate eating, portion control, and calorie counting. Eating low fat is a convenient indirect way to restrict calories because fat is calorie dense compared to protein and carbohydrates. Low-fat eating essentially involves reducing daily fat consumption by 20% to 30%, which amounts to eating only 20 to 35 grams of fat per 1,000 calories, whereas low-carbohydrate eating (e.g., Atkins, 1998) restricts carbohydrates to 20 to 30 grams per day (Paharia & Kase, 2008).

The high-protein intake of a low-carbohydrate diet may increase feelings of satiation (i.e., fullness and satisfaction), which could account for its success. However, by virtually eliminating a whole class of macronutrients that we are

TABLE **12.4** Estimated Calorie Needs per Day by Age, Gender, and Physical Activity Level[a]

Estimated calories needed to maintain weight through caloric balance

Gender	Age (years)	Physical Activity Level[b]		
		Sedentary	Moderately Active	Active
Child (female and male)	2–3	1,000–1,200[c]	1,000–1,400[c]	1,000–1,400[c]
Female[d]	4–8	1,200–1,400	1,400–1,600	1,400–1,800
	9–13	1,400–1,600	1,600–2,000	1,800–2,200
	14–18	1,800	2,000	2,400
	19–30	1,800–2,000	2,000–2,200	2,400
	31–50	1,800	2,000	2,200
	51+	1,600	1,800	2,000–2,200
Male	4–8	1,200–1,400	1,400–1,600	1,600–2,000
	9–13	1,600–2,000	1,800–2,200	2,000–2,600
	14–18	2,000–2,400	2,400–2,800	2,800–3,200
	19–30	2,400–2,600	2,600–2,800	3,000
	31–50	2,200–2,400	2,400–2,600	2,800–3,000
	51+	2,000–2,200	2,200–2,400	2,400–2,800

a. Based on Estimated Energy Requirements (EER) equations, using reference heights (average) and reference weights (healthy) for each age/gender group. For children and adolescents, reference height and weight vary. For adults, the reference man is 5 feet 10 inches tall and weighs 154 pounds. The reference woman is 5 feet 4 inches tall and weighs 126 pounds. EER equations are from the Institute of Medicine. Dietary Reference Intakes for Energy, Carbohydrate, Fiber, Fat, Fatty Acids, Cholesterol, Protein, and Amino Acids. Washington, DC: The National Academies Press; 2002.

b. Sedentary means a lifestyle that includes only the light physical activity associated with typical day-to-day life. Moderately active means a lifestyle that includes physical activity equivalent to walking about 1.5 to 3 miles per day at 3 to 4 miles per hour, in addition to the light physical activity associated with typical day-to-day life. Active means a lifestyle that includes physical activity equivalent to walking more than 3 miles per day at 3 to 4 miles per hour, in addition to the light physical activity associated with typical day-to-day life.

c. The calorie ranges shown are to accommodate needs of different ages within the group. For children and adolescents, more calories are needed at older ages. For adults, fewer calories are needed at older ages.

d. Estimates for females do not include women who are pregnant or breastfeeding.

SOURCE: U.S. Department of Agriculture and U.S. Department of Health and Human Services (USDA & HHS). (2010). *Dietary Guidelines for Americans, 2010* (7th ed.). Washington, DC: U.S. Government Printing Office.

encouraged by health authorities to consume in the greatest abundance, the low-carbohydrate diet plan has been an ongoing source of controversy. One concern is that it increases health risks. A recent research finding (Sacks et al., 2009) suggests that low-carbohydrate diets may be safe to follow for up to 2 years but more confirmatory research is needed.

Most structured behavioral weight loss programs are in alignment with the recommendation by the majority of health authorities to eat a high- rather than a low-carbohydrate diet. These programs include eating low-fat meals with a lot of fruits, vegetables, and whole grains for a total daily calorie consumption of between 1,200 (a minimum intake advisable without a physician's supervision) and 1,500 calories (Faulconbridge & Wadden, 2010).

Another strategy, using portion control, involves consuming meal replacements such as commercially prepared liquid shakes or lower calorie frozen food entrees. This method makes it easier to manage calories without having to count calories for a variety of foods, which can facilitate greater adherence to the plan. The last strategy, calorie counting, is simply a matter of recording the calories consumed to know when the maximum allotted for the day has been reached. There are no restrictions on the types of foods eaten, just the total calories consumed.

Among these four general strategies all are effective and no one method appears to be more effective than the others. Fad diets and starvation diets, however, should be avoided because they may not supply adequate nutrition and can even be dangerous (Paharia & Kase, 2008).

Physical exercise is a crucial component of weight maintenance programs. However, in order for exercise to have a meaningful impact on weight loss, the American College of Sports Medicine (Donnelly et al., 2009) recommends engaging in a minimum of 250 minutes per week or at least 100 minutes more than the standard recommended by the U.S. government to achieve general health benefits (see Chapter 11).

Finally, for maintaining weight loss four main principles are recommended. They are (1) exercise on a regular basis, (2) maintain a caloric balance, (3) keep a record of physical activity and food consumptions, and (4) weigh on a regular basis (Faulconbridge & Walden, 2010).

HEALTHY EATING

Tying it all together, we can see that the Harvard School of Public Health's (2011) "Healthy Eating Pyramid" (Figure 12.6) is a good overall guide to healthy eating. (Note: The Harvard School of Public Health's [2011] Healthy Eating Pyramid is an improvement over the U.S. government's food guide pyramid that was replaced in 2011 with ChooseMyPlate.gov.) According to any food pyramid's guidelines, we should eat more foods at the base of the pyramid and less as we move toward the top. Following the Healthy Eating Pyramid's recommendations we see that the base of the pyramid consists of daily exercise along with maintaining caloric balance for weight control. The next level of the pyramid is populated by fruits and vegetables, healthy fats and oils, and whole grains. Moving higher, we find sources of protein that emphasize "nuts, seeds, beans, tofu, fish, poultry, and eggs." Next is dairy followed by sugar, salt, high saturated fat and glycemic foods that should be eaten sparingly. A daily multivitamin is recommended for most along with extra vitamin D. Last, alcohol is optional and should only be consumed in moderation by adults with lower risk factors.

THE HEALTHY EATING PYRAMID

Department of Nutrition, Harvard School of Public Health

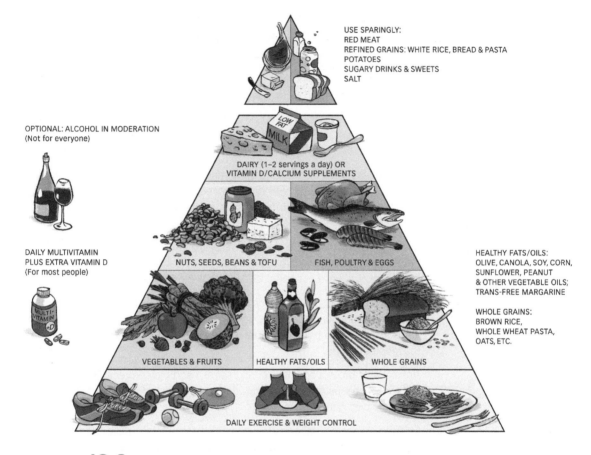

USE SPARINGLY:
RED MEAT
REFINED GRAINS: WHITE RICE, BREAD & PASTA
POTATOES
SUGARY DRINKS & SWEETS
SALT

OPTIONAL: ALCOHOL IN MODERATION
(Not for everyone)

DAIRY (1–2 servings a day) OR
VITAMIN D/CALCIUM SUPPLEMENTS

DAILY MULTIVITAMIN
PLUS EXTRA VITAMIN D
(For most people)

NUTS, SEEDS, BEANS & TOFU

FISH, POULTRY & EGGS

HEALTHY FATS/OILS:
OLIVE, CANOLA, SOY, CORN,
SUNFLOWER, PEANUT
& OTHER VEGETABLE OILS;
TRANS-FREE MARGARINE

WHOLE GRAINS:
BROWN RICE,
WHOLE WHEAT PASTA,
OATS, ETC.

VEGETABLES & FRUITS

HEALTHY FATS/OILS

WHOLE GRAINS

DAILY EXERCISE & WEIGHT CONTROL

FIGURE **12.6** The healthy eating pyramid from the Harvard School of Public Health

SOURCE: Harvard School of Public Health (2011). Food pyramids: What should you really eat? Retrieved from http://www.hsph.harvard.edu/nutritionsource/what-should-you-eat/pyramid-full-story/index.html.

CHAPTER SUMMARY AND CONCEPT REVIEW

- Most people change their eating patterns in response to stress; common patterns include eating less, emotional eating, and the night-eating syndrome.

- Eating in response to stress tends to be selective with most preferring high-fat sugar snacks.

- Components of foods include macronutrients, micronutrients, phytochemicals, fiber, and water.

- The macronutrients are carbohydrate, protein, and fat.

- Carbohydrates are sugar molecules that divide into simple and complex versions with particular forms of carbohydrate increasing the glycemic index or load.

- Highly processed foods often lack nutrient density and may contain empty calories.

- Fiber, especially cereal fiber, has health protective effects by reducing low-density lipoproteins (LDL) and reducing coronary heart disease (CHD) risk.

- Protein consists of amino acid building blocks; half of the amino acids we need must be obtained from dietary sources.

- Animal protein is considered a complete protein but is generally accompanied by saturated fat, whereas plant proteins may be incomplete but are often accompanied by fiber, carbohydrates, phytochemicals, and generally healthy fats.

- Fat is higher in calories than the other macronutrients and includes saturated fat, trans-fat, and cholesterol, which are not required in one's diet and have detrimental health effects, and monounsaturated fat and polyunsaturated fat including the essential fatty acids that have health beneficial effects.

- Micronutrients include vitamins and minerals that ideally can be obtained in food, but taking a daily multivitamin/mineral supplement is good insurance even though studies have not conclusively established its health benefits.

- Although the Food and Drug Administration (FDA) does not recognize the category of functional foods, it does allow qualified health claims for specific whole foods and supplements that may have health-protective effects beyond that of other foods.

- Antioxidants protect against oxidation stress and may protect against vulnerability to the diseases of aging; brightly colored pigmented plant foods are often saturated with antioxidants.

- Evidence indicates that consuming fruits and vegetables daily reduces the risk of heart disease and may reduce the risk of particular cancers.

- Eating patterns associated with reduced cardiovascular disease risk include the DASH plan, the Mediterranean-style, and vegetarian eating.

- The caffeine in tea and coffee can exacerbate stress reactions if too much is consumed; however, tea may contain other compounds, including phytochemicals, that aid in the recovery from stress.

- Green tea has a high concentration of beneficial polyphenols, especially EGCG.

- Moderate consumption of alcohol reduces CHD risk as well as increases longevity; although red wine has phytochemicals and other compounds that may benefit health, the evidence is suggestive but not established that it confers any additional health benefit over consuming other alcoholic beverages.

- Tobacco use has a myriad of health risks, including early mortality; there are a number of effective pharmacologically based and behaviorally oriented smoking cessation tools.

- Obesity increases the risk of morbidity and mortality and is a product of maintaining a caloric imbalance whereby more calories are consumed than expended.

- Popular and effective weight loss strategies involve the principle of calorie reduction in one form or the other.

CRITICAL THINKING QUESTIONS

1. When you are under stress, do you eat more or less? If you eat more, what type of foods are you drawn to? Does eating these foods reduce your stress? If so, what mechanisms seem to account for the stress reduction? What healthy stress management strategies could you employ instead of stress eating?

2. How does living a healthy lifestyle including maintaining good nutrition reduce stress? What are three lifestyle changes you could make based on information you learned in this chapter that would reduce your stress?

3. Given what you have read, if you served as your own eating plan consultant, what would be your recommendations? Draw up an eating plan. What is your rationale for your new plan? Explain.

4. Do you believe in the idea of "food as medicine"? What are the pros and cons of approaching food choices with this concept in mind?

5. Which food controversies are you most skeptical about? Take the devil's advocate position on a food that may promote health. What is the foundation of your skepticism? Explain.

KEY TERMS AND CONCEPTS

Alcohol	DASH (dietary approaches to stop hypertension)	Glycogen*	Minerals
Amino acid		Green tea	Monounsaturated fats*
Antioxidant*	EGCG	High-glycemic index/ load*	Nicotine
Body mass index (BMI)*	Emotional eaters		Night-eating syndrome
Calorie imbalance*	Empty calories*	Incomplete proteins	Nutrient density
Caffeine	Essential amino acids*	Insulin	Nutrients
Catechins	Essential fatty acids	Lacto-ovo vegetarians	Obese*
Cereal fiber	Fat	Leptin	Omega-3 fatty acids*
Cholesterol	Fiber	Macronutrients	Overweight
Complete proteins*	Functional foods*	Mediterranean-style eating pattern	Oxidative stress*
Complex carbohydrates*	Genetics model of obesity	Micronutrients	Phytochemicals*

Polyphenols*	Red wine	Simple carbohydrates*	Triglycerides
Polyunsaturated fats*	Restraint eaters*	Tea	Vegans
Positive incentive model	Resveratrol	Tobacco	Vitamins
Protein	Saturated fats*	Trans-fats*	Weight set point model

MEDIA RESOURCES

CENGAGE**brain**^{.com}

Access an interactive eBook, chapter-specific
interactive learning tools, including flashcards,
quizzes, videos, and more in your Psychology
CourseMate, accessed through CengageBrain.com.

13

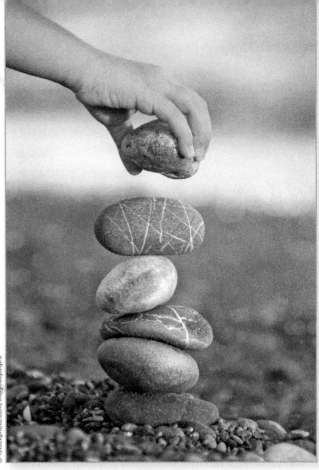

© Istockphoto.com/imagedepotpro

The time to relax is when you don't have time for it.

~SIDNEY J. HARRIS

SELF-REGULATION RELAXATION STRATEGIES

PROGRESSIVE MUSCLE RELAXATION

■ **STRESS MANAGEMENT EXERCISE 13.1**
Progressive Muscle Relaxation

■ **STRESS MANAGEMENT EXERCISE 13.2**
Brief Relaxation Exercise

AUTOGENIC TRAINING

■ **STRESS MANAGEMENT EXERCISE 13.3**
Autogenic Exercise

GUIDED IMAGERY RELAXATION

■ **STRESS MANAGEMENT EXERCISE 13.4**
Creating Your Personal Guided Imagery
Relaxation Script

April settled into the easy chair at the counseling center. Her counselor, Crystal, dimmed the lights. Soon Crystal began talking to April in a slow, soothing voice. "Imagine you have peacefully and calmly floated to a serene secluded beach. You are relaxing on the warm beach enjoying the soft breeze and the sun's rays warming your body. You hear the waves breaking in the distance as they eventually roll gently toward the warm white sandy beach. In and out . . . in and out . . . the waves flow toward you then away. Most people, if they try, can smell the salt in the air and even taste it on their lips as they take in their relaxing experience. Allow yourself to let go and relax in the warm sand, enjoying the sun's rays continuing to warm your body. . . . Slowly, the sun starts to ever so gently rest in the horizon and you notice the beginnings of yellow, orange, and red colors gradually expand to paint the sky. These now brilliant colors reflect off the waves that gently roll in and out . . . in and out . . . as you become more relaxed . . . safe and secure in your own corner of the secluded beach. As soon as you hear each gentle wave, you become more and more deeply relaxed, calm, and peaceful. . . ."

Crystal continued on with her guided imagery relaxation session until April settled into a deeply relaxed state. She knew from April's counseling sessions that April was troubled with stress and anxiety. Before April began her sessions she had never truly learned how to relax. Crystal's goal was to provide April training in a variety of strategies she could use to relax. Previously, Crystal had shown April a passive self-hypnotic strategy called autogenic training, and before that an active strategy of tensing and relaxing major muscle groups called progressive relaxation training. Today, April was learning how to use mental imagery to relax.

When a person like April says "I'm stressed," what advice do you usually hear? The advice is usually "you need to relax." Yet, do you hear that advice followed with guidance on how to relax like Crystal gave April? Although we know that the antidote to stress is relaxation, the real challenge is how to bring about relaxation. For some people, relaxing means crawling in bed and taking a nap; for others it is having a few drinks; and for yet others it is socializing, watching television, or reading a good book. However, as you experienced with April's journey, there are specific strategies that a person can use to achieve relaxation states that do not involve sleeping, drinking, socializing, or recreational activities. In fact, although sleeping and relaxation are both restorative, they are different states that serve different functions. Of course alcohol achieves its relaxation effects through its drug action, and relaxation can be an indirect by-product of social or recreational activities. However, we can employ direct self-regulation strategies to naturally reduce excessive autonomic and central nervous system activation and somatic tension while staying in a waking state of consciousness. These strategies like progressive relaxation, autogenics, and guided imagery that Crystal presented to April are known as **deep relaxation strategies.**

As discussed in Chapter 7, relaxation strategies can lower the diffuse physiological arousal that underpins the fight-or-flight emotions of anger and anxiety by helping us reduce their intensity. In addition, practicing deep relaxation exercises for 20 minutes twice a day helps to restore balance to physiological systems that are in overdrive and thus reduce the body's allostatic load. In effect, we are resetting baselines and helping to restore homeostatic balance for the cardiovascular and other systems that may be elevated by stress. For example, engaging in deep relaxation exercises lowers blood pressure (McCallie, Blum, & Hood, 2006). In addition, the practice lowers stress hormone levels; reduces fatigue, pain, headaches, and insomnia; and increases energy (Hyman, Feldman, Harris, Levin, & Malloy; 1989; McCallie et al., 2006). Engaging in deep relaxation strategies is not "goofing off" or being lazy, but rather involves making a healthy lifestyle choice for managing stress.

PROGRESSIVE MUSCLE RELAXATION

Dr. Edmund Jacobson (1888–1983), an American physician with a clinical and research interest in relaxation, developed a deep relaxation technique called *progressive relaxation* (Jacobson, 1938) in the 1920s that is also known today as **progressive muscle relaxation (PMR).** The technique consists of tensing and relaxing different muscle groups. In doing the exercise the practitioner learns **muscle sense awareness,** that is, the ability to differentiate a tense muscle from a relaxed one. In addition, Jacobson discovered that after holding a muscle contraction and then releasing the contraction, the muscle fibers elongate. These elongated muscle fibers are more relaxed and can be trained to reach a zero firing threshold (i.e., the neurons that tense these muscle fibers do not exceed their firing thresholds), a phenomenon that is verifiable with an electromyograph instrument. When a person reaches this level after contracting, holding, and releasing forearm tension, for instance, the hand goes limp like a wet dishrag.

Jacobson's original progressive relaxation method was one of the first behavioral medicine techniques created to manage health and well-being. Its historical significance is vast, especially considering that Jacobson's first published work became available in the early part of the 20th century and yet still has relevance today. Early on, Jacobson determined that a truly relaxed person with eyes closed showed no startle response to a sudden unexpected noise like the smack of a book dropping onto a floor. The startle response, of course, reflects an exaggerated somatic response. He further determined that patients

deep relaxation strategies: strategies like progressive relaxation, autogenics, and guided imagery that one can employ to reduce diffuse physiological arousal.

progressive muscle relaxation (PMR): a deep relaxation technique pioneered by Jacobson that consists of tensing and relaxing different muscle groups.

muscle sense awareness: the ability to differentiate tense muscles from relaxed ones.

who claimed to be relaxed often carried tension that they were unaware of in their muscles. Thus, he saw somatic muscular tension as a barometer of relaxation levels and interventions aimed at reducing somatic tension as the key to inducing relaxed states. In his clinical practice and research, Jacobson tirelessly and successfully applied his method both as a prevention tool and as a treatment strategy for a variety of tension-related disorders during his career, which spanned over a half a century (McGuigan & Lehrer, 2007).

By learning how to relax the somatic nervous system, Jacobson believed that the sympathetic branch of the autonomic nervous system would follow suit. Indirect evidence for this idea is found in research results showing reduced heart rate and blood pressure when using this procedure (Bernstein, Carlson, & Schmidt, 2007). Likewise, successful application of his method results in the mind and emotions becoming calm. For example, a recent meta-analytic review by Manzoni, Pagnini, Casetelnuovo, and Molinari (2008) confirms that relaxation training is especially effective for reducing anxiety. The review found an average effect size in the medium-high range of 0.57 for relaxation training (i.e., progressive muscle relaxation, applied relaxation, autogenic training, and meditation) with progressive muscle relaxation being one of the most effective strategies. The process requires no exertion of willpower to relax, but rather relaxation happens naturally as a result of tensing and then releasing the contraction of the body's different muscle groups.

Jacobson's original approach was "lengthy and painstaking" with training sometimes taking over 100 sessions (Bernstein et al., 2007, p. 88). Therefore, Joseph Wolpe (1958) later developed a condensed version for use with his now classic counterconditioning method called *systematic desensitization*. The process of systematic desensitization involves pairing increasingly fearful phobic images with relaxation in the mind's eye. Because relaxation is incompatible with anxiety, the person gradually progresses to the most feared image and learns to experience this imagined stimulus without excessive anxiety. This process is discussed in more detail later in this chapter.

This approach opened the door for use of a variety of abbreviated progressive relaxation strategies (Bernstein & Borkovec, 1978). Some of these incorporate instructions for deep breathing or relaxation along with progressive tensing and relaxing of muscle groups. Today, as Douglas Bernstein, who pioneered an early version of abbreviated progressive relaxation training, and his colleagues note (Bernstein et al., 2007, p. 88), "progressive relaxation training is not a single method but a group of techniques that vary considerably in procedural detail, complexity, and length." What they all have in common, however, is the strategy of tensing muscle groups and releasing the tension to achieve a deep relaxation state. Let us next look at an abbreviated method of progressive relaxation training.

Abbreviated Progressive Muscle Relaxation

In its abbreviated form, the Jacobson technique is easy to teach and learn. Although there are over 1,030 skeletal muscles in the body, they can be grouped together into 16 muscle groups, then 7, and, finally, 4, in progressively abbreviated versions (Bernstein et al., 2007). The 16 groups include the

"(1) dominant hand and forearm, (2) dominant upper arm, (3) nondominant hand and forearm, (4) nondominant upper arm, (5) forehead, (6) upper cheeks and nose, (7) lower face, (8) neck, (9) chest, shoulders, upper back, (10) abdomen, (11) dominant upper leg, (12) dominant calf, (13) dominant foot, (14) nondominant upper leg, (15) nondominant calf, [and] (16) nondominant foot" (Bernstein et al., 2007, p. 107). Skipping for the moment the seven-muscle group set, the final four-muscle group set involves the (1) arms and hand, (2) face and neck, (3) shoulders, chest, back, and abdomen, and (4) legs and feet. The seven-muscle group set uses the format of the four groups but splits the arms and hands into dominant and nondominant groups, the face and neck into separate groups, and the legs and feet into dominant and nondominant groups. Bernstein's (Bernstein et al., 2007) method starts with three formal sessions with the 16 muscle groups, followed by 2 weeks of practice with the 7 muscle groups, and culminates with 10-minute sessions of the 4-group method. Regular practice is required to gain proficiency.

A cue word like "now" is used throughout Bernstein's training sessions so that clients can learn how to release tension by recalling the cue word. In effect, they begin to associate the cue word with the relaxation feeling for each muscle group. After learning the four-group method, the client learns to focus consecutively on each of the four muscle groups and relax them without tensing by using the cue word. After the trainer has guided the client through the four muscle groups using the cue word, then deeper relaxation is introduced through a counting method, counting from 1 to 10 as in the following:

> OK, as you go right on relaxing, I am going to count slowly from 1 to 10. As I count, I would like for you to allow all the muscles in your body to become even more deeply and completely relaxed. Just focus on your muscles as they relax more and more on each count.
>
> OK, 1 . . . 2. Let your arms and hands relax even more. 3 . . . 4. Focus on the muscles of the neck and face as they relax. 5 . . . 6. Allow the muscles of the chest, shoulders, back, and abdomen to become even more relaxed. 7 . . . 8. Let the muscles in your legs and feet relax more and more. 9 . . . . 10. You are relaxing more and more all through your body. (Bernstein et al., 2007, p. 114)

With sufficient practice, the client may be able to simply use the cue word and the counting method to self-induce deep relaxation. This is the ultimate goal of learning how to self-regulate relaxation.

Potential Issues in Progressive Relaxation Training

There are several issues involved in learning how to do progressive muscle relaxation, including comfort, potential for cramping, sleep, anxiety, and self-consciousness. All of these can be dealt with easily.

Comfort   Get into a comfortable position either sitting or lying down and wear comfortable clothing when doing the exercise. You can listen to a recording of the exercise or have a friend read a script to you. After sufficient practice sessions, you will be able do the exercise from memory. The exercise is best done in a room with no noise or distractions.

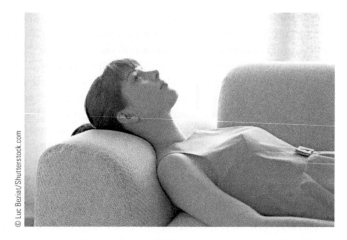

Lying down on your back with your arms resting alongside your body is a good position for doing the progressive muscle relaxation exercise, although it can also be done in a sitting position.

Cramping Generally, muscles should not be held for too long in a tense state—no more than 5 to 7 seconds to prevent any muscle cramps. Holding the tension for a count of 5 before releasing the muscle is a good rule of thumb. Avoid overstraining the muscles. For example, muscles should not be quivering when tensed. When doing the exercises, avoid tensing potential trouble spots like your abdomen if you are pregnant or any injured or strained muscles like those in your lower back if you have low back pain.

Sleep You can use progressive muscle relaxation as a method to induce sleep if that is your goal. It is very effective. However, keep in mind that if your goal is stress management, then you need to stay awake because sleep and relaxation serve different restorative functions. A very deeply relaxed state rests on the threshold between sleep and consciousness, a state known as the *hypnagogic* state, so it is very easy to slip over the threshold. If you find that you are falling asleep during the exercise when in a supine position (i.e., lying on your back) and sleep is not your goal, then you may want to change your posture to a sitting position. If you are already in a sitting position, try resting your elbow on a table so that your arm is balanced in an upright position. When you fall asleep, your arm will drop and wake you up.

Anxiety Paradoxically, clinicians report that a small percentage of clients who are given relaxation training experience anxiety problems such as disturbing sensations (4%) or anxiety about losing control (9%) (Edinger & Jacobsen, 1982). For those who suffer from excessive anxiety, the problem is even more exacerbated. For example, in one study (Heide & Borkovec, 1983) 30% of individuals with moderate to severe anxiety reported that they felt *more* rather than *less* tension during progressive relaxation. Further, it is not uncommon for individuals to experience laughing, sneezing, or restless movement during the training, which may also indicate anxiety.

It is important to keep in mind that when you undergo novel or unusual experiences you may feel some anxiety. However, in this case, if the anxiety becomes too uncomfortable, you can always stop. If you are listening to a recording, turn off the recording. Remember, you are always in control and can stop the experience at any time.

Self-Consciousness   If you are doing the exercises in front of someone else, you may feel self-conscious. For example, as you are tensing your forehead or other facial muscles, you may think that you look silly. You may even experience some embarrassment. This is natural. It will help if you feel accepted and comfortable with anyone who may see you do the exercises. If you are doing the exercise in a group, other group members will also look like you so you will not be the only one with a silly face. Have a good time and go with it. Doing the exercise with the lights out or alone also may help to reduce self-consciousness.

Progressive Muscle Relaxation Exercise

If you would like to do a brief version of progressive muscle relaxation, you are invited to explore Stress Management Exercise 13.1. You may want to first record the exercise and play the recording to guide you through the relaxation or have someone read it while you do the exercise. This brief progressive muscle relaxation exercise uses abdominal breathing as well as the tensing and relaxing of different muscle groups. Recall that abdominal breathing (otherwise known as diaphragmatic breathing), first discussed in Chapter 7, is a type of deep breathing that during inhalation involves first filling your lower lungs before your upper lungs. You know that you are doing it correctly when your abdomen expands as you take in the initial air followed by your chest expanding as you continue to fill your lungs completely.

The basic process for Stress Management Exercise 13.1 involves the following steps: (1) tensing a muscle group, (2) holding the tension for a count of 5 (5 seconds), (3) releasing the tension, (4) taking a deep abdominal breath, (5) holding it for a count of 3 (3 seconds), then (6) slowly releasing your breath. When tensing one muscle group, remember to keep the others relaxed. This exercise is an abbreviated adaptation of the procedure developed by Charlesworth and Nathan (1985).

Brief Relaxation Exercise

Practicing deep relaxation exercises twice a day is a good way to prevent adverse effects of stress. However, you may still benefit from the occasional booster, especially during a work day or school day, to keep your stress levels in the optimal zone (see Chapter 1). For example, before giving a presentation, you may want a relaxation booster to keep your stress levels in check. If you are able to find 5 minutes of alone time during your work day, try the

STRESS MANAGEMENT EXERCISE **13.1**

Progressive Muscle Relaxation

To begin, get into a comfortable position, close your eyes, and turn your attention to your forehead. As soon as you are ready, go ahead and raise your eyebrows and wrinkle your forehead. Feel the tension in your forehead and hold it. [Pause for a 5 count.] Now release the tension and feel your forehead smooth out as you take a slow deep abdominal breath. Hold it. [Pause for a 3 count.] Now slowly breathe out as your body naturally relaxes.

Next, close your eyes tightly. Feel the tension in and around your eyes. [Pause for a 5 count.] Now release the tension and let your eyelids become relaxed and heavy as you take a slow deep breath. Hold it. [Pause for a 3 count.] Slowly release your breath as your body naturally relaxes.

Continuing with the muscles in your face, go ahead and clench your jaw—not too tight, but tight enough to feel the tension. [Pause for 5 count.] Now gently release the tension and allow your lips to slightly part as your jaw slackens. Take a slow deep abdominal breath and hold it. [Pause for a 3 count.] Now slowly exhale as your body naturally relaxes.

Now slowly scan your head and face, releasing any remaining tension starting with your forehead and working down to your jaw. Forehead relaxed . . . eyes relaxed . . . cheeks relaxed . . . jaw relaxed. Your face feels smooth and relaxed. All the remaining tension is slipping away.

Next, move down to your neck and shoulders. Pull your shoulders up toward your ears, shrugging your shoulders to feel the tension in your neck and shoulders. [Pause for a count of 5.] Now gently allow your shoulders to drop. Take a slow deep breath and hold it. [Pause for a count of 3.] Now slowly release your breath as your body naturally relaxes. Notice what it's like when your shoulders and neck join your head and face as the relaxed parts of your body. It's as if your head could gently roll from side to side. As your neck and shoulders become more relaxed, your face and head become more relaxed.

Moving now to your hands and arms go ahead and make fists with both hands. Feel how your forearms and hands are tense. [Pause for a count of 5.] Now release the tension and take a slow deep breath. Hold it. [Pause for a count of 3.] Now slowly exhale as your body naturally relaxes.

Next, press your hands down onto the surface beneath them. Feel the tension in your arms. Feel your shoulders tense. [Pause for a count of 5.] Now relax the tension and take a slow deep breath. Hold it. [Pause for a count of 3.] Now slowly release your breath as your body naturally relaxes. Shoulders relaxed . . . arms relaxed . . . hands relaxed.

Now turn your focus to your chest muscles as you progressively move down your body. Go ahead and tighten your chest muscles. Feel their tension while relaxing the rest of your body. [Pause for a count of 5.] Now release the tension and take a slow deep breath. Hold it. [Pause for a count of 3.] Release your breath and the tension in your chest as you slowly exhale. Feel the tension flow out of your body each time you breathe out. Let the tension flow out. Allow your breathing to remain smooth, regular, and natural as you feel more relaxed with each breath.

Next, move to your back muscles. When you are ready, arch your back to feel the tension in your back muscles. [Pause for a count of 5.] Now release the tension and take a slow deep breath. Hold it. [Pause for a count of 3.] Now slowly breathe out as your body naturally relaxes. It's as if the relaxation is slowly spreading across your body. Relaxation is spreading from your face . . . your neck . . . your shoulders . . . your chest . . . your back, going deeper and more relaxed with each breath.

Now slowly turn your focus to your stomach area. Tighten the muscles of your stomach and hold the tension. [Pause for a count of 5.] Release the tension, allow the muscles to relax, and take a slow deep breath. [Pause for a count of 3.] Breathe out and slowly let go as your body naturally relaxes.

Moving next to your hips, legs, and feet, begin to tense your hips and legs by pressing the heels of your feet down into their resting areas. Feel the tension in your hips and legs as you press down. [Pause for a count of 5.] Release the tension. Now take a slow deep breath. [Pause for a count of 3.] Slowly exhale as your body naturally relaxes.

Next, tense your calf muscles by pointing your toes toward your head. Notice the tension in your calf muscles. [Pause for a count of 5.] Now release the tension. Take a slow deep breath. [Pause for a count of 3.] Slowly exhale as your body naturally relaxes. Allow your legs to join the rest of your deeply relaxed body as your relaxation continues to spread across your body.

Last, turn your attention to your feet. Go ahead and curl your toes gently downward. Hold the tension in your toes. [Pause for a count of 5.] Now release the curl, wiggling your toes to release any remaining tension. Take a slow deep abdominal breath. [Pause for a count of 3.] Slowly release your breath as your body naturally relaxes.

Now you have moved through all your major muscle groups. As you take each breath you find that your whole body's relaxation becomes deeper and more enjoyable. Take a moment to scan your body from your head to your toes, allowing the relaxation to spread in waves over your body. Your head . . . neck, . . . and shoulders relaxed . . . your arms . . . and hands relaxed . . . your chest . . . and back relaxed . . . your hips . . . legs, . . . and feet relaxed. Enjoy the sensations that deepen with each breath. As each wave of relaxation settles over you, you drift into a deeper and more relaxed state. Allow yourself this time of calm, serenity, and enjoyment. [Long pause.]

After a count of 5, open your eyes and feel relaxed, though refreshed and alert. Ready, 1 . . . 2 . . . more alert . . . 3 . . . 4 . . . refreshed . . . 5. Now alert and refreshed.

Stress Management Exercise 13.2. This exercise uses skills you develop through practicing abdominal breathing and progressive muscle relaxation.

Systematic Desensitization

systematic desensitization: a technique for treating phobias that involves successively pairing relaxation with imagined phobic images along a continuum that starts with the least feared and progresses to the most feared image.

As discussed earlier, Wolpe's (1958) systematic desensitization procedure uses an abbreviated version of progressive relaxation. The basic principle of **systematic desensitization** is to pair graduated imagined phobic scenarios (e.g., scenarios associated with giving a speech for a speech-anxious person) with the experience of deep relaxation. These graduated images form a hierarchy that starts with the least feared (e.g., thinking about enrolling in a speech class) and progresses to the most feared (e.g., giving a speech to a speech class that will be critically evaluated by the instructor). Progressively moving up the

STRESS MANAGEMENT EXERCISE **13.2**

Brief Relaxation Exercise

■ Find a place where you will not be disturbed, such as your office with the door closed, car, or an empty classroom, and sit in a comfortable position.

■ Close your eyes.

■ Take one slow abdominal breath, hold it briefly, and as you release your breath feel your tension slowly flow out of your body.

■ Rotate your head slowly to the left twice and then to the right twice. Make a full circular motion each time.

■ Beginning with your forehead, slowly scan your body from top to bottom, noticing and relaxing any tense areas. Focus on the major muscle groups you practiced when using progressive muscle relaxation, starting with your face and head and then moving to your neck and shoulders, arms and hands, chest and back, abdomen, hips, legs, and last your feet.

■ Take three successive slow abdominal breaths. Hold each briefly and as you release your breath feel your tension flow out of your body.

■ Focus your mind on a relaxing image for 15 seconds.

■ Take one last slow abdominal breath and let the remaining tension flow out as you release your breath.

■ Go back to your regular activities, feeling relaxed, refreshed, and alert.

hierarchy pairing threatening images with relaxation instead of anxiety counterconditions the anxiety response. In other words, the anxiety is replaced with more favorable responses. If imaginal **counterconditioning** is successful and realistic, then it should generalize to real life. Therefore, when the successfully treated individual must in reality confront a desensitized feared scenario such as public speaking, that person should be able to do so without experiencing excessive anxiety.

Is systematic desensitization effective for treating phobias? Yes, it does appear to be effective for treating some anxiety conditions (Tryon, 2005), especially simple phobias (see Chapter 7) (Head & Gross, 2008). However, research indicates that procedures like systematic desensitization that use **imaginal exposure** are not quite as effective as procedures that use in vivo (i.e. live) exposure (Choy, Fyer, & Lisitz, 2007). For example, the practice of giving a speech to a live audience more successfully desensitizes anxiety than imagining giving the speech. However, because fear can paralyze and prevent action, for some people it is more motivating to first take the transitional step through systematic desensitization on the way to confronting the real-life phobic scenario than to try to confront the feared scenario without this preparation.

imaginal exposure: a form of exposure therapy such as systematic desensitization where the client confronts phobic imagined images rather than live phobic objects or situations.

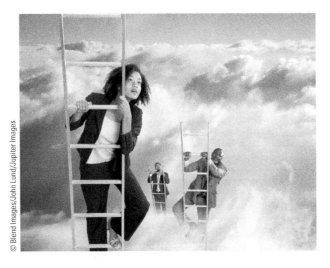

© Blend Images/John Lund/Jupiter Images

During systematic desensitization the participant climbs an imaginary fear ladder toward the image that evokes the highest level of distress.

What then is the process of systematic desensitization? The first step in systematic desensitization is to learn how to achieve deep relaxation through training in abbreviated progressive muscle relaxation. The next step is to create an anxiety hierarchy. The hierarchy can be thought of as a fear ladder with the least fearful phobic stimulus residing on the lowest rung of the ladder. Fear can be measured on a 100-point scale in units called **subjective units of distress (SUDS)**. Each rung then consists of images that provoke a gradual increase in SUDS until reaching the top rung, which contains the image that provokes the highest SUDS. Generally there are 10 to 20 rungs on the fear ladder. See Table 13.1 for an example of the types of events that can be placed on the rungs of a fear ladder for public speaking. In addition to constructing a fear hierarchy, individuals select one or two relaxing images they can use to calm them when needed while undergoing systematic desensitization.

In working with a therapist, the client is instructed to begin the first systematic desensitization session by using abbreviated progressive muscle relaxation training to go into a deep relaxation state. The therapist then starts with the image that is lowest on the fear ladder and guides the client to imagine the scene as realistically as possible. Upon experiencing any anxiety, the client is told to signal the therapist by lifting a finger. If the client gives the signal, the therapist instructs the client to change to one of the relaxing scenes. If no anxiety is elicited by the phobic scene, the client continues with the image for 10 seconds. After a pause to experience more deep relaxation, the therapist will repeat the scene before guiding the client to climb the next rung of the fear ladder. Usually, no more than three or four rungs are climbed per session. A typical desensitization session lasts no more than 15 to 30 minutes because it is difficult to sustain a state that combines concentration with relaxation for longer periods (Prochaska & Norcross, 2010). The therapist will usually end the session with a successful scene completion.

The next session begins with the successful scene and progressively climbs several more rungs up the fear ladder. With sufficient sessions, the successful

subjective units of distress (SUDS): a self-report measure used in systematic desensitization that indicates the amount of fear and distress the phobic image elicits.

TABLE **13.1**   Fear Hierarchy for Public Speaking

SUDS represent the client's estimate of subjective units of distress associated with each event.

Feared Event	SUDS
Giving the speech	100
Five minutes before the speech	90
The day before the speech	80
Practicing the speech in front of a small group of friends	70
Practicing the speech alone	60
Preparing the speech	50
Being given a speech presentation assignment	40
First day of the Speech class	30
Enrolling in a Speech class	20
Thinking about enrolling in a Speech class	10

© Cengage Learning 2013.

client reaches the top rung and is able to maintain relaxation while imagining that scene. Next, clients are encouraged to move gradually through the hierarchy in real life to reach their ultimate goal of confronting the top rung of the ladder without experiencing excessive anxiety.

AUTOGENIC TRAINING

hypnotic state: an altered state of waking consciousness with sleep-like characteristics that is distinguished by increased suggestibility.

The German psychiatrist and neurologist Johannes Heinrich Schultz (1884–1970) developed autogenic training as a novel relaxation technique derived from his work with clinical hypnosis. The **hypnotic state** is an altered state of waking consciousness with sleeplike characteristics that is distinguished by increased suggestibility. The term originates from the word *Hypnos,* the Greek god of sleep. It should be noted, however, that the "hypnotic state" is not a unique state defined by characteristic psychophysiological markers (e.g., electroencephalographic wave patterns) like the waking state or the sleep state, but rather constitutes an expectancy state, a type of cultural script that we associate with trance conditions (Karlin, 2007). The movie image of the hypnotist is of a person with almost magic powers over the patient. The hypnotist induces a trance state and then influences the patient through suggestions. The patient is totally dependent on the skills and power of the hypnotherapist to enter the hypnotic state. However, is this depiction accurate?

According to Schultz it was not. The inspiration for Schultz's belief came from Oskar Vogt's research conducted during the last decade of the 19th century. Vogt was a renowned brain physiologist working at the Berlin Institute in the areas of sleep and hypnosis. To Vogt's surprise, some of his hypnotic patients learned how to put themselves into an autohypnotic state. His patients had

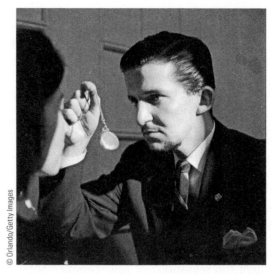

The movie image of a hypnotist suggests a person with almost magic powers over the patient. Is this image accurate?

autohypnotic state: a self-generated hypnotic state.

success doing this through applying various short-term mental exercises. The **autohypnotic state** they induced was beneficial in preventing somatic stress reactions such as muscular tension and headaches. Thus, Schultz concluded that (1) patients could engage in self-management of their stressful conditions through achieving an autohypnotic state and (2) they were always in control of this state. Ultimately then he believed that it is the patient and not the hypnotherapist who opens the door to the patient's trance state. Schultz's goal was to create a method in which the patient would be given the key to the door and use it when desired to enter into a restorative state similar to that observed in Vogt's patients. He called it *autogenic,* which combined the Greek words *autos* (i.e., *self*) and *genos* (i.e., *generation*) to indicate that his method was self-generated.

Schultz's technique is described as both a form of *self-hypnosis* and a method of *passive concentration*. The primary focus of his method is on the autonomic nervous system. When using autogenics the practitioner allows the experience to happen rather than forces it. Thus, **autogenic training** involves learning a method of deep relaxation through self-hypnosis or passive concentration that centers on the autonomic nervous system. This contrasts with Jacobson's progressive relaxation training that uses active strategies of tensing and relaxing major muscle groups of the somatic nervous system. Ultimately, both likely reach similar deep relaxation end states. In spite of their difference in focus, there is little research demonstrating overall physiological pattern differences of the relaxation states achieved by these two methods. For example, Linden (2007, p. 154) notes upon reviewing the relevant literature that "unfortunately, few published studies indicate effect specificity for AT [autogenic training]." The few studies that do show differences, however, do report greater heart rate reductions and slower breathing rates during autogenic training than achieved through progressive muscle relaxation, which is in keeping with autogenic training's greater focus on the autonomic nervous system but not sufficient to make any sweeping generalizations.

autogenic training: a deep relaxation strategy pioneered by Schultz that uses self-hypnosis/ passive concentration to center on the autonomic nervous system.

Schultz's first book, *Autogenic Training*, was published in 1932 in his native German language but his method did not reach an American audience until Wolfgang Luthe published an English language article introducing it in the *American Journal of Psychotherapy* in 1963. Thus, Schultz's method was a late-comer to America compared to progressive relaxation. Today autogenic training is much more popular in Europe and Japan than in North America where progressive relaxation with its early American origin predominates. Over the course of Schulz's prodigious professional life, he wrote over 400 publications including a co-authored work with Luthe of a six-volume book series (Linden, 2007).

Schultz developed six formulas or exercises that focus on different systems of the body. The bodily sensations the practitioner focuses on are those that occur naturally during hypnotic states. They are not theoretically derived, but rather based on reports from patients of their experiences when in trances or deeply relaxed states. For example, Schultz noted that the two types of sensations most commonly reported by his hypnotized patients were heaviness and warmth. Therefore, he incorporated into his verbal formulas self-suggestions that highlight the sensations of heaviness and warmth. The practitioner of autogenics is asked to focus on and subvocalize six formulas. These include the following (Linden, 2007, p. 163):

- Heaviness (muscular relaxation)—"Arms and legs are heavy"
- Warmth (vascular dilation)—"Arms and legs are pleasantly warm"
- Heart (heart regulation)—"The heart is beating calmly and regularly"
- Breathing (breathing regulation)—"It breathes me"
- Viscera (visceral organ regulation)—"Sun rays are streaming and warm"
- Head (cooling the forehead)—"The forehead is cool"

Each statement is repeated 6 times and followed by the word *quiet* one time. Practitioners may be encouraged by trainers to use a visual image to facilitate the process. For example, to facilitate the sensation of warmth the practitioners can imagine lying on the beach in the sun, taking a warm bath, or holding their hands over a campfire (Norris, Fahrion, & Oikawa, 2007). At the end of the autogenic session the practitioner is instructed to achieve a normal waking state by making fists, bending one's arms, breathing deeply, and opening one's eyes.

Each formula has a specific bodily target and its associated sensations. The heaviness formula focuses on muscular relaxation. Pleasant warm sensations are associated with vascular dilation that occurs in relaxation. Heart regulation is designed to emphasize regular and even heartbeats rather than slow beats. The odd phrase "it breathes me" is meant to emphasize the passive nature of the exercise, to let the breathing happen naturally rather than try to force it. For the viscera exercise, the practitioner is to focus on an image of the solar plexus (a network of nerves of the abdominal viscera located below the breastbone) with warm rays extending to the organs of the body. Last, the cooling forehead experience is meant to replicate the relaxing effect of placing a cool cloth on one's forehead. Trainees learn each exercise consecutively over the course of approximately 8 weeks, starting with the heaviness formula and then progressively adding new formulas in the order listed previously.

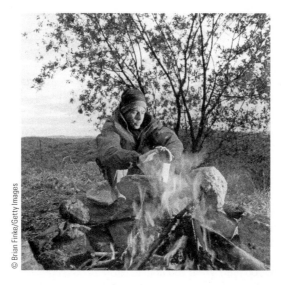

Imagining yourself holding your hands over a campfire can facilitate the process of hand warming.

© Brian Finke/Getty Images

These formulas and self-suggestions should be practiced regularly to achieve maximum relaxation benefits. Trainers often recommend that trainees keep diaries to facilitate the learning process. Autogenic training usually occurs in group settings although individual training also occurs. Like progressive muscle relaxation training, autogenic training may be introduced in abbreviated or modified forms. For example, autogenic training is sometimes combined with biofeedback (see Chapter 14) in an attempt to enhance its effectiveness (Norris et al., 2007). The specific phrases used may be altered slightly and diaphragmatic breathing may also be introduced to enhance relaxation. On the whole, is autogenic training effective?

There is a lot of variability in response to autogenic training with some people responding well to the training but others making no changes or even deteriorating (Linden, 2007). Like progressive relaxation training, some individuals have anxiety reactions. These anxiety reactions may take the form of "myoclonic jerks, spasms, twitches, or restlessness" known as "autogenic discharges" (Linden, 2007, p. 157). Anxiety issues may result from unfamiliarity with the relaxation experience or with concerns about loss of control. These issues need to be addressed if they arise in order for the training to be successful.

Stetter and Kupper (2002) conducted the most comprehensive meta-analytic review of the autogenic research to date. Their review included 60 controlled trials, including a number published in non-English languages. The authors determined that autogenic training generally resulted in a medium effect size for biological and psychological indices of change compared to controls. For stress-related disorders, Stetter and Kupper (2002) reported that several studies found medium beneficial effects for tension-type headaches, migraines, asthma, and Raynaud's disease (a circulation disorder of the hands and feet discussed in more depth in Chapter 14). They also identified autogenic training as moderately effective for treating sleep disorders and reducing anxiety.

An individual study illustrates the benefit of autogenic training for anxiety reduction. Kanji, White, and Ernst (2006) conducted a randomized controlled

STRESS MANAGEMENT EXERCISE **13.3**

Autogenic Exercise

Would you like to try two of the autogenic exercises (i.e., formulas) to sample them? This is accelerating the progression, but it will give you an idea of what the exercises are like. The recommended starting phrase in autogenic training is "My right arm is heavy" if you are right-handed or "My left arm is heavy" if you are left-handed. "My right arm is heavy" is slowly and silently repeated 6 times followed by the phrase "I feel quiet" and then repeat the cycle. Next, begin the phrase "My right arm is warm." You may also want to visualize a pleasant image of warming such as the sun's rays, a warm bath, or a campfire. Repeat the phrase "My right arm is warm" 6 times followed by the phrase "I feel quiet" and then repeat the cycle.

Now get into a comfortable position, close your eyes, and silently repeat the phrases in the "heavy" exercise for 1 minute and then the "warm" exercise for 1 minute.

How did you feel? Were you able to experience a sensation of heaviness and warmth in your arm? Did you notice any streaming or flowing sensations of warmth? If so, these could be associated with changes in blood flow to your arm. If you like the exercise, with practice you can slowly build on it by adding the other autogenic phrases when ready. As Kanji (1997, pp. 163–164) notes regarding autogenic training, "at the outset, passive concentration on a formula should not last more than 30–60 seconds and should lead only to superficial relaxation. The time span is gradually increased, with an increasing depth of relaxation, to 10–15 minutes."

trial of 93 nursing students in the United Kingdom and determined that participants in their 8-week autogenic training group showed lower anxiety, heart rate, and blood pressure than individuals in placebo and wait-list control groups.

Is autogenic training as effective as progressive muscle relaxation for reducing anxiety? A recent meta-analytic review (Manzoni et al., 2008) found that both progressive muscle relaxation and meditation (see Chapter 14) are more effective than autogenic training for anxiety reduction. So it may not be the best deep relaxation method for anxiety reduction, but is a viable alternative if the practitioner does not respond well to progressive muscle relaxation or meditation training. If you would like to sample a couple of autogenic formulas, try Stress Management Exercise 13.3.

GUIDED IMAGERY RELAXATION

guided imagery relaxation: a deep relaxation strategy that uses language to create relaxing sensory-filled images and scenarios that transport the participants to new worlds within their imagination.

If the saber-toothed tigers of our minds can create fight-or-flight stress responses, then surely the serene beaches, blue mountain lakes, and magic gardens of our minds can create relaxation responses. This is the principle of guided imagery relaxation. When we engage in **guided imagery relaxation,** we use language to create relaxing sensory-filled images and scenarios that transport us to a new world, a world of our imagination. In order to experience total immersion in this imaginative world, the language that guides us often uses scripts. These scripts contain vivid imagery that fully engages our five senses while kindling comfortable feelings.

Do you recall Crystal's script at the beginning of this chapter that transported April to a warm secluded beach? April was guided to imagine the *visual* experience of the white sandy beach, to *hear* the waves breaking in the distance as they eventually rolled gently toward the beach, to *feel* the warm sand and the sun's rays warming her body, and to *smell* the salt air and even *taste* it on her lips. Thus, Crystal presented April with a rainbow of sensory experiences that enabled April to fully immerse into a new imaginary world. In addition, she used words like *peacefully, calmly, gently, safe, secure,* and *relaxed* to add comfort and security to April's corner of the secluded beach.

The concept of using storytelling and metaphor to create helpful or healing imagery-based suggestions has a long and deep tradition in the world's major religions, in indigenous traditions such as those practiced by Native Americans, and in traditional Chinese medicine among others (Utay & Miller, 2006). Even though this method has been practiced for several millennia, psychologists were generally slow to adopt it until the mid-20th century when Joseph Wolpe incorporated the use of phobic images into his systematic desensitization method. Today, variations of *positive* guided imagery are used in counseling and psychotherapy. They also are used in behavioral medicine applications as well as sports training.

Guided imagery is used primarily in counseling contexts to promote relaxation and stress reduction. It also can be used to foster insight or help clients visualize a more positive future. In behavioral medicine applications, guided imagery is sometimes used to help medical patients reduce pain, enhance health-related quality of life, or attempt to strengthen their immune systems and promote healing. For example, King (2010) concluded from her review of the relevant literature of patients with cancer pain that there is evidence that guided imagery has potential as an adjunct to traditional treatments in reducing cancer-related pain. However, she notes that the research in the area is limited, has small sample sizes, and is generally low in methodological quality. Therefore, she is hesitant "to give concrete recommendations that GI [guided imagery] will work for all patients that suffer from cancer pain" (King, 2010, p. 105).

The following study illustrates some of these issues with a different type of pain-related medical condition. Baird and Sands (2006) randomly assigned 28 older women patients with the painful condition of osteoarthritis to two groups. In one group patients completed a 12-week program of guided imagery with relaxation. The other group served as a no treatment control. Both groups kept a daily diary in which they recorded their symptoms. Upon completion of the program, patients in the guided imagery group showed increases in health-related quality of life, a measure that included indices of pain and mobility. Even after statistically controlling for pain and mobility scores, the effect still held, suggesting that it was not limited to improvements in just these domains. This study is limited by its small sample size and lack of a placebo control. However, it is suggestive of how guided imagery with relaxation can be applied to medical patients with pain conditions to potentially improve their health-related quality of life.

There also is some suggestive evidence that guided imagery can elevate immune system responses perhaps through reducing distress (Trakhtenberg, 2008). However, the research in this area is sparse and often confounds imagery interventions with relaxation interventions. A meta-analysis (Miller & Cohen, 2001) of 85 trials found that relaxation is reliably associated with total salivary immunoglobulin A (sIgA) concentrations but not consistently related to other stress-related immunological indicators (e.g., natural killer cells). Although this meta-analytic review did not specifically address guided imagery, it revealed that hypnosis was the relaxation-related intervention most consistently related to immune system responsiveness. Hypnosis has some overlap with guided imagery in that they both typically evoke imagery-related sensory experiences. It is unknown, however, if hypnosis had its effects on the immune system through inducing relaxation or through image-specific mechanisms. On the whole, the evidence is modest at best that guided imagery can modulate the immune system. More research with higher-quality methodology is needed before any definitive conclusions can be drawn.

The use of mental imagery rehearsal to improve sports performance has a stronger base of empirical support (Taktek, 2004; Vealey & Greenleaf, 2006). For example, Vealey and Greenleaf (2006, p. 312) noted after reviewing the relevant literature that "improvements in the following sport skills has been documented through mental practice: basketball shooting, volleyball serving, tennis serving, golf, football placekicking, figure skating, swimming starts, dart throwing, alpine skiing, karate skills, driving, trampoline skills, competitive running, dance, rock climbing, and field hockey performance." A number of regional cerebral blood flow studies indicate that mental imagery and physical practice involve activation of similar regions of the brain (Taktek, 2004). The cerebellum, the area of the brain associated with motor movement in particular appears to participate "in the formation of a motor program during mental imagery and in the execution of that program during physical practice" (Taktek, 2004, p. 108). Thus, within the brain there appears to be a certain level of equivalence between mental imagery and physical practice of motor skills, which could account for improvements in athletic performance through using mental imagery.

Using Guided Imagery to Promote Deep Relaxation

If you want to relax using guided imagery, the most convenient way to do it is to get into a comfortable position and listen to a recording of a guided imagery script. You can write your own script and record it or purchase a commercially produced version. One advantage to writing your own script is that you can tailor it to your individual tastes. Scenarios that some people find relaxing others may find neutral or even stressful. Most guided imagery transports you to a tranquil natural setting such as a tropical island, remote beach, field of flowers, evergreen forest, snow-covered mountain vista, or a peaceful stream or lake. The following is an example of a lake imagery script from Charlesworth and Nathan (1985).

The water is just barely lapping along the shore of the lake. You see a small boat tied there. You enter the boat and find some blankets in the bottom. Now, lying on the soft blankets, gently untie the boat. You are floating in the quiet, shallow lake. The boat is rocking gently from the motion of the water, as it drifts on and on. The boat drifts on and on, rocking and massaging.

As the boat carries you along, the lake lazily flows into a stream. Feel the warm sunlight once again. There is a soft breeze as you continue to drift. You feel relaxed, peaceful, and calm. The gentle rocking motion massages you with feelings of peace. All is well. Your state of relaxation will become more and more profound as the boat gently tosses to and fro.

You drift deeper and deeper into your feelings of relaxation. As you continue to drift, become aware of the sounds of nature: the soft breeze, the lapping water, and the birds and animals on the shore. Smell the grass and flowers as the breeze brings you their pleasant scents. You are lazily drifting deeper and deeper into a profound feeling of peace and pleasantness until very slowly and gently, the small boat washes up against the shore. You remain in a very complete and total state of relaxation. (p. 116)

Like the guided imagery scenario just described of a relaxing experience floating on a boat in a shallow lake, most guided imagery scenarios are solitary experiences. A less common theme involves the participant relaxing with other people such as in the following scenario: "imagine yourself surrounded by one or more positive people who make you feel secure, happy, and relaxed" (La Roche, Batista, & D'Angelo, 2011, p. 50). Even though they are less common, some individuals may find people-oriented themes more comforting than solitary themes.

When you listen to a guided imagery recording or reading, allow yourself to become fully immersed in the imaginary world. If you have any unwanted

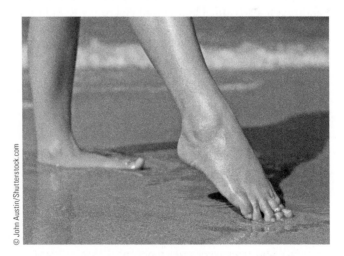

© John Austin/Shutterstock.com

When creating a guided image scenario, remember to involve as many senses as possible including touch. For example, can you imagine what it feels like to dig your toes into the warm wet sand? What does it feel like as you walk along the wet beach and the sand squishes between your toes?

STRESS MANAGEMENT EXERCISE **13.4**

Creating Your Personal Guided Imagery Relaxation Script

Select an imagery scene that is meaningful and relaxing to you. Like the boat on the shallow lake scenario, compose three paragraphs that guide you into a pleasant, serene, and relaxing world. For example, you can select a peaceful nature scene or a scene where you are surrounded by positive people. In creating your images, include as many different senses as possible. For example, consider the following:

1. Sight—"I see _____."

2. Smell—"I smell _____."

3. Sound—"I hear _____."

4. Touch—"I feel _____."

5. Taste—"I taste _____."

After you complete your script, have someone read it to you in a relaxing place. If you are happy with your script, gradually add more paragraphs until you have about 15 or 20 minutes of script. Then record your script and use it as an alternative deep relaxation strategy to progressive muscle relaxation or autogenic training.

thoughts or images, allow them to pass through your consciousness like leaves falling on a stream. There is no need to try to fight them but rather simply re-focus on the relaxing images and continue with the process. If you would like to create your own guided imagery scenario, then begin Stress Management Exercise 13.4.

CHAPTER SUMMARY AND CONCEPT REVIEW

- Progressive muscle relaxation, autogenic training, and guided imagery relaxation are known as deep relaxation strategies.

- Deep relaxation strategies can help restore homeostatic balance and lower the harmful effects of stress.

- The restorative effects of deep relaxation are different from those of sleep and, therefore, serve a different function.

- Progressive muscle relaxation is achieved through tensing and relaxing the body's major muscle groups.

- Progressive muscle relaxation is one of the most effective relaxation strategies for managing anxiety.

- Today, abbreviated forms of progressive muscle relaxation predominate.

- With sufficient progressive muscle practice, the method can be reduced from 16 muscle groups to 4, and, ultimately, cue words and countdowns can be used to achieve relaxation effects without needing to tense muscles.

- Potential issues in doing progressive relaxation training include comfort, cramping, sleep, anxiety, and self-consciousness.

- Systematic desensitization uses an abbreviated form of progressive muscle relaxation to induce deep relaxation that is then paired with graduated imagined phobic scenarios.

- Imaginal exposure techniques like systematic desensitization are effective for treating simple phobias but not as effective as in vivo exposure.

- Autogenic training achieves deep relaxation through self-hypnosis or passive concentration that centers on the autonomic nervous system.

- Autogenic training is moderately effective for reducing negative psychophysiological effects of stress, treating sleep disorders, and reducing anxiety.

- Guided imagery relaxation uses language to create relaxing sensory-filled images and scenarios.

- Guided imagery is used in counseling to promote relaxation and stress reduction; in behavioral medicine to help medical patients reduce pain, enhance health-related quality of life, or attempt to strengthen their immune systems and promote healing; and in sports to improve athletic performance.

CRITICAL THINKING QUESTIONS

1. In what ways is the deep relaxation state different from the sleep state? In what ways does each state serve different restorative functions? How are they alike and different as tools for managing stress?

2. How is the hypnotic state similar to and different from a deep relaxation state? (Hint—do some outside research on whirling dervishes and determine if they are in trance states. If so, are they relaxed?)

3. How is imagery able to achieve its relaxation effects? How important is imagery in autogenic training? Why do you think the sensations of warm and heavy arms and legs used in autogenic training are commonly associated with relaxation and hypnotic states?

4. What imagery theme do you find most relaxing? What associations do you have with this theme? What is it about this theme that makes it stand out over the others?

5. Which of the three deep relaxation strategies discussed in this chapter do you find most appealing? Why? What top three reasons might you have for doing a deep relaxation exercise on a regular basis?

KEY TERMS AND CONCEPTS

Autogenic training*

Autohypnotic state*

Counterconditioning

Deep relaxation strategies*

Guided imagery relaxation*

Hypnotic state*

Imaginal exposure*

Muscle sense awareness*

Progressive muscle relaxation (PMR)*

Subjective units of distress (SUDS)*

Systematic desensitization*

MEDIA RESOURCES

CENGAGE **brain**

Access an interactive eBook, chapter-specific interactive learning tools, including flashcards, quizzes, videos, and more in your Psychology CourseMate, accessed through CengageBrain.com.

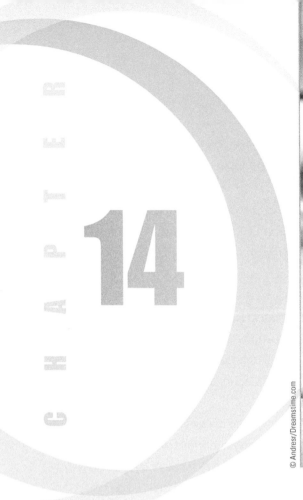

14

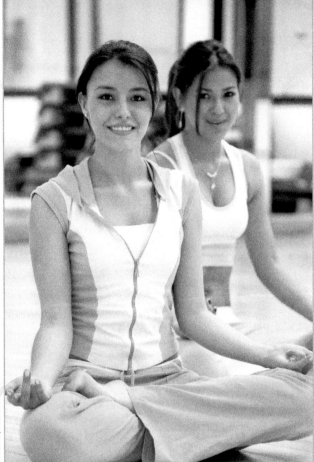

© Andresr/Dreamstime.com

Plant the seed of meditation and reap the
fruit of peace of mind.

~REMEZ SASSON

MEDITATION, YOGA, AND BIOFEEDBACK

Dr. J. Hoenig, a University of Manchester, England, physician and psychiatrist, described his investigation of an Indian Yogi named Shri S. R. Krishna Iyengar in the city of Bangalore, India, in his 1968 paper entitled "Medical Research on a Yogi." The Yogi, at the time age 48, 5 feet 6 inches tall, and weighing 120 pounds, was a practitioner of Hatha yoga. Having heard of amazing feats performed by Yogis through breathing exercises and meditation, including being buried underground for several days, Dr. Hoenig was eager to be one of the first physicians to medically document and scientifically test the accuracy of such claims.

Dr. Hoenig, the Yogi, and the All India Institute of Mental Health agreed to an experiment in which the Yogi would be monitored with physiological recording equipment while buried in an underground pit with less than 1 cubic meter of air. Although the Yogi offered to stay buried for 36 hours, the group of experimenters settled on 9 hours though even that amount of time seemed very risky.

After having been given a thorough medical examination a few days earlier, the Yogi entered the pit wearing only a leopard skin loin cloth, recording wires were attached to his body, and he assumed a supine position known in Yoga as Shavasana or the corpse pose. The pit was closed with a wooden plank and covered with dirt. He was buried alive. After 9 hours transpired, Dr. Hoenig recounts what happened next.

> *At the end of the experiment, that is, during the cooler hours of the late afternoon, the earth was removed and the plank lifted aside. There on the floor of the pit lay the Yogi, in exactly the same position he had been in the beginning. The assistants climbed in, disconnected the wires and the Yogi sat up. He got up to his feet and looked at us. He looked fresh and agile. Villagers, who stood around, gasped, then rushed forward and put a garland of flowers around his neck. The Yogi still in the pit took a coconut, broke it and sprinkled water into the pit. Then he threw a few petals of his garland into the pit, folded his hands and prayed. He appeared much fresher I dare say than any of us. He then jumped out of the pit, turned to it once more with his head bent and hands folded, then walked away with big strides, the villagers beside him and behind him in a fair crowd, trying to keep up with his stride. (Hoenig, 1968, p. 74)*

What did the recordings reveal? Amazingly, the carbon dioxide levels in his air space had risen to only 3.8%, which was far lower than the 6.6% predicted by normal breathing within a lesser time of 2 hours in an airtight

pranayama: a controlled breathing strategy used in yoga and meditation.

space. The predicted level he noted would make life "quite impossible"
(Hoenig, 1968, p. 76). Breathing rates suggested that the Yogi had em-
*ployed a controlled breathing strategy, a **pranayama,** known as Ujjaya,*
one that he had demonstrated earlier to investigators. His heart rate had
varied from 100 beats per minute (bpm) to 40 bpm in a 20- to 25-minute
cyclic pattern from fast to slow. Electroencephalogram (EEG) patterns
showed a stable alpha rhythm throughout with no indication of sleeping.
Further, there were no physiological recording artifacts suggestive of
movement other than breathing throughout the entire 9 hours.

When asked how he was able to succeed in staying buried in the pit
for the entire period, the Yogi told investigators that he had been lying
absolutely still and confirmed that he had employed the breathing strategy
of Ujjaya. He also said that he had been praying and had tried to reach
Samadhi, an intense meditative state in which one's awareness is yoked or
*fused with the focus of the meditation. Technically the word **yoga** means*
*"yoked," a form of union. In the Hindu religion it is believed that **Samadhi***
can result in the experience of union with Divine Consciousness.

asanas: different postural positions used by yoga practitioners.

Although most Westerners tend to associate yoga with **asanas,** or different postural positions popularized by Hatha yoga, Hindus use the word *yoga* to mean "meditation." In order to meditate successfully, you must turn your focus and consciousness inward. Classically, many yoga practitioners were instructed that the best way to do this is to sit in a variant of the asana we think of as the lotus position with your legs crossed. It has been speculated that this was preferred over the more comfortable repose position (*Shavasana*) because the repose position could result more easily in a sleep state rather than a meditative state. However, if you have ever tried to sit in the lotus position for any length of time, you will probably find it uncomfortable unless you have had practice. That is where training in **Hatha yoga,** the yoga of physical discipline, comes into play. A benefit of this form of yoga is that it uses *pranayama* and different asanas to limber and condition the muscles used in meditation so that you can engage in the practice of meditation more easily. Today, secularized versions of Hatha yoga are also used in the West that focus more on the asanas for their physical and psychological benefits, including relaxation, than on the practice of meditation that the asanas were designed to promote.

Hatha yoga: a form of yoga that emphasizes physical discipline through using pranayama and different asanas.

There are a number of different types of yoga besides Hatha yoga. Though not an exhaustive list, these include *Raja yoga, Karma yoga, Bhakti yoga, Jnana yoga,* and *Kundalini Tantra yoga.* Historically the *Yoga Sutras,* written by

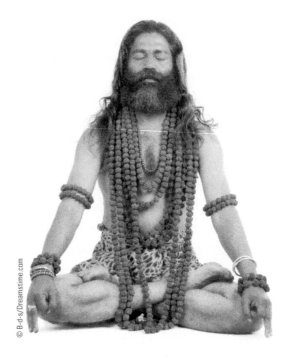

© B-d-s/Dreamstime.com

Western pioneer researchers traveled to India to determine how much control Yogis had over their psychophysiological processes.

the sage Patanjali (circa 200–500 BC), codified the asanas as part of the practice of *Raja yoga,* a type of yoga that laid the foundation for other yoga systems. *Raja yoga* (*Raja* means "king") is characterized by practitioners as the *royal path to realization* and has eight components of spiritual practice. These include *Yama*—self-restraint, *Niyana*—ethics, *Asana*—proper posture, *Pranayama*—breath control, *Pratyahara*—restriction of the senses, *Dharana*—concentration, *Dhyana*—meditation, and *Samadhi*—union with supreme consciousness.

As demonstrated by the Yogi studied by Dr. Hoenig who emerged successfully from a pit after 9 hours of burial, yoga mastery can involve an amazing degree of control over one's internal psychophysiology. The degree of control and mastery possible has direct implications for furthering our understanding of how the human nervous system functions and how to apply that understanding to the study of our health and well-being. As a result, other Western pioneer researchers in the field also traveled to India to study Yogis. One was Dr. M. A. Wenger, a physician, who embarked on a 5-month investigative journey through India in 1957. His primary mission was to determine if Yogis had direct control over autonomic functions as was often claimed. At the time, most experts believed that the autonomic nervous system was strictly involuntary and could not be consciously directed. They believed that only classically conditioned learning (an automatic involuntary stimulus-response-based learning) was possible with the autonomic nervous system.

Dr. Wenger wrote in a prelude to his coauthored paper (Wenger & Bagchi, 1961) that he was intrigued by the records of a French cardiologist, Dr. Theresa Brosse, who had taken a portable electrocardiograph to India in 1935 to measure the claim that some Yogis made that they could control their heart action. He wrote that her electrocardiogram (EKG) records indicated that the Yogis were able to reduce their heart potentials to such a low level, near zero, Dr. Brosse concluded that her Yogi subjects had direct voluntary control over the heart.

To test Dr. Brosse's conclusions, Wenger and Bagchi (1961) used physiological recording devices to measure the levels of autonomic control of 43 Indian men and 2 Indian women who were either Yogis or students of yoga. What do you think they found?

They determined that their participants were able to show "marked changes in autonomic functions" at times but believed these changes were almost always mediated by using "intervening voluntary mechanisms" (Wenger & Bagchi, 1961, p. 322). A few yoga practitioners they met who claimed they could directly stop their heart action indeed had such faint pulses when put to the test that no heart sounds could be heard through a stethoscope; however, EKG records indicated that their hearts were still beating. The authors concluded that these yoga practitioners had used a type of Valsalva maneuver that involved strongly contracting their abdominal muscles, closing their glottis, and holding their breath. This strategy causes significantly reduced blood flow to the heart so that when the heart contracts, less blood is ejected, and the pulse is imperceptible without proper recording equipment.

The investigators did find, however, one subject who seemed to have direct control over at least one autonomic function. He was a Yogi who perspired from his forehead on command. The Yogi explained that his guru taught him to voluntarily warm his body through visualizing himself in a high-temperature environment to better weather extremely cold winters he braved when meditating in Himalayan mountain caves. Later, in more temperate climates, the Yogi discovered that when he employed the same strategy, his forehead perspired.

Around the time of these investigations, other researchers were investigating the parameters of control over psychophysiological processes through the use of biofeedback. Applied biofeedback originated in the United States in the late 1950s as a convergence of a number of different approaches. Some of these included instrumental (operant) conditioning approaches to the autonomic nervous system, behavioral approaches to therapy and medicine, stress management approaches, biomedical engineering, cybernetics (the interdisciplinary study of regulatory systems), and the study of altered states of consciousness (Schwartz & Olson, 2003). **Biofeedback** involves the use of recording devices to present visual or auditory tracking information to participants of their targeted internal physiological responses. The participants use this information to guide and direct in cybernetic fashion these physiological responses. The cybernetic process is similar to how a guided missile uses tracking information to self-correct and hone in on its target.

biofeedback: the use of a physiological recording device to present visual or auditory tracking information to participants so they can learn how to regulate targeted internal physiological responses.

Can you imagine trying to learn how to shoot a basketball into a hoop if you were blindfolded and had your ears plugged? If you want to learn how to shoot a basketball so that it falls into the hoop, you have to know whether you hit or miss the hoop after each shot. If you miss it, you need to know by how much so that your next shot can correct for missing high, low, to the left, or to the right of the hoop. With practice, you should be able to make adjustments so that you use the optimum strategy for hitting the hoop. Without visual or auditory feedback, however, you would not have the information needed to make the adjustments to refine your strategies to optimize success. Biofeedback, like the feedback required to learn how to shoot a hoop, provides the needed information (feedback) to optimize success for hitting the desired biological hoop such as heart rate, muscle contraction, skin temperature, or other psychophysiological changes.

In its early use, clinicians and researchers discovered that applied biofeedback could be used to facilitate control of skeletal muscle responses by increasing awareness of underlying muscle tension (e.g., forehead muscle tension) so that the increased awareness could be used to develop strategies to self-regulate muscle activity. This discovery was not surprising because skeletal muscles have always been considered to be under conscious central nervous system (CNS) control. However, what was surprising was that biofeedback could also be used to operantly condition, that is, bring under some conscious control, visceral (i.e., organ) responses that are regulated by the autonomic nervous system and were previously thought impossible to control. Does this sound familiar? Remember the Yogi who could make his forehead perspire on command by visualizing himself in a hot environment. And though no Yogis who could stop their heart from beating were found, the Yogi buried underground showed remarkable psychophysiological control through meditation and breathing exercises to be able to survive for 9 hours in an environment that would have clearly imperiled the life of others. This is why biofeedback has sometimes been referred to affectionately by its researchers and practitioners as an *electronic guru* or *yoga of the west*.

Strategies for regulating the viscera often use cognitions such as thoughts and sensory imagery (e.g., visualizing oneself in a high-temperature environment as the Yogi had done to perspire). In effect, some believe that the strategy is cognitively mapped in the neocortex in much the same way the motor cortex maps motor movements. Stimulated by the research and concepts originating from the interplay of cognitions and internal physiology, the field of **psychophysiology** emerged in the late 1960s and early 1970s as "the scientific study of the interrelationships of physiological and cognitive processes" (Schwartz & Olson, 2003, p. 5). Applied psychophysiology is now so intricately tied to biofeedback that the original professional society for the study of biofeedback, the Biofeedback Research Society founded in 1969, was transformed 19 years later into what is today known as the Association for Applied Psychophysiology and Biofeedback (AAPB). Credentials for the practice of clinical biofeedback have been issued by the Biofeedback Certification Institute of America (BCIA) since 1981 to appropriately trained biofeedback practitioners.

As we can see, yoga and meditation have a long and venerable history in Hindu culture and religion. Biofeedback and applied psychophysiology are newcomers to the scene but share some common interests and were inspired by some of the secular components of yoga and meditation. These interests include employing cognitive strategies in ways that positively affect internal physiological processes. On the whole then, biofeedback, applied psychophysiology, yoga, and meditation all share similar interests in self-regulation. Let us now take a closer look at meditation.

psychophysiology: the study of the interplay between cognitive and physiological processes.

MEDITATION

Although Hoenig (1968) was unsure how the Yogi he studied, Shri S. R. Krishna Iyengar, was able to stay buried in a pit with only 1 cubic meter of air for 9 hours, he speculated that there may have been air leakage through the earth or more dramatically perhaps the Yogi was indeed able to directly lower his oxygen consumption and basal metabolism rate. The ability to markedly lower oxygen consumption, he noted, was reported in another study by Anand, Chhina, and Singh (1961) of a different Yogi who allowed himself to be placed in a hermetically sealed metal box. Hoenig discussed how that study found that the Yogi's baseline oxygen consumption outside the box was 19.5 liters per hour, but inside the box his oxygen consumption rate fell to as low as 10.1 liters per hour.

Cardiologist Dr. Herbert Benson (1975) also acknowledged the studies of Indian Yogis and remarked that researchers in the 1950s and 1960s found that Zen monks of Japan, too, were able to reduce their oxygen consumption or metabolism through meditation as much as 20%. These types of findings led Benson and his colleagues in the early 1970s to study practitioners of **Transcendental Meditation (TM)** in the United States. At the time TM was a newly modified transitional form of yoga meditation that was exported to the West by its Indian originator, Maharishi Mahesh Yogi. As Benson explains, the Maharishi removed many of what he considered to be *nonessential* elements of yoga and created a version that he believed could be more easily understood by Westerners. Benson attributed the burgeoning popularity of TM in the West to the spotlight the Beatles and other celebrities placed on it.

Benson and his colleagues sought to determine if TM subjects would also show some of the psychophysiological characteristics of the yoga meditators previously studied. They indeed found that oxygen consumption levels characteristic of a **hypometabolic state** (low metabolism rates) could be achieved during the typical 20- to 30-minute meditative sessions (Wallace, Benson, & Wilson, 1971). Hypometabolic states also are found during sleep, though Benson (1975) noted they occur very gradually over the course of 4 or 5 hours, whereas during meditation decreases in oxygen consumption occur during the first 3 minutes.

Early investigators also showed other physiological indicators of relaxation such as lowered blood lactate levels, indicating reduced skeletal muscle metabolism (Wallace et al., 1971); higher skin resistance, indicating less anxiety (Wallace, 1970); decreased heart rate (Wallace, 1970); and increased alpha wave activity (Wallace et al., 1971). The findings of increased alpha wave activity are in concordance with Dr. Hoenig's findings for the meditating Yogi he studied. If the fight-or-flight response could be considered the *stress response*, then the *relaxation response* (a phrase Benson coined and used in his book title by the same name) achieved during meditation would be its natural antidote. Such findings prompted a flurry of research on the psychophysiological benefits of meditation during the 1970s and 1980s that substantiated the basic findings of Benson and his fellow investigators. Since that time fewer studies have been published on this form of meditation because these benefits are now well established.

Transcendental Meditation (TM): a modified transitional form of mantra meditation originated by Maharishi Mahesh Yogi that removed what he considered to be the nonessential elements of yoga.

hypometabolic state: a state characterized by reduced oxygen consumption due to low bodily metabolism rates.

What Is the Meditative State?

A question often asked is "What is the meditative state?" "Is it different from the normal rest state?" "Is it the same or different from the sleep state?" "Is it the same as the hypnotic state?" As discussed earlier, a short period of meditation can result in a hypometabolic state. This clearly differentiates it from a normal rest state. EEG patterns also show that the person meditating is not in a sleep state. Richard Bandler, cocreator of the alternative interpersonal communication and social influence field of Neuro-Linguistic Programming (NLP) and a well-known hypnotist, sees similarities between hypnotically induced trance states and those generated through meditation in that they both are altered states that seem to reach similar relaxation end points (Bandler, 2008).

Patricia Carrington (2007, p. 265), the originator of **clinically standardized meditation (CSM)**, suggests "that meditation may be an unusually fluid state of consciousness, partaking of qualities of both sleep and wakefulness, and possibly resembling the hypnogogic or 'falling asleep' state more than any other state of consciousness." It seems to be a deeply relaxed altered state with EEG recordings showing what she calls an "alert-drowsy pattern with high alpha and occasional theta wave patterns" (p. 265). The hypnogogic state should not be confused with the hypnotic state. Though both can result in altered states, on the whole the evidence suggests that the meditative state is different from hypnotic states. For example, Wallace (1970) noted that physiological changes associated with hypnosis do not share the reduction of oxygen consumption associated with mantra meditation or the same EEG patterns. Besides the physiological differences, the perception of locus of control differs between hypnosis and meditation. In hypnosis, the subject is seen as under the influence of the hypnotist, whereas in meditation the experience is seen as self-generated. Therefore, though meditation and hypnosis may both result in altered states, the quality of the experiences differs physiologically and experientially.

Herbert Benson (1975) reported that the subjective quality of the relaxation response is one that most people describe as pleasurable, relaxing, and in some cases even ecstatic. He contends that through early religious writings we can see references to similar states of consciousness in both Eastern and Western mysticism, and these writings refer to age-old wisdoms of how to reach these states. To reach the relaxation response Benson suggests there must be four elements present, which he later reduced to two. These two are:

> (1) a mental device—a sound, word, phrase, or prayer repeated silently or aloud, or a fixed gaze at an object and (2) a passive attitude—not worrying about how well one is performing the technique and simply putting aside distracting thoughts in return to one's focus. (Benson, 1975, p. xviii, Foreword: Twenty-Fifth Anniversary Update)

mantra: a word, sound, or phrase that is repeated during concentrative meditation.

In TM, a special word called a **mantra** is given to the novitiate, and the mantra is silently repeated during meditation. Benson describes the practice of Christian mystics still found in the monasteries of Mt. Athos, Greece, who have passed on the tradition of using repetitive prayers, such as the Prayer of the Heart, since the 13th century. This prayer follows the rhythm of breathing in a form of mantra meditation. The invocation calls for one to imagine looking into one's heart and with each breath during exhalation saying "Lord Jesus Christ, have mercy on me." He also cites Judaic literature, Buddhist teachings, Sufi writings and practices as well as Taoism, and even secular writings by poets such as Wordsworth and Tennyson as describing similar processes for reaching the pleasurable state associated with the relaxation response. Benson advocates the use of mantra meditation and gives his patients a choice of using their own prayer or a secular phrase to use as a mantra as he believes that the mantra chosen should best fit the belief system of the patient.

Indicators of a Meditative State   How can a person recognize that he or she is in a meditative state? Allen (1983) discussed six indicators of an altered state that may be associated with meditation. These are time distortion, ineffability, present-centeredness, perceptual distortion, enhanced receptivity, and self-transcendence. The hypothesized underlying mechanisms for achieving these effects are purely speculative at this time.

One theory of why **time distortion** occurs is that the right hemisphere (for right-handers though for left-handers it may be the left hemisphere) is more dominant during meditation. The left hemisphere is the time keeper and the right hemisphere is believed to engage in non-time-linked thinking. Therefore, during meditation as the right hemisphere dominates, we lose our perception of time. Usually, this means that a 20-minute meditation seems much shorter, more like 5 to 10 minutes or sometimes even less.

Allen (1983) described the experience of **ineffability** as a type of experience that cannot be put into words. Because the right hemisphere is more involved in wordless thinking, it speaks to us in nonword symbols and sensations and its messages may have an ineffable quality during meditation.

Present-centeredness means that the mind is focused on what is occurring in the moment and not engaged in thinking about the past or future as we often do in our normal waking state. Tasks of meditation such as focusing on a mantra or being a passive observer of passing thoughts are very present focused.

Perceptual distortions may occur regarding bodily sensations due to the way the right hemisphere processes sensory information and the left hemisphere interprets it during right hemispheric dominance. Meditators sometimes have an experience of their body shrinking, sinking, floating, or disappearing as they *lose the self* in meditation.

As the walls of the waking self or ego become more permeable during meditation, unconscious thoughts may enter into consciousness. The result is **enhanced receptivity** to suggestions from the inner unconscious self.

Finally, during the experience of **self-transcendence,** meditation can evoke mystical or spiritual qualities. This can lead to an experience of an expanded consciousness, more positive thoughts, and a feeling of inner peace that is traditionally associated with the feelings of enlightenment many spiritually minded people seek.

Overall then there are predictable indicators that one is experiencing an altered state during meditation. Though a meditator may not experience all of the six indicators, the presence of one or more of these indicators suggests the presence of an altered state.

Meditation Experiences

Have you ever meditated? If so, did you experience any of these indicators of the meditative state? Which ones did you experience? When you found yourself experiencing them, what types of sensations and feelings did you have? If you have never meditated, imagine yourself meditating. Does it feel comfortable to you? If so, which of the meditative state experiences do you find most appealing? If not, which of the meditative state experiences, if any, could you find yourself enjoying?

How Meditation Achieves Its Effects

There are a number of theories of how meditation achieves its effects. Upon reviewing the research and theory of mantra meditation, Carrington (2007) surmised that there are four most widely accepted theories of the process. They are desensitization theory, blank-out theory, rhythm theory, and cerebral hemisphere balance theory.

Desensitization theory, based on the concept of systematic desensitization, suggests that mantra meditation induces a global desensitization of many disturbing thoughts and images. Systematic desensitization, a technique pioneered by the behavior therapist Joseph Wolpe (1958), pairs relaxation responses with a graduated hierarchy of phobic images (see Chapter 13). These mental images start with the least and proceed in a graded fashion to the most phobic. By pairing relaxation with these phobic images, the anxiety associated with them is attenuated through a process called *counterconditioning.* When encountering these same images in real life, the individual with a phobia who undergoes this counterconditioning process no longer experiences unmanageable anxiety. The desensitization theory of mantra meditation then suggests that as the meditator experiences various thoughts and images that drift in and out of consciousness, some disturbing or anxiety-provoking thoughts and images are desensitized by being paired with the relaxation-inducing mantra. It is like demagnetizing a library book before walking out of the library. The demagnetized book will not set off the alarm as it would have done had it remained magnetized.

Blank-out theory suggests that mantra meditation restricts consciousness of our external world and in effect temporarily deletes it from our active neural circuitry. The effect is achieved by turning our attention inward and recycling the stimulus input (i.e., the mantra) while blocking external stimuli. After meditation there is often a heightening or sharpening of the senses (e.g., colors appear more vivid and saturated, sounds more acute, etc.) that comes from clearing and rebooting the sensory neurological circuitry.

According to **rhythm theory,** natural rhythms are soothing, comforting, and relaxing. The rhythm of the mantra or of our own biological processes that we experience more fully during meditation, such as drawing our breath and then releasing it, creates feelings of relaxation. In fact, focusing on one's breathing is a component of many forms of meditation. It is well known by

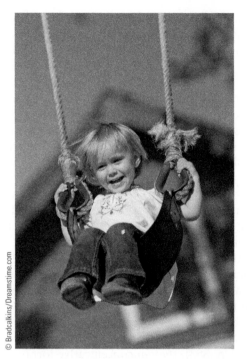

Humans enjoy rhythms, including the rhythmic activity of swinging. We often find rhythmic activity soothing and relaxing. How much do you think the rhythmic activity of repeating a mantra contributes to relaxation?

parents that distressed infants can be comforted by rocking them or engaging them in some form of rhythmic activity. Many forms of music we listen to are relaxing due to their repetitious or rhythmic patterns. Chants and rhythmic word patterns also can have trance-inducing properties. Therefore, mantra meditation may achieve its relaxation effects by tuning us in to natural rhythms we are biologically programmed to find soothing.

Carrington (2007) argues that there is suggestive research that mantra meditation leads to a **greater balance between the two cerebral hemispheres.** In most right-handed people, the left hemisphere is most responsible for analytical, logical, deductive thinking, and the right hemisphere for holistic intuitive thinking. During our everyday activities the left hemisphere is often dominant, but as discussed earlier, during meditation the right hemisphere plays a more dominant role. Therefore, with repeated meditation experiences, we strengthen the role of the right hemisphere, which ultimately leads to a greater balance of the hemispheres. According to Carrington, this balance contributes to the therapeutic effects of meditation.

A form of meditation called mindfulness meditation to be discussed in the next section probably has some overlap with mantra meditation in terms of how it achieves its beneficial effects, but as Jean Kristeller (2007) notes upon reviewing the theory and research of mindfulness meditation, there is some limited evidence suggesting there are differences in the neuropsychological processes between mantra and mindfulness meditation: "Unlike concentrative techniques, mindfulness meditation is not designed to 'block out' conscious thinking, but rather to cultivate the ability to relate to conscious awareness in a nonreactive way" (Kristeller, 2007, p. 399). Therefore, part of the therapeutic effect of mindfulness meditation may be achieved by learning the ability to **disengage** from our involuntary reactive tendencies and more fully engage our inner and outer worlds in a more conscious deliberative manner.

Although the preceding theories are interesting, they are speculative and have at this time little empirical data supporting or refuting them. Processes are more difficult to confirm than outcomes, and whereas there are good outcome studies establishing the benefits of meditation, more studies are needed before we can more definitively determine how underlying processes during meditation lead to their beneficial outcomes.

Forms of Meditation

concentrative meditation: a form of meditation that includes mantra meditation in which the strategy employed is to focus or concentrate on one stimulus.

Herbert Benson's **mantra meditation,** patterned after TM, is a form of meditation with the largest body of research findings. Most of the groundbreaking mantra meditation findings were gathered around the time Benson popularized his relaxation response, especially during the 1970s and 1980s, and there is currently minimal recent research activity in the area. This form of meditation is technically classified as **concentrative meditation** because the strategy employed is to focus or concentrate on one stimulus.

nonconcentrative meditation: a form of meditation like mindfulness meditation in which attention is kept broader along a continuum of stimuli.

mindfulness meditation: a form of nonconcentrative meditation in which practitioners adopt a detached observer style along with acceptance of the object of awareness in the present moment.

However, another form of meditation known as **nonconcentrative** has since the 1990s received increased attention from researchers. As described by Kristeller (2007, p. 393), the nonconcentrative form of meditation known as "mindfulness meditation may utilize any object of attention—whether an emotion, a breath, a physical feeling, an image, or an external object—such that there is more flexibility in the object of awareness than there is in concentrative meditation and such that the object may shift from moment to moment." Attention is kept broader along a continuum of stimuli, and there is no judgment or analysis of one's stream of consciousness during meditation. Practitioners are encouraged to adopt a detached observer style during meditation. This form of meditation has its roots in Buddhist traditions of Japan, Thailand, Burma, Tibet, Vietnam, Korea, and China.

Zen Buddhist meditation (Zazen) has many mindfulness practices (e.g., shinkantaza—just sitting). Just as Herbert Benson's work on mantra meditation forms the cornerstone of much of the applied scientific work in this area, Jon Kabat-Zinn's (1990, 2005) work in developing **mindfulness-based stress reduction (MBSR)** group programs serves as a foundation and impetus for much of the applied scientific work in this area. Thus, the two primary meditational strategies most heavily researched by Western practitioners and investigators are mantra meditation and mindfulness meditation.

Mindfulness Approaches

What is mindfulness? According to Brown, Ryan, and Creswell (2007a, p. 272), "mindfulness is essentially about waking up to what the present moment offers." Another definition suggested by Siegel (2010, p. 27) says that mindfulness is "awareness of present experience with acceptance." Definitions of mindfulness differ somewhat depending on the perspective of those doing the defining. This has frustrated some researchers who are grappling with how to

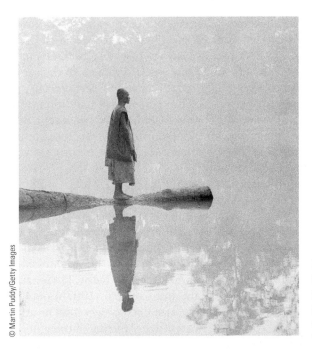

© Martin Puddy/Getty Images

Mindfulness has its roots in Buddhist traditions and involves awareness of the moment with nonjudgmental acceptance.

measure the dimensions of such a simple yet paradoxically complex construct. As such, a group of 11 researchers put their collective wisdom together to fashion an operational definition (i.e., a definition that can be independently tested or validated) of the term. They reached a consensus that mindfulness involves two components.

> The first component involves self-regulation of attention so that it is maintained on immediate experience, thereby, allowing for increased recognition of mental events in the present moment. The second component involves adopting a particular orientation toward one's experiences in the present moment, an orientation that is characterized by curiosity, openness, and acceptance. (Bishop et al., 2004, p. 230)

Looking at the primary self-report instruments used to measure mindfulness, Baer, Smith, Hopkins, Krietemeyer, and Toney (2006) found that three factors emerged when using the statistical procedure called a factor analysis (see Chapter 6) that best predicted psychological symptoms. These are (1) *act with awareness*, (2) *nonjudge*, and (3) *nonreact*.

meta-cognition: thinking about one's thinking.

As Bishop et al. (2004) note, mindfulness involves self-regulation of attention and ***meta-cognition***, in other words, sustaining attention and thinking about one's thinking. Harris (2008, p. 40) shows us how we can go from having a thought that "I am X" to "I'm having a thought that I am X" to "I notice that I am having a thought that I am X." Sometimes these thoughts are stressful or disturbing. Going from "I am incompetent" to "I'm having a thought that I am incompetent" to "I notice that I am having a thought that I am incompetent" goes from a simple stressful cognition to a more complex and less stressful meta-cognition.

observing self: the component of the self in mindfulness practice that notices thoughts.

defuse: a mindfulness process of preventing the fusing or merging of the self with disturbing or stressful thoughts.

decenter: a mindfulness practice of becoming less reactive to one's inner experiences because the mind's activity is observed and the thoughts are seen as outside the center of the self.

Mindfulness practice then encourages us to use the *observing self* (the observing self notices the thought) to notice the present moment's mental events. In doing so, we do not fuse (i.e., become one) with the disturbing or stressful thoughts. Instead we *defuse* them so that our awareness of them has a lessened emotional impact on us. This *decentering* process results in us being less reactive to our inner experiences. In addition, rather than trying to suppress unwanted thoughts or emotions, we accept them as being part of an active mind. We can thank our mind for its thought in a nonsarcastic accepting way and then continue the observation process without latching onto the thought or acting on it.

Within the last several decades, four main mindfulness-based psychological intervention approaches have emerged for dealing with human problems. Kabat-Zinn (1982) was the first pioneer in the field to implement a secular mindfulness-based psychological intervention program, one he calls MBSR, followed later by **dialectical behavior therapy (DBT)** (Linehan, 1993), **acceptance and commitment therapy (ACT)** (Hayes, Strosahl, & Wilson, 1999), and **mindfulness-based cognitive therapy (MBCT)** (Segal, Williams, & Teasdale, 2002). As Brown, Ryan, and Creswell (2007b) note, all four approaches are multidimensional, involve sustained observation or attention to present experiences and conscious awareness or labeling of thoughts and feelings, and the development of an attitude of acceptance. DBT is somewhat different from the rest in that it only uses a nonmeditative approach to mindfulness. See Table 14.1 for a comparison of these four mindfulness-based psychological interventions.

Let us now take a closer look at one of these approaches, ACT. As Hayes, Luoma, Bond, Masuda, and Lillis (2006) explain, ACT is based on six core principles: (1) *Self as Context*, (2) *Defusion*, (3) *Acceptance*, (4) *Contact with the Present Moment*, (5) *Values*, and (6) *Committed Action*. The first four are part of the *Mindfulness Acceptance Processes* and the last four are part of the *Commitment and Behavior Change Processes*. These lead to a general formula

TABLE **14.1**   Four Main Mindfulness-Based Psychological Intervention Approaches

Mindfulness Approach	Primary Populations	Use of Meditation	Average Duration
Mindfulness-Based Stress Reduction (MBSR)	Psychological disorders Medical conditions Stressed but healthy	Yes	8 to 10 weeks
Acceptance and Commitment Therapy (ACT)	Psychological disorders Medical conditions Stressed but healthy	Yes	1 day to 16 weeks
Mindfulness-Based Cognitive Therapy (MBCT)	Clinical depression relapse prevention	Yes	8 to 10 weeks
Dialectical Behavior Therapy (DBT)	Borderline personality disorder Impulse control disorders	No	1 year for first stage

© Cengage Learning 2013.

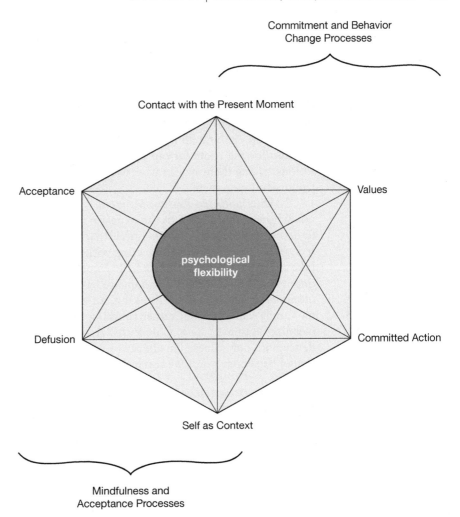

Commitment and Behavior
Change Processes

Contact with the Present Moment

Acceptance

Values

psychological
flexibility

Defusion

Committed Action

Self as Context

Mindfulness and
Acceptance Processes

FIGURE **14.1**   Acceptance and commitment therapy (ACT) is based on six core principles. Some of these are subsumed under the umbrella of Commitment and Behavior Change Processes and others under Mindfulness and Acceptance Processes. Together they determine psychological flexibility.   SOURCE: Hayes, S. C., Luoma, J. B., Bond, F. W., Masuda, A., & Lillis, J. (2006), Acceptance and commitment therapy: Model, processes and outcomes, *Behavior Research and Therapy, 44*, 1–25. Reproduced with permission of PERGAMON via Copyright Clearance Center.

for psychological health that is *Mindfulness + Commitment and Behavior Change = Psychological Flexibility. **Psychological flexibility*** enables us to adapt to the demands of daily living more successfully and hence to experience better mental health (Figure 14.1).

Upon examining Figure 14.1, we can see that the *Mindfulness and Acceptance Process* involves the *Self as Context, Defusion, Acceptance,* and *Contact with the Present Moment;* and the *Commitment and Behavior Change Process* involves *Contact with the Present Moment, Values, Committed Action,* and *Self as Context.*

The *Self as Context* refers to the observing self, discussed earlier, that when engaged, allows us to notice or label our thoughts in a nonjudgmental way so that our experiences are noted without investing in them. This promotes *defusion* and *acceptance*. *Defusion* involves the *decentering* process where we maintain separateness from unhelpful or disturbing thoughts rather than fusing with them. It refers to how we interact with these thoughts. By maintaining separateness from these thoughts while still engaging them we can weaken our attachment to them and not let them define us. *Acceptance* means allowing room for our unpleasant thoughts, images, feelings, and sensations, giving them space rather than ignoring, suppressing, or trying to control or eliminate them.

Contact with the Present Moment is part of the process of engaging our nonjudgmental attention to the experience of the now. Our thoughts are used to describe momentary events rather than to judge or predict them. *Values* refers to the importance of connecting with our values, which in turn leads us to take more purposive actions and to experience a more meaningful life. It is important that the values we adopt are based on our own choices and not those of others so that we are not thinking, for example, "I should value this because my family values it" but rather thinking "I value this because it is personally meaningful to me." Last, *Committed Action* refers to taking action in concordance with our values. This in turn leads us to establish a purposeful life pattern of behaviors where we can feel good about our self, others, and our world.

Applications and Benefits of Meditation

Richard Bandler, an advocate for the benefits of hypnosis and hypnotic-induced trance states, also has high praise for the practice of meditation.

> I've studied many different kinds of meditation in many different countries. I've been to hundreds of sacred temples and spoken to every guru I could find. Their methods might have differed, but they all said more or less the same thing: learn to meditate and practice it regularly and your problems will float away. You'd become more enlightened as a person, more functional as a businessperson. You'd be better for your family, a better spouse and parent, a better partner and friend.
>
> I don't think this is unrealistic, however far-fetched some people might think it is. People who meditate are simply more evenly balanced. Instead of letting the stress of everyday life snowball into chaos, they have a place to go that brings them peace, comfort, and regeneration. (Bandler, 2008, pp. 159–160)

Although Bandler's conclusions may seem hyperbolic, in many ways his contentions are supported by research findings. In general, regular meditation seems to improve mood, affect, and well-being, including helping the meditator cope with anxiety, stress, and some forms of mild depression while cultivating more positive emotional experiences. It also seems to reduce the severity of some conditions of illness and enhance the ability to cope with illness. Furthermore, it appears to facilitate personal growth and improve interpersonal relationships.

Mood, Affect, and Well-Being Empirical findings consistently indicate that regular mantra meditation leads to lessened anxiety. For example, Alexander,

Robinson, Orme-Johnson, Schneider, and Walton (1994) reported in their summary of meta-analyses encompassing several hundred individual studies that mantra meditation decreased both physiological arousal levels and trait anxiety. Because anxiety is one of the primary emotions associated with the fight-or-flight response (i.e., the flight component), and physiological arousal is reduced by mantra meditation, it seems natural that anxiety also is lessened.

What about using meditation for the treatment of anxiety disorders? Mindfulness-based approaches have indeed been used for the treatment of these disorders. For example, Kabat-Zinn et al. (1992) and Miller, Fletcher, and Kabat-Zinn (1995) found that in their 8-week group MBSR program participants with anxiety disorder reported significantly reduced anxiety and panic symptoms. The majority of participants continued to engage in meditation practice at 3-year follow-up, and significant symptom reductions were still present at that time.

Mantra meditation can elevate mood states in those experiencing mild forms of depression (Carrington et al., 1980) though it is probably not beneficial for most other types of depression. John Teasdale and his associates (2000) successfully used MBCT approaches for the prevention of relapse/reoccurrence of major depression episodes over a 60-week period in individuals who had already undergone treatment. Their mindfulness approach was designed to help patients cultivate a "detached, decentered relationship to depression-related thoughts and feelings" and develop skills "to prevent the escalation of negative thinking patterns at times of potential relapse/recurrence (Teasdale et al., 2000, p. 616). Although the study's validity could be questioned due to an absence of a comparison group, its findings were later replicated by Ma & Teasdale (2004), thus adding more support for the findings.

In a review of the literature of the benefits of mindfulness interventions, Brown et al. (2007b) reported that numerous randomized clinical trial studies determined that MBSR leads to reductions in stress symptoms (including self-reports of distress) and mood disturbances in both healthy and patient groups. Likewise, ACT results in reduced psychological symptoms in healthy-stressed groups and burnout in counselors. Brown and his colleagues (2007b) also noted that DBT is successful in reducing symptoms of depression (when combined with antidepressants) or distress in certain clinical populations such as older adults with depression and individuals with borderline personality disorder.

Although these results are encouraging, Toneatto and Nguyen (2007) reviewed all the controlled studies they could identify (15 studies) that used MBSR with clinical populations and concluded that the results were mixed for symptoms of anxiety and depression. Specifically, they noted that the better controlled studies found no evidence of MBSR effectiveness. They further suggested that the studies that put participants on a waiting list as a control condition, a weaker form of control, were more likely to find effects than those with stronger controls. The authors speculated that the effects found when using weaker control conditions could be due to nonspecific effects (i.e., placebo effects) like the extra attention the experimental groups received rather than to the MBSR intervention.

More recently, Hofmann, Sawyer, Witt, and Oh (2010) conducted a meta-analysis of 39 studies that included 1,140 participants and determined that mindfulness-based therapy showed large pre-post effect sizes for anxiety reduction in patients with anxiety disorders (effect size = 0.97) and for depression symptoms in patients with depression (effect size = 0.95). In their overall sample that included participants in both clinical and nonclinical populations the pre-post effect size for anxiety (effect size = 0.63) and depression (effect size = 0.59) reduction was moderate. Like Toneatto and Nguyen (2007), they acknowledged that more randomized controlled studies are needed with placebo controls because only 16 of the 39 studies they examined had control groups. However, they concluded that "the pre-post treatment effects were robust and were unlikely to be the result of a psychological placebo because the observed effect size is greater than what would be expected from a psychological placebo" (Hoffman et al., 2010, p. 180).

Using functional magnetic resonance imaging, Creswell, Way, Eisenberger, and Lieberman (2007) determined that the amygdalas of those scoring high in trait mindfulness were less reactive to threatening emotional stimuli during an affect labeling task probably because they had greater prefrontal cortical activation that could inhibit amygdala responses. Thus, mindful individuals seem to be better at self-regulating emotional responses to threat and there are brain area studies that can account for this.

Investigators (Shapiro, Schwartz, & Bonner, 1998) reported increased empathy and increased psychological as well as spiritual well-being in premedical and medical students who participated in a mindfulness meditation program. In addition, state mindfulness is associated with higher levels of daily positive affect and lower levels of negative affect (Carlson & Brown, 2005).

In sum, the research findings generally support the contention that meditation practice leads to a reduction in stress and anxiety symptoms. However, better controlled studies are still needed to unravel and quantify the specific effects of mindfulness from nonspecific factors when treating anxiety disorders with mindfulness-based interventions. There is evidence to suggest that meditation and mindfulness-based practices lead to a reduction in depression and mood disturbances and an overall elevation of positive affect. Mindfulness-based approaches also have been successful at preventing treatment relapses in people struggling with clinical depression. In addition, higher levels of mindfulness are associated with an overall heightened sense of well-being.

Health Conditions and Behaviors   Numerous studies document the positive effects of meditation on health conditions and the stress associated with them. For example, studies indicate that mantra meditation reduces the symptoms associated with cardiovascular disease such as preventricular contractions (Benson, Alexander, & Feldman, 1975) and angina pectoris (Tulpule, 1971) in patients with ischemic heart disease, blood pressure in patients with hypertension (Benson, 1977) and young adults at risk for hypertension (Nidich et al., 2009), and serum cholesterol in patients with hypercholesterolemia (Cooper & Aygen, 1979). Studies also document its effectiveness in reducing symptoms of health conditions exacerbated by stress such as asthma (Honsberger &

Wilson, 1973), psoriasis (Gaston, 1988–1989), and irritable bowel syndrome (IBS) (Keefer & Blanchard, 2002). Besides mantra meditation, psoriasis also seems to respond well to mindfulness meditation when used as an adjunctive treatment to phototherapy and photochemotherapy (Bernhard, Kristeller, & Kabat-Zinn, 1988).

MBSR appears to aid in the self-regulation of pain in patients with chronic pain immediately following treatment and long term (Kabat-Zinn, Lipworth, & Burney, 1985; Kabat-Zinn, Lipworth, Burney, & Sellers, 1986). ACT seems to be effective in reducing the need for medical care in certain at-risk populations. For example, one study (Dahl, Wilson, & Nilsson, 2004) observed that adults with chronic stress and pain who were at risk of developing a long-term disability who received ACT reduced their use of medical treatment resources and sick days posttreatment and at a 6-month follow-up.

Women with cancer demonstrated reduced distress symptoms and better health quality of life following a mindfulness-based art therapy treatment (Monti et al., 2006). In a randomized controlled study (Foley, Baillie, Huxter, Price, & Sinclair, 2010), patients with cancer receiving MBCT reported significant reductions in anxiety, depression, and distress, suggesting that this form of mindfulness-based treatment may also help to improve symptoms of negative affect associated with the diagnosis and treatment of cancer.

There also is evidence suggesting that MBSR may improve immune response in patients with breast and prostate cancer. For example, Carlson, Speca, Patel, and Goodey (2003) found changes in cytokine (e.g., increased interleukin, IL-4, levels) profiles in patients in MBSR treatment diagnosed with these cancers, suggesting improved immunity. They noted that theirs was the first study of its kind to find changes in production of cancer-related cytokines related to MBSR program participation. A meta-analysis (Grossman, Niemann, Schmidt, & Walach, 2004, p. 39) of 20 studies that met strict methodological inclusion standards for MBSR health benefit research determined that "the consistent and relatively strong level of effect sizes across very different types of sample indicates that mindfulness training might enhance general features of coping with distress and disability in everyday life, as well as under more extraordinary conditions of serious disorder or stress."

Brain meditation researcher Richard J. Davidson and his colleagues (2003) discovered that an 8-week program of MBSR resulted in brain changes in meditators (more left-sided anterior activation) associated with a greater experience of positive affect. They also detected a better antibody response to an influenza vaccine than they found in their nonmeditator controls. Even more remarkable, using magnetic resonance imaging, Lazar and her associates (2005) determined that regular meditators who were extensively trained in what she called *insight meditation* had thicker prefrontal cortexes and right anterior insulas than matched controls. Her group uncovered a direct positive correlation between the amount of the practice of meditation and the thickness of these regions of the brain. The authors of the study concluded that "our initial results suggest that mediation may be associated with structural changes in areas of the brain that are important for sensory, cognitive and emotional processing" (p. 1896).

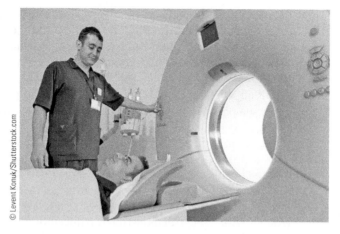

© Levent Konuk/Shutterstock.com

Magnetic resonance imaging research suggests that regular meditation leads to positive brain changes that slow age-related declines in cognitive function.

Pagnoni and Cekic (2007) also used magnetic resonance imaging on experienced Zen meditators (more than 3 years of daily practice) and found that their cerebral gray matter volume did not show the normal negative correlation to age (an age-related decline) that the matched control subjects showed. They noted that "the effect of meditation on gray matter volume was most prominent in the putamen, a structure strongly implicated in attentional processing. These findings suggest that the regular practice of meditation may have neuroprotective effects and reduce cognitive decline associated with normal aging" (p. 1623).

The practice of meditation also seems to be associated with decreased substance use. For example, among marijuana users, the longer they practiced mantra meditation, the more likely they were to report reductions or cessation in marijuana use (Shafi, Lavely, & Jaffe, 1974). Reduction or cessation of cigarette use among smokers (Royer, 1994) and reduction of alcohol use among heavy social drinkers who began and continued the practice of mantra meditation also are reported (Murphy, Pagano, & Marlatt, 1986).

Likewise, ACT shows promise as a smoking cessation treatment in a study (Hernandez-Lopez, Luciano, Bricker, Roales-Nieto, & Montesinos, 2009) that compared it to the gold standard for the field, cognitive-behavioral treatment. Further, researchers (Bowen et al., 2006) reported that incarcerated subjects who engaged in a form of mindfulness meditation called **Vipassana meditation** (based on Buddhist practice) showed significantly reduced substance use of alcohol, marijuana, and crack cocaine after release from jail.

In summary, it appears that the regular practice of meditation can assist in reducing some types of health symptoms for a number of medical conditions. Mindfulness approaches also seem to benefit patients with chronic pain and improve the immune response in patients with certain types of cancers. Regular meditation also may increase the volume of cerebral gray matter and slow age-related declines in cognitive function. In addition, meditation practice

Vipassana meditation: a form of mindfulness meditation based on Buddhist practice.

is associated with reduced substance use. On the whole then, meditation seems to have many health-related benefits and is a worthwhile component to programs promoting health, wellness, and stress reduction.

Personal Growth and Interpersonal Relations   Self-acceptance is an important component of personal growth. Although of limited generalizability due to its small sample (eight health care professionals), Shapiro, Astin, Bishop, and Cordova (2005) reported that subjects who were randomly assigned to an 8-week MBSR program showed improvements in self-compassion and increased quality of life compared to control subjects. Similarly, Easterlin and Cardena (1998) found greater positive mood, self-acceptance, and self-awareness among more experienced Vipassana mindfulness meditators than their less experienced counterparts. Additionally, a type of mindfulness meditation program called **loving kindness meditation therapy** was found to improve satisfaction of marital relationships even in happy relationships (Carson, Carson, Gil, & Baucom, 2004). Thus, mindfulness meditation seems to promote many positive qualities associated with awareness and compassion for self and others.

The Practice of Meditation

Although the practice of meditation has established beneficial effects, Rice (1999) argues that it is not a panacea and is not for everyone. Carrington (2007) likewise cautions that it has its limitations. Some individuals can actually become more anxious when meditating because they may have fear of change or think that the practice of meditation somehow threatens their belief systems. Others who are unfamiliar with deep relaxation may have feelings of anxiety as they push the boundaries of their normal experiences. A person who has never truly relaxed may find the sensations of relaxation strange or unsettling.

Driven Type A personalities may see meditation as unproductive and lose patience with it because there are no immediate concrete outcomes. Sitting still for long periods may seem like a waste of time to people who feel that they need to be on the go. Also, to the Type A person who is only familiar with two states, full speed and sleep, it may seem inconceivable that there is a middle ground state of relaxation that can actually recharge a person and help that person become more productive.

Meditation is not an established treatment or adjunct for certain types of psychological disorders (i.e., schizophrenia) and, therefore, may not be indicated unless recommended by a therapist. For the great majority of people, however, meditation can be an effective way to manage stress and experience some of the beneficial physiological and psychological changes discussed earlier.

Mantra Meditation Practice   Cardiologist Herbert Benson reduced mantra meditation to its most basic elements in a form called **secular meditation** or **relaxation response meditation**. Benson (1975) recommends that beginners simply use the word *One* or some other neutral word as their mantra. By repeating the word *One* over and over again for about 20 minutes twice daily, Benson states that the same results can be achieved with this mantra method as with TM. As noted earlier in the chapter, the steps are:

1. Repeat a word, sound, prayer, phrase, or muscular activity.

2. Passively disregard everyday thoughts that come to mind, and return to your repetition. (Benson, 1996; p. 134)

Benson recommends that the word or phrase be consistent with the meditator's belief system. For those preferring a secular word, Benson (1996, p. 135) suggests *One, Ocean, Love, Peace, Calm,* and *Relaxed.* For those with a religious focus he suggests for Christians (Protestant or Catholic) *Our Father who art in heaven* or *The Lord is my shepherd;* for Catholics *Hail, Mary, full of grace* or *Lord Jesus Christ, have mercy on me;* for Jewish *Sh'ma Yisroel, Shalom, Echod,* and *The Lord is my shepherd;* for Muslims, *Insha'allah;* and for Hindus, *Om.*

Patricia Carrington's (1978, 1998, 2007) clinically standardized meditation (CSM) method is usually taught via compact discs (CDs) and a programmed instruction workbook. The beginning meditator selects a mantra from a list of 16 included in her workbook. The mantras included in the workbook are believed to have a calming effect and have no English language meaning. They include sounds such as *ahnam, shi-rim,* and *ra-mah.* During training the beginner first repeats the word out loud, next whispers it, then is instructed to (with eyes closed) silently think it. The goal is to reach a 20-minute mantra meditation practice, though for some who are uncomfortable with this length of time, a series of 2- to 3-minute **mini-meditations** may substitute. Her research suggests that a person can achieve many of the beneficial effects of mantra meditation without necessarily adhering to the strict 20-minute twice-a-day routine (strongly advocated by TM's founder Maharishi Mahesh Yogi) as long as the person practices meditation on a fairly regular schedule.

Carrington advises that the training program not be taken lightly because it is an important moment in a person's life to learn to meditate and that inadequately trained meditators are more likely to later abandon its practice. For more information on Carrington's approach, refer to her book called *The Book of Meditation: The Complete Guide to Modern Meditation* (Carrington, 1998).

Mindfulness Meditation Practice Jean Kristeller (2007) suggests that the practice of mindfulness meditation can be divided into three aspects that she calls (1) breath awareness, (2) open awareness, and (3) guided mindfulness meditation. **Breath awareness** is associated with many types of meditation practices, including some concentrative techniques. The idea is to focus your attention on the breathing process—inspiration, in-between, and expiration. Slowing your breath to very low respiration rates can also have very powerful relaxation benefits.

During **open awareness** meditation, the meditator disengages the analytical mind, suspends judgment, and becomes a passive observer of the images, sensations, feelings, and cognitions that stream through consciousness. As these elements pass through the mind, the meditator makes a mental note of them but does not react or get swept away with them. Instead, the mediator

STRESS MANAGEMENT EXERCISE **14.1**

Mantra Meditation

Now that you know the basics of mantra meditation, you are encouraged to select a mantra that feels right to you. Did you select one? Now notice what it feels like when you get in a comfortable position, close your eyes, and begin to silently repeat the mantra over and over again. You may find yourself drifting into a meditative state even as you allow yourself a 2- or 3-minute mini-meditation.

Did you try it? If so, what did it feel like? Did you experience any of the meditative state qualities that we discussed earlier? If you didn't, you may be wondering if you could. A person can with practice learn to meditate and experience its benefits. If meditation is not for you, other approaches including the relaxation strategies discussed in Chapter 13 are also beneficial. However, if meditation is something that feels comfortable to you, you are encouraged to continue your meditation practices.

lets what floats by get carried like a leaf on a stream out of consciousness and then observes what comes next. In a combined practice of breath awareness and mindfulness meditation Kristeller (2007) instructs,

> As you continue, you will notice that the mind will become caught up in thoughts and feelings. It may become attached to noises or bodily sensations. You will find yourself remembering something from your past or thinking about the future. This is to be expected. This is the nature of the mind. If the thought or experience is particularly powerful, without self-judgment, simply observe the process of the mind. You might note to yourself the nature of the thought or experience: "worry," "planning," "pain," "sound." Then gently return your attention to the breath. (p. 409)

In **guided meditation** the idea is to focus on aspects of the self that are relevant to your aspirations and to do so in a **mindful way** that suspends judgment and analysis. The focus may be on stress, for example, for persons who aspire to have a more balanced approach to stress. In therapeutic applications, the guided meditation may be scripted. For example, loving kindness scripts may be used by couples who wish to increase their intimacy levels.

The practice of mindfulness meditation should be for 20 to 40 minutes, once or twice a day. A goal of practice is the integration of the meditative experiences or of mini-meditations into daily living as the practitioner becomes more focused on the moment, more mindful, and less reactive. The person is instructed at times throughout the day to shift attention to one's current activity in a mindful way or to one's breathing as a form of breath awareness. In that way, there is a seamless generalization of the process and of its beneficial experiences.

As you know meditation has many psychological and physiological benefits related to self-regulation. Historically, biofeedback, too, has been seen as an even more target-specific mechanism for self-regulating the physiological underpinnings of stress and disease states. Let us next take a closer look at biofeedback and examine its benefits and shortcomings.

STRESS MANAGEMENT EXERCISE **14.2**

Mindfulness Meditation

Are you ready to try a mindfulness meditation exercise, maybe a mini-mediation or longer? You may be wondering about breath awareness meditation. This breath awareness meditation exercise is an adaptation of an exercise by Ronald Siegel (2010) in which he uses the metaphor of puppy training to describe what happens when your puppy wanders off during training just as our mind wanders during meditation. What do you do with the puppy? You gently bring it back each time it wanders.

If you would like to try this exercise, get into a comfortable position, close your eyes, and begin to observe your breath. As you allow your breathing to be comfortable and natural, notice the rise in your belly as you breathe in and its fall as you breathe out. Rising and falling with each breath. Some breaths are short and shallow and others are deep and long.

If your attention begins to wander, you can allow your observing mind to note the types of thoughts, images, or sensations you have. Thoughts may be worry, judging, planning, fantasizing, criticizing, or whatever label your observing mind wants to give them. These are natural. You could say silently to yourself "worrying" to note the thought, or say "I notice I am having a thought that I can't be mindful enough" should this thought or others like it occur.

Like a curious puppy, it's only natural that your mind will wander. As it wanders gently bring it back. Be kind and loving to your curious puppy mind as I know you will. Bring your focus to your belly rising and falling with each breath. As your puppy mind wanders off again, note the thought, then gently bring your puppy mind back again. Allow your puppy to wander off as much as it wants, that's what puppies do. And puppy trainers bring their puppies back again and again in a loving and kind way.

If you feel a sensation, have your observing self note the sensation, like "itch," and then move your focus back to your belly rising and falling. When you find yourself hearing a noise, have your observing self note that as "noise" or "sound." As you have an image, note the image, perhaps it is a "fantasy." Return once again to your belly rising and falling, rising and falling, rising and falling. Continue on for 20 minutes.

Did you try your mindfulness exercise? If you did, what was it like? Did you experience the defusion associated with the observing self? Did you feel decentered? Is the practice of mindfulness meditation something you could imagine yourself doing on a regular basis? Could this help you with stressful thoughts, feelings, and images? Suppose you were to practice it and get better and better at it. As you practice, you could become more comfortable with mindfulness and make it a regular part of your daily routine.

BIOFEEDBACK

As discussed previously, biofeedback uses technology to provide visual or auditory feedback to facilitate the process of learning degrees of control over the monitored physiological systems. Though biofeedback is sometimes used for broad relaxation training, its main appeal is its ability to target specific physiological responses and, therefore, focus more precisely on health conditions that

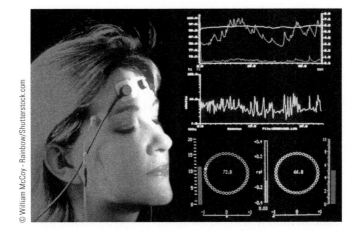

Biofeedback electrodes are placed on the frontalis muscle to measure electromyograph (EMG) forehead tension.

electromyograph (EMG): a measure of electrical activity of the skeletal muscles.

relate to these responses. For example, electrodes can be placed on the frontalis muscle to measure **electromyograph** (EMG) forehead tension that might relate to the onset or intensity of tension-type headaches. Through feeding information back to the patients, they can learn to control muscle tension in this area to better manage the frequency and intensity of headaches.

Biofeedback, usually in combination with other treatments, is successfully applied to a wide variety of disorders and health conditions. Schwartz (2003, p. 107) lists the use of biofeedback as "best efficacy" for symptom relief in the following conditions: tension-type headache, migraine headache, nocturnal enuresis, fecal or urinary incontinence or other pelvic floor disorders, essential hypertension, and phantom limb pain.

A lesser but still important category of biofeedback efficacy called "good efficacy" includes application to the conditions of certain types of insomnia, anxiety disorders (generalized anxiety disorder, phobias, and posttraumatic stress disorder), attention-deficit hyperactivity disorder, epilepsy, nausea and vomiting, IBS, asthma, temporomandibular disorders and bruxism, tinnitus, Raynaud's disease and Raynaud's phenomenon, chronic pain, fibromyalgia, and hyperventilation. Schwartz states, however, the following cautions and contraindications for biofeedback:

> Most practitioners consider the following disorders and conditions as outright contraindications to biofeedback, or at least as indicating the need for caution. These include severe depression; acute agitation; acute or fragile schizophrenia (or a strong potential for psychotic decompensation); mania; paranoid disorders with delusions of influence; severe obsessive-compulsive disorder (OCD); delirium; acute medical decompensation; or a strong potential for a dissociative reaction, fugue state, or depersonalization. There is very little or no literature on biofeedback or other applied psychophysiological interventions for patients with these disorders, as logic has precluded such interventions with these patients. (p. 107)

It is beyond the scope of this book to examine all the research in the area of biofeedback. Instead, several areas of research are highlighted that exemplify how clinical biofeedback is successfully applied. The painful condition of headache is examined first, then Raynaud's disease, and last, the application of biofeedback to essential hypertension.

Headache

Andrasik (2007) explains that there are three primary behavioral approaches to the treatment of chronic headache disorders. The first approach attempts to facilitate overall relaxation, the second targets the physiological systems that are believed to contribute most directly to the pathophysiology of the headache, and the third approach focuses on how to best manage reactions to stress.

Methods for promoting **general relaxation** include progressive relaxation training, autogenic training, meditation, and **biofeedback-assisted relaxation training**. For headache, the **direct targeted approach** generally uses biofeedback of muscle tension for tension-type headache and biofeedback of physiological indicators of blood flow for migraine. Finally, for learning how to cope with stress, some form of cognitive therapy or **stress management training** is used. Andrasik notes that after nearly four decades of research, the evidence indicates that all three approaches are successful in reducing headache activity and that studies report an average 30% to 60% reduction in headache symptom scores.

biofeedback-assisted relaxation training: using biofeedback to promote a state of general relaxation.

Tension-Type Headache   Nestoriuc, Rief, and Martin (2008) conducted a meta-analysis that included a total of 53 biofeedback treatment studies of tension-type headache. The studies they selected were carefully screened for their higher methodological quality. Most of the studies used EMG feedback with the electrodes placed bifrontal (over the frontalis muscle, the one at the forehead), though some also placed electrodes over other muscle areas (trapezius muscle or masseter muscle). Their results were impressive with medium-to-large magnitude effects for biofeedback treatment (improvement on the order of one standard deviation). These effects were obtained over an average of 11 sessions with patients who had suffered with tension-type headache activity for an average of 14 years.

Nestoriuc et al. (2008) noted also that this was the first meta-analytic study with sufficient power to find that the treatments led to significantly reduced muscle tension. Why is this important? It is important because it establishes a missing physiological link between the theory of muscle tension reduction and its relation to headache symptom reduction. The link had been hypothesized but never firmly established in previous meta-analyses. This had caused some earlier researchers to speculate that EMG biofeedback-mediated headache symptom reductions were probably wholly *psychologically* driven rather than at least partly related to reductions in muscle tension that were presumed to more directly underlie the pathophysiology of the tension-type headache. Now there appears to be good evidence establishing the *physiological* link for biofeedback efficacy in treating tension-type headache.

These investigators also found that biofeedback was more effective than general relaxation therapies for the treatment of tension-type headache, though EMG biofeedback combined with general relaxation therapy was found to be

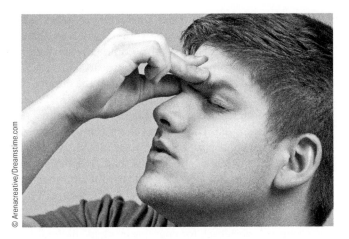

Tension-type headache responds best to EMG biofeedback when it is combined with general relaxation therapy. However, EMG biofeedback alone is more effective than general relaxation therapy.

more effective than EMG biofeedback alone. Also, there were a number of corollary benefits such as greater self-efficacy, reduced anxiety, reduced depression, and reduced use of analgesic medications associated with the biofeedback treatments. Finally, it should be noted that children and adolescents showed greater improvements with biofeedback than adults, which is similar to other studies showing that these populations are particularly responsive to biofeedback training. Overall, given the documented magnitude and scope of the findings, Nestoriuc and her associates (2008) concluded that biofeedback meets the criteria established by the American Psychological Association for being an **empirically supported therapy** for tension-type headache.

Migraine Headache   Unlike tension-type headache's relation to skeletal muscle tension, migraine headache appears to be vascular in origin. Migraine pain is likely caused by the extracranial cephalic blood vessels (i.e., the blood vessels of the head that are outside the skull) dilating and becoming inflamed. Schwartz and Andrasik (2003, p. 326) noted that "it is more than 30 years since the incidental finding of an association between hand warming and reduced migraines."

In order to **hand warm** (i.e., to use cognitive strategies that increase the skin temperature of the hand), the vessels in the hands must dilate and allow more blood flow to this peripheral region of the body. Somehow learned hand warming generally has a beneficial effect on migraines. To this day, however, Schwartz and Andrasik admit, "we are still unsure of the mechanism(s) involved" (p. 326). Possible mechanisms include changes in blood flow, the CNS, the autonomic nervous system, or neurotransmitters disrupting the migraine's pathophysiology.

In order to take advantage of the hand-warming phenomenon, biofeedback clinicians and investigators use peripheral skin temperature feedback (a sensitive

blood-volume-pulse feedback: biofeedback in which changes in skin blood volume are measured with a noninvasive instrument called a photoelectric plethysmograph.

resistor known as a thermister is usually placed on a finger that is sensitive to temperature changes) or **blood-volume-pulse feedback** (i.e., changes in skin blood volume are measured with a noninvasive procedure called a photoelectric plethysmograph from a recording device attached to the area measured like the superficial temporal artery that runs from the neck to the temple).

Nestoriuc and Martin (2007) conducted a meta-analysis of the use of biofeedback for migraine that involved 55 studies out of a possible 86 that met their inclusion standards. They found a medium effect size (improvement on the order of more than half a standard deviation) with blood-volume-pulse feedback leading to greater effect sizes than peripheral skin temperature or EMG feedback. Further, they determined that the treatments had long-term effectiveness (more than 1 year documented by follow-ups). The authors concluded that

> The meta-analysis documents medium effect sizes for short- and long-term outcome of biofeedback for migraine in adults. Biofeedback significantly and substantially reduces the pain and psychological symptoms of highly chronified patients within the scope of only 11 sessions. Thus, biofeedback can be recommended as an evidence-based behavioral treatment option for the prevention of migraine. (Nestoriuc & Martin, 2007, p. 123)

Although Nestoriuc and Martin's (2007) findings were limited to *adults* with migraine, it should be noted that Trautmann, Lackschewitz, and Kroner-Herwig (2006) conducted a meta-analysis that excluded adults and included only children and adolescents who suffered from reoccurring headache (including migraine) and found that biofeedback patients in the 23 studies who met their inclusion criteria showed significant reductions in headache symptoms (greater than 50% improvement) and that the benefits were long term (present at 1-year follow-up).

Raynaud's Disease and Raynaud's Phenomenon

Raynaud's phenomenon (RP): a painful condition triggered by cold exposure or emotional stress involving vasoconstriction of the arteries and arterioles of the fingers and toes.

Raynaud's phenomenon (RP) involves spasms (vasoconstriction) of the arteries and arterioles of the fingers and toes. The spasms, typically induced by cold exposure or emotional stress, cause reduced blood flow to the area, which leads first to skin blanching (i.e., reduced coloration), then cyanosis (i.e., a bluish color due to lack of oxygen), and finally redness upon reperfusion (i.e., blood restoration) of the digits. Spasmodic episodes may last minutes or hours and may involve burning or cold sensations in the affected areas. Although many factors are involved in RP, current research supports the theory that attacks occur because of hypersensitivity of blood vessel alpha-2 adrenergic receptors to cold or to catecholamines elevated during emotional stress.

As with migraine treatments, behavioral treatments for RP mainly use voluntary hand-warming strategies. Though some practitioners use nonbiofeedback approaches to hand warming, Schwartz and Sedlacek (2003, p. 371) contend, "in our view, however, biofeedback appears to result in improved acquisition of hand-warming skills." Just as with treatments for migraine, most typically, the treatment for Raynaud's involves using a thermister on a digit to measure skin temperature changes.

In a review of the biofeedback literature for the treatment of RP, Karavidas, Tsai, Yucha, McGrady, and Lehrer (2006) point to two studies in particular by Freedman and associates (Freedman, Ianni, & Wenig, 1983; Freedman et al., 1988) that used rigorous controls in which subjects learned hand-warming skills through biofeedback training under cold stress that resulted in 67% to 92% reductions in symptom frequency; and symptom reductions were still present at a 3-year follow-up.

Likewise, Schwartz and Sedlacek (2003) praised Freedman's two studies as the best controlled studies of the effects of skin temperature biofeedback for the treatment of RP. As a result of these and a handful of other studies, Karavidas et al. (2006) contend that the evidence suggests that the use of temperature biofeedback for the treatment of RP was demonstrated by independent laboratories as *efficacious* (level IV), which is a higher level of treatment confidence than *probably efficacious* (level III) but not as high as the top level of *efficacious and specific* (level V).

Essential Hypertension

Essential hypertension (also known as primary hypertension) is a disease of unknown etiology characterized by chronically elevated blood pressure. It is believed to be related to overactivity of the sympathetic branch of the autonomic nervous system. There have been a number of behavioral approaches to the treatment of hypertension that follow either a single-component or multicomponent protocol. The single component biofeedback approach typically uses a constant blood pressure cuff procedure to directly feedback this targeted physiological response.

On the other hand, the multicomponent approach typically uses biofeedback-assisted relaxation training (usually temperature feedback or EMG feedback) augmented with nonbiofeedback approaches such as training in progressive muscle relaxation, autogenic approaches, or meditation. Home practice of relaxation and home monitoring of blood pressure also are typical components of the multicomponent approach. As noted by Fahrion, Norris, Green, Green, and Snarr (1986), in general the multicomponent indirect approach is more effective than the single component direct approach in the use of biofeedback to treat essential hypertension.

Two studies, both conducted in 1986, are illustrative of the early findings of the effectiveness of the multicomponent approach. Fahrion and his associates (1986) used a biofeedback-assisted relaxation approach (thermal and EMG biofeedback) to train 77 patients with essential hypertension how to warm their hands and feet and engage in muscle relaxation. They also trained subjects in diaphragmatic breathing and the use of autogenic phrases as well as employed home practice of relaxation sessions and home monitoring of blood pressure. Their approach resulted in patients significantly reducing their blood pressure to the point where 58% of the medicated patients were able to discontinue using blood pressure medication and another 35% were able to cut their medication dosage in half. In their nonmedicated patients, 70% were able to reduce their blood pressure below 140/90 millimeters of mercury (the target goal). Their results were still clinically significant at a 33-month follow-up.

Blanchard et al. (1986) also obtained significant results using thermal biofeedback combined with the use of autogenic phrases. In their study of

87 patients who were on at least two antihypertensive medications, Blanchard's group found that thermal biofeedback was successful in reducing blood pressure levels following treatment and at 1-year follow-up. They reported that 35% of their patients were able to discontinue use of their second-stage medication for at least 1 year.

In a review article, Blanchard (1990) discussed the previous 15 years of his research in the area and remarked that his studies consistently found a posttreatment reduction in tonic levels of blood pressure but never a reduction of cardiovascular reactivity. So whereas the treatments are effective in lowering basal blood pressure, they appear not to be effective in reducing sympathetically mediated cardiovascular reactivity to stress.

More recently, a meta-analytic review study (Nakao, Yano, Nomura, & Kuboki, 2003) of 22 randomized controlled studies that included 905 patients with hypertension confirmed that only relaxation-assisted biofeedback (not simple biofeedback) was successful in reducing blood pressure. Relaxation-assisted biofeedback combines biofeedback with other forms of deep relaxation training. The reductions were modest, averaging 7.3 mm Hg for systolic and 5.8 mm Hg for diastolic blood pressure.

However, even though many studies find some beneficial impact of using relaxation-assisted biofeedback, the current consensus among clinicians is that in spite of the early encouraging studies, the clinical impact is not sufficient to recommend it over drug treatment. For example, authors of a current review of the research in the area (Greenhalgh, Dickson, & Dundar, 2010) conclude that "we found no convincing evidence that consistently demonstrates the effectiveness of the use of any particular biofeedback treatment in the control of essential hypertension when compared to pharmacotherapy, placebo, no intervention or other behavioural therapies." At best, the authors suggest, it should be used as an adjunct to drug treatment.

Biofeedback Conclusions and Recommendations

Biofeedback showed great promise during its inception as a vehicle for directly targeting underlying pathophysiological mechanisms of certain health conditions and diseases. In some cases, for example, in EMG feedback for the treatment of tension-type headache, it has lived up to its promise. However, in other cases, for example, in treatment of essential hypertension, it seems to be effective primarily by assisting in increasing general levels of relaxation. As a result, some have argued that in many cases alternative less expensive methods such as meditation or deep relaxation training can produce similar relaxation mediated benefits and are more cost effective than biofeedback.

Therefore, it is important when considering behavioral approaches to the treatment of health conditions to examine the efficacy of different approaches and to weigh the cost against the efficacy. Biofeedback can be very cost effective and efficacious for the behavioral treatment of a restricted range of health conditions, though for other health conditions alternative relaxation-oriented approaches may be the optimal treatments of choice.

CHAPTER SUMMARY AND CONCEPT REVIEW

- Western researchers studying Indian Yogis in the 1950s and 1960s were intrigued by the idea that a person could apply conscious control to the autonomic nervous system, a component of the overall nervous system, that was previously thought involuntary.

- From these early investigations and other factors spawned the fields of applied psychophysiology and biofeedback.

- Interests in meditation from Indian yoga practices and Asian Buddhist traditions prompted researchers such as Dr. Herbert Benson to study and apply the benefits of mantra meditation and Jon Kabat-Zinn to do the same for mindfulness meditation.

- Benson developed a form of mantra meditation that involves repetition of a mental device while adopting a passive attitude, whereas mindfulness meditation often involves breath awareness, open awareness, and/or guided meditation.

- There are four main mindfulness-based psychological intervention approaches: mindfulness-based stress reduction (MBSR), dialectical behavior therapy (DBT), acceptance and commitment therapy (ACT), and mindfulness-based cognitive therapy (MBCT).

- ACT involves increasing psychological flexibility through mindfulness plus a commitment to behavior change.

- During the practice of meditation a person can experience changes in consciousness, and there are a number of indicators of this state.

- Although there may be some overlap between normal resting states, sleeping states, hypnotic states, and meditative states, meditation seems to differ from these other states and has been characterized as an alert-drowsy state that is in between the sleep and normal waking states of consciousness.

- Research supports the contention that meditation practice leads to a reduction in stress and anxiety symptoms.

- Mindfulness-based psychological interventions have been successful at treating anxiety disorders, though better controlled studies are needed to determine the degree that mindfulness as opposed to extraneous factors plays in the outcome; these interventions also have been successful in reducing distress, mood disturbances, and elevating positive affect in clinical and healthy-stressed populations.

- The regular practice of meditation can reduce some types of health symptoms in a number of medical conditions, including chronic pain, as well as improve the immune response in patients with certain types of cancers.

- Regular practice of meditation may increase the volume of cerebral gray matter and slow age-related declines in cognitive function.

- Regular meditation practice may lead to reduced substance use, including less use of alcohol and tobacco.

- There is suggestive evidence that mindfulness meditation can lead to personal growth, improvements in self-compassion, and improved satisfaction in marital relationships.

- Biofeedback has been successfully applied to a wide variety of disorders and health conditions though its empirically validated best efficacy applications are limited to a narrow number of conditions.

- The use of EMG biofeedback for tension-type headache and blood-volume-pulse feedback or hand warming for migraine headache are some of biofeedback's best success stories.

- Other interesting applications of biofeedback include hand-warming feedback for Raynaud's disease and Raynaud's phenomenon and biofeedback-assisted relaxation training for essential hypertension.

- In considering biofeedback treatment, one should weigh cost and efficacy factors in relation to other behavioral treatments.

CRITICAL THINKING QUESTIONS

1. In what ways do you think the state achieved during mantra meditation is similar or different from the state achieved during a deep relaxation exercise such as progressive muscle relaxation training?

2. Of the different theories of how mantra meditation achieves its effects, which one do you believe is most plausible? Why? Which one do you believe is most implausible? Why?

3. What do you consider to be the key differences between mindfulness-based approaches to dealing with stress and mantra meditation approaches? How are they similar?

4. If you were to adopt a regular practice of meditation, which approach would you use, mantra or mindfulness? Why?

5. Why would biofeedback be affectionately called the *electronic guru*? What are its advantages and disadvantages over the practice of meditation?

KEY TERMS AND CONCEPTS

Acceptance and commitment therapy (ACT)

Asanas*

Biofeedback*

Biofeedback-assisted relaxation training*

Blank-out theory

Blood-volume-pulse feedback*

Breath awareness

Clinically standardized meditation (CSM)

Concentrative meditation*

Decenter*

Defuse*

Desensitization theory

Dialectical behavior therapy (DBT)

Direct targeted approach

Disengage

Efficacious

Electromyograph (EMG)*

Empirically supported therapy

Enhanced receptivity

General relaxation

Greater balance between the two cerebral hemispheres

Guided meditation

Hand warming

Hatha yoga*

Hypometabolic state*

Ineffability

Loving kindness meditation therapy

Mantra*

Mantra meditation

Meta-cognition*

Mindful way

Mindfulness meditation*

Mindfulness-based cognitive therapy (MBCT)

Mindfulness-based stress reduction (MBSR)

Mini-meditations

Nonconcentrative meditation*

Observing self*

Open awareness

Perceptual distortions

Pranayama*

Present-centeredness

Psychological flexibility

Psychophysiology*

Raja yoga

Raynaud's phenomenon (RP)*

Relaxation response

Relaxation response meditation

Rhythm theory

Samadhi

Secular meditation

Self-transcendence

Stress management training

Time distortion

Transcendental Meditation (TM)*

Vipassana meditation*

Yoga

Zen Buddhist meditation (Zazen)

MEDIA RESOURCES

CENGAGE**brain**.com

Access an interactive eBook, chapter-specific interactive learning tools, including flashcards, quizzes, videos, and more in your Psychology CourseMate, accessed through CengageBrain.com.

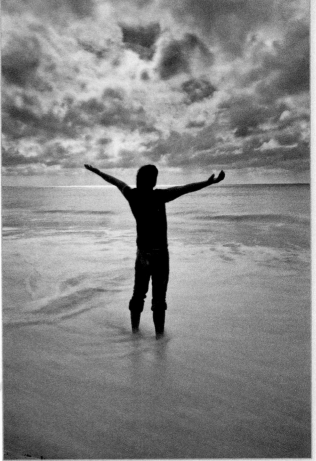

© Istockphoto.com/Maria Pavlova

"One day your life will flash before your eyes.
Make sure it's worth watching."

~ANONYMOUS

GUIDELINES FOR STRESS MANAGEMENT AND WELL-BEING ENHANCEMENT

LIVING A HEALTHY LIFESTYLE

USE EFFECTIVE COPING AND
SELF-REGULATION STRATEGIES

FOSTERING POSITIVE RELATIONSHIPS

ENHANCING HAPPINESS
AND WELL-BEING

■ STRESS MANAGEMENT EXERCISE 15.1
Seligman's (2011) What-Went-Well Exercise

Imagine, just imagine that you are 90 years old. How do you feel? Do you feel vibrant, energetic, and full of life? If so, what are your secrets? How did you live your life to reach this milestone while maintaining a high quality of life? Did you live a health-conscious life? Did you use effective coping and self-regulation strategies to manage your stress? Has your life been filled with purpose and meaning? Have you experienced your share of flow? How about mindfulness and savoring? Have you been able to hold on to those positive moments of enjoyment and satisfaction and savor them? Have you fostered positive relationships? Do you feel loved? Have you loved in return? Do you give social support and feel it from those around you? Are gratitude, forgiveness, and compassion important to you? Do you forgive yourself and others for missteps? Can you show compassion to yourself when you stumble? Have you been able to seek help and guidance from others when you could benefit, and help others in turn who seek your counsel? Have you consistently nourished your body and spirit? Has your life been well lived?

LIVING A HEALTHY LIFESTYLE

health-conscious living: to live with full awareness of how the choices we make affect our health.

When you imagine living a health-conscious life, what does it look like? What do you see yourself doing? What did you do in the past that you are no longer doing? **Health-conscious living** means being fully aware of the choices we make and how they affect our health. It involves taking responsibility for both our good and bad health-related choices. Just like caring for a car, when our vehicle has low mileage we can neglect or even abuse it without adversely affecting its performance or structural integrity. However, in time, the cumulative damage of redlining the engine and neglecting oil changes begins to show. Your car will start to run a little rougher. One day you may notice a few drops of shiny oil under your car. When you crank up the engine you see wisps of white smoke blowing out the tailpipe. Likewise, as we put some real miles on our bodies, we may start to experience them running a little rougher and slower. You notice you have lower energy, some creeping joint or back pains, and easy fatigue. If you smoke, you will likely feel plagued by an annoying hack each morning that does not go away until later in the day. These are the early warning signs that portend more serious problems. We can trade in our used car and get a new one, but what do we do with a worn-out body?

Luckily, our bodies are remarkably forgiving and will rebound to better health if given half a chance. Our bodies come with no owner's manual or recommended maintenance schedule. However, if we follow a few basic principles we can keep our endowments, these amazing gifts of nature, in optimal running condition. What are these principles? A body needs proper fuel, exercise, and restoration as well as protection from abuse and unnecessary damage. Doing this is a lifetime commitment. Just as we would not change our car oil once or twice and forget about it, we would not follow our body's maintenance schedule once or twice and then throw in the towel.

You may be thinking, "I'll be okay because I had an Uncle Charlie who outlived everyone around him in spite of his bad habits." Every family has an Uncle Charlie who ate a bowl of nails for breakfast, smoked unfiltered cigarettes, knocked back a fifth of Jack Daniels every day, and lived to a ripe old age to tell us about it. He was one lucky guy. He beat the odds. Most of us will not. Rather than depend exclusively on Uncle Charlie's exceptional luck, we can make choices that boost our odds to favorable levels through health-conscious living.

What this entails is following a healthy lifestyle. It does not mean *perfectly* following a prescriptive life, but rather allowing for our human imperfections with self-compassion while giving our best effort to make responsible choices. It may involve a lot of stumbles before we figure out what works best for us. That is okay. Ultimately, each person is unique, and, therefore, each person's healthy lifestyle manual is unique. If we can discern the blueprint of our unique manual we are ahead of the game. Then implementing the maintenance plan becomes part of daily living.

Health-conscious daily living involves a process of replacing counterproductive habits with new productive ones. As Aristotle said, "We are what we repeatedly do. Excellence then is not an act, but a habit." This process takes time. In time and with a lot of practice, the new habits become part of your identity. Be patient, be persistent, and you will get there. It may involve some effort and sacrifice—as do most worthwhile things in life. However, this endeavor has positive qualities and payoffs. Be mindful of the fun, the good feelings, and the payoffs, and it will all be worthwhile.

Nutrition

When it is time to fill your car's tank with gasoline, do you fill it with diesel? Why not? Although the answer is obvious, many people eat foods their bodies are not designed to burn when they would never treat their vehicles the same way. Yes, high-fat sugar snacks taste good, and we may be entitled to a little indulgence. However, if we have a steady diet of these foods, we may temporarily feel good but our body's engine will feel sorely used. The right fuel can reduce low-density lipoproteins (LDL), increase high-density lipoproteins (HDL), reduce coronary heart disease and cancer risk, and generally afford some protection against the diseases of aging. What general dietary principles then can we follow to maximize our health benefits?

- **Maintain good nutrition.** Follow the most current guidelines of the Institute of Medicine's Food and Nutrition Board (2002): For optimal health you should consume 45% to 65% of your total dietary intake from carbohydrates, 10% to 35% from protein, and 20% to 35% from fats; and take a daily multivitamin/multimineral to provide you with a

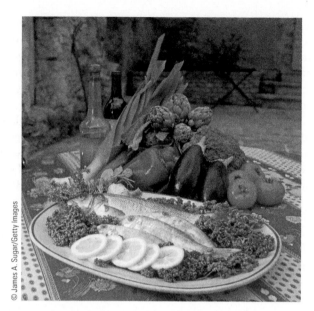

© James A. Sugar/Getty Images

A pescovegetarian eating plan consists primarily of a plant-based diet that includes fish but excludes red meat and poultry.

micronutrient insurance policy. Pay special attention to selenium, folic acid, vitamin B$_{12}$, and vitamin D.

- **Eat more functional foods.** Consume a "rainbow diet" of multicolored fruits and vegetables to increase your fiber, beneficial phytochemicals, and antioxidants. Eat more nuts and whole grains containing cereal fiber. Use monounsaturated and polyunsaturated fats to satisfy your body's dietary fat needs. Eat more fatty marine fish, selecting those with low mercury content, or take fish oil supplements. Consider a plant-based diet that includes marine fish, a *pescovegetarian diet,* if you want to maximize your health through diet (Walsh, 2011). Remember, other empirically documented healthy eating plans include the DASH (dietary approaches to stop hypertension), Mediterranean-style, and strict vegetarian patterns. Add foods like tomatoes; green tea; garlic; onions; soy; turmeric; grapes and berries such as strawberries, raspberries, and blueberries; citrus; and cruciferous vegetables such as cabbage, broccoli, kale, and Brussels sprouts to your diet for their potential anticancer properties.

- **Eat less of foods that can harm your health.** Reduce animal (saturated) fats, red and processed meats, and foods with added sugar and excess sodium. Limit white rice, refined grains, pasta, bread, potatoes, sugary drinks, and desserts. Avoid altogether foods that contain trans-fats. If you drink, keep alcohol consumption to moderate levels—no more than one drink per day for women and two per day for men. Remember, it is unlikely that you have Uncle Charlie's iron constitution or luck even if you were born under a shamrock.

pescovegetarian diet: a plant-based eating plan that also includes fish.

- **Reduce caffeine to reduce the physiological effects of stress.** Drink beverages like water, natural fruit juices, or green tea. Remember green tea is low in caffeine and high in beneficial polyphenols. It also is available in a decaffeinated form.

- **Reduce excess calorie intake.** Maintain a caloric balance to reduce long-term accumulation of fat stores. Excess fat is proinflammatory. Because many of the diseases of aging are stoked by the "fire inside," why fan the flames with unnecessary fat deposits? Reducing weight means dropping 500 calories a day from your menu. For some, that is a matter of giving up two 20-ounce colas a day and substituting them with water or green tea. Dropping 500 calories a day will result in a loss of 1 pound per week. That is 52 pounds in a year!

- **Give up tobacco use.** If you use tobacco in any form, select a quit day and do not look back. If you relapse, try again. The more times you quit, the better you get. Ultimately, you will figure out how to quit for good.

Physical Exercise

Move it or lose it. Our muscles are made for use. As we age, we lose about a half pound of muscle each year unless we exercise. The less muscle we have, the less calorie-burning mass we have. This, in turn, leads to a greater tendency toward weight gain. There are numerous health and psychological benefits of physical exercise. These include reduced risk for all-cause mortality, cardiovascular disease, breast and colon cancer, type 2 diabetes, stroke, hypertension, osteoporosis, stress, anxiety, and depression. In addition, cardiorespiratory fitness enhances psychological well-being. A combination of moderate aerobic exercise and light resistance training is the antidote. To keep our bodies fit, we can do the following:

- **Engage in moderate-intensity aerobic exercise.** If you are a *sedentarian,* become an *activarian*—rouse your active vibrant self. Select an activity that you like the most and that you are likely to continue. Start slow and work up to 150 minutes of moderate-intensity aerobic exercise a week. Alternatively, if you meet the health requirements, cut the time in half by engaging in 75 minutes of vigorous activity per week.

- **Start a 10,000-step program.** If you feel more comfortable weaving your activity throughout your day rather than through scheduled physical exercise sessions, try the daily 10,000 steps program. The first thing to do is buy a step counter or pedometer. Take your baseline during week 1 and then gradually work up to a 10,000-step-per-day goal after several weeks.

- **Engage in light resistance training.** Twice a week engage in light resistance training to keep your upper body muscles toned and active. These muscles tend to get less of a workout during most types of aerobic exercise so engaging the upper body muscles helps to prevent their age-related muscle loss.

Restoration

Our bodies need time to recharge and restore. We can accomplish this primarily through getting adequate sleep and sufficient relaxation. Sleep and relaxation have different restorative functions. For example, a person can sleep 10 hours a day and still be stressed-out when awake.

An inverse situation is when we are sleep deprived but relaxed. Eventually, we will nod off even as we try to stay awake. No amount of deep relaxation will substitute for the hours of missed sleep. Sleep deprivation is associated with increased blood pressure, appetite and weight gain (through reducing the hunger-suppressing hormone leptin), sympathetic nervous system activation, inflammation, and elevation of evening cortisol levels; epidemiological studies also indicate that it may be linked to early mortality, cardiovascular disease, and diabetes (Sigurdson & Ayas, 2007). Recall that shift work is linked to higher cardiovascular risk, and night work with an elevated risk of breast cancer and colorectal cancer. One of the restorative functions of sleep appears to be to regulate the immune system. Chronic sleep deprivation leads to proinflammatory cytokine production and expression. What then is a good lifestyle practice for getting sufficient restoration?

- **Get between 7 and 8 hours of sleep a night.** Epidemiological studies indicate that the Goldilocks amount of sleep is between 7 and 8 hours (Sigurdson & Ayas, 2007). Too much or too little sleep increases mortality and morbidity risk. See Table 15.1 for a list of good sleep hygiene practices by sleep experts Pigeon and Perlis (2008).

- **Practice deep relaxation exercises at least 20 minutes twice a day.** Practicing deep relaxation exercises reduces stress hormone levels, blood pressure, fatigue, headaches, and insomnia as well as increases energy. The ideal amount of time is 20 minutes twice a day, but some find it difficult to weave this into their daily routines, especially if they are already engaged in daily physical exercise. If you are pressed for time, you may first need to employ time management strategies. At a minimum, aim for a once a day deep relaxation session. However, if you find that even your best efforts do not succeed, try doing the exercise at night when you are lying in bed getting ready to sleep. Stay awake during the practice. However, once you finish, you have the added benefit of your deep relaxation easing you into your night's sleep.

- **Meditate.** A viable alternative to practicing deep relaxation strategies is meditation. Like deep relaxation, meditation ideally involves 20 minutes twice a day. Mini-meditations throughout the day also can be useful. Similar to deep relaxation, the practice of meditation can reduce stress and anxiety symptoms. It also may reduce chronic pain, improve immune responses, increase the volume of cerebral gray matter, and slow declines in age-related cognitive function.

TABLE **15.1**   Pigeon and Perlis's (2008) recommendations for good sleep hygiene practices

1. *Sleep only as much as you need to feel refreshed during the following day.* Restricting your time in bed helps to consolidate and deepen your sleep. Excessively long tiimes in bed lead to fragmented and shallow sleep. Get up at your regular time the next day, no matter how little you slept.

2. *Get up at the same time each day, 7 days a week.* A regular wake time in the morning leads to regular times of sleep onset, and helps to set your "biological clock."

3. *Exercise regularly.* Schedule exercise times so that they do not occur within 3 hours of when you intend to go to bed. Exercise makes it easier to initiate sleep and deepen sleep.

4. *Make sure your bedroom is comfortable and free from light and noise.* A comfortable, noise-free sleep environment will reduce the likelihood that you will wakeup during the night. Noise that does not awaken you may also disturb the quality of your sleep. Carpeting, insulated curtains, and closing the door may help.

5. *Make sure that your bedroom is at a comfortable temperature during the night.* Excessively warm or cold sleep environments may disturb sleep.

6. *Eat regular meals and do not go to bed hungry.* Hunger may disturb sleep. A light snack at bedtime (especially carbohydrates) may help sleep, but avoid greasy or "heavy" foods.

7. *Avoid excessive liquids in the evening.* Reducing liquid intake will minimize the need for nighttime trips to the bathroom.

8. *Cut down on all caffeine products.* Caffeinated beverages and foods (coffee, tea, cola, chocolate) can cause difficulty falling asleep, awakenings during the night, and shallow sleep. Even caffeine early in the day can disrupt nighttime sleep.

9. *Avoid alcohol, especially in the evening.* Although alcohol helps tense people fall asleep more easily, it causes awakenings later in the night.

10. *Smoking may disturb sleep.* Nicotine is a stimulant. Try not to smoke during the night when you have trouble sleeping.

11. *Don't take your problems to bed.* Plan some time earlier in the evening for working on your problems or planning the next day's activities. Worrying may interfere with initiating sleep and produce shallow sleep.

12. *Train yourself to use the bedroom only for sleeping and sexual activity.* This will help condition your brain to see bed as the place for sleeping. Do *not* read, watch TV, or eat in bed.

13. *Do not try to fall asleep.* This only makes the problem worse. Instead, turn on the light, leave the bedroom, and do something different like reading a book. Don't engage in stimulating activity. Return to bed only when you are sleepy.

14. *Put the clock under the bed or turn it so that you can't see it.* Clock watching may lead to frustration, anger, and worry, which interfere with sleep.

15. *Avoid naps.* Staying awake during the day helps you to fall asleep at night.

SOURCE: Pigeon, W. R., & Perlis, M. L. (2008), Cognitive behavioral treatment of insomnia in W. O'Donohue & J. E. Fisher (Eds.), *Cognitive Behavior Therapy: Applying Empirically Supported Techniques in Your Practice*, 2nd ed., p. 289, table 36.1. Hoboken, NJ: John Wiley & Sons. Used by permission of John Wiley & Sons, Inc.

USE EFFECTIVE COPING AND SELF-REGULATION STRATEGIES

Most of us would like to cope more effectively with stress, experience less distress and more eustress. Yet, like lifestyle concerns, we were not born with a personalized stress management manual. We have had to figure it out on our own. As you know, there are many factors that influence how we respond to stressors, including temperament and personality variables. As Antonovsky

(1987) proposed, stressors are not inherently pathogenic but rather create tension. Depending on how we manage this tension, we will move toward the negative entropic end of the health continuum or the positive salutary end. Our challenge then is to learn to accept and adapt to our stress-filled environments so that we can move toward the salutary end of the health continuum. In order to do this, we need to be able to recognize what stresses us, step outside ourselves and observe our reactions, and develop coping skills for dealing with these stressors.

Part of learning how to cope with stressors is learning how to self-regulate. The process of **self-regulation** involves setting standards and goals and then guiding yourself toward these goals while maintaining your internal standards. If your goal is to manage your stress better, then learning your unique stressors and applying the tools described in this book to determine what works will begin the process. Approaching it as an active participant rather than just an intellectual exercise is the only way to get the feedback you need to determine what works. Failure and setbacks are a normal part of this experiential learning process but so is success. Success comes with persistence and ongoing learning through feedback. As you become more successful, you will see yourself as a more competent and resourceful stress manager. Your self-efficacy will increase when you can get the saber-toothed tigers of your mind to purr occasionally and even roll over for a belly rub.

What then are some of the core strategies you can apply to cope with stress and improve self-regulation? Laying a good foundation with the lifestyle factors of sound nutrition, physical exercise, and restorative practices is essential. Upon this platform you can build a number of stress-busting approaches. What follows are some of the core elements.

self-regulation: setting standards and goals and then guiding oneself toward these goals while maintaining one's internal standards.

- **Self-monitor.** Keep a stress log and record your stress intensity levels 3 times a day (morning, afternoon, and evening) for several weeks. Identify your primary stressors. Record any physiological, emotional, mental, or behavioral reactions you may experience to these stressors. For example, you may note in the morning that your stress level is an 8 on a 10-point scale because you will be giving a speech in the afternoon. You notice that you have a queasy stomach and a tense neck, you are feeling anxious, worried, and are fidgeting.

  Once you identify how you respond to your stressors, use the information to cue you when to employ specific stress management strategies. For example, you could implement a plan where when your stress level reaches a 5, you will do a minimum of 2 minutes of abdominal breathing. Alternatively, when you notice a particular physiological signal such as a tense neck, it is time to do a 5-minute brief relaxation exercise (see Chapter 13).

- **Use abdominal (diaphragmatic) breathing.** Breathing is a powerful yet underestimated self-regulatory tool. Abdominal breathing helps reduce diffuse physiological arousal associated with the fight-or-flight response. When you feel the day's stress start to build, use this strategy to unwind some of the tension you feel.

- **Challenge negative thinking.** Why unnecessarily multiply the number of saber-toothed tigers in your mind? Get a handle on how many there are, how big they are, and how dangerous they are with the triple column method. They may be pussycats that are easy to deal with once you see them more realistically.

- **Be flexible when using coping strategies.** Think of your coping strategies as a collection of tools you carry in your toolbox. Keep a lot of tools in your toolbox and learn how and when to use them.

  As a general rule, in most situations reach for approach coping tools (engagement coping) before avoidance coping tools (disengagement coping). Recall that dispositional optimists are more prone to use approach strategies over avoidance strategies (Nes & Segerstrom, 2006). This tendency may account for some of the many positive health and well-being benefits associated with optimism.

- **Learn how to be a realistic optimist.** As Seligman (1990) demonstrated, optimism can be learned. Optimism has many advantages over pessimism for coping with stress and promoting subjective and physical well-being. It also may protect against our biological inflammatory response to stress. Realistic optimism (Schneider, 2001) is expecting good things to happen while employing appropriate reality checks.

- **Manage hostility and anger.** There is little doubt that chronic excess hostility and anger damage interpersonal relationships and raise the risk of adverse health consequences, including coronary heart disease (CHD) and early death. Use anger management strategies such as taking responsibility, using humor, examining intentions, practicing deep breathing and relaxation exercises, taking time-outs, challenging anger-building cognitions, empathizing, being assertive, and practicing forgiveness.

- **Get treatment for clinical depression.** Depression not only adversely affects psychological well-being, but also physical health. It seems to stimulate the promotion of proinflammatory cytokines and also increases the risk of cardiovascular disease and cardiac death.

  See your physician to first rule out any underlying medical conditions that can cause depression symptoms. There are many effective pharmacological and psychological treatments for major depressive disorder. Remember also to engage in aerobic exercise, reduce or eliminate alcohol, get social, and challenge negative thinking.

- **Deal with work stress and burnout.** There is substantial evidence that work stress and burnout contribute to the development of cardiovascular risk including myocardial infarction (MI). Working nights and long-hour schedules also increases risk of an MI. Night work is associated with an increased risk of developing some types of cancer. Therefore, when feasible, it is prudent to change schedules away from the night shift, reduce work hours if they are excessive, and deal with work stress using the tools we use for other types of stress. If all else fails, look for another job. Your health is too important, and without it you will not have a job.

Employ good self-care strategies to prevent burnout, including staying self-aware, using humor, sharing quality time with friends and family, setting limits and boundaries, engaging in wellness behaviors, enjoying leisure activities such as vacations, and practicing spiritual beliefs.

- **Use time management.** When you feel overwhelmed by demands, remember to go back to the basics of good time management. Prioritize, follow the Pareto principle, set boundaries, manage technostresss, and delegate when feasible and appropriate. Use assertiveness to say "no" more often to reduce piling on of new tasks. Remember, the idea is to work more efficiently rather than harder.

- **Take time for recreation.** As Walsh (2011) notes, recreation involves play, playfulness, humor, art, music, relaxation, exercise, time in nature, and social interaction—activities that mitigate stress and cultivate positive feelings. Find what you enjoy doing and spend time doing it.

FOSTERING POSITIVE RELATIONSHIPS

Love, compassion, empathy, altruism, forgiveness, and gratitude all serve to bring us closer together, to forge bonds, and to strengthen connections. These are ageless themes taken up recently by positive psychologists that add greater meaning and purpose to the stress and health construct of social support. Social support is a vital source of sustenance that protects our health and nourishes our well-being. Even a man as hardy as Uncle Charlie probably would not survive to a ripe old age without the love and support of his family. As *National Geographic*'s author of the *Blue Zones*, Dan Buettner (2008, p. 52) writes concerning the high number of centenarians living in Sardinia, "all the centenarians I met told me *la famiglia* was the most important thing in their lives—their purpose in life." Steger (2009, p. 683) similarly concludes from reviewing the research on life's meaning that "most people have indicated that relationships with others are the most important source of meaning in their lives."

That said, we also know that relationships can be a double-edged sword if they engender more social strain than social support. How, then, can we foster positive healthy relationships?

- **Promote good feelings through positive reciprocity.** Genuinely expressing how much we like each other's positive qualities and behaviors promotes good feelings. We all enjoy being recognized for our positive contributions. Acknowledging these contributions engenders good feelings, which in turn increases feelings of closeness.

- **Convey empathy.** Empathy can be conveyed through active listening. Actively feeding back what you believe the message is from the communicator helps that person feel understood. This may include attempting to identify the emotions the other person is feeling. When we feel understood, we also feel a sense of connection and closeness.

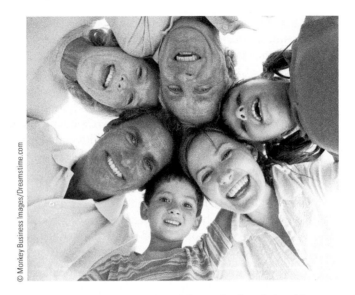

Our social relationships, especially our family relationships, are an important source of purpose and meaning in life.

- **Use whole clear messages.** A whole clear message is not contaminated by subtext. It respectfully conveys your observations, thoughts, feelings, and needs. Whole clear messages use clean communication and are conducive to working through differences and getting your needs met.

- **Define boundaries and set limits.** Use assertiveness skills to define what you will agree to or accept from others and what you will not. In some cases the broken record technique is an appropriate response to a perceived boundary infringement. Setting limits often means saying "no" more often in a respectful and diplomatic way.

- **Use minimally effective responses.** When standing your ground and communicating assertively, use minimally effective responses. Consider the minimal level of assertion that can accomplish your objectives. Then if this is not effective, gradually escalate from there. Keep your response proportional to the event. There is no need to drive a nail with a sledge-hammer. A regular hammer will do just fine and is less likely to splinter the wood you are driving the nail into.

- **Negotiate.** Informal negotiations are a normal part of all close relation-ships. Negotiations help to resolve differences and facilitate the various parties getting their needs met. If you reach an impasse, remember to take a time-out and revisit the issue later. Taking a time-out helps to cool frustrations and provides space for perspective taking. Persistence is a key ingredient to success.

- **Detriangulate.** If you find yourself being pulled into the drama triangle, step out of it. Do not become a participant in someone else's game. Recognize the different roles involved and be yourself rather than follow a game script. Deal with parties directly rather than through a third person. Expect others to do the same and assertively stand your ground when they try to pull you into the middle of their conflict.

- **Express gratitude.** Expressing gratitude is a prosocial behavior that promotes good feelings, enhances social relationships, and increases your well-being. It enables you to savor more fully the benefits of positive actions taken by others on your behalf. In addition, people tend to like grateful people and are more likely to give them social rewards. So people who express appreciation and gratitude give social rewards and are more likely to receive them in kind.

     To illustrate the positive benefits of expressing gratitude we can look at a study (Seligman, Steen, Park, & Peterson, 2005) that found that nonclinical participants who wrote a letter of gratitude and delivered it in person to someone who had not been properly thanked felt happier and less depressed than placebo controls. The gains persisted for up to 1 month.

- **Practice forgiveness.** Forgiveness is a prosocial tool for relationship restoration. People who practice forgiveness are better able to derive benefits from social support. They also are more likely to experience higher levels of well-being. In addition, more forgiving personalities are less likely to experience negative affect such as anger, anxiety, and depression. Remember to practice self-forgiveness as well.

- **Help others.** The practice of helping others benefits both the person giving and the person receiving the help. As Walsh (2011, p. 9) notes, "altruism is said to reduce unhealthy mental qualities such as greed, jealousy, and egocentricity while enhancing healthy qualities such as love, joy, and generosity." Just as Ebenezer Scrooge experienced greater buoyancy and health after becoming more generous, research indicates that practicing kindness, compassion, and generosity often leads to greater health, well-being, and longevity (Post, 2005). In fact, engaging in acts of altruism can be so rewarding that it can lead to a "helper's high" (Luks, 1988). Even small acts of kindness may be uplifting.

     A caveat regarding altruism is that if the effort and time spent helping is too overtaxing it will cancel out the beneficial effects for the giver (Post, 2005). Further, service motivated by duty or obligation may not result in improved well-being for the helper (Walsh, 2011). Some forms of long-term caregiving (e.g., long-term care for a loved one with dementia) can even result in health impairment and diminished well-being (see Chapter 4). This is not to discourage some forms of altruism because altruism in the form of long-term caregiving, for example, is the ultimate form of virtuous giving, but rather to highlight the potential risks and benefits involved when undertaking altruistic endeavors.

- **Allow others to help you.** The ability to receive love is just as important as the ability to give it. Everyone at times needs help and compassion whether it is from a family member, a friend, or someone else; the capacity to accept help is an important attribute for reducing stress and fostering

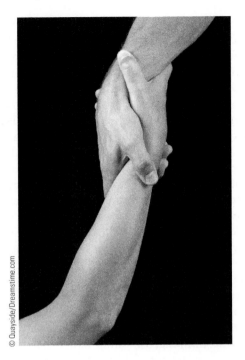

© Quayside/Dreamstime.com

Helping others and allowing others to help you promotes greater reciprocal well-being. Can you think of a time when you experienced a "helper's high" as a result of your act of kindness or altruism?

positive relationships. If needed, allowing others to help you may involve seeking and receiving professional counseling. Reaching out for professional counseling is not a sign of weakness, but rather shows courage and strength of character. It is not easy to acknowledge vulnerability, but doing so is the first step toward establishing a supportive positive relationship with a professional who can help you through a life difficulty.

ENHANCING HAPPINESS AND WELL-BEING

If we want to live the *good life*, is it sufficient to minimize the effects of stress in our life? If we minimize negative affect, does it necessarily follow that we will experience happiness and well-being? As you know, subtracting negative affect at best brings us to a neutral state. We have to add positive affect and build on those good feelings if we want to achieve happiness and well-being. As Seligman (2011, p. 57) states, "if we want to flourish and if we want to have well-being, we must indeed minimize our misery; but in addition, we must have positive emotion, meaning, accomplishment, and positive relationships." He further notes that before the advent of positive psychology, as a psychotherapist he had success helping his patients get rid of many of their feelings of sadness, anxiety, and anger, but he did not necessarily get a happy patient. As he laments, "I got an empty patient. That is because the skills of enjoying positive emotions, being engaged with people you care about, having meaning in life, achieving your work goals, and maintaining good relationships are entirely different from the skills of not being depressed, not being anxious, and not being angry" (Seligman, 2011, p. 168). What then are these skills and how can we develop them?

Many of these skills and behaviors are the ones we previously covered in the sections of this chapter that dealt with lifestyle, coping and self-regulation, and positive relationships. Noticeable standouts that promote good feelings or positive relationships are physical exercise, optimism, recreation, positive reciprocity, empathy, gratitude, forgiveness, and altruism. By employing these and other similar skills and behaviors, we can influence up to 40% of our overall happiness, or what Sonja Lyubomirsky (2007, p. 20) calls "the 40% solution." Recall that empirical findings suggest that 40% of our happiness is determined by intentional activity, 10% from life circumstances, and 50% from our happiness set point. What then do the positive psychology experts suggest we do to enhance our happiness and well-being?

Pioneer Michael Fordyce (1977, 1981, 1983), one of the first researchers to develop a program designed to increase personal happiness, attempted to answer this question. Based on his research, Fordyce (1983, p. 517) recommends practicing what he calls the "14 fundamentals of personal happiness": "(a) spend more time socializing, (b) strengthen your closest relationships, (c) develop an outgoing, social personality, (d) be a better friend, (e) work on a healthy personality, (f) lower expectations and aspirations, (g) develop positive, optimistic thinking, (h) value happiness, (i) become more active, (j) become involved in meaningful work, (k) get better organized and plan things out, (l) develop your 'present orientation,' (m) reduce negative feelings, and (n) stop worrying." In a series of studies, Fordyce (1977, 1983) found that compared to placebo controls, students who participated in his program showed greater elevations in happiness.

In her book *The How of Happiness: A New Approach to Getting the Life You Want*, Sonja Lyubomirsky (2007, Foreword, pp. 2–3) spells out 12 activities for boosting happiness including (1) "expressing gratitude," (2) "cultivating optimism," (3) "avoiding overthinking and social comparison," (4) "practicing acts of kindness," (5) "nurturing social relationships," (6) "developing strategies for coping," (7) "learning to forgive," (8) "increasing flow experiences," (9) "savoring life's joys," (10) "committing to your goals," (11) "practicing religion and spirituality," and (12) "taking care of your body."

Positive psychology's initiator and organizer Martin E. P. Seligman also weighs in with ideas for boosting happiness and well-being through first delineating their core elements. In 2002 Seligman proposed a theory of **authentic happiness** consisting of three elements: (1) positive emotion, (2) engagement, and (3) meaning. By 2011 he broadened his focus and formulated a new perspective he labels **well-being theory.** As Seligman (2011, p. 23) states, "I used to think that the topic of positive psychology was happiness, that the gold standard for measuring happiness was life satisfaction, and that the goal of positive psychology was to increase life satisfaction. I now think that the topic of positive psychology is well-being, that the gold standard for measuring well-being is flourishing, and that the goal of positive psychology is to increase flourishing."

Seligman's (2011) well-being theory retains the three elements of (1) positive emotion, (2) engagement, and (3) meaning that define authentic happiness,

authentic happiness: Seligman's theory that happiness consists of positive emotions, engagement, and meaning.

well-being theory: Seligman's theory that well-being consists of positive emotions, engagement, meaning, positive relationships, and accomplishment.

but he adds two additional elements of (4) positive relationships and (5) accomplishment to his more broadly defined construct of well-being. *Positive emotion* is self-explanatory. *Engagement* refers to experiencing *flow*, of losing oneself in a challenging activity. Seligman defines *meaning* and *purpose in life* as factors that bring about service or belonging to something beyond the self. *Positive relationships* involve our connections with other people. Last, *accomplishment* refers to the act of achieving. Seligman believes that people often pursue achievements just to experience achieving, rather than necessarily using achievement as a means toward experiencing good feelings, flow, or meaning.

flourishing: a state of optimal functioning.

According to Seligman (2011), a person is **flourishing** when the five elements of positive emotion, engagement, meaning, positive relationships, and accomplishment are experienced in the upper range. To increase well-being, then, one must enhance these five elements.

Seligman's (2011) authentic happiness and well-being theories are anchored by his construct of **signature strengths.** These strengths are positive personality characteristics such as curiosity, judgment, integrity, fairness, self-control, spirituality, forgiveness, humor, and others that are central to our identities. Seligman (2002, p. 159) lists 24 signature strengths grouped into 6 virtue clusters of "wisdom and knowledge," "courage," "humanity and love," "justice," "temperance," and "transcendence" (Table 15.2). Each of us has a unique pattern of signature strengths.

signature strengths: personality characteristics that represent one's virtues such as curiosity, integrity, fairness, self-control, spirituality, forgiveness, and humor that are measured by the Values in Action Scale.

Once we know our strengths, Seligman recommends that we deploy them toward mastering life's challenges rather than exert too much energy shoring up our weaknesses. The process involves, first, identifying our signature strengths and, second, applying them toward reaching our goals, overcoming challenges, and building strong relationships. Seligman's Signature Strengths Test can be taken at http://www.authentichappiness.sas.upenn.edu. The test results present you with a rank order of your signature strengths. What then are some of the primary ways we can enhance happiness and well-being? Beyond promoting well-being, how can we move toward flourishing and thriving in the 21st century?

- **Play to your strengths.** Determine your unique virtues and strengths and use them to overcome challenges and reach your goals. For example, Seligman (2011) recounts that a sergeant was able to use his strengths of wisdom, love, and gratitude to help a soldier who created interpersonal conflicts because of problems the troubled soldier had in his marital relationship. The sergeant helped the soldier see his wife's perspective and encouraged him to send her a letter of gratitude thanking her for handling the challenges she experienced during his three deployments.

- **Practice mindfulness.** Mindfulness involves being attentive and aware of the present with acceptance. It means living life fully in the now— appreciating the moment. High mindfulness participants in studies exhibit less depression, anxiety, and negative affect; more positive affect; and higher self-esteem than their low mindfulness counterparts. Mindfulness practice encourages us to use our observing self to *decenter* disturbing or stressful thoughts so they have less emotional impact on

Table **15.2** Seligman's 24 signature strengths grouped into their 6 virtue clusters

Virtue and Strength	Definition
1. Wisdom and knowledge	Cognitive strengths that entail the acquisition and use of knowledge
Creativity	Thinking of novel and productive ways to do things
Curiosity	Taking an interest in all of ongoing experience
Open-mindedness	Thinking things through and examining them from all sides
Love of learning	Mastering new skills, topics, and bodies of knowledge
Perspective	Being able to provide wise counsel to others
2. Courage	Emotional strengths that involve the exercise of will to accomplish goals in the face of opposition, external or internal
Authenticity	Speaking the truth and presenting oneself in a genuine way
Bravery	*Not* shrinking from threat, challenge, difficulty, or pain
Persistence	Finishing what one starts
Zest	Approaching life with excitement and energy
3. Humanity	Interpersonal strengths that involve "tending and befriending" others
Kindness	Doing favors and good deeds for others
Love	Valuing close relations with others
Social intelligence	Being aware of the motives and feelings of self and others
4. Justice	Civic strengths that underlie healthy community life
Fairness	Treating all people the same according to notions of fairness and justice
Leadership	Organizing group activities and seeing that they happen
Teamwork	Working well as a member of a group or team
5. Temperance	Strengths that protect against excess
Forgiveness	Forgiving those who have done wrong
Modesty	Letting one's accomplishments speak for themselves
Prudence	Being careful about one's choices; *not* saying or doing things that might later be regretted
Self-regulation	Regulating what one feels and does
6. Transcendence	Strengths that forge connections to the larger universe and provide meaning
Appreciation of beauty and excellence	Noticing and appreciating beauty, excellence, and/or skilled performance in all domains of life
Gratitude	Being aware of and thankful for the good things that happen
Hope	Expecting the best and working to achieve it
Humor	Liking to laugh and tease; bringing smiles to other people
Religiousness	Having coherent beliefs about the higher purpose and meaning of life

Source: Seligman, M. E. P., Steen, T. A., Park, N., & Peterson, C. (2005), Positive psychology progress: Empirical validation of interventions. *American Psychologist, 60,* 410–421. Copyright American Psychological Association.

us. Mindfulness meditation practice is associated with a robust number of health and well-being benefits.

- **Savor the joys of life.** The more we savor, the more we develop the capacity to embrace the joys of life. Holding on to our positive experiences welcomes our positive emotions so that they stay longer to provide us with more happiness and life satisfaction. People with a strong capacity for savoring have more self-esteem and optimism as well as less neuroticism, depression, and guilt. Savoring involves not only

STRESS MANAGEMENT EXERCISE **15.1**

Seligman's (2011) What-Went-Well Exercise

This final stress management exercise is one of the most important because this simple exercise will strengthen your well-being muscles. Seligman (2011) calls this the What-Went-Well exercise. Set aside a few minutes each night for the next week and list three things that went well during that day. Next to each, write down why you think it went well.

Seligman (2011, p. 41) provides the following examples: "if you wrote that your husband picked up the ice cream, write 'because my husband is really thoughtful sometimes' or 'because I remembered to call him from work and remind him to stop by the grocery store.' Or if you wrote, 'My sister just gave birth to a healthy baby boy,' you might have picked as a cause 'God was looking out for her' or 'She did everything right during her pregnancy.'"

Seligman et al. (2005) found in a randomized placebo-controlled study that this simple exercise boosted happiness and reduced depression symptoms for up to 6 months. If you like the exercise and it works for you, continue to make it part of your daily routine and reap the benefits.

SOURCE: Seligman, M. E. P. (2011), *Flourish: A Visionary New Understanding of Happiness and Well-Being.* New York: Simon & Schuster.

appreciating positive moments when they happen, but also anticipating them in advance and reminiscing about them when they are over.

- **Achieve.** Set goals and pursue them. Lyubomirsky (2007) describes six benefits of pursuing your personal goals. Pursuing goals (1) provides us a sense of purpose and control, (2) boosts our self-esteem and increases our self-efficacy, (3) adds meaning and structure to our lives, (4) teaches us how to master use of our time, (5) develops our capacity to cope with challenges, and (6) connects us to other people and consequently forges social bonds. The Big Five personality trait of conscientiousness embodies the spirit and habit of goal pursuit and accomplishment and is associated with higher levels of well-being and longevity.

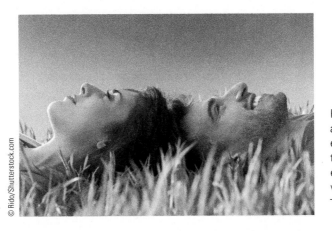

© Rido/Shutterstock.com

Practicing mindfulness as well as savoring enables us to embrace the joys of life and enhance our overall well-being.

- **Embrace flow experiences.** When we pursue goals, especially challenging ones that we are able to master through deploying our greatest strengths, we experience flow. This process of *engagement* leads to merging our consciousness with the event. The flow experience is intrinsically rewarding and presents a sense of deep satisfaction when we are done.

- **Cultivate your meaning and purpose.** Find your meaning and purpose in life. Recall that Antonovky's (1979, 1987) sense of coherence (SOC) model considers *meaning* the most important component of our worldview. Developing a strong SOC promotes resilience and positive mental and physical health. It also is associated with a reduced risk of early mortality.

  Meaning is the thread that ties the fabric of our life together into a coherent pattern. How you weave the tapestry and form the pattern is up to you. Whether it is through spirituality, religion, family, politics, or a cause that gives you a larger purpose and sense of transcendence, significance, and overarching aim in life, the key is to cultivate your meaning and purpose.

  Applying meaning to your coping repertoire through meaning-making coping is a valuable strategy for dealing with life's inevitable losses and tragedies. Reexamining life's meaning issues also plays a vital role in fostering posttraumatic growth if we have had the misfortune of encountering a traumatic stressor.

  It is worth revisiting Victor Frankl's (1992, p. 116) poignant counsel that, "we must never forget that we may also find meaning in life even when confronted with a hopeless situation, when facing a fate that cannot be changed. For what then matters is to bear witness to the uniquely human potential at its best, which is to transform personal tragedy into triumph, to turn one's predicament into a human achievement."

One final thought—remember, it is never too late to make important changes in your life. As Dr. Dale Turner (1989, p. C9) so eloquently expressed, "Dreams are renewable. No matter what our age or condition, there are still untapped possibilities within us and new beauty waiting to be born."

May you enjoy the journey of pursuing your dreams so that when you look back you can indeed answer, "yes, my life was well lived."

CHAPTER SUMMARY AND CONCEPT REVIEW

- Health-conscious living involves being fully aware of how our choices affect our health and taking responsibility for them.

- Living a healthy lifestyle involves maintaining good nutrition, eating more functional foods, eating fewer foods that can harm your health, reducing caffeine, consuming a caloric balance, discontinuing any tobacco use, engaging in moderate-intensity aerobic exercise or a 10,000-step program, engaging in light resistance training, getting between 7 and 8 hours of sleep a night, practicing deep relaxation exercises daily, and meditating.

- Self-regulation is the process of setting standards and goals and then guiding yourself toward these goals while maintaining your internal standards.

- Core strategies for coping with stress and improving self-regulation include self-monitoring, using abdominal breathing, challenging negative thinking, using coping strategies flexibly, learning to be a realistic optimist, managing hostility and anger, getting treatment for depression, dealing with work stress and burnout, using time management, and taking time for recreation.

- Strategies for fostering positive relationships include using positive reciprocity, conveying empathy, using whole clear messages, defining boundaries and setting limits, using minimally effective responses, negotiating, detriangulating, expressing gratitude, practicing forgiveness, helping others, and allowing others to help you.

- Both Michael Fordyce and Sonja Lyubomirsky offer a number of strategies for how to increase personal happiness.

- Martin E. P. Seligman's authentic happiness theory involves three elements, and his well-being theory, five elements; he suggests that reaching high levels of the five elements of positive emotion, engagement, meaning, positive relationships, and accomplishment leads to a state of flourishing.

- Seligman also stresses the importance of identifying and using your signature strengths.

- Strategies for enhancing happiness and well-being include playing to your strengths, practicing mindfulness, savoring the joys of life, achieving, embracing flow experiences, and cultivating your sense of meaning and purpose.

CRITICAL THINKING QUESTIONS

1. From which lifestyle strategy do you believe you could derive the most benefit? How? What is the first step you would need to take to implement this strategy?

2. What is the most important positive change you can make for coping with stress and improving your self-regulation? How could you go about implementing this change?

3. Of the different methods for fostering positive relationships, which one do you currently practice the most? Which one the least? What additional skill in fostering positive relationships would you most like to develop? How could you best develop this skill?

4. Do you agree with Seligman's theory that states there are five elements of well-being that include positive emotion, engagement, meaning, positive relationships, and accomplishment? Are there any elements you would add or subtract? Why? Explain. Do you agree that the goal of positive psychology should be to increase flourishing? If so, why? If not, why not?

5. If you were to write your personal prescription for flourishing and thriving, what would be your top five recommendations? Why would you select these five? Explain.

KEY TERMS AND CONCEPTS

Authentic happiness*	Health-conscious living*	Self-regulation*	Well-being theory*
Flourishing*	Pescovegetarian diet*	Signature strengths*	

MEDIA RESOURCES

CENGAGE**brain**.com

Access an interactive eBook, chapter-specific interactive learning tools, including flashcards, quizzes, videos, and more in your Psychology CourseMate, accessed through CengageBrain.com.

Abdominal breathing* Also known as diaphragmatic breathing; breathing that involves drawing the first part of the breath into the lower part of the lungs, which results in the abdomen expanding, and then the remaining breath into the upper part of the lungs, which results in the chest expanding.

Abstinence violation effect* A process whereby a person experiences a temporary relapse back to a previous habit or lifestyle and then uses all-or-nothing thinking to justify abandonment of the newly adopted habit or lifestyle.

Acceptance and commitment therapy (ACT) A mindfulness-based psychological intervention program designed to promote defusion, acceptance, experience of the present moment, connecting to values, and committed action to cultivate psychological flexibility.

Accommodation The process of changing the larger organizing schema so that the smaller one can fit within the new schema.

Acetylcholine The neurotransmitter used by all preganglionic neurons of the autonomic nervous system as well as the postganglionic neurons of the parasympathetic branch of the autonomic nervous system.

ACTH* Adrenocorticotropic hormone; released by the anterior pituitary and responsible for stimulating the adrenal cortex to release glucocorticoids.

Activating event The first phase of Ellis's ABC model that represents the stimulus event.

Active listening* A collaborative process of attending the message being conveyed by the communicator and then feeding back an understanding of the message.

Acute coronary syndrome (ACS) An umbrella term that refers to a range of sudden heart conditions such as myocardial infarction that result from restricted blood flow to the heart.

Adaptive immune system* Also known as the acquired or specific immune system, this slower but more advanced line of defense against antigens remembers past invaders and other antigens and consists of T-cytotoxic, T-helper, and B lymphocytes as well as immunoglobulins.

Adrenal cortex* The outer covering of the adrenal glands responsible for secreting corticosteroids.

Adrenal medulla* The inner core of the adrenal glands responsible for secreting the catecholamines epinephrine and norepinephrine.

Adrenals Cone-shaped glands that sit atop the kidneys that secrete the catecholamines epinephrine and norepinephrine as well as corticosteroids.

Aerobic* With air/oxygen.

Aerobic fitness Also known as cardiorespiratory fitness; refers to the ability of the body's heart, blood vessels, and lungs to supply oxygen-rich blood to the muscles during sustained physical activity.

Afferent Neural pathways that send signals from the periphery to the brain.

Affiliate According to the tend-and-befriend model, it is the process of seeking out others in order to form groups for joint protection against threat.

Agency A component of Snyder's hope model that refers to the motivational trait-like perception that a wide range of goals will be pursued.

Agoraphobia An anxiety disorder characterized by a fear of being in a public place or outside the home to the extent that it might be difficult to leave without embarrassment or to get help in the event of experiencing a panic attack.

Agreeableness* One of the Big Five traits with soft-hearted, trusting, and good-natured characteristics.

Alarm stage Selye's first stage of the general adaptation syndrome characterized by the fight-or-flight reaction.

Alcohol A drug found in beer, wine, and spirits that acts as a central nervous system depressant.

All cause mortality Indicates that death can be from any cause.

Allergic rhinitis (AR)* Also known as hay fever; involves allergic reactions to certain pollens, dust particles, or airborne chemicals.

Allostatic load* The cost the organism pays when subjected to chronic stressors.

Altruism The act of helping unselfishly.

Amino acids Molecular building blocks of proteins.

Amygdala* Region of the cerebral hemispheres and part of the limbic system responsible for mediating emotional responses, particularly fear and anxiety.

Anaerobic Without air/oxygen.

Anger The feeling state associated with (a) the "fight" component of the fight-or-flight response that can range from irritation to rage and (b) harm and blame appraisals in Lazarus's model.

Anger expression The behaviors associated with the feeling of anger.

Anger management Application of cognitive, relaxation, and social skills training to regulate anger.

Angina pectoris* Severe chest pain resulting from the heart receiving inadequate oxygen.

Anterior cingulate Region of the limbic system that plays a major role in the emotional control system because of its extensive connections with the thalamus and its connections with other parts of the limbic system.

Anterior pituitary Region of the pituitary that secretes beta-endorphin and adrenocorticotropic hormone (ACTH).

Antibodies Also known as immunoglobulins; soluble proteins produced by B cells that circulate in the bloodstream and bind to viruses and other antigens to neutralize them.

Antigens Toxins, substances, particles, cells, and organisms that pose a threat to one's physical well-being.

Antioxidants* Chemicals found in particular vitamins, minerals, and phytochemicals that reduce oxidative stress.

Anxiety Diffuse feelings of uneasiness related to perceived impending threats.

Anxiety disorder* A psychological disorder such as generalized anxiety disorder, panic disorder, phobic disorders, obsessive-compulsive disorder, and posttraumatic stress disorder in which anxiety is excessive and disabling.

Anxiety sensitivity* Fear and worry that one will experience anxiety or panic.

Appraisal A judgment about the relative significance of an event.

Approach coping* Using strategies to reduce or eliminate the stressor or its effects.

Arousal pathway system The neural network involving the reticular activating system responsible for vigilance and excitement of higher brain centers.

Arteriosclerosis A hardening and thickening of the arteries due to progressive degenerative arterial disease such as atherosclerosis.

Asanas* Different postural positions used by yoga practitioners.

Assimilation The process of adding new information to an already existing schema.

Asthma A chronic condition that has acute phases in which the respiratory system becomes inflamed and bronchial airways constrict.

Atherosclerosis* A progressive degenerative arterial disease characterized by a narrowing of blood flow through affected arteries due to the formation of arterial fibrous plaque layers.

Atopic dermatitis A condition characterized by a hypersensitivity of the skin to particular foods or environmental allergens that results in the skin becoming inflamed, feeling itchy, scaling, or flaking.

Atopic disorders* Health disorders characterized by biological hypersensitivity and inflammation such as asthma, allergic rhinitis, atopic dermatitis, and conjunctivitis.

Attributional retraining (AR)* Programs designed to change attributional explanatory styles to cultivate learned optimism or a greater sense of personal control over outcomes.

Attributions* Cognitions people use to explain why a person behaves a certain way.

Authentic happiness* Seligman's theory that happiness consists of positive emotions, engagement, and meaning.

Autogenic training* A deep relaxation strategy pioneered by Schultz that uses self-hypnosis/passive concentration to center on the autonomic nervous system.

Autohypnotic state* A self-generated hypnotic state.

Automatic negative thoughts* Distorted cognitions that occur almost reflexively and sometimes without awareness.

Autonomic nervous system The nervous system responsible for enervating the organ systems of the body.

Avoidance coping* Disengaging from the stressor or its effects.

Basal energy conservation and restoration state The body's state when it is harboring and resupplying its energy reserves.

B cells* Lymphocytic cells ("B" for bone marrow cells) of the adaptive immune system that produce antibodies.

Bedford College Life Events and Difficulties Schedule (LEDS) An assessment tool that measures cumulative life change stress with a semistructured interview and a panel of trained raters.

Behavioral approach system (BAS)* The system in Gray's reinforcement sensitivity theory that is sensitive to reward and fueled by the dopamine areas and circuits of the brain.

Behavioral inhibition system (BIS)* The system in Gray's reinforcement sensitivity theory that is sensitive to punishment or nonreward and is driven by the norepinephrine systems of the brain.

Behavioral medicine The field of study that applies elements of the behavioral sciences to illness prevention and treatment.

Beliefs The cognitive filters through which the activating event is perceived in Ellis's ABC model.

Benign-positive appraisals Primary appraisals in Lazarus's model that the event is neutral or pleasant.

Beta-endorphin The body's natural opiate that reduces pain sensations and creates feelings of euphoria.

Bicultural* Belonging to two cultures.

Big Five Also known as the Five Factor Model; the five relatively independent factors of neuroticism, extraversion, openness, conscientiousness, and agreeableness.

Big Three Eysenck's three independent factors known as supertraits or personality types of psychoticism, extraversion, and neuroticism.

Biofeedback* The use of a physiological recording device to present visual or auditory tracking information to participants so they can learn how to regulate targeted internal physiological responses.

Biofeedback-assisted relaxation training* Using biofeedback to promote a state of general relaxation.

Biological predisposition model Genetic or constitutional factors influence a person's physiological, emotional, behavioral, and cognitive responses to stress.

Biomedical model* A traditional model of health that assumes health is primarily a product of biological factors.

Biopsychosocial model* A newer model of health that assumes health is a product of biological, psychological, and social influences.

Blank-out theory A theory that mantra meditation achieves its beneficial effects by clearing and rebooting the sensory neurological circuitry.

Blood-volume-pulse feedback* Biofeedback in which changes in skin blood volume are measured with a noninvasive instrument called a photoelectric plethysmograph.

Body mass index (BMI)* An estimate of body fat based on a formula that uses height and weight.

Bottom-up theories of happiness The sum of our positive experiences determines our happiness levels.

Boundaries* One's physical and psychological space.

Brain stem Region of the brain consisting of the medulla oblongata, the pons, and the midbrain responsible for many of the vegetative functions of the body.

Breath awareness An object of focus of many types of meditation practices in which the focus of attention is on the breathing process.

Broaden-and-build* Fredrickson's model that explains the adaptive and evolutionary value of our positive emotions.

Broken record technique An assertiveness technique of making a statement repeatedly.

Bruxism* Involuntary habit of excessive teeth clenching or grinding that can lead to abrasive wear on the teeth, headaches, and/or temporomandibular pain and dysfunction syndrome.

Buffer The concept that a third variable such as a personality trait can reduce the impact of stressors.

Burnout* Emotional exhaustion and depletion due to ongoing stress with corollary physical and mental fatigue.

Caffeine A phytochemical that stimulates the body by lowering its neurons' thresholds of excitability.

Calorie imbalance* Consuming more calories than one expends or vice versa.

Cancer* An umbrella category of around 200 diseases involving endogenous abnormal cells developing, proliferating, and then invading the body's healthy tissues.

Cardiac muscle The heart muscle.

Cardiorespiratory fitness* Also known as aerobic fitness; refers to the ability of the body's heart, blood vessels, and lungs to supply oxygen-rich blood to the muscles during sustained physical activity.

Cardiovascular system Also known as the circulatory system; includes the heart and blood vessels of the body.

Catastrophize* To cognitively maximize the perceived negative consequences of an event.

Catechins Also known as flavonols; the primary polyphenols found in green tea.

Catecholamines Hormones that affect the cardiovascular system such as epinephrine and norepinephrine.

Catharsis theory* A discredited theory of anger management based on the concept that to reduce anger one should ventilate it periodically.

Causal attributions Cognitions people use to explain why a person behaves a certain way.

CD4 The molecule on the surface of T-helper cells that enables them to respond to the targeted antigen.

CD8 The molecule on the surface of T-cytotoxic cells that enables them to lock on to the targeted antigen.

Cellular-mediated immunity* The defense strategy employed by the human immune system involving the natural killer cells, the granulocytes, the macrophages, and T cells inflaming, phagocytosing, and releasing toxic substances.

Central nervous system (CNS) The spinal cord and the brain.

Cereal fiber A type of fiber found in whole grains.

Cerebral hemispheres Consist of the neocortex and the white matter beneath it, the basal ganglia, the amygdala, and the hippocampus; the two hemispheres are connected by the corpus callosum.

Challenge (a) An appraisal in Lazarus's model that potential harm-loss can be successfully met with one's coping abilities; (b) a component of the hardiness construct that concerns a sense that stress and change are catalysts for growth and personal development.

Cholesterol A sterol compound the body manufactures and uses as a component of its cell membranes and steroidal hormones.

Circadian rhythm* The 24-hour biological cycle linked to the light-dark cycle that regulates one's internal physiological processes.

Clarifying The process in active listening of asking for more information from the communicator in order to get a better understanding of the message being communicated.

Clinically standardized meditation (CSM) A programmed instruction in mantra meditation developed by Carrington.

Cognitive-behavioral therapy* A short-term cognitively oriented therapeutic approach that also uses behavioral strategies that is designed to challenge dysfunctional automatic thoughts, assumptions, and beliefs that sustain a particular disorder and to replace them with healthier realistic thinking patterns.

Cognitive model A model applied to the construct of stress that postulates that one's stress reactions are a result of the mental filters one uses to think about the stressors.

Cognitive primacy* The idea that cognitions influence how one responds to stress.

Cognitive restructuring* A technique used in cognitive-behavioral therapy of challenging dysfunctional automatic thoughts, assumptions, and beliefs and replacing them with healthier realistic thinking patterns.

Commitment A component of the hardiness construct indicating the degree to which one is deeply involved in one's life endeavors and true to one's self and values.

Compassion A feeling of sympathy people have when they witness suffering.

Complete mental health Keyes's system that characterizes good mental health as a combination of the absence of mental illness and presence of hedonia/positive functioning.

Complete proteins* Proteins that contain all the essential amino acids.

Complex carbohydrates* Also known as starches; consist of macronutrient long-chain glucose molecules.

Comprehensibility One of three factors that comprise Antonovsky's construct of sense of coherence that indicates the degree to which one can make cognitive sense of stimuli that one perceives.

Compulsions Behaviors or mental acts that are ritualistic and designed to reduce anxiety.

Concentrative meditation* A form of meditation that includes mantra meditation in which the strategy employed is to focus or concentrate on one stimulus.

Conscientiousness* One of the Big Five traits with characteristics such as ambitious, responsible, and hardworking.

Consequences The emotional and behavioral outcomes in Ellis's ABC model.

Constructive anger expression Assertively discussing one's upset in an

attempt to resolve the situation while considering the target of the anger's point of view.

Control (a) To exert influence or mastery; (b) a component of the hardiness construct that refers to one's ability to cope with difficulties and to have an influence on outcomes.

Control group The comparison group in an experimental study.

Coping* Effectively using resources and strategies to deal with potentially harmful or stressful internal or external demands.

Coping humor* Using humor to cope with stress.

Core relational meaning The meaning attached to an appraisal that is linked to a specific emotional response.

Coronary heart disease (CHD)* Also known as coronary artery disease; a progressive degenerative inflammatory disease involving atherosclerosis of the heart's arteries.

Coronary vascular disease (CVD) Also known as coronary heart disease; a progressive degenerative inflammatory disease involving atherosclerosis of the heart's arteries.

Correlational studies Also called observational studies; research studies that can determine the strength and direction of relationships between two or more variables but not their causal relationships.

Cortisol* The body's primary glucocorticoid secreted by the adrenal cortex during the fight-or-flight response that raises glucose levels in the bloodstream, increases catecholamine synthesis, and reduces inflammation.

Counterconditioning A learning process of replacing an unfavorable response with a favorable one represented in systematic desensitization by pairing threatening images with relaxation so that anxiety is replaced with a more benign response.

Crohn's disease (CD) An autoimmune disease characterized by swollen joints, skin rash, eye inflammation, and gastrointestinal inflammatory symptoms.

Cross-sectional design* A study that observes cohorts at only one point in time.

Cultures Interwoven fabric of values, beliefs, words, and customs reflected

in art, music, stories, and behaviors that are distinctive for groups.

Cynicism One of Maslach's three dimensions of burnout characterized by experiences of disillusionment, loss of idealism, negativity, detachment, hostility, and lack of concern.

Cytokines* Chemical messenger molecules sometimes thought of as hormones of the immune system that stimulate immune responses.

DASH (dietary approaches to stop hypertension) An eating pattern that emphasizes eating healthy foods and avoiding foods that sustain chronic high blood pressure.

Decenter* A mindfulness practice of becoming less reactive to one's inner experiences because the mind's activity is observed and the thoughts are seen as outside the center of the self.

Declarative memory Memory of events that can be consciously discussed.

Deep relaxation strategies* Strategies like progressive relaxation, autogenics, and guided imagery that one can employ to reduce diffuse physiological arousal.

Defuse* A mindfulness process of preventing the fusing or merging of the self with disturbing or stressful thoughts.

Demand-withdraw pattern* A destructive interaction pattern identified by Gottman and Gottman in which demands from one party ultimately lead to withdrawal and stonewalling from the other party.

Dependent variable The variable that is measured in an experimental study.

Dermal system The body's skin.

Desensitization theory A theory that mantra meditation achieves its beneficial effects by counterconditioning disturbing thoughts and images that drift in and out of consciousness.

Destructive anger justification Blaming others for one's anger and expressing self-justification and desire for vindication.

Destructive anger rumination Holding grudges, brooding, and discussing one's anger repetitiously in a way that magnifies animosity.

Diagnostic and Statistical Manual (DSM) A manual published by the

American Psychiatric Association developed by psychiatrists to guide psychiatric diagnoses.

Dialectical behavior therapy (DBT) A mindfulness-based psychological intervention program designed primarily to treat individuals with a borderline personality disorder or impulse control disorders.

Diathesis-stress model* Illness results from environmental stressors having an adverse impact on an individual's most vulnerable biological systems.

Diathesis stress model of depression* Stress leads to depression in vulnerable individuals.

Diencephalon The region of the brain that lies above the midbrain and contains the brain structures called the thalamus and the hypothalamus.

Direct effect model of social support Social support has beneficial health and well-being effects independent of the level of stress.

Direct targeted approach Using biofeedback to directly target the physiological systems that support the symptoms such as muscle tension biofeedback for tension-type headache.

Discrimination* Behaviors motivated by prejudice that range from social exclusion to aggression.

Disease A pathological health condition with a recognized pattern of signs and symptoms.

Disengage The idea that mindfulness meditation achieves some of its beneficial effects by the practitioner learning to let go of tendencies to react automatically to stimuli.

Disengagement coping A form of coping in which the stressor or the emotions it evokes are not dealt with directly but are instead avoided or escaped from.

Dispositional optimism* An enduring tendency to have global expectations of positive outcomes.

Dispositions Also known as traits; the particular characteristics or structural elements of personality that predispose a person to respond in certain ways.

Dispute The act of challenging irrational beliefs in REBT.

Distal stressors* Stressors that occurred in the more distant past.

Distress Selye's term for the negative effects of stressors.

Divine command theory Following the commands of a supreme being is the path to happiness.

Divorce-stress-adjustment perspective The stress and adjustment trajectory of divorce depends on the person, the stressors associated with the divorce, and the factors that moderate the impact of the divorce.

Dopamine One of the "feel good" neurotransmitters that can elevate mood states; in the brain it also is important for regulating motor movements.

Drama triangle* A game played that involves a persecutor, victim, and rescuer.

Duchenne smile* A genuine smile that is characterized by the skin crinkling around the corners of the eyes.

Effect size* An indicator of the strength of the relationship of the independent variable on the dependent variable.

Efferent Neural pathways that send signals from the brain to the periphery.

Efficacious Empirical findings support the use of a specific intervention to treat a particular disorder.

Efficacy expectation Belief that one can successfully execute the actions that lead to the desired outcome.

Effort-reward imbalance (ERI) model* A model of organizational stress that states that high-cost low-gain work efforts are stressful.

EGCG Epigallocatechin-3-gallate; the primary polyphenol found in green tea.

Electromyograph (EMG)* A measure of electrical activity of the skeletal muscles.

Emotional eaters Individuals who attempt to regulate their negative affect through eating.

Emotional exhaustion One of Maslach's three dimensions of burnout characterized by feeling emotionally depleted, drained, and lacking in emotional resources.

Emotion-focused coping* Managing the distress caused by the problem.

Empathy The experience of identifying and understanding another person's emotions and perceptions.

Empirically supported therapy An efficacious therapeutic approach for a particular disorder.

Empty calories* The food consumed has calories but very little nutritional value.

Endocrine system A system of organs and glands that secrete hormones into our bloodstream that act as biochemical messengers to their respective target cells and organs.

Endorphins The body's natural opiates that reduce pain sensations and create feelings of euphoria.

Energy mobilization and expenditure state The body's state when it is activating or using its energy reserves such as during the fight-or-flight response.

Engagement* Represents in Maslach's model of burnout the positive polarity of her three dimensions characterized by high energy, involvement, and sense of efficacy.

Engagement coping* The stressor or the emotions it evokes are dealt with directly.

Enhanced receptivity A characteristic of an altered or meditative state in which the waking self or ego becomes more permeable to unconscious thoughts.

Epinephrine* Also known as adrenaline; a catecholamine hormone secreted by the adrenal medulla that has a marked effect on the cardiovascular system, stimulates the release of glucose into the bloodstream, and increases the body's metabolic rate.

Epstein Barr virus (EBV) A virus within the herpes family that is associated with mononucleosis in adolescence and young adulthood but is typically asymptomatic in adults by the age of 40.

Errors of thinking Cognitive processing styles that are distorted, biased, or illogical.

Essential amino acids* Amino acids needed by the body that must come from dietary sources because the body cannot synthesize them.

Essential fatty acids Long-chain polyunsaturated fats the body requires from food because it cannot manufacture them.

Essential hypertension (HTN)* Also known as high blood pressure; a chronic condition with no known organic cause that is characterized by systolic blood pressure of 140 mm Hg or higher or diastolic blood pressure of 90 mm Hg or higher.

Ethnic identity* Defining a person through culture, language, or national origin.

Eudaimonia* Aristotle's concept of happiness possessed of true well-being that is a by-product of living the virtuous life.

Eustress* Selye's term for positive stress.

Executive control* Cognitive tasks associated with memory and higher cortical functions such as working memory, planning, and scheduling.

Exhaustion stage Selye's third and final stage of the general adaptation syndrome characterized by the body's organ systems failing from chronic stress exposure.

Existential anxiety A form of anxiety associated with awareness of ultimate concerns such as death, meaning, freedom, and isolation.

Expectancy effects Placebo and other nonspecific factors that influence outcomes in intervention studies.

Experimental group The group that receives the manipulation in an experimental study.

Experimental studies Research studies that hold the extraneous variables constant, manipulate the independent variables, and measure the dependent variables.

Explanatory style The patterns of causal inferences people make about why things happen to them.

Exposure therapy* A form of therapy in which the person in treatment systematically confronts the feared event or stimulus in a safe and controlled environment.

Expressive writing* A therapeutic writing exercise in which participants are asked to write their thoughts and feelings about their most upsetting and traumatic experiences.

Externalizing disorders Psychological disorders like substance abuse or dependence that are characterized by an outward expression of pathology.

External locus of control A general disposition to expect that reinforcements and other outcomes are the result of outside forces such as luck, fate, coincidence, or powerful others.

External unstable attribution Causal attributions that the target person's behavior is due to temporary situational factors.

External validity The ability of the study to generalize its results to relevant populations.

Extraversion* One of the Big Three and Big Five traits; attributes include being warm, friendly, social, active, and passionate.

Eysenck's PEN model* Eysenck's three supertraits of psychoticism, extraversion, and neuroticism that define an individual's personality.

Facets Subcomponents of each of the factors of the Five Factor Model measured by the NEO-PI.

Factor analysis A multivariate statistic that uses multiple correlations to determine which variables cluster together to form unifying themes.

Fat A macronutrient that consists of fatty acids and their related organic compounds.

Fear The emotion we feel when there is a perception of concrete danger.

Feedback The process in active listening of the communicator providing information to the listener about the listener's accuracy of understanding of the message.

Fiber A plant's indigestible cellulose components.

Fight-or-flight* Cannon's term for the body's physiological activation response when it prepares to fight off or flee from a threat.

FITT principle* Fitness is a product of frequency, intensity, time, and type of physical activity.

Five Factor Model (FFM)* Also known as the Big Five; the five relatively independent factors of neuroticism, extraversion, openness, conscientiousness, and agreeableness.

Flourishing* A state of optimal functioning.

Flow* An experience of merging one's consciousness with an event in the present moment.

Forgiveness An act of giving up resentments toward those we perceive to have harmed us or another and letting go of claims for retribution and restitution.

Functional disorder* A health condition with a diagnosable pattern that has no known organic cause.

Functional foods* Foods that have added health benefits beyond their nutritional value.

Functional syndrome A health condition with no detectable organic cause.

GABA* Gamma aminobutyric acid; an inhibitory neurotransmitter that reduces neuronal excitation.

Gastrointestinal (GI) system The mouth, pharynx, esophagus, stomach, small intestine, large intestine, liver, gallbladder, and pancreas, which work in concert to ingest and digest food.

General adaptation syndrome (GAS)* Selye's three-stage model of the effects of chronic stress.

Generalized anxiety disorder (GAD) An anxiety disorder characterized by excessive uncontrollable anxiety and worry that persists for at least 6 months and causes clinically significant distress or impairment.

Generalized resistance resources (GRRs) The factors in Antonovsky's salutogenic model that reduce stress-induced pressure to move toward the entropic direction of the health continuum.

General relaxation A restorative waking state that can be achieved through progressive relaxation training, autogenic training, guided imagery, meditation, or biofeedback-assisted relaxation training.

Genetics model of obesity It is evolutionarily adaptive to the human species to genetically predispose some members of the human gene pool to retain more fat stores so that these individuals can survive famines when others perish.

Global beliefs Construct systems that cover broad areas like predictability, justice, and control.

Global goals Broad states, ideals, or objects that one pursues such as work, knowledge, and relationships.

Global meaning A product of one's core values, beliefs, and goals used to interpret one's experiences of the world.

Glucocorticoids A family of steroid compounds secreted by the adrenal cortex during the fight-or-flight response that raise glucose levels in the bloodstream.

Gluconeogenesis The process of converting noncarbohydrate energy stores into glucose.

Glucose Sugar molecules.

Glycogen* Also known as animal starch; a long-chain glucose molecule stored in the body's liver and muscles.

Good life Living an optimal life full of meaning and satisfaction.

Goodness of fit hypothesis Suggests that coping is most effective when there is a good match between the coping strategy and the amount of control one can exert over the stressor.

Gratitude A feeling of appreciation for something good that another is responsible for bringing about.

Greater balance between the two cerebral hemispheres The theory that mantra meditation achieves its beneficial effects by strengthening the role of the brain's less dominant right hemisphere, which ultimately leads to a greater balance of the two hemispheres.

Green tea A tea developed from fresh tea leaves that are steamed or dried in a way that minimizes oxidation and therefore preserves the green pigment.

Guided imagery relaxation* A deep relaxation strategy that uses language to create relaxing sensory-filled images and scenarios that transport the participants to new worlds within their imagination.

Guided meditation A form of mindfulness meditation that may be scripted in which the participant focuses on aspects of the self that are relevant to his or her aspirations such as managing stress or increasing intimacy levels.

Habituation The process whereby repeated exposure to a stimulus elicits less responsiveness.

Hand warming Using cognitive strategies to voluntarily increase skin temperature of the hands.

Happiness Positive affect combined with high life satisfaction.

Happiness set point* The idea that happiness levels are fixed, stable across time, and somewhat impervious to control.

Hardiness* A construct described as a stress-resistant personality that exhibits existential courage through a synergy of the three cognitive elements of control, challenge, and commitment.

Harm-loss appraisals Primary appraisals in Lazarus's model that the event involves damage or a loss.

Hassles* Small irritants and pressures experienced in everyday life.

Hatha yoga* A form of yoga that emphasizes physical discipline through using pranayama and different asanas.

Health* A positive physical, mental, and social state of well-being.

Health-conscious living* To live with full awareness of how the choices we make affect our health.

Health psychology* A specialty area of psychology that uses the scientific and professional knowledge base of the discipline of psychology to promote and maintain health as well as to treat illnesses.

Health-related behavior models Personality influences our stress-motivated health behaviors in the positive or negative direction, which, in turn, increases our chance of developing improved health or impaired health.

Heart muscles The cardiac muscles.

Heavy control communication Use of communication patterns that involve power and control tactics and language.

Hedonic adaptation* The concept that happiness due to circumstances tends to be temporary because we generally adjust fairly soon to our new circumstances.

Hedonic definition of happiness The concept that happiness is a product of positive feelings, good moods, and pleasurable experiences.

Hedonic treadmill A metaphor for hedonic adaptation that suggests that no matter how slow or fast we move, our happiness levels stay the same.

Helicobacter pylori (H. pylori) bacteria* Bacterial microorganisms that are usually benign but can sometimes inflame the mucosal layer of the stomach or duodenum, leading to the development of an ulcer.

Herpes simplex virus (HSV) A virus that goes through dormant states followed by active states, which during an active state can produce a cold sore around the mouth or genital area.

High-glycemic index/load* Foods that spike blood sugar levels.

Hippocampus* Region of the cerebral hemispheres involved in encoding declarative memories.

Homeostasis* The biological self-regulation process that enables an organism to adapt to life's demands.

Hope The concept in Snyder's model that refers to the ability to envision one or more routes toward reaching a desired goal combined with a motivational trait-like perception that a wide range of goals will be pursued.

Hormonal system Also known as the endocrine system; a system of organs and glands that secrete biochemical messengers, the hormones, into the bloodstream that act on their respective target cells and organs.

Hormones Biochemical messengers secreted into the bloodstream by organs and glands that act on their respective target cells and organs.

Hostility* An attitudinal disposition of cynicism, suspicion, and resentment toward others.

Human-animal interaction Term used to describe the type of bonding and behavior of animals toward humans that may provide social support.

Human immunodeficiency virus (HIV-1) A virus that infects cells such as the CD4 helper T lymphocytes that can start a process that eventually leads to acquired immunodeficiency disease syndrome (AIDS).

Humoral immunity* The second-line strategy employed by the human immune system after cellular immunity involving Type 2 T-helper cells partnering with B cells to stimulate antibody production.

Hypnotic state* An altered state of waking consciousness with sleeplike characteristics that is distinguished by increased suggestibility.

Hypometabolic state* A state characterized by reduced oxygen consumption due to low bodily metabolism rates.

Hypothalamic-pituitary-adrenal (HPA) axis* A primary system of the fight-or-flight response that involves the hypothalamus influencing the pituitary gland to secrete ACTH, which, in turn, stimulates the adrenal cortex to release glucocorticoids.

Hypothalamus* Region of the diencephalon that exerts control over fight-or-flight activities, fear and anger states, and a host of other functions.

Illness An unhealthy state caused by a disease.

Illness behavior A characteristic pattern of behavior associated with the sick role in which a person evaluates symptoms, seeks medical care, and asks for support from close others.

Imaginal exposure* A form of exposure therapy such as systematic desensitization where the client confronts phobic imagined images rather than live phobic objects or situations.

Immune dysregulation* An impaired immune system that overreacts or underreacts to antigens.

Immune system The body's system of organs, tissues, and cells designed to protect itself against infections and harmful substances.

Immunoglobulins (Igs)* Also known as antibodies; soluble proteins produced by B cells that circulate in the bloodstream and bind to viruses and other antigens to neutralize them.

Incomplete proteins Proteins that are missing one or more of the essential amino acids.

Independent variable The variable that is manipulated in an experimental study.

Ineffability A characteristic of an altered or meditative state described as a type of experience that cannot be put into words.

Infection An invasion of the body by a harmful microorganism.

Inflammation* An immune response of the body to damaged tissue or infection characterized by swelling, pain, heat, and/or redness.

Inflammatory bowel disease (IBD) A broad term that incorporates both Crohn's disease and ulcerative colitis involving visible inflammation of the intestinal lining.

Innate immune system* Also known as the natural immune system, this more primitive but rapid system consists of phagocytic cells, natural killer cells, and various enzymes and serum proteins that are involved in the inflammation process.

Innate protective system The skin and the innate immune system.

Insulin A hormone secreted by the pancreas used to transport glucose to the body's cells.

Interferon One of several families of cytokine molecules.

Interleukin One of several families of cytokine molecules.

Intermittent explosive disorder (IED) A psychological disorder characterized by episodes of extreme anger and acting out the anger through assaults or the destruction of property.

Internalizing disorders Psychological disorders like mood or anxiety disorders that are characterized by an inward expression of pathology.

Internal locus of control A general disposition to expect that one's actions will lead to predictable outcomes and reinforcements.

Internal stable attributions Causal attributions that the target person's behavior is due to personality, traits, or other internal enduring factors.

Internal validity The study's ability to discern causal relationships.

Interoceptive sensitivity* Having a high conscious awareness of one's internal physiological activity such as one's heartbeat activity.

Interpersonal psychotherapy A form of psychotherapy used successfully to treat depression that addresses its social context.

Introverts Possessing attributes on the low end of the extraversion scale.

Irrelevant appraisals Primary appraisals in Lazarus's model that the event has no bearing on one's health or well-being.

Irritable bowel syndrome (IBS)* A functional disorder characterized by episodes of abdominal pain or tenderness along with bowel disruptions in the form of diarrhea and/or constipation.

Ischemia Insufficient blood flow to bodily tissues.

Job demands-control* A model of organizational stress that states that when a worker experiences high psychological demands paired with minimal control then job strain occurs.

Job strain* The harmful consequences that result from exposure to job stressors.

Job stress The roles, tasks, or demands of one's work exceeding one's capacities.

Lacto-ovo vegetarians People who eat a plant-based diet that also includes milk and eggs.

Learned helplessness* A passive state analogous to depressed states in which one's efforts are perceived as not affecting outcomes.

Learned optimism* Acquiring an ability to generally expect positive outcomes.

Leptin When fat stores fall this appetite-suppressing hormone found in adipose tissues drops, signaling the hypothalamus to induce hunger.

Leukocytes White blood cells.

Life change units (LCUs) A quantitative indicator of the cumulative life change events experienced.

Life satisfaction* A global judgment about how good one's life is.

Limbic system* The brain's neural circuit for emotion that includes the hippocampus, the thalamus, parts of the hypothalamus, the amygdala, the prefrontal cortex, and other structures such as the cingulated gyrus.

Limit setting Delineating what one will agree to or accept from others and what one will not.

Lipolysis The liberation of fat stores for use as a fuel source.

Locus ceruleus (LC) A small cluster of norepinephrine synthesizing cell bodies residing in the dorsal brain stem region of the reticular formation that plays an important role in vigilance and arousal.

Locus of control* General expectancies about the connections between one's actions and the outcomes and reinforcements that follow them.

Longitudinal designs* A study in which cohorts are tracked across time.

Loving kindness meditation therapy A guided mindfulness meditation intervention designed to promote intimacy.

Low decision latitude* A worker's experience of having insufficient skills or authority over one's job to autonomously complete the assigned job tasks.

Lymphocytes* A category of immune system cells that includes the natural killer cells, the T cells, and the B cells.

Macronutrients The nutrients we consume in large quantities to fulfill our energy requirements.

Macrophages* Monocytes of the innate immune system that become enlarged upon leaving the bloodstream and entering bodily tissue.

Major depressive disorder* A mood disorder characterized by experiencing depressed moods or the loss of pleasure that stretch throughout the day almost every day for a least 2 weeks.

Maladaptive attitudes Enduring dysfunctional cognitive structures in Beck's model that serve as wellsprings for automatic negative thoughts.

Manageability One of three factors that comprise Antonovsky's construct of sense of coherence that refers to one's ability to access internal and external coping resources and use them when needed.

Mantra* A word, sound, or phrase that is repeated during concentrative meditation.

Mantra meditation A form of concentrative meditation in which a word, sound, or phrase is repeated during the meditative session.

Meaningfulness One of three factors that comprise Antonovsky's construct of sense of coherence that refers to one's ability to emotionally make sense of demands and to perceive these demands as worthwhile investments of energy.

Meaning in life* The larger understanding, significance, and purpose one sees in one's life.

Meaning-making coping* To use one's values, beliefs, and goals to shape meaning in stressful situations that are generally not conducive to the use of problem-focused coping.

Meanings made Cognitive products that are the result of meaning-making coping's assimilation and accommodation processes.

Mediterranean-style eating pattern A healthy eating plan that emphasizes eating fruits, vegetables, nuts, whole grains, olive oil, and fish; it may also include drinking wine with meals.

Medulla Region of the brain stem that contains the vital life support centers that control autonomic processes such as heart rate, blood pressure, respiration, and digestion.

Melatonin* A hormone released by the pineal gland that lowers one's body temperature and causes drowsiness.

Meta-analytic studies* Also known as meta-analytic reviews; studies that use statistical procedures to determine average effect sizes of multiple studies.

Metabolic rate The amount of energy expended by the body.

Meta-cognition* Thinking about one's thinking.

Micronutrients The essential substances we need in very small quantities, the vitamins and minerals.

Midbrain Region of the brain stem that controls and coordinates many sensory and motor activities such as the auditory and visual systems as well as voluntary motor movement.

Migraine headaches* Head pain believed to be neurovascular in origin that is typically felt more on one side of the head and may be accompanied by feelings of nausea and auras such as unusual lights and odors.

Mind Human consciousness represented by the brain's cognitions, perceptions, memory, and feelings.

Mindfulness Being fully aware and accepting in the present.

Mindfulness-based cognitive therapy (MBCT) A mindfulness-based psychological intervention program designed to prevent relapses for individuals who have been successfully treated for clinical depression.

Mindfulness-based stress reduction (MBSR) A mindfulness-based psychological intervention program pioneered by Kabat-Zinn designed to treat stress and some types of psychological disorders and medical conditions.

Mindfulness meditation* A form of nonconcentrative meditation in which practitioners adopt a detached observer style along with acceptance of the object of awareness in the present moment.

Mindful way Suspending judgment and analysis.

Minerals Essential inorganic elements the body needs in minute amounts to support growth, to maintain bodily tissues, and to metabolize food.

Minimally effective response* The least threatening assertive response that can accomplish the objective.

Mini-meditations A series of 2- to 3-minute meditation sessions practiced throughout the day.

Moderate-intensity activity* Bodily movement such as brisk walking that produces a sustained heart rate of around 60% of one's maximum capacity.

Moderation models* Assume that personality or other factors are intervening variables between stress and health and can serve as an intensifier of stress or a buffer that reduces the impact of stressors.

Monoamine oxidase inhibitors (MAOIs) An older class of antidepressants believed to increase the brain's serotonin, norepinephrine, and dopamine levels.

Monoamines The family of "feel good" neurotransmitters present in the brain such as serotonin, norepinephrine, and dopamine.

Monocytes Mononuclear phagocytes of the innate immune system involved in the inflammatory process.

Monounsaturated fats* Plant-based fatty acids that have one double-carbon bond that are liquid at room temperature.

Muscle sense awareness* The ability to differentiate tense muscles from relaxed ones.

Muscular system Skeletal muscles of the body.

Music In the context of stress management, music is a vocal or instrumental sound used for enjoyment and mood regulation.

Myocardial infarction (MI)* Also known as a heart attack; when the heart has insufficient blood supply usually due to occlusion of a coronary artery, which results in cardiac tissue death.

Natural killer (NK) cells* Lymphocytic cells of the innate immune system programmed to recognize other cells that are nonself, such as tumor cells and cells infected with viruses, and to release cytotoxic chemicals that lyse these cells.

Negative affect* Unpleasant emotions such as sadness, anger, fear, and anxiety.

Negative cognitive triad* A tendency among depressed people in Beck's model of depression to view the self, the world, and the future in a negative light.

Negative correlation Variables have an inverse relationship such that a large value of x is associated with a small value of y and a small value of x is associated with a large value of y.

Negative feedback loop A homeostatic mechanism for damping down responses.

Negative life stress events Life change experiences associated with distress.

Negative reciprocity* One person directs a hostile, angry, or accusatory remark toward the other, which prompts a negative response in kind from the targeted person, leading to rounds of verbal attacks and counterattacks.

Negotiations A series of communication exchanges made with the objective of reaching a mutually satisfying outcome.

Neocortex The gray matter outside covering of the brain responsible for higher order functions related to sensation, perception, emotion, movement, cognition, memory, organization, planning, language, and conscious awareness.

Neuropeptides Endogenous protein molecules such as endorphins.

Neurosis A psychiatric diagnostic category no longer in use that refers to an anxiety or depression condition in which there is adequate reality testing.

Neurotic cascade A proposed set of predictable interlocking negative events associated with neuroticism.

Neuroticism* One of the Big Three and Big Five traits characterized by a disposition to experience emotional lability, a general sense of vulnerability, and negative affect.

Neurotransmitter A chemical messenger that travels across the synaptic junction and affects neuronal impulses.

Neutrophils The most common leukocyte of the natural immune system.

Nicotine A bioactive substance found in the tobacco leaf that affects the "feel good" neurotransmitters in the brain, such as norepinephrine, serotonin, and dopamine, while also increasing heart rate and blood pressure.

Night-eating syndrome A problematic eating pattern often leading to weight gain in which a person eats very little in the morning but overeats at night.

Nonconcentrative meditation* A form of meditation like mindfulness meditation in which attention is kept broader along a continuum of stimuli.

Nonevaluative social support A type of social support in which the receiver perceives no criticism or judgment from the giver.

Nonspecific action tendencies Represent the propensity in Fredrickson's broaden-and-build model for positive emotions to evoke a wide range of behavioral options.

Nonspecific responses The general physiological response pattern in Selye's model that occurs to a broad band of stressful stimuli.

Nonsteroidal anti-inflammatory drugs (NSAIDs) A class of medications that includes aspirin that reduces inflammatory responses without using steroids.

Norepinephrine* Also known as noradrenaline; a catecholamine hormone and neurotransmitter that excites the fight-or-flight systems.

Nutrient density The quantity of nutrients packed into the calories consumed.

Nutrients Ingredients in food that provide energy or that sustain cells and tissues.

Obese* Having a body mass index of 30 or above.

Observing self* The component of the self in mindfulness practice that notices thoughts.

Obsessions Thoughts, images, or impulses that are intrusive or inappropriate enough to cause a marked elevation of anxiety.

Obsessive-compulsive disorder An anxiety disorder characterized by having recurrent intrusive or inappropriate thoughts, images, or impulses that cause a marked elevation of anxiety along with engaging in behaviors or mental acts that are ritualistic and designed to lower anxiety.

Omega-3 fatty acids* Long-chain polyunsaturated essential fatty acids found primarily in fatty marine fish and some plant sources known for their cardiovascular and anti-inflammatory benefits.

Open awareness A mindfulness meditation practice in which the meditator disengages the analytical mind; suspends judgment; and becomes a passive observer of the images, sensations, feelings, and cognitions that stream through consciousness.

Openness* Also known as openness to experience; one of the Big Five traits associated with being creative, imaginative, and enjoying variety.

Optimal experiences Living life fully and in the moment.

Organizational injustice model A model of organizational stress that assumes that stress occurs when the organization's interpersonal transactions, procedures, or outcomes are perceived as unfair.

Organizational role stress Concept of organizational stress that includes role conflict, role ambiguity, and role overload.

Organizational stress Refers to how the structure and processes of the organization bring about stress for the workers.

Osteoporosis* A skeletal disease involving loss of bone density.

Outcome expectations One's belief that a particular action will lead to a particular outcome.

Overweight Having a body mass index of 25 to 29.9.

Oxidative stress* The adverse effects of oxygen free radicals on cells.

Oxytocin* A hormone found in high concentrations in nursing women that is believed to facilitate maternal-infant bonding.

Panic attacks* Acute episodes of intense fear with prominent physiological features.

Panic disorder An anxiety disorder characterized by repeated and unexpected panic attacks along with worry and concern about reoccurrence of attacks.

Paraphrasing The simplest form of active listening that involves rephrasing the communicator's message.

Parasympathetic branch* The branch of the autonomic nervous system that damps down the fight-or-flight response and is responsible for the body's basal energy conservation and restoration state.

Pareto principle* The principle that only 20% of one's goals contain 80% of the total value; therefore, good time management involves spending most of one's time on the most important 20% of one's goals.

Passive-aggressive behavior* A form of resistance to others through procrastination, excuse-making, obstructionism, or poor or destructive performance of tasks where the person engaging in the behavior does not take responsibility for his or her actions or inactions.

Pathways A component of Snyder's hope model that refers to the ability to envision one or more routes toward reaching a desired goal.

Pearson Product Moment Correlation Coefficient A type of bivariate correlation coefficient designated as r that ranges from -1.0 to $+1.0$.

Pedometer* A measuring device that can be clipped to a person's waist that counts the person's steps and distance traveled by foot.

Peptic ulcers* Erosions in the lining of the esophagus, stomach, or duodenum.

Perceived racism* Subjectively experiencing that one is the target of prejudice or discrimination.

Perceptual distortions Characteristics of an altered or meditative state in which bodily sensations are experienced as unusual or out of the ordinary.

Peripheral nervous system Consists of the somatic nervous system and the autonomic nervous system.

Personality The overall enduring pattern of thoughts, emotions, and behaviors that define an individual.

Personality disorder An enduring personality pattern associated with distress or impairment.

Personality types Qualitative categories of personality within a particular domain that define the person according to the construct's characteristics, such as Type A.

Person-environment (P-E) fit* A model of organizational stress that states that stress occurs when there is a poor match between the worker and the work environment.

Pescovegetarian diet* A plant-based eating plan that also includes fish.

Pessimists People who generally have global expectations for negative outcomes.

Phagocytes* Cells of the immune system that eat the antigens they attack.

Phobia An anxiety disorder characterized by unreasonable or excessive fear of a particular object, situation, or activity.

Physical activity* Health-enhancing bodily movement.

Physical Activity Readiness Questionnaire (PAR-Q) A paper and pencil screening tool used to determine if a person has a low enough health risk to begin a physical activity program.

Physical exercise* Planned physical activity designed to exert one's body for health and fitness benefits.

Physical fitness An umbrella term that encompasses elements such as muscular strength, cardiorespiratory endurance, and flexibility.

Phytochemicals* Bioactive compounds found in plants that are not essential nutrients for sustaining life.

Pineal gland A tiny pine cone shaped gland in the center of the brain that releases melatonin during the dark phase and inhibits its release during the light phase of the light-dark circadian cycle.

Pituitary gland The pea-sized master gland at the base of the brain.

Pituitary portal system Pathway through which the hypothalamus secretes peptide messengers called releasing factors into the anterior pituitary to stimulate the pituitary's secretion of beta-endorphin and adrenocorticotropic hormone (ACTH) into the bloodstream.

Placebo pills Inert pills that control for expectancy effects because participants believe these pills may contain active medicinal ingredients.

Polyphenols* Antioxidant phytochemicals consisting of over 4,000 currently identified compounds.

Polyunsaturated fats* Fatty acids found in plant-based foods and fish with more than one double-carbon bond that are liquid at room temperature.

Pons Region of the brain stem that serves as a transmitting bridge for motor information sent from the cerebral hemisphere to the cerebellum.

Positive affect* Pleasant emotions such as joy, love, and amusement.

Positive correlation Variables are related such that a large value of x is associated with a large value of y and a small value of x is associated with a small value of y.

Positive growth Development in a beneficial direction.

Positive illusions Unrealistic positive beliefs.

Positive incentive model Obesity is a result of a motivation to eat pleasurable foods that are in abundance in modern societies.

Positive mental health models* Focus on how positive therapy and interventions can maximize flourishing and other optimal positive functioning experiences.

Positive psychology* The field of study in psychology that focuses on examining and promoting well-being and optimal human functioning.

Positive reciprocity The flip side of negative reciprocity involves expressing how much individuals like each other's positive qualities and behaviors.

Postganglionic neurons Nerve fibers that are stimulated by preganglionic neurons.

Posttraumatic growth* A positive response to trauma usually characterized by strengthening of relationships and development of more positive self and worldviews.

Posttraumatic stress disorder (PTSD)* A psychological disorder stemming from a reaction to traumatic stressors characterized by persistently reexperiencing the traumatic event, avoiding stimuli correlated with the event, experiencing a general response numbing, and having persistent increased arousal.

Pranayama* A controlled breathing strategy used in yoga and meditation.

Preganglionic neurons Nerve fibers that exit the spinal cord.

Prejudice Negative attitudes and beliefs about a particular group.

Present-centeredness A characteristic of an altered or meditative state in which the mind is focused on what is occurring in the moment.

Primary appraisal* A judgment in Lazarus's model about the relative significance of an event regarding its potential benefit or harm-loss.

Primary prevention Within an organizational stress intervention context, primary prevention refers to strategies that attempt to minimize the source of stress and to promote a supportive organizational culture.

Problem-focused coping* Dealing with the perceived cause of the distress.

Progressive muscle relaxation (PMR)* A deep relaxation technique pioneered by Jacobson that consists of tensing and relaxing different muscle groups.

Projection* A defense mechanism in which a person sees in others disowned elements of his or her own personality.

Prospective research design Also known as a longitudinal design; involves research in which participants are evaluated at baseline and then tracked across time.

Protein A macronutrient that consists of building blocks called amino acids.

Proximal stressors* Stressors that occurred in the more recent past.

Psychoendocrinology* The study of the relationship between psychological processes and endocrine function.

Psychological flexibility The desired goal of acceptance and commitment therapy that represents mindfulness plus commitment/behavior change.

Psychological well-being* Ryff's model that contends that well-being is a product of the six dimensions of self-acceptance, positive relations with others, autonomy, environmental mastery, purpose in life, and personal growth.

Psychoneuroimmunology (PNI) The study of the relationship among psychological, neurological, and immunological variables.

Psychophysiology* The study of the interplay between cognitive and physiological processes.

Psychosomatic medicine A medical orientation that assumes some physical illness symptoms are the result of mental and emotional processes and approaches treatment accordingly.

Psychoticism A supertrait in Eysenck's model that broadly reflects traits often associated with nonconformity or social deviance.

Qualitative overload* A term used within the role episode model of organizational stress, indicating that the employee does not have the required competencies to complete the tasks.

Quantitative overload* A term used within the role episode model of organizational stress, indicating that there are insufficient resources to complete the tasks assigned in the time provided.

Racism Disparaging beliefs, attitudes, and behaviors directed toward individuals or groups based on their phenotypic characteristics or ethnicity.

Raja yoga A type of yoga that is believed to be the foundation for the other yoga systems.

Randomized controlled trial* The gold standard experimental study in medicine in which participants are randomly assigned to groups and then the group that receives the intervention being tested is compared to one or more control groups.

Rational-emotive behavior therapy (REBT)* A cognitive therapy developed by Ellis that involves active disputation of irrational beliefs.

Raynaud's phenomenon (RP)* A painful condition triggered by cold exposure or emotional stress involving vasoconstriction of the arteries and arterioles of the fingers and toes.

Realistic optimism Having a general expectation of positive outcomes without using self-deception.

Reappraisal The use of ongoing feedback in Lazarus's model to make new judgments about the stressful situation.

Reduced efficacy One of Maslach's three dimensions of burnout characterized by feelings of diminished self-efficacy, personal competency, and productivity.

Red wine A type of wine that gets its coloring from the red skin of the grapes used in the fermentation process.

Reinforcement sensitivity theory Gray's theory that proposes two functionally independent motivational systems called the behavioral approach system and the behavioral inhibition system.

Relapse prevention* The process of identifying high-risk relapse situations and then avoiding the risks, making alternative plans, or planning how to best deal with these risks if encountered.

Relaxation response Benson's term for a state achieved during meditation that he considered to be the natural antidote to the stress response.

Relaxation response meditation Also called secular meditation; a form of mantra meditation pioneered by Benson.

Reliability A measure of consistency of an instrument.

Religion The practice of spirituality within the context of formal institutions.

Religious-based coping* The use of religious methods such as prayer to reduce stress.

Resilient* The ability to recover or respond positively to a negative event.

Resistance stage Selye's second stage of the general adaptation syndrome characterized by depletion or injury of the body's systems due to exposure to chronic stress.

Respiratory system The lungs and airways that enable breathing.

Response prevention* Refers to the planned practice of inhibiting compulsive behaviors when exposed to a feared event or stimulus.

Restraint eaters* Individuals who normally limit their food intake to maintain or lose weight.

Resveratrol A plant hormone polyphenol found in high concentrations in red wine.

Reticular formation (RF)* A network of neurons through which the hypothalamus sends descending signals to the brain stem and the viscera to activate the fight-or-flight response; also serves as an ascending pathway of sensory information from the periphery to the thalamus.

Retrospective research design A research design in which people are asked to recall past events that are recorded as variables under study.

Rheumatoid arthritis (RA) A chronic autoimmune disorder characterized by inflammation of and sometimes damage to the joints and surrounding tissues.

Rhythm theory The theory that mantra meditation achieves its beneficial effects by tuning people in to natural rhythms that they are biologically programmed to find soothing.

Role ambiguity A term within the role episode model of organizational stress indicating that the duties, responsibilities, and performance expectations of the job are not clearly defined by organizational leaders.

Role conflict A term within the role episode model of organizational stress indicating that two or more role demands are incompatible with each other.

Role overload A term within the role episode model of organizational stress indicating that there is either quantitative or qualitative overload.

Ruminative thinking Repeated cognitions aimed at uncovering the causes and implications of one's depressed or anxious feelings.

Runner's high A phenomenon in which a runner experiences euphoria precipitated by the act of running.

Salutogenic model* Antonovsky's model of health that proposes that health resides on a continuum from an entropic end to a salutary end; how one manages stress can move a person toward either end of the continuum.

Samadhi The term in the Hindu religion that refers to an intense meditative state in which one's awareness is yoked or fused with Divine Consciousness.

Saturated fats* A form of fat that is solid at room temperature and is found primarily in animal sources such as meat and dairy.

Savoring* Applying conscious awareness to enjoyment experiences.

Secondary appraisal* The judgment in Lazarus's model about how well one can deal or cope with a given stressful situation.

Secondary gains Rewards associated with adopting a sick role and exhibiting illness behavior.

Secondary prevention Within an organizational stress intervention context refers to educational strategies such as teaching stress management skills.

Secular meditation Also called relaxation response meditation; a form of mantra meditation pioneered by Benson.

Selective serotonin reuptake inhibitors (SSRIs)* A newer class of antidepressants designed to increase the brain's serotonin levels.

Self-care A strategy whereby each individual takes personal responsibility for using strategies that prevent or minimize burnout and other forms of professional impairment.

Self-determination theory* When one is intrinsically motivated to move toward realistic goals one chooses, one has a better chance of experiencing well-being.

Self-efficacy* The belief in one's abilities and skills to bring about a successful outcome in a given situation.

Self-forgiveness The process of letting go of a desire to punish, retaliate, or act destructively toward oneself due to one's perceived transgressions.

Self-regulation* Setting standards and goals and then guiding oneself toward these goals while maintaining one's internal standards.

Self-talk* The silent internal dialogue people have with themselves.

Self-transcendence A characteristic of an altered or meditative state in which a person experiences expanded consciousness, more positive thoughts, and a feeling of inner peace associated with feelings of enlightenment.

Sense of coherence (SOC)* One's worldview according to Antonovsky that is comprised of the three integrated factors of comprehensibility, manageability, and meaningfulness.

Sense of entitlement An attitude of expecting special rights and privileges.

Sensory projection system* The circuit from a sense organ moving through the thalamus to its specific region in the neocortex responsible for the experience of sensation.

Sensory systems The body's systems that detect stimuli in its inner and outer environment to enable vision, hearing, and pain, for example.

Serotonin norepinephrine reuptake inhibitors (SNRIs) One of the newest classes of antidepressants designed to increase the brain's serotonin and norepinephrine levels.

Sexual coercion A form of pressure for sexual involvement tied to job outcomes.

Sexual harassment* The engagement in gender-based insulting or hostile behaviors, sexual coercion, or the application of unwanted attention or pressure of a sexual nature not tied to job outcomes by one worker to another worker.

Shift work* A type of work schedule that involves large periods of work outside the normal daylight hours.

Sickness An unhealthy state caused by a disease.

Sick role A role people may adopt when they are ill in which they evaluate symptoms, seek medical care, and ask for support from close others.

Signal-to-noise ratio The degree to which a stimulus event stands out against background stimuli.

Signature strengths* Personality characteristics that represent one's virtues such as curiosity, integrity, fairness, self-control, spirituality, forgiveness, and humor that are measured by the Values in Action Scale.

Simple carbohydrates* Macronutrient sugars that consist of single or double glucose units.

Sixteen Personality Factor (16 PF) Questionnaire An objective personality test based on Cattell's factor analyses that measures 16 distinct correlated personality factors.

Skeletal muscles Also known as the striated muscles or the voluntary muscles; the muscles of the body attached to the bone that facilitate voluntary movement.

Smooth muscles Noncardiac muscles of the organs and blood vessels.

Social comparison The process of evaluating oneself by comparing oneself with others on relevant dimensions.

Social phobia An anxiety disorder characterized by a fear of being engaged in interpersonal activity with unfamiliar people that might cause the person with the disorder to feel scrutinized and embarrassed.

Social Readjustment Rating Scale (SRRS) A self-report instrument created by Holmes and Rahe to measure the magnitude of positive and negative life change events experienced by the participant.

Social strain* Refers to social interactions within a network of social relationships that are a source of stress because they drain resources or provide assistance in an unhelpful manner.

Social support* Refers to social interactions embedded within a network of social relationships that provide a person with potential access to or receipt of actual or perceived resources from others who are perceived as caring.

Somatic nervous system Component of the peripheral nervous system that innervates the skeletal muscles, the skin, and the sense organs.

Specific action tendencies The propensity of negative emotions in Fredrickson's broaden-and-build model to narrow behavioral options.

Specific phobia An anxiety disorder characterized by feeling intense and exaggerated fears of specific objects or situations; does not include phobias of public places or social contexts.

Spirituality* A search for self-transcendence or to form connections with a higher power, divine being, or ultimate reality.

States Temporary internal phenomena.

Stonewalling* The fourth step in the demand-withdraw pattern when the withdrawing person withholds attention and puts up a wall that blocks communication and cooperation as a way to punish the demanding person.

Stress* The constellation of cognitive, emotional, physiological, and behavioral reactions the organism experiences as it transacts with perceived threats and challenges.

Stress audits Organizational assessments designed to identify organizational stress issues and areas.

Stress buffer model of social support Social support lessens the effects of exposure to stressors.

Stress inoculation Novaco's multicomponent program designed to build coping abilities and skills for use in stressful situations and to manage anger.

Stress inoculation training (SIT)* Meichenbaum's cognitive-behavior modification training program designed to prepare individuals for stressful future encounters or treat current excess stress.

Stress management Application of strategies to regulate stress.

Stress management training A multimodal program designed to teach participants a variety of strategies for dealing with stress.

Stressor The event or stimulus that causes a stress response.

Striated muscles Also known as the skeletal muscles; muscles that facilitate voluntary movement.

Stroke volume The amount of blood ejected during the heart's contraction.

Subculture An embedded culture within a superculture.

Subcutaneous fat Adipose tissue found just beneath the skin.

Subjective units of distress (SUDS)* A self-report measure used in systematic desensitization that indicates the amount of fear and distress the phobic image elicits.

Subjective well-being* Represents the concept that happiness is determined by one's appraisal of life satisfaction and positive feelings.

Substantia nigra Region of the brain stem's midbrain that transmits important information to the basal ganglia that is necessary for regulating voluntary motor movement.

Sudden cardiac death (SCD)* Cardiac arrest that occurs very shortly after symptom onset that results in death.

Superculture The predominate culture that has embedded subcultures.

Sympathetic-adrenal-medulla (SAM) axis* A primary system of the fight-or-flight response that involves the hypothalamus commanding the sympathetic nervous system to stimulate the adrenal medulla to secrete the catecholamines epinephrine and norepinephrine.

Sympathetic branch* The branch of the autonomic nervous system that is responsible for the fight-or-flight response and supports the energy mobilization and expenditure state.

Sympathetic nervous system The branch of the autonomic nervous system associated with enervating and activating the organ systems of the body that are involved in the fight-or-flight response.

Systematic desensitization* A technique for treating phobias that involves successively pairing relaxation with imagined phobic images along a continuum that starts with the least feared and progresses to the most feared image.

Systemic autoimmune disorders* Disorders characterized by the immune system broadly attacking the body's own cells and tissues.

Systemic lupus erythematosus (SLE) A relatively rare chronic multisystemic autoimmune disease whereby the immune system targets the body's organs and tissues, resulting in symptoms such as fatigue, fever, skin rash, weight loss, various inflammation responses, and lowered resistance to infections.

T cells* Lymphocytic cells that develop in the thymus that are part of the adaptive immune system.

T-cytotoxic cells Also known as CD8 cells; lymphocytic cells that are components of the adaptive immune system that specialize in lysing unwanted cells, especially the body's own cells that are infected with virus or otherwise compromised to become tumor or cancer cells.

Tea A beverage made from the leaves of the plant *Camellia sinensis*.

Technostress* The pressure to adapt to serious and fundamental changes in job roles that are driven by new technology; may also relate to general difficulty adapting to new technology.

Temperament Biologically based influences on personality.

Temporomandibular pain and dysfunction syndrome (TMPDS)* A syndrome characterized by myofascial pain, particularly in the temporomandibular joint and the muscles involved in chewing.

Tend-and-befriend* Taylor's theory that biobehavioral mechanisms influenced by oxytocin influence women toward engaging in affiliative behaviors when under stress.

Tension-type headache (TTH)* The most common type of headache, characterized by head pain that often has corollary pain in the neck, back, or other related muscle areas.

Tertiary prevention Within an organizational stress intervention context, tertiary prevention refers to providing rehabilitation and recovery assistance to individuals who have developed mental or physical health conditions related to stress.

Thalamus Region of the diencephalon that gates information from the sense organs to the neocortex.

T-helper cells Also known as CD4 cells; lymphocytic cells that are components of the adaptive immune system that direct and amplify the immune response through the use of chemical messengers.

Thought-action repertoires Represented in Fredrickson's broaden-and-build model, the range of potential cognitions and behaviors available to a person.

Threat appraisals Appraisals in Lazarus's model that the events have potential to result in harm or loss.

Thrive* To flourish and show vigorous growth.

Thyroid gland A gland shaped like a butterfly that sits just below the larynx that releases thyroxine.

Thyroid-stimulating hormone (TSH) A biochemical messenger released by the anterior pituitary into the bloodstream that stimulates the thyroid gland to release thyroxine.

Thyroxine A thyroid gland hormone that regulates cellular metabolic rates.

Time distortion A characteristic of an altered or meditative state in which normal perception of time is lost.

Time management Using one's time efficiently to accomplish one's goals.

Time-out Taking a break from the negotiation process before resuming negotiations.

Tobacco A plant that contains nicotine whose leaves can be used in a smokeless form such a snuff and chewing tobacco or by burning them and inhaling their smoke through puffing on cigarettes, cigars, or pipes.

Top-down theories of happiness Theories that suggest that individuals' happiness levels are determined by how they view their circumstances.

Traits* Also known as dispositions; the particular characteristics or structural elements of personality that predispose a person to respond in certain ways.

Transcendental Meditation (TM)* A modified transitional form of mantra meditation originated by Maharishi Mahesh Yogi that removed what he considered to be the nonessential elements of yoga.

Trans-fats* Generally vegetable oils that have been chemically modified to make them solid through a process called partial hydrogenation.

Traumatic stressors Highly distressing experiences that can result in feelings of terror, extreme fright, or helplessness.

Triangulation* The process whereby two people in dispute pull in a third person.

Tricyclic antidepressants (TCAs) An older class of antidepressants believed to increase the brain's norepinephrine levels.

Triglycerides The fatty acid form of fat generally stored in fat cells and later burned for energy.

Triple column method* A daily exercise used for cognitive restructuring designed to identify, challenge, and replace automatic negative thoughts.

Tumor necrosis factor One of several types of cytokine molecules.

Type A* A behavior pattern characterized by an exaggerated sense of time urgency, competitiveness, hostility, and an inordinate drive that Friedman and Rosenman proposed as a predictor of coronary heart disease.

Type B A relaxed, easy-going behavior pattern; the opposite of the Type A behavior pattern.

Type D* A distressed personality type that has high negative affectivity and social inhibition; the construct was proposed as an indicator of a poor prognosis for patients with heart disease.

Ulcerative colitis (UC) A serious inflammatory bowel disease that is characterized by gastrointestinal symptoms and ulcers of the colon.

Undoing hypothesis Fredrickson's concept that one of the purposes of positive emotions is to help a person recover more quickly from detrimental effects of negative emotions.

Uplifts* Positive encounters and experiences.

Validity An indicator of the accuracy an instrument.

Values in Action (VIA) Peterson and Seligman's classification system of signature strengths.

Vegans Vegetarians who do not consume any food from animal sources.

Vigor* Represents the positive pole on a burnout continuum in Shirom's model of burnout characterized by emotional, physical, and cognitive vibrancy.

Vigorous activity* Bodily movement such as running that produces a sustained heart rate of at least 70% of one's maximum capacity.

Vipassana meditation* A form of mindfulness meditation based on Buddhist practice.

Virtue theory Aristotle's approach that happiness is not a goal to pursue but rather a by-product of living the virtuous life.

Viscera The body's organs, ducts, and glands.

Visceral fat* The internal fat that pads the liver and abdominal organs.

Vital exhaustion A concept related to burnout that involves a low energy state, sleep disturbances, extreme fatigue, irritability, and feelings of demoralization.

Vitamins Essential organic substances the body needs in minute amounts to support growth, to maintain bodily tissues, and to metabolize food.

Weight bearing exercise* A form of exercise like walking and weight lifting in which the muscles work against the full effect of gravity.

Weight set point model A model that maintains that weight loss is difficult to maintain because the body's internal regulating mechanisms drive the body's weight back to its natural predetermined level.

Well-being theory* Seligman's theory that well-being consists of positive emotions, engagement, meaning, positive relationships, and accomplishment.

Wellness A global concept of health that promotes physical, mental, emotional, and spiritual well-being.

Whole clear message A form of clean communication that involves four elements: the communicator's observations, thoughts, feelings, and needs.

Workplace discrimination* Hostile behaviors directed toward workers by other employees because of the target persons' identity group characteristics.

Workplace harassment Workers receiving adverse employment opportunities because of their identity group's characterisitics.

Work stress A generic term that applies to all manner of work-related contexts including the stress of informal work, self-employment, a formal job, or work in an organization.

Worldview Assumptions and beliefs about oneself, others, and the world.

Worry The process of recycling one's anxiety-driven thoughts.

Yerkes-Dodson Curve Optimal task performance occurs at the midlevel of diffuse physiological arousal.

Yoga A form of meditation practiced in the Hindu religion; secular versions of Hatha yoga emphasize learning aspects of physical discipline.

Zen Buddhist meditation (Zazen) A form of Buddhist meditation that involves mindfulness practices.

Aan het Rot, M., Collins, K. A., & Fitterling, H. L. (2009). Physical exercise and depression. *Mount Sinai Journal of Medicine, 76,* 204–214.

Aberg, M. A. I., Pedersen, N. L., Toren, K., Svantengren, M., Backstrand, B., Johnsson, T., . . . Kuhn, G. (2009). Cardiovascular fitness is associated with cognition in young adulthood. *Proceedings of the National Academy of Sciences, 106*(49). Retrieved from http://www.pnas.org_cgi_doi_10.1073_pnas.0905307106.

Abramson, L. Y., Seligman, M. E. P., & Teasdale, J. (1978). Learned helplessness in humans: Critique and reformulation. *Journal of Abnormal Psychology, 87,* 32–48.

Ackerman, K. D., Heyman, R., Rabin, B. S., Anderson, B. P., Houck, P. R., Frank, E., & Baum, A. (2002). Stressful life events precede exacerbations of multiple sclerosis. *Psychosomatic Medicine, 64,* 916–920.

Adams, S. G., Dammers, P. M., Saia, T. I., Brantley, P. J., & Gaydos, G. R. (1994). Stress, depression, and anxiety predict average symptom severity and daily fluctuation in systemic lupus erythematosus. *Journal of Behavioral Medicine, 17,* 459–477.

Affleck, G., Tennen, H., Urrows, S., & Higgins, P. (1994). Person and contextual features of daily stress reactivity: Individual differences in relations of undesirable daily events with mood disturbance and chronic pain intensity. *Journal of Personality and Social Psychology, 66,* 329–340.

Ahola, K., Vaananen, A., Koskinen, A., Kouvonen, A., & Shirom, A. (2010). Burnout as a predictor of all-cause mortality among industrial employees: A 10-year prospective register-linkage study. *Journal of Psychosomatic Research, 69,* 51–57.

Akehurst, R., & Kaltenthaler, E. (2001). Treatment of irritable bowel syndrome: A review of randomised controlled trials. *Gut, 48,* 272–282.

Albee, E. (1962). *Who's afraid of Virginia Woolfe?* New York: H. Wolff.

Aldana, S. G., Greenlaw, R., Salberg, A., Merrill, R. M., Hager, R., & Jorgensen, R. B. (2007). The effects of intensive lifestyle modification program on carotid artery intima-media thickness: A randomized trial. *American Journal of Health Promotion, 21,* 510–516.

Aldwin, C., Levenson, M. R., Spiro, A., III, & Bosse, R. (1989). Does motionality predict stress? Findings from the Normative Aging Study. *Journal of Personality and Social Psychology, 56,* 618–624.

Alexander, C. N., Robinson, P., Orme-Johnson, D. W., Schneider, R. H., & Walton, K. G. (1994). The effects of transcendental meditation compared to other methods of relaxation and meditation in reducing risk factors, morbidity, and mortality. *Homeostasis, 35,* 243–263.

Alexander, F. (1950). *Psychosomatic medicine: Its principles and applications.* New York: Norton.

Allen, R. J. (1983). *Human stress: Its nature and control.* Minneapolis, MN: Burgess.

Allport, G. W. (1937). *Personality: A psychological interpretation.* New York: Holt, Rinehart & Winston.

Amaral, D. G. (2000). The anatomical organization of the nervous system. In E. R. Kandel, J. H. Schwartz, & T. M. Jessell (Eds.), *Principles of neural science* (4th ed., pp. 317–336). New York: McGraw-Hill.

Amato, P. R. (2000). The consequences of divorce for adults and children. *Journal of Marriage and Family, 62,* 1269–1287.

American Cancer Society. (2010). *Cancer facts and figures 2010.* Atlanta, GA: Author. Retrieved from http://www.cancer.org/acs/groups/content/@nho/documents/document/acspc-024113.pdf.

American Cancer Society. (2011a). *Guidelines on nutrition and physical activity for cancer prevention.* Retrieved from http://www.cancer.org/acs/groups/cid/documents/webcontent/002577-pdf.pdf.

American Cancer Society. (2011b). *Stay healthy: Healthy living information to help you stay well.* Retrieved from http://www.cancer.org/Healthy/index.

American College of Sports Medicine (ACSM). (2005). *Guidelines for exercise testing and prescription* (7th ed.). Baltimore: Lippincott Williams & Wilkins.

American College of Sports Medicine and the American Diabetes Association. (2010). Joint position statement: Exercise and type 2 diabetes. *Medicine & Science in Sports & Exercise, 42,* 2282–2303.

American Diabetes Association. (2004). Nutrition principles and recommendations in diabetes. *Diabetes Care, 27,* S36–S46.

American Dietetic Association. (2009). Position of the American Dietetic Association: Functional foods. *Journal of the American Dietetic Association, 109,* 735–746.

American Heart Association. (2010). *Heart disease and stroke statistics—2010 update.* Dallas, TX: Author.

American Heart Association. (2011a). *Know your fats.* Retrieved from http://www.heart.org/HEARTORG/Conditions/Cholesterol/PreventionTreatmentofHighCholesterol/Know-Your-Fats_UCM_305628_Article.jsp.

American Heart Association (2011b). *Alcohol, wine and cardiovascular disease.* Retrieved from http://www.heart.org/HEARTORG/GettingHealthy/NutritionCenter/Alcohol-Wine-and-Cardiovascular-Disease_UCM_305864_Article.jsp.

American Psychiatric Association, (1952). *Diagnostic and statistical manual of mental disorders.* Washington, DC: Author.

American Psychiatric Association, (1968). *Diagnostic and statistical manual of mental disorders* (2nd ed.). Washington, DC: Author.

American Psychiatric Association. (1987). *Diagnostic and statistical manual of mental disorders* (3rd ed.). Washington, DC: Author.

American Psychiatric Association. (2000). *Diagnostic and statistical manual of mental disorders* (4th ed., text rev.). Washington, DC: Author.

Ames, B. N., McCann, J. C., Stampfer, M. J., & Willett, W. C. (2007). Evidence-based decision making on micronutrients and chronic disease: Long-term randomized controlled trials are not enough. *American Journal of Clinical Nutrition, 86,* 522–525.

Amirkhan, J. H. (1990). A factor analytically derived measure of coping: The coping strategy indicator. *Journal of Personality and Social Psychology, 59,* 1066–1074.

Anand, B. K., Chhina, G. S., & Singh, B. (1961). Studies of Shri Rananand Yogi during his stay in an airtight box. *Indian Journal of Medical Research, 49,* 82–89.

Andel, R., Crowe, M., Pedersen, N. L., Fratiglioni, L., Johansson, B., & Gatz, M. (2008). Physical exercise at midlife and risk of dementia three decades later: A population-based study of Swedish twins. *Journals of Gerontology Series A, Biological Sciences and Medical Sciences, 63,* 62–66.

Andersen, L. F., Jacobs, D. R., Jr., Carlsen, M. H., & Blomhoff, R. (2006). Consumption of coffee is associated with reduced risk of death attributed to inflammatory and cardiovascular diseases in the Iowa Women's Health Study. *American Journal of Clinical Nutrition, 83,* 1039–1046.

Andrasik, F. (2007). What does the evidence show? Efficacy of behavioural treatments for recurrent headaches in adults. *Neurological Sciences, 28,* S70–S77.

Angevaren, M., Aufdemkampe, G., Verhaar, H. J., Aleman, A., & Vanhees, L. (2008). Physical activity and enhanced fitness to improve cognitive function in older people without known cognitive impairment. *Cochrane Database System Review* (3). CD005381.

Anglem, N., Lucas, S. J. E., Rose, E. A., & Cotter, J. D. (2008). Mood,

illness and injury responses and recovery with adventure racing. *Wilderness and Environmental Medicine, 19,* 30–38.

Antonovsky, A. (1979). *Health, stress, and coping.* San Francisco: Jossey-Bass.

Antonovsky, A. (1987). *Unraveling the mystery of health: How people manage to stay well.* San Francisco: Jossey-Bass.

Armstrong, J. F., Wittrock, D. A., & Robinson, M. D. (2006). Implicit associations in tension-type headaches: A cognitive analysis based on stress reactivity processes. *Headache, 46,* 1281–1290.

Arnold, M. B. (1960). *Emotion and personality: Vol. I, Psychological aspects.* New York: Columbia University Press.

Arnow, B., Kenardy, J., & Agras, W. S. (1995). The Emotional Eating Scale: The development of a measure to assess coping with negative affect by eating. *International Journal of Eating Disorders, 18,* 79–90.

Aronson, E., Wilson, T. D., & Akert, R. M. (2010). *Social psychology* (7th ed.). New York: Prentice Hall.

Arthur, H. M. (2002). High trait anger increased stroke in people ≤ 60 years and those with high density lipoprotein cholesterol concentration > 47 mmol/l. *Evidence-Based Mental Health, 5,* 94.

Asher, I., Bawna-Cagnani, C. B., Boner, A, Canonica, G. W., Chuchalin, A., Custovic, A., . . . Zhong, N. S. (2004). World Allergy Organization guidelines for prevention of allergy and allergic asthma. *International Archives of Allergy and Immunology, 135,* 83–92.

Atkins, R. C. (1998). *Dr. Atkins' new diet revolution.* New York: Avon Books.

Ax, A. F. (1953). The physiological differentiation of fear and anger in humans. *Psychosomatic Medicine, 15,* 433–442.

Baer, R. A., Smith, G. T., Hopkins, J., Krietemeyer, J., & Toney, L. (2006). Using self-report assessment methods to explore facets of mindfulness. *Assessment, 13,* 27–45.

Baird, C. L., & Sands, L. P. (2006). Effect of guided imagery with relaxation on health-related quality of life in older women with osteoarthritis. *Research in Nursing and Health, 29,* 442–451.

Bandler, R. (2008). *Richard Bandler's guide to trance-formation: How to harness the power of hypnosis to ignite effortless and lasting change.* Deerfield Beach, FL: Health Communications Inc.

Bandura, A. (1977). Self-efficacy: Toward a unifying theory of behavioral change. *Psychological Review, 84,* 191–215.

Bandura, A. (1989). Human agency in social cognitive theory. *American Psychologist, 44,* 1175–1184.

Barlow, D. H., Allen, L. B., & Basden, S. L. (2007). Psychological treatments for panic disorders, phobias, and generalized anxiety disorder. In P. E. Nathan & J. M. Gorman (Eds.), *A guide to treatments that work* (3rd ed., pp. 351–394). New York: Oxford University Press.

Baron, R. S., Cutrona, C. E., Hicklin, D., Russell, D. W., & Lubaroff, D. M. (1990). Social support and immune function among spouses of cancer patients. *Journal of Personality and Social Psychology, 59,* 344–352.

Bassett, D. R., Schneider, P. L., & Huntington, G. E. (2004). Physical activity in an Old Order Amish community. *Medicine & Science in Sports & Exercise, 36,* 79–85.

Bassuk, S. S., & Manson, J. E. (2005). Epidemiological evidence for the role of physical activity in reducing risk of type 2 diabetes and cardiovascular disease. *Journal of Applied Physiology, 99,* 1193–1204.

Bassuk, S. S., & Manson, J. E. (2010). Physical activity and cardiovascular disease prevention in women: A review of the epidemiologic evidence. *Nutrition, Metabolism, & Cardiovascular Diseases, 20,* 467–473.

Batson, C. D., Ahmad, N., & Lishner, D. A. (2009). Empathy and altruism. In S. J. Lopez & C. R. Snyder (Eds.), *Handbook of positive psychology* (2nd ed., pp. 417–426). New York: Oxford University Press.

Baum, A. (1990). Stress, intrusive imagery, and chronic distress. *Health Psychology, 9,* 653–675.

Beck, A. T. (1967). *Depression: Clinical, experimental, and theoretical aspects.* New York: Harper & Row.

Beck, A. T. (1991). Cognitive therapy: A 30-year retrospective. *American Psychologist, 46,* 368–375.

Beck, A. T., Emery, G., & Greenberg, R. L. (1985). *Anxiety disorders and phobias: A cognitive perspective.* New York: Basic Books.

Beck, A. T., Rush, A. J., Shaw, B. F., & Emery, G. (1979). *Cognitive therapy of depression.* New York: The Guilford Press.

Beehr, T. A., & Glazer, S. (2005). Organizational role stress. In J. Barling, E. K. Kelloway, & M. R. Frone (Eds.), *Handbook of work stress* (pp. 7–33). Thousand Oaks, CA: Sage.

Beliveau, R., & Gingras, D. (2007). *Foods to fight cancer: Essential foods to help prevent cancer.* New York: DK.

Bellg, A. J. (2008). Cardiovascular disease. In B. A. Boyer & M. I. Paharia (Eds.), *Comprehensive handbook of clinical health psychology* (pp. 127–152). Hoboken, NJ: John Wiley & Sons.

Benedittis, G. D., & Lorenzetti, A. (1992). The role of stressful life events in the persistence of primary headache: Major events vs. daily hassles. *Pain, 51,* 35–42.

Benishek, L. A., & Lopez, F. G. (1997). Critical evaluation of hardiness theory: Gender differences, perception of life events, and neuroticism. *Work and Stress, 11,* 33–45.

Benson, H. (1975). *The relaxation response.* New York: Avon Books.

Benson, H. (1977). Systemic hypertension and the relaxation response. *The New England Journal of Medicine, 296,* 1152–1156.

Benson, H. (1996). *Timeless healing.* New York: Scribner.

Benson, H., Alexander, S., & Feldman, C. L. (1975). Decreased premature ventricular contractions through the relaxation response in patients with stable ischaemic heart disease. *Lancet, 2,* 380.

Benton, G. Cordiano, R., Palmieri, R., Cavuto, F., Buttazzi, P., & Palatini, P. (2010). Comparison of C-reactive protein and albumin excretion as prognostic markers for 10-year mortality after myocardial infarction. *Clinical Cardiology, 33,* 508–515.

Berghofer, A., Pischon, T., Reinhold, T., Apovian, C. M., Sharma, A. M., & Willich, S. N. (2008). Obesity prevalence from a European perspective: A systematic review. *BMC Public Health, 8,* 200–209.

Berk, L. E. (2007). *Development through the lifespan* (4th ed.). New York: Allyn and Bacon.

Berkman, L. F., & Syme, S. L. (1979). Social networks, host resistance, and mortality: A nine-year follow-up study of Alameda county residents. *American Journal of Epidemiology, 109,* 186–204.

Berne, E. (1964). *Games people play.* New York: Grove.

Bernhard, J. D., Kristeller, J., & Kabat-Zinn, J. (1988). Effectiveness of relaxation and visualization techniques as an adjunct to phototherapy and photochemotherapy of psoriasis. *Journal of the American Academy of Dermatology, 19,* 572–574.

Bernstein, D. A., & Borkovec, T. D. (1978). *Progressive relaxation training: A manual for the helping professions.* Champaign, IL: Research Press.

Bernstein, D. A., Carlson, C. R., & Schmidt, J. E. (2007). Progressive relaxation: Abbreviated methods. In P. M. Lehrer, R. L. Woolfolk, & W. E. Sime (Eds.), *Principles and practice of stress management* (3rd ed., pp. 88–122). New York: The Guilford Press.

Berscheid, E., & Reis, H. T. (1998). Attraction and close relationships. In D. T. Gilbert, S. T. Fiske, & G. Lindzey (Eds.), *The handbook of social psychology* (Vol. 2, 4th ed., pp. 193–281). New York: McGraw-Hill.

Berscheid, E., & Walster, E. H. (1978). *Interpersonal attraction* (2nd ed.). Reading, MA: Addison-Wesley.

Bhagat, R. S., McQuaid, S. J., Lindholm, H., & Segovis, J. (1985). Total life tress: A multimethod validation of the construct and its effects on organizationally valued outcomes and withdrawal behaviors. *Journal of Applied Psychology, 70,* 202–214.

Bhaskaram, P. (2002). Micronutrient malnutrition, infection, and immunity: An overview. *Nutrition Reviews, 60,* S40–S45.

Biasucci, L. M., Liuzzo, G., Fantuzzi, G., Caliguiuri, G., Rebuzzi, A. G., Ginnetti, F., . . . Maseri, A. (1999). Increasing levels of interleukin (IL)-1Ra and IL-6 during the first 2 days of hospitalization in unstable angina are associated with increased risk of in-hospital coronary events. *Circulation, 99,* 2079–2084.

Billings, A. G., & Moos, R. H. (1981). The role of coping responses and social resources in attenuating the impact of stressful life events. *Journal of Behavioral Medicine, 4,* 139–157.

Billings, A. G., & Moos, R. H. (1984). Coping, stress, and social resources among adults with unipolar depression. *Journal of Personality and Social Psychology, 46,* 877–891.

Biondi, M., & Picardi, A. (1993). Temporomandibular joint pain dysfunction syndrome and bruxism: Etiopathogenesis and treatment from a psychosomatic integrative viewpoint. *Psychotherapy and Psychosomatics, 59,* 84–98.

Bishop, S. R., Lau, M., Shapiro, S., Carlson, L., Anderson, N. D., Carmody, J., . . . Devins, G. (2004). Mindfulness: A proposed operational definition. *Clinical Psychology Science and Practice, 11,* 230–241.

Biswas, S. Ghoshal, P. K., Mandal, S. C., & Mandal, N. (2010). Relation of anti- to pro-inflammatory cytokine ratios with acute myocardial infarction. *The Korean Journal of Internal Medicine, 25,* 44–50.

Blake, C. S., & Hamrin, V. (2007). Current approaches to the assessment and management of anger and aggression in youth: A review. *Journal of Child and Adolescent Psychiatric Nursing, 20,* 209–221.

Blanchard, E. B. (1990). Biofeedback treatments of essential hypertension. *Biofeedback and Self-Regulation, 15,* 209–228.

Blanchard, E. B., Lackner, J. M., Jaccard, J., Roswell, D., Caresella, A. M., Powell, C., . . . Kuhn, E. (2008). The role of stress in symptom exacerbation among IBS patients. *Journal of Psychosomatic Research, 64,* 119–128.

Blanchard, E. B., McCoy, G. C., Musso, A., Gerardi, M. A., Pallmeyer, T. P., Gerardi, R. J., . . . Andrasik, F. (1986). A controlled comparison of thermal biofeedback and relaxation training in the treatment of essential hypertension: Short-term and long-term outcome. *Behavior Therapy, 17,* 563–579.

Blumenthal, J. A., Babyak, M. A., Doraiswamy, M., Watkins, L., Hoffman, B. M., Barbour, K. A., . . . Sherwood, A. (2007). Exercise and pharmacotherapy in the treatment of major depressive disorder. *Psychosomatic Medicine, 69,* 587–596.

Blumenthal, J. A., Sherwood, A., Babyak, M. A., Watkins, L. L., Waugh, R., Georiades, A., . . . Hinderliter, A. (2005). Effects of exercise and stress management training on markers of cardiovascular risk in patients with ischemic heart disease: A randomized controlled trial. *Journal of the American Medical Association, 293,* 1626–1634.

Boecker, H., Sprenger, T., Spilker, M. E., Henriksen, G., Koppenhoefer, M., Wagner, K. J., . . . Tolle, R. R. (2008). The runner's high: Opioidergic mechanisms in the human brain. *Cerebral Cortex, 18,* 2523–2531.

Bogg, T., & Roberts, B. W. (2004). Conscientiousness and health-related behaviors: A meta-analysis of the leading behavioral contributors to mortality. *Psychological Bulletin, 130,* 887–919.

Boggild, H., & Knutsson, A. (1999). Shift work, risk factors and cardiovascular disease. *Scandinavian Journal of Work, Environment and Health, 25,* 85–99.

Bolger, N., & Schilling, E. A. (1991). Personality and the problems of everyday life: The role of neuroticism in exposure and reactivity to daily stressors. *Journal of Personality, 59,* 355–386.

Bolger, N., & Zuckerman, A. (1995). A framework for studying personality and health behavior. *Journal of Personality and Social Psychology, 69,* 890–902.

Bonanno, G. A. (2004). Loss, trauma, and human resilience: Have we underestimated the human capacity to thrive after extreme aversive events? *American Psychologist, 59,* 20–28.

Bonneau, R. H. (1994). Experimental approaches to identify mechanisms of stress-induced modulation of immunity to herpes simplex virus infection. In R. Glaser & J. K. Kiecolt-Glaser (Eds.), *Handbook of human stress and immunity* (pp. 125–160). New York: Academic Press.

Bono, G., McCullough, M. E., & Root, L. M. (2008). Forgiveness, feeling connected to others, and well-being: Two longitudinal studies. *Personality and Social Psychology Bulletin, 34,* 182–195.

Booth-Kewley, S., & Vickers, R. R., Jr. (1994). Associations between the major domains of personality and health behavior. *Journal of Personality, 62,* 281–298.

Borg, G. (1998). *Borg's perceived exertion and pain scales.* Champaign, IL: Human Kinetics.

Bourdouxhe, M. A., Queinnec, Y., Granger, D., Baril, R. H., Guertin, S. C., Massicotte, P. R., . . . Lemay, F. L. (1999). Aging and shiftwork: The effects of 20 years of rotating 12-hour shifts among petroleum refinery operators. *Experimental Aging Research, 25,* 323–329.

Bowen, D., & Boehmer, U. (2010). The role of behavior in cancer prevention. In J. M. Suls, K. W. Davidson, & R. M. Kaplan (Eds.), *Handbook of health psychology and behavioral medicine* (pp. 370–380). New York: The Guilford Press.

Bowen, M. (1978). *Family therapy in clinical practice.* New York: Jason Aronson.

Bowen, S., Witkeiwitz, K., Dillworth, T., Chawla, N., Simpson, T., Ostafin, B., . . . Marlatt, A. (2006). Mindfulness meditation and substance use in an incarcerated population. *Psychology of Addictive Behaviors, 20,* 343–347.

Bradbury, T. N., & Fincham, F. D. (1990). Attributions in marriage: Review and critique. *Psychological Bulletin, 107,* 3–33.

Brand-Miller, J. C. (2003). Glycemic load and chronic disease. *Nutrition Reviews, 61,* S49–S55.

Bricker, J. B. (2010). Theory-based behavioral interventions for smoking cessation: Efficacy, processes, and future directions. In J. M. Suls, K. W. Davidson, & R. M. Kaplan (Eds.), *Handbook of health psychology and behavioral medicine* (pp. 544–566). New York: The Guilford Press.

Brickman, P., & Campbell, D. T. (1971). Hedonic relativism and planning the good society. In M. H. Appley (Ed.), *Adaptation level theory: A symposium*. New York: Academic Press.

Brickman, P., Coates, D., & Janoff-Bulman, R. (1978). Lottery winners and accident victims: Is happiness relative? *Journal of Personality and Social Psychology, 36*, 917–927.

Bricou, O., Taieb, O., Baubet, T., Gal, B., Guillevin, L., & Moro, M. R. (2006). Stress and coping strategies in systemic lupus erythematosus: A review. *Neuroimmunomodulation, 13*, 283–293.

Brod, C. (1982). Managing technostress: Optimizing the use of computer technology. *Personnel Journal, 61*, 753–757.

Brod, C. (1988). *Technostress: Human cost of the computer revolution*. Reading, MA: Addison-Wesley.

Brody, S. (1956). Psychological factors associated with the disseminated lupus erythematosus and effects of cortisone and ACTH. *Psychiatric Quarterly, 30*, 44–60.

Brondolo, E., Gallo, L. C., & Myers, H. F. (2009). Race, racism and health: Disparities,mechanisms, and interventions. *Journal of Behavioral Medicine, 32*, 1–8.

Brondolo, E., Rieppi, R., Kelly, K. P., & Gerin, W. (2003). Perceived racism and blood pressure: A review of the literature and conceptual and methodological critique. *Annals of Behavioral Medicine, 25*, 55–65.

Broocks, A., Bandelow, B., Pekrun, G., George, A., Myer, T., Barmann, M. A., . . . Ruther, E. (1998). Comparison of aerobic exercise, clomipramine, and placebo in the treatment of panic disorder. *American Journal of Psychiatry, 155*, 603–609.

Brown, D. E., James, G. D., & Mills, P. S. (2006). Occupational differences in job strain and physiological stress: Female nurses and school teachers in Hawaii. *Psychosomatic Medicine, 68*, 524–530.

Brown, G. W., & Harris, T. (1978). *Social origins of depression*. London, England: Tavistock.

Brown, J. D. (1998). *The self*. New York: Routledge.

Brown, K. W., & Ryan, R. M. (2003). The benefits of being present: Mindfulness and its role in psychological well-being. *Journal of Personality and Social Psychology, 84*, 822–848.

Brown, K. W., Ryan, R. M., & Creswell, J. D. (2007a). Reply: Addressing fundamental questions about mindfulness. *Psychological Inquiry, 18*, 272–281.

Brown, K. W., Ryan, R. M., & Creswell, J. D. (2007b). Mindfulness: Theoretical foundations and evidence for its salutary effects. *Psychological Inquiry, 18*, 211–237.

Brown, L., Rosner, B., Willett, W. W., & Sacks, F. M. (1999). Cholesterol-lowering effects of dietary fiber: A meta-analysis. *American Journal of Clinical Nutrition, 69*, 30–42.

Brown, R. P. (2003). Measuring individual differences in the tendency to forgive: Construct validity and links with depression. *Personality and Social Psychology Bulletin, 29*, 759–771.

Bruggemann, J. M., & Barry, R. J. (2002). Eysenck's P as a modulator of affective and electrodermal responses to violent and comic film. *Personality and Individual Differences, 32*, 1029–1048.

Bruininks, P., & Malle, B. F. (2005). Distinguishing hope from optimism and related affective states. *Motivation and Emotion, 29*, 327–355.

Brunstein, J. C., Schultheiss, O. C., & Grassman, R. (1998). Personal goals and emotional well-being: The moderating role of motive dispositions. *Journal of Personality and Social Psychology, 75*, 494–508.

Bryant, F. B. (1989). A four-factor model of perceived control: Avoiding, coping, obtaining, and savoring. *Journal of Personality, 57*, 773–797.

Bryant, F. B. (2003). Savoring Beliefs Inventory (SBI): A scale for measuring beliefs about savouring. *Journal of Mental Health, 12*, 175–196.

Bryant, F. B., & Veroff, J. (2006). *Savoring: A new model of positive experience*. Mahwah, NJ: Erlbaum.

Brydon, L., Walker, C., Wawrzyniak, A. J., Chart, H., & Steptoe, A. (2009). Dispositional optimism and stress-induced changes in immunity and negative mood. *Brain, Behavior, and Immunity, 23*, 810–816.

Buchanan, G. M., & Seligman, M. E. P. (Eds.). (1995). *Explanatory style*. Hillsdale, NJ: Erlbaum.

Buckworth, J. (2007). Behavior modification. In E. T. Howley & B. D. Franks (Eds.), *Fitness professional's handbook* (5th ed., pp. 329–342). Champaign, IL: Human Kinetics.

Buettner, D. (2008). *The blue zones: Lessons for living longer from the people who've lived the longest*. Washington, DC: National Geographic.

Bukowski, C. (1980). The shoelace. On *Bukowski reads his poetry*. Santa Monica, CA: Takoma Records.

Burns, D. D. (1993). *Ten days to self-esteem*. New York: Quill William Morrow.

Butki, B. D., Rudolph, D. L., & Jacobsen, H. (2001). Self-efficacy, state anxiety, and cortisol responses to treadmill running. *Perceptual and Motor Skills, 92*, 1129–1138.

Butler, A. C., Chapman, J. E., Forman, E. M., & Beck, A. T. (2006). The empirical status of cognitive-behavioral therapy: A review of meta-analyses. *Clinical Psychology Review,26*, 17–31.

Butow, P. N., Hiller, J. E., Price, M. A., Thackway, S. V., Kricker, A., & Tennant, C. C. (2000). Epidemiological evidence for a relationship between life events, coping style, and personality factors in the development of breast cancer. *Journal of Psychosomatic Research, 49*, 169–181.

Butt, M. S., & Sultan, M. T. (2009). Green tea: Nature's defense against malignancies. *Critical Reviews in Food Science and Nutrition, 49*, 463–473.

Caccioppo, J. T., Kiecolt-Glaser, J. K., Malarkey, W. B., Laskowski, B. F., Rozlog, L. A., Poehlmann, K. M., . . . Glaser, R. (2002). Autonomic and glucocorticoid associations with the steady-state expression of latent Epstein-Barr virus. *Hormones and Behavior, 42*, 32–41.

Campbell, A. (1981). *The sense of well-being in America*. New York: McGraw-Hill.

Campbell-Sills, L., Cohan, S. L., Stein, M. B. (2006). Relationship of resilience to personality, coping, and psychiatric symptoms in young adults. *Behaviour Research and Therapy, 44,* 585–599.

Cannon, W. B. (1932). *The wisdom of the body.* New York: W.W. Norton.

Capuron, L., Ravaud, A., Miller, A. H., & Danzer, R. (2004). Baseline mood and psychosocial characteristics of patients developing depressive symptoms during interleukin-2 and/or interferon-alpha cancer therapy. *Brain, Behavior, and Immunity, 18,* 205–213.

Carlson, L. E., & Brown, K. W. (2005). Validation of the Mindful Attention Awareness Scale in a cancer population. *Journal of Psychosomatic Research, 58,* 29–33.

Carlson, L. E., Speca, M., Faris, P., & Patel, K. (2007). One year pre-post intervention follow-up of psychological, immune, endocrine and blood pressure outcomes of mindfulness-based stress reduction (MBSR) in breast and prostate cancer outpatients. *Brain, Behavior, and Immunity, 21,* 1038–1049.

Carlson, L. E., Speca, M., Patel, K. D., & Goodey, E. (2003). Mindfulness-based stress reduction in relation to quality of life, mood, symptoms of stress, and immune parameters in breast and prostate cancer outpatients. *Psychosomatic Medicine, 5,* 571–581.

Carney, R. M., & Freedland, K. E. (2007). The management of depression in patients with coronary heart disease. In A. Steptoe (Ed.), *Depression and physical illness* (pp. 109–124). New York: Cambridge University Press.

Carrington, P. (1978). *Clinically standardized meditation (CSM) professional pack.* Kendall Park, NJ: Pace Educational Systems.

Carrington, P. (1998). *The book of meditation.* Kendall Park, NJ: Pace Educational Systems.

Carrington, P. (2007). Modern forms of mantra meditation. In P. W. Lehrer, R. L. Woolfolk, & W. E. Sime (Eds.), *Principles and practice of stress management* (3rd ed., pp. 363–392). New York: The Guilford Press.

Carrington, P., Collings, G. H., Benson, H., Robinson, H., Wood, L. W., Lehrer, P. M. . . . Cole, J. W.

(1980). The use of meditation-relaxation techniques for the management of stress in a working population. *Journal of Occupational Medicine, 22,* 221–231.

Carroll, L. (2004). *Alice's adventures in wonderland and through the looking glass.* New York: Barnes & Noble Classics.

Carson, J. W., Carson, K. M., Gil, K. M., & Baucom, D. H. (2004). Mindfulness-based relationship enhancement. *Behavior Therapy, 35,* 471–494.

Cartwright, S., & Cooper, C. (2005). Individually targeted interventions. In J. Barling, E. K. Kelloway, & M. R. Frone (Eds.), *Handbook of work stress* (pp. 149–188). Thousand Oaks, CA: Sage.

Carver, C. S. (1989). How should multifaceted personality constructs be tested? Issues illustrated by self-monitoring, attributional style, and hardiness. *Journal of Personality and Social Psychology, 56,* 577–585.

Carver, C. S., & Connor-Smith, J. (2010). Personality and coping. *Annual Review of Psychology, 61,* 679–704.

Carver, C. S., Scheier, M. F., & Weintraub, J. K. (1989). Assessing coping strategies: A theoretically based approach. *Journal of Personality and Social Psychology, 56,* 267–283.

Carver, C. S., Scheier, M. F., Miller, C. J., & Fulford, D. (2009). Optimism. In S. J. Lopez & C. R. Snyder (Eds.), *Oxford handbook of positive psychology* (2nd ed., pp. 303–311). New York: Oxford University Press.

Cassell, E. J. (2009). Compassion. In S. J. Lopez & C. R. Snyder (Eds.), *Oxford handbook of positive psychology* (2nd ed., pp. 393–403). New York: Oxford University Press.

Cathcart, S. Petkov, J., Winefield, A. H., Lushington, K., & Rolan, P. (2010). Central mechanisms of stress-induced headache. *Cephalalgia, 30,* 285–295.

Cathcart, S., & Prichard, D. (2008). Daily stress and pain sensitivity in chronic tension-type headache sufferers. *Stress and Health: Journal of the International Society for the Investigation of Stress, 24,* 123–127.

Cattell, R. B., & Eber, H. W. (1962). *Handbook for the Sixteen P. F. Test.* Champaign, IL: IPAT.

Centers for Disease Control and Prevention. (2010a). Recommended adult immunization schedule—United States, 2010. *MMWR, 59*(1). Retrieved from http://www.cdc.gov/mmwr/PDF/wk/mm5901-Immunization.pdf.

Centers for Disease Control and Prevention (CDC). (2010b). *Tobacco use: Targeting the nation's leading killer: At a glance 2010.* Retrieved from http://www.cdc.gov/chronicdisease/resources/publications/aag/osh.htm.

Centers for Disease Control and Prevention. (2011a). *Arthritis-related statistics.* Retrieved from http://www.cdc.gov/arthritis/data_statistics/arthritis_related_stats.htm#2.

Centers for Disease Control and Prevention. (2011b). *Eliminate disparities in lupus.* Retrieved from http://www.cdc.gov/omhd/amh/factsheets/lupus.htm.

Centers for Disease Control and Prevention (CDC). (2011c). *Faststats: Smoking.* Retrieved from http://www.cdc.gov/nchs/fastats/smoking.htm.

Centers for Disease Control and Prevention (CDC). (2011d). *Frequently asked questions about calculating obesity-related risk.* Retrieved from http://www.cdc.gov/PDF/Frequently_Asked_Questions_About_Calculating_Obesity-Related_Risk.pdf.

Centers for Disease Control and Prevention. (2011e). *Growing stronger—strength training for older adults.* Retrieved from http://www.cdc.gov/physicalactivity/growingstronger/why/index.html.

Centers for Disease Control and Prevention (CDC). (2011f). *Obesity and overweight.* Retrieved from http://www.cdc.gov/nchs/fastats/overwt.htm.

Chacko, S. M., Thambi, P. T., Kuttan, R., & Nishigaki, I. (2010). Beneficial effects of green tea: A literature review. *Chinese Medicine, 5,* 1–9.

Chandola, T., Britton, A., Brunner, E., Hemingway, H., Malik, M., Kumari, M., . . . Marmot, M. (2008). Work stress and coronary heart disease: What are the mechanisms? *European Heart Journal, 29,* 640–648.

Chandrashekara, S., Jayashree, K., Veeranna, H. B., Vadiraj, H. S., Ramesh, M. N., Shobha, A., . . . Vikram, Y. K. (2007). Effects of anxiety on TNF-α levels during psychological stress. *Journal of Psychosomatic Research, 63,* 65–69.

Chaouloff, F. (1997). Effects of acute physical exercise on central serotonergic systems. *Medicine & Science in Sports & Exercise, 29,* 58–62.

Charlesworth, E. A., & Nathan, R. G. (1985, 2004). *Stress management: A comprehensive guide to wellness.* New York: Atheneum.

Charnetski, C. J., Brennan, F. X., Jr., & Harrison, J. (1998). Effects of music and auditory stimuli on secretory immunoglobulin A (IgA). *Perceptual and Motor Skills, 87,* 1163–1170.

Charney, D. S. (2004). Psychobiological mechanisms of resilience and vulnerability. *American Journal of Psychiatry, 161,* 195–216.

Cherlin, A. J. (1992). *Marriage, divorce, remarriage.* Cambridge, MA: Harvard University Press.

Chida, Y., & Hamer, M. (2008). Chronic psychosocial factors and acute physiological responses to laboratory induced stress in the healthy populations: A quantitative review of 30 years of investigations. *Psychological Bulletin, 134,* 829–885.

Chida, Y., & Steptoe, A. (2009). The association of anger and hostility with future coronary heart disease: A meta-analytic review of prospective evidence. *Journal of the American College of Cardiology, 53,* 936–946.

Chida, Y., Hamer, M., & Steptoe, A. (2008). A bidirectional relationship between psychosocial factors and atopic disorders: A systematic review and meta-analysis. *Psychosomatic Medicine, 70,* 102–116.

Chida, Y., Steptoe, A., & Powell, L. H. (2009). Religiosity/spirituality and mortality. *Psychotherapy and Psychosomatics, 78,* 81–90.

Chodzko-Zajko, W. J., Proctor, D. N., Singh, M. A. F., Minson, C. T., Nigg, C. R., Salem, G. J., & Skinner, J. S. (2009). American College of Sports Medicine position stand: Exercise and physical activity for older adults. *Medicine & Science in Sports & Exercise, 41,* 1510–1530.

Choy, Y., Fyer, A. J., & Lipsitz, J. D. (2007). Treatment of specific phobia in adults. *Clinical Psychology Review, 27,* 266–286.

Church, T. S., Earnest, C. P., Skinner, J. S., & Blair, S. N. (2007). Effects of different doses of physical activity on cardiorespiratory fitness among sedentary, overweight or obese postmenopausal women with elevated blood pressure: A randomized controlled trial. *Journal of the American Medical Association, 297,* 2081–2091.

Claessens, B. J. C., van Eerde, W., & Rutte, C. G. (2007). A review of the time management literature. *Personnel Review, 36,* 255–276.

Clark, M. S., & Oswald, A. J. (1996). Satisfaction and comparison income. *Journal of Public Economics, 61,* 359–381.

Clark, R., Anderson, N. B., Clark, V. R., & Williams, D. R. (1999). Racism as a stressor forAfrican Americans: A biopsychosocial model. *American Psychologist, 54,* 805–816.

Clarke, J. H., MacPherson, B. V., & Holmes, D. R. (1982). Cigarette smoking and external locus of control among young adolescents. *Journal of Health and Social Behavior, 23,* 253–259.

Clarke, S., & Robertson, I. T. (2005). A meta-analytic review of the Big Five personality factors and accident involvement in occupational and non-occupational settings. *Journal of Occupational and Organizational Psychology, 78,* 355–376.

Cloninger, S. (2008). Theories of personality: *Understanding persons* (5th ed.). Upper Saddle River, NJ: Pearson Prentice Hall.

Coe, C. L. (2010). All roads lead to psychoneuroimmunology. In J. M. Suls, K. W. Davidson, & R. M. Kaplan (Eds.), *Handbook of health psychology and behavioral medicine* (pp. 182–199). New York: The Guilford Press.

Cohen, J. (1992). A power primer. *Psychological Bulletin, 112,* 155–159.

Cohen, S. (2004). Social relationships and health. *American Psychologist, 59,* 676–684.

Cohen, S., Hamrick, N., Rodriguez, M. S., Feldman, P. J., Rabin, B. S., & Manuck, S. B. (2002). Reactivity and vulnerability to stress-associated risk for upper respiratory illness. *Psychosomatic Medicine, 64,* 302–310.

Cohen, S., Janicki-Deverts, D., & Miller, G. E. (2007). Psychological stress and disease. *Journal of the American Medical Association, 14,* 1685–1687.

Cohen, S., Tyrrell, D. A. J., & Smith, A. P. (1991). Psychological stress and susceptibility to the common cold. *The New England Journal of Medicine, 325,* 606–612.

Cohen, S., Tyrrell, D. A. J., & Smith, A. P. (1993). Negative life events, perceived stress, negative affect, and susceptibility to the common cold. *Journal of Personality and Social Psychology, 64,* 131–140.

Cohn, M. A., & Fredrickson, F. (2009). Positive emotions. In S. J. Lopez & C. R. Snyder (Eds.), *Oxford handbook of positive psychology* (2nd ed., pp. 13–24). New York: Oxford University Press.

Colcombe, S. J., & Kramer, A. F. (2003). Fitness effects on the cognitive function of older adults: A meta-analytic study. *Psychological Science, 14,* 125–130.

Colcombe, S. J., Erickson, K. I., Raz, N., Webb, A. G., Cohen, N. J., McAuley, E., & Kramer, A. F. (2003). Aerobic fitness reduces brain tissue loss in aging humans. *Journals of Gerontology, Series A, Biological Sciences and Medical Sciences, 58,* 176–180.

Compton, W. C. (2005). *An introduction to positive psychology.* Belmont, CA: Wadsworth.

Congreve, W. (1967). The mourning bride. In H. Davis (Ed.), *The complete plays of William Congreve* (pp. 326–384). Chicago: The University of Chicago Press.

Conner-Smith, J. K., & Flachsbart, C. (2007). Relations between personality and coping: A meta-analysis. *Journal of Personality and Social Psychology, 93,* 1080–1107.

Conrad, C. (2010). The art of medicine: Music for healing: From magic to medicine. *Lancet, 376,* 1980–1981.

Conrad, C., Niess, H., Jauch, K.-W., Bruns, C. J., Hartl, W., & Welker, L. (2007). Overture for growth hormone, requiem for interleukin-6? *Critical Care Medicine, 35,* 2709–2713.

Consedine, N. S., Magai, C., & Chin, S. (2004). Hostility and anxiety differentially predict cardiovascular disease in men and women. *Sex Roles, 50,* 63–77.

Cooper, C. L., Dewe, P. J., & O'Driscoll, M. P. (2001). *Organizational stress: A review and critique of theory, research, and applications.* Thousand Oaks, CA: Sage.

Cooper, C. L., Dewe, P. J., & O'Driscoll, M. P. (2011). Employee assistance programs: Strengths, challenges, and future roles. In J. C. Quick & L. E. Tetrick (Eds.), *Occupational health psychology* (2nd ed., pp. 337–356). Washington, DC: American Psychological Association.

Cooper, K. (1968). *Aerobics.* New York: Bantam Books.

Cooper, M. J., & Aygen, M. M. (1979). A relaxation technique in the management of hypercholestolemia. *Journal of Human Stress, 5,* 24–27.

Corah, W. L., & Boffa, J. (1970). Perceived control, self-observation and response to aversive stimulation. *Journal of Personality and Social Psychology, 16,* 1–4.

Costa, G. (1996). The impact of shift and night work on health. *Applied Ergonomics, 27,* 9–16.

Costa, G., Haus, E, & Stevens, R. (2010). Shift work and cancer: Considerations on rationale, mechanisms, and epidemiology. *Scandinavian Journal of Work and Environmental Health, 36,* 163–179.

Costa, P. T., Jr., & McCrae, R. R. (1980). Influence of extraversion and neuroticism on subjective well-being: Happy and unhappy people. *Journal of Personality and Social Psychology, 38,* 668–678.

Costa, P. T., Jr., & McCrae, R. R. (1980). Somatic complaints in males as a function of age and neuroticism: A longitudinal analysis. *Journal of Behavioral Medicine, 3,* 245–257.

Costa, P. T., Jr., & McCrae, R. R. (1985). *The NEO Personality Inventory manual.* Odessa, FL: Psychological Assessment Resources.

Costa, P. T., Jr., & McCrae, R. R. (1987). Neuroticism, somatic complaints, and disease: Is the bark worse than the bite? *Journal of Personality, 55,* 299–316.

Costa, P. T., Jr., & McCrae, R. R. (1992). *Revised NEO Personality Inventory (NEO-PI-R) and NEO Five-Factor Inventory (NEO-FFI) professional manual.* Odessa, FL: Psychological Assessment Resources.

Costa, P. T., Jr., McCrae, R. R., & Zonderman, A. B. (1987). Environmental and dispositional influences on well-being: Longitudinal follow-up on an American national sample. *British Journal of Psychology, 78,* 299–306.

Costanzo, E. S., Lutgendorf, S. K., Sood, A. K., Anderson, B., Sorosky, J., &Lubaroff, D. M. (2005). Psychosocial factors and interleukin-6 among women with advanced ovarian cancer. *Cancer, 104,* 305–313.

Council on Scientific Affairs. (1987). Results and implications of the AMA-APA Physician Mortality Project, Stage II. *Journal of the American Medical Association, 257,* 2949–2953.

Cousins, N. (1976). *Anatomy of an illness.* New York: Norton.

Cousins, N. (1978). Anatomy of an illness (as perceived by the patient). *The New England Journal of Medicine, 295,* 1458–1463.

Coyle, Y. M. (2008). Physical activity as a negative modulator of estrogen-induced breast cancer. *Cancer Causes Control, 19,* 1021–1029.

Coyne, J. C., & Holroyd, K. (1982). Stress, coping, and illness: A transactional perspective. In T. Millon, C. Green, & R. Meagher, *Handbook of clinical health psychology* (pp. 103–127). New York: Plenum.

Coyne, J. C., Stefanek, M., & Palmer, S. C. (2007). Psychotherapy and survival in cancer: The conflict between hope and evidence. *Psychological Bulletin, 133,* 367–394.

Craighead, W. E., Sheets, E. S., Brosse, A. L., & Ilardi, S. S. (2007).

Psychosocial treatments for major depressive disorder. In P. E. Nathan & J. M. Gorman (Eds.), *A guide to treatments that work* (3rd ed., pp. 289–322). New York: Oxford University Press.

Creswell, J. D., Way, B. M., Eisenberger, N. I., & Lieberman, M. D. (2007). Neural correlates of dispositional mindfulness during affect labeling. *Psychosomatic Medicine, 69,* 560–565.

Cropanzano, R., Goldman, B. M., & Benson, L. (2005). Organizational justice. In J. Barling, E. K. Kelloway, & M. R. Frone (Eds.), *Handbook of work stress* (pp. 63–87). Thousand Oaks, CA: Sage.

Csikszentmihalyi, M. (1975). Play and intrinsic rewards. *Journal of Humanistic Psychology, 15,* 41–63.

Csikszentmihalyi, M. (1990). *Flow: The psychology of optimal experience.* New York: Harper & Row.

Csikszentmihalyi, M., & LeFevre, J. (1989). Optimal experience in work and leisure. *Journal of Personality and Social Psychology, 56,* 815–822.

Dahl, J., Wilson, K. G., & Nilsson, A. (2004). Acceptance and commitment therapy and the treatment of persons at risk for long-term disability resulting from stress and pain symptoms: A preliminary randomized trial. *Behavior Therapy, 35,* 785–801.

Damjanovic, A. K., Yang, Y., Glaser, R., Kiecolt-Glaser, J. K., Nguyen, H., Laskowski, B., . . . Weng, N. P. (2007). Accelerated telomere erosion is associated with a declining immune function of caregivers of Alzheimer's patients. *Journal of Immunology, 179,* 4249–4254.

Danese, A., Pariante, C. M., Caspi, A., Taylor, A, & Poulton, R. (2007). Childhood maltreatment predicts adult inflammation in a life-course study. *Proceedings from the National Academy of Sciences, 104,* 1319–1324.

Danesh, J., Wheeler, J. G., Hirschfield, G. M., Edna, S., Eiriksdottir, G., Rumley, A., . . . Gudnason, V. (2004). C-reactive protein and other circulating markers of inflammation in the prediction of coronary heart disease. *The New England Journal of Medicine, 350,* 1387–1397.

Daubenmier, J. J., Weidner, G., Sumner, M. D., Mendell, N., Merritt-Worden, T., Studley, J., & Ornish, D. (2007). The contribution of changes in diet, exercise, and stress management to changes in coronary risk in women and men in the Multisite Cardiac Lifestyle Intervention Program. *Annals of Behavioral Medicine, 33,* 57–68.

Davidson, K. W., & Mostofsky, E. (2010). Anger expression and risk of coronary heart disease: Evidence from the Nova Scotia health survey. *American Heart Journal, 159,* 199–206.

Davidson, R. J., Kabat-Zinn, J., Schumacher, J., Rosenkranz, M., Muller, D., Santorelli, S. F., . . . Sheridan, J. F. (2003). Alterations in brain and immune function produced by mindfulness meditation. *Psychosomatic Medicine, 65,* 564–570.

Davila, J., Bradbury, T. N., Cohan, C. L., & Tochluk, S. (1997). Marital functioning and depressive symptoms: Evidence for a stress generation model. *Journal of Personality and Social Psychology, 73,* 849–861.

Davis, C., & Cowles, M. (1985). Type A behavior assessment: A critical comment. *Canadian Psychology, 26,* 39–42.

Deary, I. J., Ramsay, H., Wilson, J. A., & Raid, M. (1988). Stimulated salivation: Correlations with personality and time of day effects. *Personality and Individual Differences, 9,* 903–909.

Deci, E. L., & Ryan, R. M. (1985). *Intrinsic motivation and self-determination in human behavior.* New York: Plenum.

Deffenbacher, J. L., Oetting, E. R., Huff, M. E., & Thwaites, G. A. (1995). Fifteen-month follow-up of social skills and cognitive-relaxation approaches to general anger reduction. *Journal of Consulting Psychology, 42,* 400–405.

Deffenbacher, J. L., Oetting, E. R., Huff, M. E., Cornell, G. R., & Dallager, C. J. (1996). Evaluation of two cognitive-behavioral approaches to general anger reduction. *Cognitive Therapy and Research, 20,* 551–573.

Deffenbacher, J. L., Story, D. A., Stark, R. S., Hogg, J. A., & Brandon, A. D. (1987). Cognitive-Relaxation and social skills interventions in the treatment of general anger. *Journal of Counseling Psychology, 34,* 171–176.

Deffenbacher, J. L., Thwaites, G. A., Wallace, T. L., & Oetting, E. R. (1994). Social skills and cognitive-relaxation approaches to general anger reduction. *Journal of Counseling Psychology, 41,* 386–396.

DeLong, M. R. (2000). The basal ganglia. In E. R. Kandel, J. H. Schwartz, & T. M. Jessell (Eds.), *Principles of neural science* (4th ed., pp. 853–867). New York: McGraw-Hill.

DeLongis, A., Coyne, J. C., Dakof, G., Folkman, S., & Lazarus, R. S. (1982). Relationship of daily hassles, uplifts, and major life events to health status. *Health Psychology, 1,* 119–136.

Dembroski, T. M., MacDougall, J. M., Williams, R, Haney, T. L., & Blumenthal, J. A. (1985). Components of Type A, hostility, and anger-in: Relationship to angiographic findings. *Psychosomatic Medicine, 47,* 219–233.

DeNeve, K. M., & Cooper, H. (1998). The happy personality: A meta-analysis of 137 personality traits and subjective well-being. *Psychological Bulletin, 124,* 197–229.

Denollet, J., Sys, S. U., & Brutsaert, D. L. (1995). Personality and mortality after myocardial infarction. *Psychosomatic Medicine, 57,* 582–591.

Depue, R. A., & Collins, P. F. (1999). Neurobiology of the structure of personality: Dopamine, facilitation of incentive motivation, and extraversion. *Behavioral and Brain Sciences, 22,* 491–517.

Dhabhar, F. S. (2009). Enhancing versus suppressive effects of stress on immune function: Implications for immunoprotection and immunopathology. *Neuroimmunomodulation, 16,* 300–317.

Di Castelnuovo, A., Rotondo, S., Iacoviello, L., Donati, M. B., & de Gaetano, G. (2002). Meta-analysis of wine and beer consumption in relation to vascular risk. *Circulation, 105,* 2836–2844.

Dickinson, H. O., Beyer, F. R., Ford, G. A., Nicolson, D., Campbell, F., Cook, J. V., & Mason, J. (2008). Relaxation therapies for the management of primary hypertension in adults. *Cochrane Database Systematic Review* (1). doi: 10.1002/14651858.CD004935.pub2.

Diener, E. (1984). Subjective well-being. *Psychological Bulletin, 95,* 542–575.

Diener, E. (1994). Assessing subjective well-being: Progress and opportunities. *Social Indicators Research, 31,* 103–157.

Diener, E. (2009). Positive psychology: Past, present, and future. In S. J. Lopez & C. R. Snyder (Eds.), *Oxford handbook of positive psychology* (2nd ed., pp. 7–11). New York: Oxford University Press.

Diener, E., & Seligman, M. E. P. (2002). Very happy people. *Psychological Science, 13,* 81–84.

Diener, E., Diener, M., & Diener, C. (1995). Factors predicting the subjective well-being of nations. *Journal of Personality and Social Psychology, 69,* 851–864.

Diener, E., Emmons, R. A., Larsen, R. J., & Griffin, S. (1985). The satisfaction with life scale. *Journal of Personality Assessment, 49,* 71–75.

Diener, E., Sandvik, E., Seidlitz, L., & Diener, M. (1993). The relationship between income and subjective well-being: Relative or absolute? *Social Indicators of Research, 28,* 195–223.

Diener, E., Suh, E. M., Lucas, R. E., & Smith, H. L. (1999). Subjective well-being: Three decades of progress. *Psychological Bulletin, 125,* 276–302.

Dimsdale, J. (2008). Psychological stress and cardiovascular disease. *Journal of the American College of Cardiology, 51,* 1237–1246.

Dishman, R. K., & O'Connor, P. J. (2009). Lessons in exercise neurobiology: The case of endorphins. *Mental Health and Physical Activity, 2,* 4–9.

Dohrenwend, B. P., Raphael, K. G., Schwartz, S., Stueve, A., & Skodol, A. (1993). The structured event probe and narrative rating method for measuring life events. In L. Goldberger and S. Breznitz (Eds.), *Handbook of stress: Theoretical and clinical aspects* (pp. 174–184). New York: Free Press.

Dohrenwend, B. S., Dohrenwend, B. P., Dodson, M., & Shrout, P. E.

(1984). Symptoms, hassles, social supports, and life events: Problem of confounded measures. *Journal of Abnormal Psychology, 93,* 222–230.

Dohrenwend, B. S., Krasnoff, L., Askenasy, A. R., & Dohrenwend, B. P. (1982). The Psychiatric Epidemiology Research Interview Life Events Scale. In L. Goldberger & S. Bresnitz (Eds.), *Handbook of stress: Theoretical and clinical aspects.* New York: Free Press.

Domschke, K., Stevens, S., Pfleiderer, B., & Gerlach, A. L. (2010). Interoceptive sensitivity in anxiety and anxiety disorders: An overview and integration of neurobiological findings. *Clinical Psychology Review, 30,* 1–11.

Dong, M., Giles, W. H., Flitti, V. J., Dube, S. R., Williams, J. E., Chapman, D. P., & Anda, R. F. (2004). Insights into causal pathways for ischemic heart disease: Adverse childhood experiences study. *Circulation, 110,* 1761–1766.

Donnelly, J. E., Blair, S. N., Jakicic, J. M., Manore, M. M., Rankin, J. W., & Smith, B. K. (2009). American College of Sports Medicine position stand: Appropriate physical activity intervention strategies for weight loss and prevention of weight regain for adults. *Medicine & Science in Sports & Exercise, 41,* 459–471.

Donovan, M. R., Glue, P., Kolluri, S., & Emir, B. (2010). Comparative efficacy of antidepressants in preventing relapse in anxiety disorders—A meta-analysis. *Journal of Affective Disorders, 123,* 9–16.

Dube, S. R., Fairweather, D., Pearson, W. S., Felitti, V. J., Anda, R. F., & Croft, J. B. (2009). Cumulative childhood stress and autoimmune diseases in adults. *Psychosomatic Medicine, 71,* 243–250.

Duijts, S. F. A., Zeegers, M. P. A., & Borne, B. V. (2003). The association between stressful life events and breast cancer risk: A meta-analysis. *International Journal of Cancer, 107,* 1023–1029.

Dunn, A. L., Trivedi, M. H., Kampert, J. B., Clark, C. G., & Chambliss, H. O. (2005). Exercise treatment for depression: Efficacy and dose response. *American Journal of Preventive Medicine, 28,* 1–8.

Dunn, D. S., Uswatte, G., & Elliot, T. R. (2009). Happiness, resilience, and positive growth following physical disability: Issues for understanding, research, and therapeutic intervention. In S. J. Lopez & C. R. Snyder (Eds.), *Oxford handbook of positive psychology* (2nd ed., pp. 651–664). New York: Oxford University Press.

Dusseldorp, E., van Elderen, T., Maes, S., Meulman, J., & Kraaij, V. (1999). A meta-analysis of psychoeducational programs for coronary heart disease patients. *Health Psychology, 18,* 506–519.

Easterlin, B. L., & Cardena, E. (1998). Cognitive and emotional differences between short- and long-term Vipassana meditators. *Imagination, Cognition and Personality, 18,* 69–81.

Edinger, J. D., & Jacobsen, R. (1982). Incidence and significance of relaxation treatment side effects. *Behavior Therapist, 5,* 137–138.

Edlin, G., & Golanty, E. (1992). *Health and wellness: A holistic approach.* Boston: Jones & Bartlett.

Edwards, J. R., Caplan, R. D., & Harrison, R. V. (1998). Person-environment fit theory: Conceptual foundations, empirical evidence, and directions for future research. In C. L. Cooper (Ed.), *Theories of organizational stress* (pp. 28–67). New York: Oxford University Press.

Egan, S. J., Wade, T. D., & Shafran, R. (2011). Perfectionism as a transdiagnostic process: A clinical review. *Clinical Psychology Review, 31,* 203–212.

Ehlers, A., Bisson, J., Clark, D. M., Creamer, M., Pilling, S., Richards, D., . . . Yule, W. (2010). Do all psychological treatments really work the same in posttraumatic stress disorder? *Clinical Psychology Review, 30,* 269–276.

Ekman, P. (1993). Facial expressions and emotion. *American Psychologist, 48,* 384–392.

Elenkov, I. J., Iezzoni, D. G., Daly, A., Harris, A. G., & Chrousos, G. P. (2005). Cytokine dysregulation, inflammation and well-being. *Neuroimmunomodulation, 12,* 255–269.

Elfenbein, H. A., & Ambady, N. (2002). On the universality of and cultural specificity of emotion recognition: A meta-analysis. *Psychological Bulletin, 128,* 203–235.

Ellis, A., & Dryden, W. (2007). *The practice of rational-emotive behavior therapy* (2nd ed.). New York: Springer.

Emmons, R. A., & McCullough, M. E. (2003). Counting blessings versus burdens: An empirical investigation of gratitude and subjective well-being in daily life. *Journal of Personality and Social Psychology, 84,* 377–389.

Endler, N. S., & Parker, J. D. A. (1990). Multidimensional assessment of coping: A critical evaluation. *Journal of Personality and Social Psychology, 58,* 844–854.

Eng, P. M., Fitzmaurice, G., Kubzansky, L. D., Rimm, E. B., & Kawachi, I. (2003). Anger expression and risk of stroke and coronary heart disease among male health professionals. *Psychosomatic Medicine, 65,* 100–110.

Engel, G. L. (1971). Sudden and rapid death during psychological stress: Folklore or folk wisdom? *Annals of Internal Medicine, 74,* 771–782.

Engel, G. L. (1977). The need for a new medical model: A challenge for bio-medicine. *Science, 196,* 129–135.

Engel, G. L. (1980). The clinical application of the biopsychosocial model. *American Journal of Psychiatry, 137,* 535–544.

Ensel, W. M., & Lin, N. (2004). Physical fitness and the stress process. *Journal of Community Psychology, 32,* 81–101.

Erickson, K. I., Prakash, R. S., Voss, M. W., Chaddock, L., Hu, L., Morris, K. S., . . . Kramer, A. F. (2009). Aerobic fitness is associated with hippocampal volume in elderly humans. *Hippocampus, 19,* 1030–1039.

Eriksson, M., & Lindstrom, B. (2005). Validity of Antonovsky's Sense of Coherence Scale: A systematic review. *Journal of Epidemiology and Community Health, 59,* 460–466.

Erlanson-Albertsson, C. (2005). How palatable food disrupts appetite regulation. *Basic and Clinical Pharmacology and Toxicology, 97,* 61–73.

Eskelinen, M., & Ollonen, P. (2010). Life stress and losses and deficit in adulthood as breast cancer risk factor: A prospective case-control study in Kuopio, Finland. *In Vivo, 24,* 899–904.

Evans, D. L., Leserman, J., Perkins, D. O., Stern, R. A., Murphy, C., Zheng, B., . . . Petitto, J. M. (1997). Severe life stress as a predictor of early disease progression in HIV infection. *American Journal of Psychiatry, 154,* 630–634.

Evans, G. W., Johansson, G., & Rydstedt, L. (1999). Hassles on the job: A study of a job intervention with urban bus drivers. *Journal of Organizational Behavior, 20,* 199–208.

Evers, A. W. M., Kraaimaat, F. W., van Riel, P. L. C. M., & de Jong, A. J. L. (2002). Tailored cognitive behavioral therapy in early rheumatoid arthritis for patients at risk: A randomized controlled trial. *Pain, 100,* 141–153.

Eyler, A. A., Brownson, R. C., Donatelle, R. J., King, A. C., Brown, D., & Sallis, J. F. (1999). Physical activity social support and middle- and older-aged minority women: Results from a US survey. *Social Science and Medicine, 49,* 781–789.

Eysenck, H. J. (1967). *The biological basis of personality.* Springfield, IL: Thomas.

Eysenck, H. J. (1990). Biological dimensions of personality. In L. A. Pervin (Ed.), *Handbook of personality: Theory and research* (pp. 244–276). New York: The Guilford Press.

Eysenck, H. J., & Eysenck, M. W. (1985). *Personality and individual differences: A natural science approach.* New York: Plenum.

Fahrion, S., Norris, P., Green, A., Green, E., & Snarr, C. (1986). Behavioral treatment of essential hypertension: A group outcome study. *Biofeedback and Self-Regulation, 11,* 257–277.

Faigenbaum, A., & McInnis, K. (2007). Exercise prescription for resistance training. In E. T. Howley & B. D. Franks (Eds.), *Fitness professional's handbook* (5th ed., pp. 189–223). Champaign, IL: Human Kinetics.

Fang, C. Y., & Myers, H. F. (2001). The effects of racial stressors and hostility on cardiovascular reactivity in African American and Caucasian men. *Health Psychology, 20,* 64–70.

Farmer, M. E., Locker, B. Z., Moscicki, E. K., Danneberg, A. L., Larsson, D. B., & Radloff, L. S. (1988). Physical activity and depressive symptoms: The NHANES 1 epidemiologic follow-up study. *American Journal of Epidemiology, 128,* 1340–1351.

Farrell, P. A., Gates, W. K., Maksud, M. G., & Morgan, W. P. (1982). Increases in plasma β-endorphin/β-lipotropin immunoreactivity after treadmill running in humans. *Journal of Applied Physiology: Respiratory, Environmental and Exercise Physiology, 52,* 1245–1249.

Fassina, G., Vene, R., Morini, M., Minghelli, S., Benelli, R., Noonan, D. M., & Albini, A. (2004). Mechanisms of inhibition of tumor angiogenesis and vascular tumor growth by epigallocatechin-3-gallate. *Clinical Cancer Research, 10,* 4865–4873.

Faulconbridge, L. F., & Wadden, T. A. (2010). Managing the obesity epidemic. In J. M. Suls, K. W. Davidson, & R. M. Kaplan (Eds.), *Handbook of health psychology and behavioral medicine* (pp. 508–526). New York: The Guilford Press.

Felmingham, K., Kemp, A., Williams, L., Das, P, Hughes, G, Peduto, A, & Bryant, R. (2007). Changes in anterior cingulated and amygdala after cognitive behavior therapy of posttraumatic stress disorder. *Psychological Science, 18,* 127–129.

Ferguson, M. A., Alderson, N. L., Trost, S. G., Essig, D. A., Burke, J. R., & Durstine, J. L. (1998). Effects of four different single exercise sessions on lipids, lipoproteins, and lipoprotein lipase. *Journal of Applied Physiology, 85,* 1169–1174.

Fernandez, E., & Scott, S. (2009). Anger treatment in chemically-dependent inpatients: Evaluation of phase effects and gender. *Behavioural and Cognitive Psychotherapy, 37,* 431–447.

Feskanich, D., Willett, W., & Colditz, G. (2002). Walking and leisure-time activity and risk of hip fracture in postmenopausal women. *Journal of the American Medical Association, 288,* 2300–2306.

Ficek, S. K., & Wittrock, D. A. (1995). Subjective stress and coping in recurrent tension-type headache. *Headache, 35,* 455–460.

Fisher, M. L., & Exline, J. J. (2006). Self-forgiveness versus excusing: The roles of remorse, effort, and acceptance of responsibility. *Self and Identity, 5,* 127–146.

Fitzgerald, T. E., Tennen, H., Affleck, G., & Pransky, G. S. (1993). The relative importance of dispositional optimism and control appraisals in quality of life after coronary artery bypass surgery. *Journal of Behavioral Medicine, 16,* 25–43.

Flor, H., & Birbaumer, N. (1993). Comparison of the efficacy of electromyographic biofeedback, cognitive-behavioral therapy, and conservative medical interventions in the treatment of chronic musculoskeletal pain. *Journal of Consulting and Clinical Psychology, 61,* 653–658.

Foley, E., Baillie, A., Huxter, M., Price, M., & Sinclair, E. (2010). Mindfulness-based cognitive therapy for individuals whose lives have been affected by cancer: A randomized controlled trial. *Journal of Consulting and Clinical Psychology, 78,* 72–79.

Folkman, S. (1984). Personal control and stress and coping processes: A theoretical analysis. *Journal of Personality and Social Psychology, 46,* 839–852.

Folkman, S., & Lazarus, R. S. (1980). An analysis of coping in a middle-aged community sample. *Journal of Health and Social Behavior, 21,* 219–239.

Folkman, S., & Lazarus, R. S. (1988a). Coping as a mediator of emotion. *Journal of Personality and Social Psychology, 54,* 466–475.

Folkman, S., & Lazarus, R. S. (1988b). *Ways of Coping Questionnaire.* Palo Alto, CA: Consulting Psychologists Press.

Folkman, S., & Moskowitz, J. T. (2004). Coping: Pitfalls and promise. *Annual Review of Psychology, 55,* 745–774.

Food and Drug Adminstration (FDA). (2011). *Health claims: Fruits and vegetables and cancer.* Retrieved from http://ecfr.gpoaccess.gov/cgi/t/text/text-idx?c=ecfr;sid=502078d8634923edc695b394a357d189;rgn=div8;view=text;node=21%3A2.0.1.1.2.5.1.9;idno=21;cc=ecfr.

Ford, J. D. (2008). Posttraumatic adaptation. In G. Reyes, J. D. Elhai, & J. D. Ford (Eds.), *The encyclopedia of psychological trauma,* (pp. 475–480). Hoboken, NJ: John Wiley & Sons.

Fordyce, M. W. (1977). Development of a program to increase personal happiness. *Journal of Counseling Psychology, 24,* 511–521.

Fordyce, M. W. (1981). *The psychology of happiness: A brief version of the fourteen fundamentals.* Ft. Myers, FL: Cypress Lake Media.

Fordyce, M. W. (1983). A program to increase happiness: Further studies. *Journal of Counseling Psychology, 30,* 483–498.

Fordyce, M. W. (1988). A review of research on the Happiness Measures: A sixty second index of happiness and mental health. *Social Indicators Research, 20,* 355–381.

Foster-Powell, K., Holt, S. H. A., & Brand-Miller, J. C. (2002). International table of glycemic index and glycemic load values: 2002. *American Journal of Clinical Nutrition, 76,* 5–56.

Foster, G., Taylor, S. J. C., Eldridge, S., Ramsay, J., & Griffiths, C. J. (2007). Self-management education programmes by lay leaders for people with chronic conditions. *Cochrane Database of Systematic Reviews* (4). doi: 10.1002/14651858.CD005108. pub2.

Frances, A., & Ross, R. (2001). *DSM-IV-TR case studies: A clinical guide to differential diagnosis.* Washington, DC: American Psychiatric Association.

Frankenhaeuser, M., & Rissler, A. (1970). Effects of punishment on catecholamine release and efficiency of performance. *Psychopharmacologica, 17,* 378.

Frankenhaeuser, M., Nordheden, B., Myrsten, A. L., & Post, B. (1971). Psychophysiological reactions to understimulation and overstimulation. *Acta Psychologica, 35,* 298.

Frankl, V. (1992). *Man's search for meaning* (4th ed.). Boston: Beacon Press.

Frattaroli, J. (2006). Experimental disclosure and its moderators: A meta-analysis. *Psychological Bulletin, 132,* 823–865.

Fredrickson, B. L. (1998). What good are positive emotions? *Review of General Psychology, 2,* 300–319.

Fredrickson, B. L., & Branigan, C. (2005). Positive emotions broaden thought-action repertoires. *Cognition and Emotion, 19,* 313–332.

Fredrickson, B. L., Cohn, M. A., Coffey, K., Pek, J., & Finkel, S. M. (2008). Open hearts build lives: Positive emotions induced through meditation build consequential resources. *Journal of Personality and Social Psychology, 95,* 1045–1062.

Fredrickson, B. L., Mancuso, R. A., Branigan, C., & Tugade, M. (2000). The undoing effect of positive emotions. *Motivation and Emotion, 24,* 237–258.

Fredrikson, M., & Matthews, K. A. (1990). Cardiovascular responses to behavioral stress and hypertension: A meta-analytic review. *Annals of Behavioral Medicine, 12,* 30–39.

Freedman, R. R., Ianni, P., & Wenig, P. (1983). Behavioral treatment of Raynaud's disease. *Journal of Consulting and Clinical Psychology, 151,* 539–549.

Freedman, R. R., Sabharwal, S. C., Ianni, P., Desai, N., Wenig, P., & Mayes, M. (1988). Nonneural beta-adrenergic vasodilating mechanism in temperature biofeedback. *Psychosomatic Medicine, 50,* 394–401.

Friedman, E. M., Hayney, M. S., Love, G. D., Urry, H. L., Rosenkranz, M. A., Davidson, R. J., . . . Ryff, C. D. (2005). Social relationships, sleep quality, and interleukin-6 in aging women. *Proceedings of the National Academy of Sciences, 102,* 18757–18762.

Friedman, H. S., Tucker, J. S., Tomlinson-Keasey, C., Schwartz, J. E., Wingard, D. L., & Criqui, M. H. (1993). Does childhood personality predict longevity? *Journal of Personality and Social Psychology, 65,* 176–185.

Friedman, L. C., Romero, C., Elledge, R., Chang, J., Kalidas, M., Dulay, M. F., . . . Osborne, C. K. (2007). Attribution of blame, self-forgiving attitude and psychological adjustment in women with breast cancer. *Journal of Behavioral Medicine, 30,* 351–357.

Friedman, M., & Rosenman, R. H. (1974). *Type A behavior and your heart.* New York: Knopf.

Friedman, M., Rosenman, R. H., & Carroll, V. (1958). Changes in serum cholesterol and blood-clotting time in men subjected to cyclic variation of occupational stress. *Circulation, 17,* 852–861.

Froh, J. J., Sefick, W. J., & Emmons, R. A. (2008). Counting blessings in early adolescents: An experimental study of gratitude and subjective well-being. *Journal of School Psychology, 46,* 213–233.

Fujita, F., Diener, E., & Sandvik, E. (1991). Gender differences in negative affect and well-being: The case for emotional intensity. *Journal of Personality and Social Psychology, 61,* 427–434.

Fumal, A., & Schoenen, J. (2008). Tension-type headache: Current and clinical management. *Lancet Neurology, 7,* 70–83.

Funch, D. P., & Gale, E. N. (1980). Factors associated with nocturnal bruxism and its treatment. *Journal of Behavioral Medicine, 3,* 385–397.

Funk, S. C. (1992). Hardiness: A review of theory and research. *Health Psychology, 11,* 335–345.

Funk, S. C., & Houston, B. K. (1987). Critical analysis of the hardiness scale's validity and utility. *Journal of Personality and Social Psychology, 53,* 572–578.

Futterman, L. G. (2002). Anger and acute coronary events. *American Journal of Critical Care, 11,* 574–576.

Gable, S. L, Reis, H. T., & Elliot, A. J. (2000). Behavioral activation and inhibition in everyday life. *Journal of Personality and Social Psychology, 78,* 1135–1149.

Gale, C. R., Batty, G. D., & Deary, I. J. (2008). Locus of control at age 10 years and health outcomes and behaviors at age 30 years: The 1970 British cohort study. *Psychosomatic Medicine, 70,* 397–403.

Gallo, L., Bogart, L. M., Vranceanu, A.-M., & Walt, L. C. (2004). Job characteristics, occupational status, and ambulatory cardiovascular activity in women. *Annals of Behavioral Medicine, 28,* 62–73.

Galper, D., Trivedi, M. H., Barlow, C. E., Dunn, A. L., & Kampert, J. B. (2006). Inverse association between physical inactivity and mental health in men and women. *Medicine & Science in Sports & Exercise, 38,* 173–178.

Gaston, L. (1988–1989). Efficacy of imagery and meditation techniques in treating psoriasis. *Imagination, Cognition and Personality, 8,* 25–38.

Gattis, K. S., Berns, S., Simpson, L. E., & Christensen, A. (2004). Birds of a feather or strange birds? Ties among personality dimensions, similarity, and marital quality. *Journal of Family Psychology, 18,* 564–574.

Geary, D. C., & Flinn, M. V. (2002). Sex differences in behavioral and hormonal response to social threat: Commentary on Taylor et al. (2000). *Psychological Review, 109,* 745–750.

George, L. K., Larson, D. B., Koenig, H. G., & McCullough, M. E. (2000). Spirituality and health: What we know, what we need to know. *Journal of Social and Clinical Psychology, 19,* 102–116.

Gill, J. M., Saligan, L., Woods, S., & Page, G. (2009). PTSD is associated with an excess of inflammatory immune activities. *Perspectives in Psychiatric Care, 45,* 262–277.

Giltay, E. J., Kamphuis, M. H., Kalmijn, S., Zitman, F. G., & Kromhout, D. (2006). Dispositional optimism and the risk of cardiovascular death: The Zutphen Elderly Study. *Archives of Internal Medicine, 166,* 431–436.

Giluk, T. L. (2009). Mindfulness, Big Five personality, and affect: A meta-analysis. *Personality and Individual Differences, 47,* 805–811.

Giraki, M., Schneider, C., Schafer, R., Singh, P., Franz, M., Raab, W. H. M., & Ommerborn, M. A. (2010). Correlation between stress, stress-coping and current sleep bruxism. *Head and Face Medicine, 6,* 2.

Glaser, R., Kiecolt-Glaser, J. K., Speicher, C. E., & Holliday, J. E. (1985). Stress, loneliness, and changes in herpesvirus latency. *Journal of Behavioral Medicine, 8,* 249–260.

Glaser, R., Kutz, L. A., MacCallum, R. C., & Malarkey, W. B. (1995). Hormonal modulation of Epstein-Barr virus replication. *Neuroendocrinology, 62,* 356–361.

Glaser, R., Rice, J., Sheridan, J., Fertel, R., Stout, J., Speicher, C., . . . Kiecolt-Glaser (1987). Stress-related immune suppression: Health implications. *Brain, Behavior, and Immunity, 1,* 7–20.

Gmelch, W. H., Lovrich, N. P., & Wilke, P. K. (1984). Sources of stress in academe: A national perspective. *Research in Higher Education, 20,* 477–490.

Golden, S. H., Williams, J. E., Ford, D. E., Yeh, H. C., Sanford, C. P., Nieto, F. J., . . .Brancati, F. L. (2006). Anger temperament is modestly associated with the risk of type 2 diabetes mellitus: The Atherosclerosis Risk in Communities Study. *Psychoneuroendocrinology, 31,* 325–332.

Goldstein, D. S. (1983). Plasma catecholamines and essential hypertension: An analytical review. *Hypertension, 5,* 86–99.

Goral, J., Karavitis, J, & Kovacs, E. J. (2008). Exposure-dependent effects of ethanol on the innate immune system. *Alcohol, 42,* 237–247.

Gottman, J. M., & Gottman, J. S. (1999). The marriage survival kit: A research-based marital therapy. In R. Berger & M. T. Hannah (Eds.), *Preventive approaches to couples therapy* (pp. 304–330). Philadelphia: Brunner/Mazel.

Gottman, J. M., & Levenson, R. W. (2000). The timing of divorce: Predicting when a couple will divorce over a 14-year period. *Journal of Marriage and the Family, 62,* 737–745.

Govil, S. R., Weidner, G., Merritt-Worden, T. A., & Ornish, D. (2009). Socioeconomic status and improvements in lifestyle, coronary risk factors, and quality of life: The Multisite Cardiac Lifestyle Intervention Program. *American Journal of Public Health, 99,* 1263–1270.

Graham, J., Christian, L. M., & Kiecolt-Glaser, J. K. (2007). Close relationships and immunity. In R. Ader (Ed.), *Psychoneuroimmunology* (Vol II, 4th ed., pp. 781–798). New York: Elsevier.

Granato, J. E. (2008). *Living with coronary heart disease: A guide for patients and families.* Baltimore: The Johns Hopkins University Press.

Gray, J. A. (1987). *The psychology of fear and stress.* Cambridge, UK: Cambridge University Press.

Graziano, W. G., Feldesman, A. B., & Rahe, D. F. (1985). Extraversion, social cognition, and the salience of aversiveness in social encounters. *Journal of Personality and Social Psychology, 49,* 971–980.

Greenhalgh, J., Dickson, R., & Dundar, Y. (2010). Biofeedback for hypertension: A systematic review. *Journal of Hypertension, 28,* 644–652.

Grossman, P., Niemann, L., Schmidt, S., & Walach, H. (2004). Mindfulness-based stress reduction and health benefits: A meta-analysis. *Journal of Psychosomatic Research, 57,* 35–43.

Gruska, M., Gaul, G. B., Winkler, M., Levnaic, S., Reiter, C., Voracek, M., & Kaff, A. (2005). Increased occurrence of out-of-hospital cardiac arrest on Mondays in a community based study. *Chronobiology International, 22,* 107–120.

Guest, C. B., Gao, Y., O'Connor, J. C., & Freund, G. G. (2007). Obesity and immunity. In R. Ader (Ed.), *Psychoneuroimmunology* (Vol. II, 4th ed., pp. 993–1011). New York: Elsevier Academic Press.

Gutek, B. A., & Koss, M. P. (1993). Changed women and changed organizations: Consequences of and coping with sexual harassment. *Journal of Vocational Behavior, 42,* 1–21.

Guthrie, B. J., Young, A. M., Williams, D. R., Boyd, C. J., & Kintner, E. (2002).African American girls' smoking habits and day-to-day experiences with racial discrimination. *Nursing Research, 51,* 183–190.

Guyton, A. C., & Hall, J. E. (2006). *Textbook of medical physiology* (11th ed.). Philadelphia: Elsevier Saunders.

Hajjar, I., & Kotchen, T. A. (2003). Trends in prevalence, awareness, treatment, and control of hypertension in the United States, 1988–2000. *Journal of the American Medical Association, 290,* 199–206.

Hall, J. H., & Fincham, F. D. (2005). Self-forgiveness: The stepchild of forgiveness research. *Journal of Social and Clinical Psychology, 24,* 621–637.

Hall, J. H., & Fincham, F. D. (2008). The temporal course of self-forgiveness. *Journal of Social and Clinical Psychology, 27,* 174–202.

Hamer, M., & Steptoe, A. (2007). Association between physical fitness, parasympathetic control, and pro-inflammatory responses to mental stress. *Psychosomatic Medicine, 69,* 660–666.

Hamer, M., Taylor, A., & Steptoe, A. (2006). The effect of acute aerobic exercise on stress related blood pressure responses: A systematic review and meta-analysis. *Biological Sciences, 71,* 183–190.

Hammen, C. (1991). Generation of stress in the course of unipolar depression. *Journal of Abnormal Psychology, 100,* 555–561.

Handwerger, K., & Shin, L. M. (2008). Limbic system. In G. Reyes, J. D. Elhai, & J. D. Ford (Eds.), *The encyclopedia of psychological trauma* (pp. 386–391). Hoboken, NJ: John Wiley & Sons.

Hankin, B. L., Abramson, L. Y., Moffitt, T. E., Silva, P. A., McGee, R., & Angell, K. E. (1998). Development of depression from preadolescence to young adulthood: Emerging gender differences in a 10-year longitudinal study. *Journal of Abnormal Psychology, 197,* 128–140.

Hansen, C. J., Stevens, L. C., & Coast, R. (2001). Exercise duration and mood state: How much is enough to feel better? *Health Psychology, 20,* 267–275.

Harburg, E., Julius, M., Kaciroti, N., Gleiberman, L., & Schork, M. A. (2003). Expressive/suppressive anger-coping responses, gender, and types of mortality: A 17-year follow-up (Tecumseh, Michigan, 1971–1988). *Psychosomatic Medicine, 65,* 588–597.

Harlapur, M., Abraham, D., & Shimbo, D. (2010). Cardiology. In J. M. Suls, K. W. Davidson, & R. M. Kaplan (Eds.), *Handbook of health psychology and behavioral medicine* (pp. 411–441). New York: The Guilford Press.

Harmon-Jones, E., & Allen, J. J. B. (1997). Behavioral activation sensitivity and resting frontal EEG asymmetry: Covariation of putative indicators related to risk for mood disorders. *Journal of Abnormal Psychology, 106,* 159–163.

Harper, G. (2004). *The joy of conflict resolution.* Gabriola Island, British Columbia, Canada: New Society.

Harrell, S. P. (2000). A multidimensional conceptualization of racism-related stress: Implications for the well-being of people of color. *American Journal of Orthopsychiatry, 70,* 42–57.

Harrington, R., & Loffredo, D. A. (2001). The relationship between life satisfaction, self-consciousness and the Myers-Briggs Type Inventory (MBTI) dimensions. *The Journal of Psychology: Interdisciplinary and Applied, 135,* 439–450.

Harris, R. (2008). *The happiness trap: How to stop struggling and start living.* Boston: Trumpeter.

Harrison, J., Maguire, P., & Pitceathly, C. (1995). Confiding in crisis: Gender differences in pattern of confiding among cancer patients. *Social Science and Medicine, 41,* 1255–1260.

Hart, P. M. (1999). Predicting employee life satisfaction: A coherent model of personality, work and nonwork experiences, and domain satisfactions. *Journal of Applied Psychology, 84,* 564–584.

Harvard Heart Letter. (2010). Resveratrol for a longer life—If you're a yeast: The promise of this red wine compound has not been confirmed in humans. *Harvard Health Letter, 21,* 4.

Harvard Men's Health Watch. (2010). Aspirin and your heart: Many questions, some answers. *Harvard Men's Health Watch, 15*(5), 1–5.

Harvard School of Public Health. (2011). *Food pyramids: What should you really eat?* Retrieved from http://www.hsph.harvard.edu/nutritionsource/what-should-you-eat/pyramid-full-story/index.html.

Hashizume, H., & Takigawa, M. (2006). Anxiety in allergy and atopic dermatitis. *Current Opinion in Allergy and Clinical Immunology, 6,* 335–339.

Hatfield, E. (1988). Passionate and companionate love. In R. J. Sternberg & M. L. Barnes (Eds.), *The psychology of love* (pp. 191–217). New Haven, CT: Yale University Press.

Hayes, N., & Joseph, S. (2003). Big 5 correlates of three measures of subjective well-being. *Personality and Individual Differences, 34,* 723–727.

Hayes, S. C., Luoma, J. B., Bond, F. W., Masuda, A., & Lillis, J. (2006). Acceptance and commitment therapy: Model, processes and outcomes. *Behaviour Research and Therapy, 44,* 1–25.

Hayes, S. C., Strosahl, K., & Wilson, K. G. (1999). *Acceptance and commitment therapy: An experiential approach to behavior change.* New York: The Guilford Press.

Haynes, S. G., & Feinleib, M. (1980). Women, work and coronary heart disease: Prospective findings from the Framingham Heart Study. *American Journal of Public Health, 70,* 133–141.

Hazaleus, S. L., & Deffenbacher, J. L. (1986). Relaxation and cognitive treatments of anger. *Journal of Consulting and Clinical Psychology, 54,* 222–226.

He, F. J., Nowson, C. A., Lucas, M., & MacGregor, G. A. (2007). Increased consumption of fruit and vegetables is related to a reduced risk of coronary heart disease: Meta-analysis of cohort studies. *Journal of Human Hypertension, 21,* 717–728.

Head, L. S., & Gross, A. M. (2008). Systematic desensitization. In W. O'Donohue & J. E. Fisher (Eds.), *Cognitive behavior therapy: Applying empirically supported techniques to your practice* (2nd ed., pp. 542–549). Hoboken, NJ: John Wiley & Sons.

Headey, B, Veenhoven, R., & Wearing, A. (1991). Top-down versus bottom-up theories of subjective well-being. *Social Indicators of Research, 24,* 81–100.

Heide, F. J., & Borkovec, T. D. (1983). Relaxation-induced anxiety: Paradoxical anxiety enhancement due to relaxation training. *Journal of Consulting and Clinical Psychology, 51,* 171–182.

Heinrichs, M., Baumgartner, T., Kirschbaum, C., & Ehlert, U. (2003). Social support and oxytocin interact to suppress cortisol and subjective responses to psychosocial stress. *Biological Psychiatry, 54,* 1389–1398.

Hemenover, S. H. (2003). Individual differences in rate of affect change: Studies of affective chronometry. *Journal of Personality and Social Psychology, 85,* 121–131.

Hendrick, C., & Hendrick, S. S. (1986). A theory and method of love. *Journal of Personality and Social Psychology, 50,* 392–402.

Hendrick, S. S., & Hendrick, C. (2002). Linking romantic love and sex: Development of the Perceptions of Love and Sex Scale. *Journal of Social and Personal Relationships, 19,* 361–378.

Herbert, J., Moore, G. F., de la Riva, C., & Watts, F. N. (1986). Endocrine responses and examination anxiety. *Biological Psychology, 22,* 215–226.

Herbert, T. B., & Cohen, S. (1993). Stress and immunity in humans: A meta-analytic review. *Psychosomatic Medicine, 55,* 364–379.

Herbst-Damm, K. L., & Kulik, J. A. (2005). Volunteer support, marital status, and survival times of terminally ill patients. *Health Psychology, 24,* 225–229.

Hermann, G., Beck, F. M., & Sheridan, J. F. (1995). Stress-induced glucocorticoid response modulates mononuclear cell trafficking during an experimental influenza viral infection. *Journal of Neuroimmunology, 56,* 179–186.

Hernandez-Lopez, M., Luciano, C., Bricker, J. B., Roales-Nieto, J. G., & Montesinos, F. (2009). Acceptance and commitment therapy for smoking cessation: A preliminary study of its effectivenss in comparison with cognitive behavioral therapy. *Psychology of Addictive Behaviors, 23,* 723–730.

Hertig, V. L., Cain, K. C., Jarrett, M. E., Burr, R. L., & Heitkemper, M. M. (2007). Daily stress and gastrointestinal symptoms in women with irritable bowel syndrome. *Nursing Research, 55,* 399–406.

Hinkle, L. E. (1973). The concept of stress in the biological and social sciences. *Science, Medicine, and Man, 1,* 31–48.

Hirano, R., Momiyama, Y., Takahashi, R., Taniguchi, H., Kondo, K., Nakamura, H., & Ohsuzu, F. (2002). Comparison of green tea intake in Japanese patients with and without angiographic coronary artery disease. *The American Journal of Cardiology, 90,* 1150–1153.

Hockemeyer, J., & Smyth, J. (2002), Evaluating the feasibility and efficacy of a self-administered manual-based stress management intervention for individuals with asthma: Results from a controlled study. *Behavioral Medicine, 27,* 161–172.

Hoenig, J. (1968). Medical research on yoga. *Confinia Psychiatrica, 11,* 69–89.

Hofmann, S. G., Sawyer, A. T., Witt, A. A., & Oh, D. (2010). The effect of mindfulness-based therapy on anxiety and depression: A meta-analytic review. *Journal of Consulting and Clinical Psychology, 78,* 169–183.

Holahan, C. J., & Moos, R. H., (1987). Personal and contextual determinants of coping strategies. *Journal of Personality and Social Psychology, 52,* 946–955.

Holahan, C. J., Moos, R. H., Holahan, C. K., Brennan, P. L., & Schutte, K. K. (2005). Stress generation, avoidance coping, and depressive symptoms: A 10-year-model. *Journal of Consulting and Clinical Psychology, 73,* 658–666.

Holmes, D. S. (1967). Pupillary response, conditioning, and personality. *Journal of Personality and Social Psychology, 5,* 98–103.

Holmes, T. H., & Masuda, M. (1974). Life change and illness susceptibility. In B. S. Dohrenwend & B. R. Dohrenwend (Eds.), *Stressful life events: Their nature and effect* (pp. 45–72). New York: Wiley.

Holmes, T. H., & Rahe, R. H. (1967). The social readjustment rating scale. *Psychosomatic Medicine, 11,* 213–218.

Honsberger, R. W., & Wilson, A. F. (1973). Transcendental meditation in treating asthma. *Respiratory Therapy: The Journal of Inhalation Technology, 3,* 79–80.

Howell, A. J., & Watson, D. (2008). Judgments of impairment and distress associated with symptoms of internalizing and externalizing disorders. *Anxiety, Stress, and Coping, 21,* 143–154.

Howley, E. T., & Franks, B. D. (2007). *Fitness professional's handbook* (5th ed.). Champaign, IL: Human Kinetics.

Hu, F. B., & Willett, W. C. (2002). Optimal diets for prevention of coronary heart disease. *Journal of the American Medical Association, 288,* 2569–2578.

Hu, F. B., Manson, J. E., Stampfer, M. J., Colditz, G., Liu, S., Solomon, C. G., & Willett, W. C. (2001). Diet, lifestyle, and risk of type 2 diabetes mellitus in women. *The New England Journal of Medicine, 345,* 790–797.

Hultquist, C. N., Albright, C., & Thompson, D. L. (2005) Comparison of walking recommendations in previously inactive women. *Medicine & Science in Sports & Exercise, 37,* 676–683.

Hurrell, J. J., Jr. (2005). Organizational stress intervention. In J. Barling, E. K. Kelloway, & M. R. Frone (Eds.), *Handbook of work stress* (pp. 623–645). Thousand Oaks, CA: Sage.

Hyman, R. B., Feldman, H. R., Harris, R. B., Levin, R. F., & Malloy, G. B. (1989). The effects of relaxation training on clinical symptoms: A meta-analysis. *Nursing Research, 38,* 216–220.

Institute of Medicine. (2002). *Dietary reference intakes for energy, carbohydrate, fiber, fat, fatty acids, cholesterol, protein, and amino acids.* Washington, DC: National Academies Press.

International Food Information Council Foundation Media Guide on Food Safety and Nutrition. (2004–2006). (2011). *Functional foods fact sheet: Antioxidants.* Retrieved from http://www.foodinsight.org/Resources/Detail.aspx?topic=Functional_Foods_Fact_Sheet_Antioxidants.

Ioannou, Y., & Isenberg, D. A. (2002). Current concepts for the management of systemic lupus erythematosus in adults: A therapeutic challenge. *Postgraduate Medical Journal, 78,* 599–606.

Ironson, G. H., O'Cleirigh, C., Weiss, A., Schneiderman, N., & Costa, P. T., Jr. (2008). Personality and HIV disease progression: Role of NEO-PI-R Openness, Extraversion, and profiles in engagement. *Psychosomatic Medicine, 70,* 245–253.

Ironson, G., Whynings, C., Schneiderman, N., Baum, A., Rodriguez, M., Greenwood, D., . . . Fletcher, M. A. (1997). Posttraumatic stress symptoms, intrusive thoughts, loss, and immune function after Hurricane Andrew. *Psychosomatic Medicine, 59,* 128–141.

Irwin, M. R. (2008). Human psychoneuroimmunology: 20 years of discovery. *Brain, Behavior, and Immunity, 22,* 129–139.

Irwin, M. R., & Miller, A. H. (2007). Depressive disorders and immunity: 20 years of progress and discovery. *Brain, Behavior, and Immunity, 21*, 374–383.

Iverson, S., Kupfermann, I., & Kandel, E. R. (2000). Emotional states and feelings. In E. R. Kandel, J. H. Schwartz, & T. M. Jessell (Eds.), *Principles of neural science* (4th ed., pp. 982–997). New York: McGraw-Hill.

Jacobsen, P. B., & Jim, H. S. (2008). Psychosocial interventions for anxiety and depression in adult cancer patients: Achievements and challenges. *CA: A Cancer Journal for Clinicians, 58*, 214–230.

Jacobson, E. (1938). *Progressive relaxation.* Chicago: University of Chicago Press.

Jenkins, C. D., Zyzanski, S. J., & Rosenman, R. H. (1979). *Jenkins Activity Survey.* New York: The Psychological Corporation.

John, O. P., & Srivastava, S. (1999). The Big Five trait taxonomy: History, measurement, and theoretical perspectives. In L. A. Pervin & O. P. John (Eds.), *Handbook of personality: Theory and research* (2nd ed., pp. 102–138). New York: The Guilford Press.

Johnson, B., Harrington, R., & Perz, C. (2004). Validation of the Scale of Allergic Rhinitis. *Psychology, Health & Medicine, 9*, 217–225.

Johnson, S. L., Cuellar, A. K., Ruggero, C., White, R., Winett-Perlman, C., Goodnick, P., Miller, I. (2008). Life events as predictors of mania and depression in bipolar disorder. *Journal of Abnormal Psychology, 117*, 268–277.

Jolliffe, J., Rees, K., Taylor, R. R. S., Thompson, D. R., Oldridge, N., & Ebrahim, S. (2001). Exercise-based rehabilitation for coronary heart disease. *Cochrane Database of Systematic Reviews* (1). doi: 10.1002/14651858.CD001800.

Jonassaint, C. R., Boyle, S. H., Williams, R. B., Mark, D. B., Siegler, I. C., & Barefoot, J. C. (2007). *Psychosomatic Medicine, 69*, 319–322.

Jones, J. M. (1997). *Prejudice and racism* (2nd ed.). New York: McGraw-Hill.

Jones, J. R., & Hodgson, J. T. (1998). *Self-reported work-related illness in 1995: Results from a household survey.* London, UK: HSE Books.

Jones, M. D. (2006). The role of psychosocial factors in peptic ulcer disease: Beyond *Helicobacter pylori* and NSAIDS. *Journal of Psychosomatic Research, 60*, 407–412.

Jylha, P., & Isometsa, E. (2006). The relationship of neuroticism and extraversion to symptoms of anxiety and depression in the general population. *Depression and Anxiety, 23*, 281–289.

Kabat-Zinn, J. (1982). An outpatient program in behavioral medicine for chronic pain patients based on the practice of mindfulness meditation: Theoretical considerations and preliminary results. *General Hospital Psychiatry, 4*, 33–47.

Kabat-Zinn, J. (1990). *Full catastrophe living.* New York: Delacorte Press.

Kabat-Zinn, J. (2005). *Coming to our senses: Healing ourselves and the world through mindfulness.* New York: Hyperion.

Kabat-Zinn, J., Lipworth, L., Burney, R., & Sellers, W. (1986). Four-year follow-up of a meditation-based program for the self-regulation of chronic pain: Treatment outcomes and compliance. *Clinical Journal of Pain, 2*, 159–173.

Kabat-Zinn, J., Lipworth, L., & Burney, R. (1985). The clinical use of mindfulness meditation for the self-regulation of chronic pain. *Journal of Behavioral Medicine, 8*, 163–190.

Kabat-Zinn, J., Massion, A. O., Kristeller, J., Peterson, L. G., Fletcher, K. E., Pbert, L., . . . Santorelli, S. F. (1992). Effectiveness of a meditation-based stress reduction program in the treatment of anxiety disorders. *American Journal of Psychiatry, 149*, 936–943.

Kahn, H. A. (1963). The relationship of reported coronary heart disease mortality to physical activity of work. *American Journal of Public Health, 53*, 1058–1067.

Kahn, R. L., Wolfe, D. M., Quinn, R. P., Snoek, J. D., & Rosenthal, R. A. (1964). *Organizational stress: Studies in role conflict and ambiguity.* New York: Wiley.

Kamarck, T., & Jennings, J. R. (1991). Biobehavioral factors in sudden cardiac death. *Psychological Bulletin, 109*, 42–75.

Kandel, E. R., Schwartz, J. H., & Jessell, T. M. (Eds.) (2000). *Principles of neural science* (4th ed.). New York: McGraw-Hill.

Kaniasty, K. (2008). Social support. In G. Reyes, J. D. Elhai, & J. D. Ford (Eds.), *The encyclopedia of psychological trauma* (pp. 607–612). Hoboken, NJ: John Wiley & Sons.

Kanji, N. (1997). Autogenic training. *Complementary Therapies in Medicine, 5*, 162–167.

Kanji, N., White, A., & Ernst, E. (2006). Autogenic training to reduce anxiety in nursing students: randomized controlled trial. *Journal of Advanced Nursing, 53*, 729–735.

Kanner, A. D., Coyne, J. C., Schaefer, C., & Lazarus, R. S. (1981). Comparison of two modes of stress management: Daily hassles and uplifts versus major life events. *Journal of Behavioral Medicine, 4*, 1–39.

Karasek, R. A. (1979). Job demands, job decision latitude, and mental strain: Implications for job redesign. *Administrative Science Quarterly, 24*, 285–308.

Karavidas, M. K., Tsai, P., Yucha, C., McGrady, A., & Lehrer, P. M. (2006). Thermal biofeedback for primary Raynaud's phenomenon: A review of the literature. *Applied Psychophysiological and Biofeedback, 31*, 203–216.

Kark, J. D., Goldman, S., & Epstein, L. (1995). Iraqi missile attacks on Israel: The association of mortality with a life threatening stressor. *Journal of the American Medical Association, 273*, 1208–1210.

Karl, A., Schaefer, M., Malta, L. S., Dorfel, D., Rohleder, N., & Werner, A. (2006). A meta-analysis of structural brain abnormalities in PTSD. *Neuroscience and Biobehavioral Reviews, 30*, 1004–1031.

Karlin, R. A. (2007). Hypnosis in the management of pain and stress: Mechanisms, findings, and procedures. In P. M. Lehrer, R. L. Woolfolk, & W. E. Sime (Eds.), *Principles and practice of stress management* (3rd ed., pp. 125–150). New York: The Guilford Press.

Karpman, S. B. (1968). Fairy tales and script drama analysis.

Transactional Analysis Bulletin, 26, 39–40.

Kawachi, I., Colditz, G. A., Stampfer, M. J., Willett, W. C., Manson, J. E., Speizer, F. E., & Hennekens, C. H. (1995). Prospective study of shift work and risk of coronary heart disease in women. *Circulation, 92,* 3178–3182.

Kay, S. J., & Fiatarone Singh, M. A. (2006). The influence of physical activity on abdominal fat: A systematic review of the literature. *Obesity Reviews, 7,* 183–200.

Keefer, L., & Blanchard, E. B. (2002). A one-year follow-up of relaxation response meditation as a treatment for irritable bowel syndrome. *Behaviour Research and Therapy, 40,* 541–546.

Keesee, N. J., Currier, J. M., & Neimeyer, R. A. (2008). Predictors of grief following the death of one's child: The contribution of finding meaning. *Journal of Clinical Psychology, 64,*1145–1163.

Keicolt-Glaser, J. K., Garner, W. Speicher, C., Penn, G. M., Holliday, J., & Glaser, R. (1984). Psychosocial modifiers of imunocompetence in medical students. *Psychosomatic Medicine, 46,* 7–14.

Keicolt-Glaser, J. K., Malarkey, W. B., Cacioppo, J. T., & Glaser, R. (1994). Stressful personal relationships: Immune and endocrine function. In R. Glaser & J. K. Kiecolt-Glaser (Eds.), *Handbook of human stress and immunity* (pp. 321–339). San Diego: Academic Press.

Keicolt-Glaser, J. K., Marucha, P. T., Malarkey, W. B., Mercado, A. M., & Glaser, R. (1995). Slowing of wound healing by psychological stress. *Lancet, 346,* 1194–1196.

Kemeny, M. E. (1994). Stressful events, psychological responses, and progression of HIV infection. In R. Glaser & J. K. Kiecolt-Glaser (Eds.), *Handbook of human stress and immunity* (pp. 245–266). New York: Academic Press.

Kemeny, M. E., Cohen, F., Zegans, L. S., & Conant, M. A. (1989). Psychological and immunological predictors of genital herpes recurrence. *Psychosomatic Medicine, 51,* 195–208.

Kemeny, M. E., Weiner, H., Duran, R., Taylor, S. E., Visscher, B., & Fahey, J. L. (1995). Immune

system changes after the death of a partner in HIV-positive gay men. *Psychosomatic Medicine, 57,* 547–554.

Kern, M. L., & Friedman, H. S. (2008). Do conscientious individuals live longer? A quantitative review. *Health Psychology, 27,* 505–512.

Kesebir, P., & Diener, E. (2008). In pursuit of happiness: Empirical answers to philosophical questions. *Perspectives on Psychological Science, 3,* 117–125.

Kessler, R. C., Berglund, P., Demler, O., Jin, R., Merikangas, K. R., & Walters, E. E. (2005). Lifetime prevalence and age-of-onset distributions of DSM-IV disorders in the National Comorbidity Survey Replication. *Archives of General Psychiatry, 62,* 593–602.

Key, T. J. (2011). Fruit and vegetables and cancer risk. *British Journal of Cancer, 104,* 6–11.

Keyes, C. L. M. (2005). Mental illness and/or mental health? Investigating axioms of the complete state model of health. *Journal of Consulting and Clinical Psychology, 73,* 539–548.

Keyes, C. L. M. (2009). Toward a science of mental health. In S. J. Lopez & C. R. Snyder (Eds.), *Handbook of positive psychology* (2nd ed., pp. 89–95). New York: Oxford University Press.

Kiecolt-Glaser, J. K., & Newton, T. (2001). Marriage and health: His and hers. *Psychological Bulletin, 127,* 472–503.

Kiecolt-Glaser, J. K., Dura, J. R., Speicher, C. E., Trask, O. J., & Glaser, R. (1991). Spousal caregivers of dementia victims: Longitudinal changes in immunity and health. *Psychosomatic Medicine, 53,* 345–362.

Kiecolt-Glaser, J. K., Heffner, K. L., Glaser, R., Porter, K., Laskowski, B., Gailen, D., . . . Malarkey, W. B. (2009). How stress and anxiety can alter immediate and late phase skin test responses in allergic rhinitis. *Psychoneuroendocrinology, 34,* 670–680.

Kiecolt-Glaser, J. K., Kennedy, S., Malkoff, S., Fisher, L., Speicher, C. E., & Glaser, R. (1988). Marital discord and immunity in males. *Psychosomatic Medicine, 50,* 213–229.

Kilpelainen, M., Koskenvuo, M., Helenius, H., & Terho, E. O. (2002). Stressful life events promote the manifestation of asthma and atopic diseases. *Clinical and Experimental Allergy, 32,* 256–263.

King, K. (2010). A review of the effects of guided imagery on cancer patients with pain. *Complementary Health Practice Review, 15,* 98–107.

Kivimaki, M., Virtanen, M., Elovainio, M., Kouvonen, A., Vaananen, A., & Vahtera, J. (2006). Work stress in the etiology of coronary heart disease—a meta-analysis. *Scandanavian Journal of Work, Environment, and Health, 32,* 431–442.

Klag, S., & Bradley, G. (2004). The role of hardiness in stress and illness: An exploration of the effect of negative affectivity and gender. *British Journal of Health Psychology, 9,* 137–161.

Kleinke, C. L. (2007). What does it mean to cope? In A. Monat, R. S. Lazarus, & G. Reevy (Eds.), *The Praeger handbook of stress and coping* (Vol. 2, pp. 289–308). Westport, CT: Praeger.

Klerman, G. L., & Weissman, M. M. (1992). Interpersonal psychotherapy. In E. S. Paykel (Ed.), *Handbook of affective disorders* (2nd ed., pp. 501–510). New York: The Guilford Press.

Knight, J. A. (2000). The biochemistry of aging. *Advanced Clinical Chemistry, 35,* 1–62.

Kobasa, S. C. (1979). Personality and resistance to illness. *American Journal of Community Psychology, 7,* 413–423.

Koch, F.-S., Sepa, A., & Ludvigsson, J. (2008). Psychological stress and obesity. *The Journal of Pediatrics, 153,* 839–844.

Koehler, T. (1985). Stress and rheumatoid arthritis: A survey of empirical evidence in human and animal studies. *Journal of Psychosomatic Research, 29,* 655–663.

Kop, W. J., & Cohen, N. (2007). Psychoneuroimmunological pathways involved in acute coronary syndromes. In R. Ader (Ed.), *Psychoneuroimmunology* II (4th ed., pp. 921–943). Boston: Elsevier Academic Press.

Kop, W. J., Hamulyak, K., Pernot, C., & Appels, A. (1998). Relationship of blood coagulation and fibrinolysis to vital exhaustion. *Psychosomatic Medicine, 60,* 353–358.

Korotkov, D. (1998). The sense of coherence: Making sense out of chaos. In P. T. P. Wong & P. S. Fry (Eds.), *The human quest for meaning: A handbook of psychological research and clinical applications* (pp. 51–70). Mahwah, NJ: Lawrence Erlbaum Associates.

Kricker, A., Price, M., Butow, P., Goumas, C., Armes, J. E., & Armstrong, B. K. (2009). Effects of life event stress and social support on the odds of a ≥2 cm breast cancer. *Cancer Causes Control, 20,* 437–447.

Kristeller, J. L. (2007). Mindfulness meditation. In P. W. Lehrer, R. L. Woolfolk, & W. E. Sime (Eds.), *Principles and practice of stress management* (3rd ed., pp. 393–427). New York: The Guilford Press.

Kroenke, K., & Mangelsdorff, A. D. (1989) Common symptoms in ambulatory care: Incidence, evaluation, therapy, and outcome. *American Journal of Medicine, 86,* 262–266.

Krueger, R. F. (1999). The structure of common mental disorders. *Archives of General Psychiatry, 56,* 921–926.

Kubitz, K. A., Landers, D. M., Petruzzello, S. J., & Han, M. (1996) The effects of acute and chronic exercise on sleep. A meta-analytic review. *Sports Medicine, 21,* 277–291.

Kuiper, N. A., Grimshaw, M., Leite, C., & Kirsh, G. (2004). Humor is not always the best medicine: Specific components of sense of humor and psychological well-being. *Humor: International Journal of Humor Research, 17,* 135–168.

Kujala, U. M., Kaprio, J., Kannus, P., Sarna, S., & Koskenvuo, M. (2000). Physical activity and osteoporotic hip fracture risk in men. *Archives of Internal Medicine, 160,* 705–708.

Kuk, J. L., Katzmarzyk, P. T., Nichaman, M. Z., Church, T. S., Blair, S. N., & Ross, R. (2006). Visceral fat is an independent predictor of all-cause mortality in men. *Obesity, 14,* 336–341.

Kullowatz, A., Rosenfield, D., Bernhard, D., Magnussen, H.,

Kanniess, F., & Thomas, R. (2008). Stress effects on lung function in asthma are mediated by changes in airway inflammation. *Psychosomatic Medicine, 70,* 468–475.

Kupper, N., & Denollet, J. (2007). Type D personality as a prognostic factor in heart disease: Assessment and mediating mechanisms. *Journal of Personality Assessment, 89,* 265–276.

Kwate, N. A., Valdimarsdottir, H. B., Guevarra, J. S., & Bovbjerg, D. H. (2003). Experiences of racist events are associated with negative health consequences for African American women. *Journal of the National Medical Association, 95,* 450–460.

Kyrou, I., Chrousos, G. O., & Tsigos, C. (2006). Stress, visceral obesity, and metabolic complications. *Annals of the New York Academy of Sciences, 1083,* 77–110.

La Forge, R. (2007). Mindful exercises for fitness professionals. In E. T. Howley & B. D. Franks (Eds.), *Fitness professional's handbook* (5th ed., pp. 343–356). Champaign, IL: Human Kinetics.

La Roche, M. J., Batista, C., & D'Angelo, E. (2011). A content analyses of guided imagery scripts: A strategy for the development of cultural adaptations. *Journal of Clinical Psychology, 67,* 45–57.

LaFromboise, T., Coleman, H. L. K., & Gerton, J. (1993). Psychological impact of biculturalism: Evidence and theory. *Psychological Bulletin, 114,* 395–412.

Lahey, B. B. (2009). Public health significance of neuroticism. *American Psychologist, 64,* 241–256.

Lambert, V. A., & Lambert, C. E. (2001). Literature review of role stress/strain on nurses: An international perspective. *Nursing and Health Sciences, 3,* 161–172.

Landsbergis, P. A., Schnall, P. L., Belkie, K. L., Baker, D., Schwartz, J., & Pickering, T. G. (2001). Work stressors and cardiovascular disease. *Work, 17,* 191–208.

Langer, E. J. (1989). *Mindfulness.* Reading, MA: Perseus.

Lara, D. R. (2010). Caffeine, mental health, and psychiatric disorders. *Journal of Alzheimer's Disease: JAD, 20,* S239–S248.

Larkin, M. (2002). Can flossing teeth foil heart disease? *The Lancet, 360,* 147.

Larsen, R. J., & Kasimatis, M. (1990). Individual differences in entrainment of mood to the weekly calendar. *Journal of Personality and Social Psychology, 58,* 164–171.

Laughlin, H. P. (1967). *The neuroses.* Washington, DC: Butterworth.

Lawlor, D., & Hopker, S. E. (2001). The effectiveness of exercise as an intervention in the management of depression: Systematic review and meta-regression analysis of randomized controlled trials. *British Medical Journal, 322,* 1–8.

Lazar, S. W., Kerr, C. E., Wasserman, R. H., Gray, J. R., Greve, D. N., Treadway, M. T., . . . Fischl, B. (2005). Meditation experience is associated with increased cortical thickness. *NeuroReport, 16,* 1893–1897.

Lazarus, R. S. (1966). *Psychological stress and the coping process.* New York: McGraw-Hill.

Lazarus, R. S. (1993). From psychological stress to the emotions: A history of changing outlooks. *Annual Review of Psychology, 44,* 1–21.

Lazarus, R. S. (1998). *Fifty years of the research and theory of R.S. Lazarus: An Analysis of historical and perennial issues.* Mahwah, NJ: Lawrence Erlbaum Associates.

Lazarus, R. S. (1999). *Stress and emotion: A new synthesis.* New York: Springer.

Lazarus, R. S. (2001). Relational meaning and discrete emotions. In K. R. Scherer, A. Schorr, & T. Johnstone (Eds.), *Appraisal processes in emotion: Theory, methods, research* (pp. 37–67). Oxford, UK: Oxford University Press.

Lazarus, R. S., & Folkman, S. (1984). *Stress, appraisal, and coping.* New York: Springer.

Leaf, A. (2007). Prevention of sudden cardiac death by n-3 polyunsaturated fatty acids. *Journal of Cardiovascular Medicine, 8,* S27–S29.

Lee, I. M. (2003). Physical activity and cancer prevention—data from epidemiological studies. *Medicine & Science in Sports & Exercise, 35,* 1823–1827.

Lee, I. M., & Buchner, D. M. (2008). The importance of walking to public health. *Medicine &*

Science in Sports & Exercise, 40, S512–S518.

Lenze, S. N., Cyranowski, J. M., Thompson, W. K., Anderson, B., & Frank, E. (2008). The cumulative impact of nonsevere life events predicts depression recurrence during maintenance treatment with interpersonal psychotherapy. *Journal of Consulting and Clinical Psychology, 76,* 979–987.

Leonardi, F., Spazzafumo, L., Marcellini, F., & Gagliardi, C. (1999). A top-down/bottom-up controversy from a constructionist approach: A method for measuring top-down effects applied to a sample of older people. *Social Indicators Research, 48,* 187–216.

Leor, J., Poole, W. K., & Kloner, R. A. (1996). Sudden cardiac death triggered by an earthquake. *The New England Journal of Medicine, 334,* 413–419.

Leserman, J., Jackson, E. D., Petitto, J. M., Golden, R. N., Silva, S. G., Perkins, D. O., . . . Evans, D. L. (1999). Progression to AIDS: The effects of stress, depressive symptoms, and social support. *Psychosomatic Medicine, 61,* 397–406.

Leserman, J., Petitto, J. M., Gu, H., Gaynes, B. N., Barroso, J., Golden, R. N., . . . Evans, D. L. (2002). Progression to AIDS, a clinical AIDS condition and mortality: Psychosocial and physiological predictors. *Psychological Medicine, 32,* 1059–1073.

Lett, H. S., Blumenthal, J. A., Babyak, M. A., Sherwood, A., Strauman, T., Robins, C., & Newman, M. F. (2004). Depression as a risk factor for coronary artery disease: Evidence, mechanisms, and treatment. *Psychosomatic Medicine, 66,* 305–315.

Levenson, J. L., & Bemis, C. (1991). The role of psychological factors in cancer onset and progression. *Psychosomatics, 32,* 124–132.

Lewinsohn, P. M., Antonuccio, D. O., Steinmetz, J. L., & Teri, L. (1984). *The coping with depression course.* Eugene, OR: Castalia.

Li, J., Hansen, D., Mortensen, P. B., & Olsen, J. (2002). Myocardial infarction in parents who lost a child: A nationwide prospective cohort study in Denmark. *Circulation, 106,* 1634–1639.

Libby, C. J., & Glenwick, D. S. (2010). Protective and exacerbating factors in children and adolescents with fibromyalgia. *Rehabilitation Psychology, 55,* 151–158.

Lin, J. K., Kelsberg, G., & Safranek, S. (2010). Does red wine reduce cardiovascular risk? *The Journal of Family Practice, 59,* 406–407.

Linden, W. (2005). *Stress management: From basic science to better practice.* Thousand Oaks, CA: Sage.

Linden, W. (2007). The autogenic training method of J. H. Schultz. In P. M. Lehrer, R. L. Woolfolk, & W. E. Sime (Eds.), *Principles and practice of stress management* (3rd ed., pp. 151–174). New York: The Guilford Press.

Linden, W., & Moseley, J. V. (2006). The efficacy of behavioral treatments for hypertension. *Applied Psychophysiology and Biofeedback, 31,* 51–63.

Lindley, P. A., & Joseph, S. (2004). Positive change following trauma and adversity: A review. *Journal of Traumatic Stress, 17,* 11–21.

Lindley, P. A., & Joseph, S. (2008). Posttraumatic growth. In G. Reyes, J. D., Elhai, & J. D. Ford (Eds.), *The encyclopedia of psychological trauma* (pp. 481–483). Hoboken, NJ: John Wiley & Sons.

Linehan, M. (1993). *Cognitive-behavioral treatment of borderline personality disorder.* New York: The Guilford Press.

Liu, Y., & Tanaka, H. (2002). Overtime work, insufficient sleep, and risk of non-fatal acute myocardial infarction in Japanese men. *Occupational and Environmental Medicine, 59,* 447–451.

Lovallo, W. R. (2005). *Stress & health: Biological and psychological interactions* (2nd ed.). Thousand Oaks, CA: Sage.

Lovallo, W. R., Whitsett, T. L., Al'Absi, M., Sung, B. H., Vincent, A. S., & Wilson, M. F. (2005). Caffeine stimulation of cortisol secretion across the waking hours in relation to caffeine intake levels. *Psychosomatic Medicine, 67,* 734–739.

Lucas, R. E. (2007a). Adaptation and the set-point model of subjective well-being: Does happiness change after major life events? *Current Directions in Psychological Science, 16,* 75–79.

Lucas, R. E. (2007b). Long-term disability is associated with lasting changes in subjective well-being: Evidence from two nationally representative longitudinal studies. *Journal of Personality and Social Psychology, 92,* 717–730.

Lucas, R. E., Clark, A. E., Georgellis, Y., & Diener, E. (2003). Reexamining adaptation and the set point model of happiness: Reactions to changes in marital status. *Journal of Personality and Social Psychology, 84,* 527–539.

Luks, A. (1988, October). Helper's high: Volunteering makes people feel good, physically and emotionally. And like "runner's calm," it's probably good for your health. *Psychology Today, 22,* 34–42.

Lull, C., Wichers, H. J., & Savelkoul, H. F. J. (2005). Antiinflammatory and immunomodulating properties of fungal metabolites. *Mediators of Inflammation, 2,* 63–80.

Lundberg, U., & Frankenhaeuser, M. (1980). Pituitary-adrenal and sympathetic-adrenal correlates of distress and effort. *Journal of Psychosomatic Research, 24,* 125–130.

Lutgendorf, S. K., Anderson, B., Sorosky, J. I., Buller, R. E., & Lubaroff, D. M. (2000). Interleukin-6 and use of social support in gynecologic cancer patients. *International Journal of Behavioral Medicine, 7,* 127–142.

Luthe, W. (1963). Autogenic training: Method, research and application in medicine. *American Journal of Psychotherapy, 17,* 174–195.

Lykken, D., & Tellegen, A. (1996). Happiness is a stochastic phenomenon. *Psychological Science, 7,* 186–189.

Lyubomirsky, S. (2001). Why are some people happier than others? The role of cognitive and motivational processes in well-being. *American Psychologist, 56,* 239–249.

Lyubomirsky, S. (2007). *The how of happiness: A new approach to getting the life you want.* New York: Penguin Books.

Lyubomirsky, S., & Lepper, H. S. (1999). A measure of subjective happiness: Preliminary reliability and construct validation. *Social Indicators Research, 46,* 137–155.

Lyubomirsky, S., Sheldon, K. M., & Schkade, D. (2005). Pursuing happiness: The architecture of sustainable change. *Review of General Psychology, 9,* 111–131.

Lyubomirsky, S., Tucker, K. L., Caldwell, N. D., & Berg, K.

(1999). Why ruminators are poor problem solvers: Clues from the phenomenology of dysphoric rumination. *Journal of Personality and Social Psychology, 77,* 1041–1060.

Ma, S. H., & Teasdale, J. D. (2004). Mindfulness-based cognitive therapy for depression: Replication and exploration of differential relapse prevention effects. *Journal of Consulting and Clinical Psychology, 72,* 31–40.

Macht, M., Haupt, C., Ellgring, H. (2005). The perceived function of eating is changed during examination stress: A field study. *Eating Behaviors, 6,* 109–112.

MacLean, P. D. (1949). Psychosomatic disease and the "visceral brain": Recent developments bearing on the Papez theory of emotion. *Psychosomatic Medicine, 11,* 338–353.

Macrodimitris, S. D., & Endler, N. S. (2001). Coping control and adjustment to type 2 diabetes. *Health Psychology, 20,* 208–216.

MADD. (2010). *In honor of . . .* Retrieved from http://www.madd.org/about-us/history/cari-lightner-and-laura-lamb-story.pdf.

Madden, K. S., & Livnat, S. (1991). Catecholamine action and immunological reactivity. In R. Ader, D. L. Felton, & N. Cohen (Eds.), *Psychoneuroimmunology* (2nd ed., pp. 283–310). New York: Academic Press.

Maddi, S. R. (2002). The story of hardiness: Twenty years of theorizing, research, and practice. *Consulting Psychology Journal: Practice and Research, 54,* 175–185.

Maddi, S. R. (2006). Hardiness: The courage to grow from stresses. *The Journal of Positive Psychology, 1,* 160–168.

Maddi, S. R., & Khoshaba, D. M. (1994). Hardiness and mental health. *Journal of Personality Assessment, 63,* 265–274.

Maddux, J. E. (2009). Stopping the "madness": Positive psychology and deconstructing the illness ideology and the DSM. In S. J. Lopez & C. R. Snyder (Eds.), *Handbook of positive psychology* (2nd ed., pp. 61–69). New York: Oxford University Press.

Malach-Pines, A. (2005). The Burnout Measure, Short Version.

International Journal of Stress Management, 12, 78–88.

Malouff, J. M., Thorsteinsson, E. B., & Schutte, N. S. (2005). The relationship between the five-factor model of personality and symptoms of clinical disorders: A meta-analysis. *Journal of Psychopathology and Behavioral Assessment, 27,* 101–114.

Malouff, J. M., Thorsteinsson, E. B., & Schutte, N. S. (2006). The five-factor model of personality and smoking: A meta-analysis. *Journal of Drug Education, 36,* 47–58.

Malouff, J. M., Thorsteinsson, E. B., Rooke, S. E., & Schutte, N. S. (2007). Alcohol involvement and the five-factor model of personality: A meta-analysis. *Journal of Drug Education, 37,* 277–294.

Malouff, J. M., Thorsteinsson, E. B., Schutte, N. S., Bhullar, N., & Rooke, S. E. (2010). The five-factor model of personality and relationship satisfaction of intimate partners: A meta-analysis. *Journal of Research in Personality, 44,* 124–127.

Manson, J. E., Skerrett, P. J., Greenland, P., & VanItallie, T. B. (2004). The escalating pandemics of obesity and sedentary lifestyle: A call to action for clinicians. *Archives of Internal Medicine, 164,* 249–258.

Manzoni, G. M., Pagnini, F., Castelnuovo, G., & Molinari, E. (2008). Relaxation training for anxiety: A ten-year systematic review with meta-analysis. *BMC Psychiatry, 8,* 41. Retrieved from http://www.biomedcentral.com/1471-244X/8/41.

Marbach, J. J., & Raphael, K. G. (1997). Future directions in the treatment of chronic musculoskeletal facial pain: The role of evidence-based care. *Oral Surgery, Oral Medicine, Oral Pathology, Oral Radiology and Endodontology, 83,* 170–176.

Markus, C. R., Panhuysen, G., Tuiten, A., Koppeschaar, H., Fekkes, D., & Peters, M. L. (1998). Does carbohydrate-rich, protein-poor food prevent the deterioration of mood and cognitive performance of stress-prone subjects when subjected to a stressful task? *Appetite, 31,* 49–65.

Marlatt, G. A., & Gordon, J. R. (1985). *Relapse prevention: Maintenance strategies in the*

treatment of addictive behaviors. New York: The Guilford Press.

Marshall, G. D., & Agarwal, S. K. (2000). Stress, immune regulation, and immunity: Applications for asthma. *Allergy and Asthma Proceedings, 21,* 241–246.

Martin, L. R., & Friedman, H. S. (2000). Comparing personality scales across time: An illustrative study of validity and consistency in life-span archival data. *Journal of Personality, 68,* 85–110.

Martin, R. A. (2002). Is laughter the best medicine? Humor, laughter, and physical health. *Current Directions in Psychological Science, 11,* 216–220.

Maslach, C. (1998). A multidimensional theory of burnout. In C. L. Cooper (Ed.), *Theories of organizational stress.* New York: Oxford University Press.

Maslach, C., & Jackson, S. E. (1986). *The Maslach Burnout Inventory.* Palo Alto, CA: Consulting Psychologist Press.

Mason, J. W. (1971). A re-evaluation of the concept of non-specificity in stress theory. *Journal of Psychiatric Research, 8,* 323.

Mason, J. W. (1975a). A historical view of the stress field. *Journal of Human Stress, 1*(2), 22–36.

Mason, J. W. (1975b). A historical view of the stress field. *Journal of Human Stress, 1*(3), 22–26.

Masten, A. S., Cutuli, J. J., Herbers, J. E., & Reed, M.-G. J. (2009). Resilience in development. In S. J. Lopez & C. R. Snyder (Eds.), *Oxford handbook of positive psychology* (2nd ed., pp. 117–131). New York: Oxford University Press.

Matarazzo, J. D. (1980). Behavioral health and behavioral medicine: Frontiers in the new health psychology. *American Psychologist, 35,* 807–817.

Materazzo, F., Cathcart, S., & Pritchard, D. (2000). Anger, depression, and coping interactions in headache activity and adjustment: A controlled study. *Journal of Psychosomatic Research, 49,* 69–75.

Maunder, R. G., & Levenstein, S. (2008). The role of stress in the development and clinical course of inflammatory bowel disease: Epidemiological evidence. *Current Molecular Medicine, 8,* 247–252.

Mayo Clinic Staff. (2011). *Caffeine content for coffee, tea, soda and more.* Retrieved from http://www.mayoclinic.com/health/caffeine/AN01211.

McAuley, E., Kramer, A. F., & Colcombe, S. J. (2004). Cardiovascular fitness and neurocognitive function in older adults: A brief review. *Brain, Behavior, and Immunity, 18,* 214–230.

McCallie, M. S., Blum, C. M., & Hood, C. J. (2006). Progressive muscle relaxation. *Journal of Human Behavior in the Social Environment, 13,* 51–66.

McCann, B. S., Benjamin, A. H., Wilkinson, C. W., Retzlaff, B. M., Russo, J., & Knopp, R. H. (1999). Plasma concentrations during episodic occupational stress. *Annals of Behavioral Medicine, 21,* 103–110.

McCloskey, M. S., Kleabir, K., Berman, M. E., Chen, E. Y., & Coccaro, E. F. (2010). Unhealthy aggression: Intermittent explosive disorder and adverse physical health outcomes. *Health Psychology, 29,* 324–332.

McClure, H. H., Martinez, C. R., Snodgrass, J. J., Eddy, J. M., Jimeniz, R. A., Isiordia, L. E., & McDade, T. W. (2010). Discrimination-related stress, blood pressure and Epstein-Barr virus antibodies among Latin American immigrants in Oregon, U.S. *Journal of Biosocial Science, 42,* 433–461.

McCrae, R. R. (1982). Consensual validation of personality traits: Evidence from self-reports and ratings. *Journal of Personality and Social Psychology, 43,* 293–303.

McCrae, R. R., & Costa, P. T. (1991). Adding liebe und arbeit: The full five-factor model and well-being. *Personality and Social Psychology Bulletin, 17,* 227–232.

McCullough, M. E., Emmons, R. A., & Tsang, J. (2002). The grateful disposition: A conceptual and empirical topography. *Journal of Personality and Social Psychology, 82,* 112–127.

McCullough, M. E., Lindsey, M. R., Tabak, B. A., & van Oyen Witvliet, C. (2009). Forgiveness. In S. J. Lopez and C. R. Snyder (Eds.), *Handbook of positive psychology* (2nd ed., pp. 427–435). New York: Oxford University Press.

McGregor, B. A., Antoni, M. H., Boyers, A., Alferi, S. M., Blomberg, B. B., & Carver, C. S. (2004). Cognitive-behavioral stress management increases benefit finding and immune function among women with early-stage breast cancer. *Journal of Psychosomatic Research, 56,* 1–8.

McGuigan, F. J., & Lehrer, P. M. (2007). Progressive relaxation: Origins, principles, and clinical applications. In P. M. Lehrer, R. L. Woolfolk, & W. E. Sime (Eds.), *Principles and practice of stress management* (3rd ed., pp. 57–87). New York: The Guilford Press.

McKay, M., Fanning, P., &Paleg, K. (2006).*Couple skills: Making your relationship work* (2nd ed.). Oakland, CA: New Harbinger.

McKenna, M. C., Zevon, M. A., Corn, B., & Rounds, J. (1999). Psychosocial factors and the development of breast cancer: A meta-analysis. *Health Psychology, 18,* 520–531.

McKeown, N. M., Meigs, J. B., Liu, S., Wilson, P. W., & Jacques, P. F. (2002). Whole grain intake is favorably associated with metabolic risk factors for type 2 diabetes and cardiovascular disease in the Framingham Offspring Study. *American Journal of Clinical Nutrition, 76,* 390–398.

McKinnon, W., Weisse, C. S., Reynolds, C. P., Bowles, C. A., & Baum, A. (1989). Chronic stress, leukocyte subpopulations, and humoral response to latent viruses. *Health Psychology, 8,* 389–402.

McLean, C. P., & Anderson, E. R. (2009). Brave men and timid women? A review of the gender differences in fear and anxiety. *Clinical Psychology Review, 29,* 496–505.

McNeilly, M. D., Robinson, E. L., Anderson, N. B., Pieper, C. F., Shah, A., Toth, P. S., . . . Gerin, W. (1995). Effects of racist provocation and social support on cardiovascular reactivity in African American women. *International Journal of Behavioral Medicine, 2,* 321–338.

McPherson, M., Smith-Lovin, L., & Cook, J. M. (2001). Birds of a feather: Homophily in social networks. *Annual Review of Sociology, 27,* 415–444.

Mechanic, D. (1966). Response factors in illness: The study of illness behavior. *Social Psychiatry, 1,* 11–20.

MedlinePlus. (2011). *Alcohol and diet.* Retrieved from http://www.nlm.nih.gov/medlineplus/ency/article/002446.htm.

Meichenbaum, D. (1977). *Cognitive behavior modification: An integrative approach.* New York: Plenum Press.

Meichenbaum, D. (1985). *Stress inoculation training.* New York: Pergamon.

Meichenbaum, D. (1996). Stress inoculation training for coping with stressors. *The Clinical Psychologist, 49,* 4–10.

Meichenbaum, D. (2007). Stress inoculation training: A preventative and treatment approach. In P. M. Lehrer, R. L. Woolfolk, & W. E. Sime (Eds.), *Principles and practice of stress management* (3rd ed., pp. 497–516). New York: The Guilford Press.

Melamed, S. (2009). Burnout and risk of regional musculoskeletal pain: A prospective study of apparently healthy employed adults. *Stress and Health, 25,* 313–321.

Melamed, S., Shirom, A., Toker, S., Berlliner, S., & Shapira, I. (2006a). Burnout and risk of cardiovascular disease: Evidence, possible causal paths, and promising research directions. *Psychological Bulletin, 132,* 327–353.

Melamed, S., Shirom, A., Toker, S., & Shapira, I. (2006b). Burnout and risk of type 2 diabetes: A prospective study of apparently healthy employed persons. *Psychosomatic Medicine, 68,* 863–869.

Mensink, R. P., Zock, P. L., Kester, A. D., & Katan, M. B. (2003). Effects of dietary fatty acids and carbohydrates on the ratio of serum total to HDL cholesterol and on serum lipids and apolipoproteins: A meta-analysis of 60 controlled trials. *American Journal of Clinical Nutrition, 77,* 1146–1155.

Milagros, R. C., King, J., Ma, Y., & Reed, G. W. (2004). Stress, social support, and cortisol: Inverse associations? *Journal of Behavioral Medicine, 30,* 11–21.

Miller, G. E., & Cohen, S. (2001). Psychological interventions and the immune system: A meta-analytic review and critique. *Health Psychology, 20,* 47–63.

Miller, J., Fletcher, K., & Kabat-Zinn, J. (1995). Three-year follow-up and clinical implications of a mindfulness meditation-based stress reduction intervention in the treatment of anxiety disorders. *General Hospital Psychiatry, 17,* 192–200.

Miller, S. C., Kennedy, C., DeVoe, D., Hickey, M., Nelson, T., & Kogan, L. (2009). An examination of changes in oxytocin levels in men and women before and after interaction with a bonded dog. *Anthrozoos, 22,* 31–42.

Miller, S., Wackman, D., Nunnally, E., & Saline, C. (1982). *Straight talk: A new way to get closer to others by saying what you really mean.* New York: Rawson, Wade.

Mitchell, T., Church, T., & Zucker, M. (2008). *Move yourself: The Cooper Clinic medical director's guide to all the healing benefits of exercise (even a little).* Hoboken, NJ: John Wiley & Sons.

Miyazaki, T., Ishikawa, T., Hirofumi, I., Akiko, M., Wenner, M., Fukunishi, I., & Kawamura, N. (2003). Relationship between perceived social support and immune function. *Stress and Health, 19,* 3–7.

Monninkhof, E. M., Elias, S. G., Vlems, F. A., Tweel van der, I., Schuit, A. J., Voskuil, D. W., & Leeuwen, F. E. (2007). Physical activity and breast cancer: A systematic review. *Epidemiology, 18,* 137–157.

Monroe, S. M., & Simons, A. D. (1991). Diathesis-stress theories in the context of life stress research: Implications for depressive disorders. *Psychological Bulletin, 110,* 406–425.

Monti, D. A., Peterson, C., Shakin Kunkel, E. J., Hauck, W. W., Pequignot, E., Rhodes, L., & Brainard, G. C. (2006). A randomized controlled trial of mindfulness-based art therapy (MBAT) for women with cancer. *Psycho-Oncology, 14,* 1–11.

Moos, R. H. (1993). *Coping Response Inventory.* Odessa, FL: Psychological Assessment Resources.

Morris, J. N., Heady, J. A., Raffle, P. A. B., Roberts, C. G., & Parks, J. W. (1953). Coronary heart disease and physical activity of work. *Lancet, 2,* 1053–1057, 1111–1120.

Morse, D. R., Martin, J., & Moshonov, J. (1992). Stress induced sudden cardiac death: Can it be prevented? *Stress and Illness, 8,* 35–46.

Mosges, R., & Klimek, L. (2007). Today's allergic rhinitis patients are different: New factors that may play a role. *Allergy, 62,* 969–975.

Moulton, R. E. (1955). Oral and dental manifestations of anxiety. *Psychiatry, 18,* 261–273.

Mountcastle, V. B. (1979). An organizing principle for cerebral function: The unit module and the distributed system. In F. O. Schmitt & F. G. Worden (Eds.), *The neurosciences: Fourth study program.* Cambridge, MA: MIT Press.

Mozaffarian, D., Ascherio, A, Hu, F. B., Stampfer, M. J., Willet, W. C., Siscovick, D. S., & Rimm, E. B. (2005). Interplay between different polyunsaturated fatty acids and the risk of coronary heart disease in men. *Circulation, 111,* 157–164.

Murphy, T. J., Pagano, R. R., & Marlatt, G. A. (1986). Lifestyle modification with heavy alcohol drinkers: Effects of aerobic exercise and meditation. *Addictive Behaviors, 11,* 175–186.

Myer, G. J., Finn, S. E., Eyde, L. D., Kay, G. G., Moreland, K. L., Dies, R. R., . . . Reed, G. M. (2001). Psychological testing and psychological assessment— a review of evidence and issues. *American Psychologist, 56,* 128–165.

Myers, D. G. (2000). The funds, friends, and faith of happy people. *American Psychologist, 55,* 56–67.

Myers, D. G., & Diener, E. (1995). Who is happy? *Psychological Science, 6,* 10–19.

Myers, H. F. (2009). Ethnicity- and socio-economic status-related stresses in context: An integrative review and conceptual model. *Journal of Behavioral Medicine, 32,* 9–19.

Myin-Germeys, I., Krabbendam, L., Delespaul, P., & van Os, J. (2003). Can cognitive deficits explain differential sensitivity to life events in psychosis? *Social Psychiatry Psychiatric Epidemiology, 38,* 262–268.

Myrteck, M. (2001). Meta-analyses of prospective studies of coronary heart disease, Type A personality, and hostility. *International Journal of Cardiology, 79,* 245–251.

Nakamura, J., & Csikszentmihalyi, M. (2009). Flow theory and research. In S. J. Lopez & C. R. Snyder (Eds.), *Oxford handbook of positive psychology* (2nd ed., pp. 195–206). New York: Oxford University Press.

Nakao, M., Yano, E., Nomura, S., & Kuboki, T. (2003). Blood pressure-lowering effects of biofeedback treatment in hypertension: A meta-analysis of randomized controlled trial. *Hypertension Research: Official Journal of the Japanese Society of Hypertension, 26,* 37–46.

Nakaya, N., Hansen, P. E., Schapiro, I. R., Saito-Nakay, K., Uchitomi, Y, & Johansen, C. (2006). Personality traits and cancer survival: A Danish cohort study. *British Journal of Cancer, 95,* 146–152.

Narayanan, L., Menon, S., & Spector, P. E. (1999). Stress in the workplace: A comparison of gender and occupations. *Journal of Organizational Behavior, 20,* 63–73.

Nasir, A., & Burgess, P. (2005). *Eczema free for life.* New York: HarperCollins.

Natella, F., Nardini, M., Belelli, F., & Scaccini, C. (2007). Coffee drinking induces incorporation of phenolic acids into LDL and increases the resistance of LDL to ex vivo oxidation in humans. *American Journal of Clinical Nutrition, 86,* 604–609.

National Cancer Institute, U.S. National Institutes of Health. (2011). *Tobacco statistics snapshot.* Retrieved from http://www.cancer.gov/cancertopics/tobacco/statisticssnapshot.

National Cholesterol Education Program. (2002). *Detection, evaluation, and treatment of high blood cholesterol in adults (adult treatment panel III): Final report* (NIH Publication No. 02-5215). Retrieved from http://www.nhlbi.nih.gov/guidelines/cholesterol/atp3full.pdf.

National Heart Lung and Blood Institute. (2011). *Calculate your body mass index.* Retrieved from http://www.nhlbisupport.com/bmi/bminojs.htm.

National Task Force on the Prevention and Treatment of Obesity. (2000). Overweight, obesity, and health risk. *Archives of Internal Medicine, 160,* 898–904.

Navarrete-Navarrete, N., Pralta-Ramirez, M. I., Sabio-Sanchez,

J. M., Coin, M. A., Robles-Ortega, H., Hidalgo-Tenorio, C., . . . Jimenez-Alonso, J. (2010). Efficacy of cognitive behavioural therapy for the treatment of chronic stress in patients with lupus erythematosus: A randomized controlled trial. *Psychotherapy and Psychosomatics, 79,* 107–115.

Nelson, D. L., & Simmons, B. L. (2011). Savoring eustress while coping with distress: The holistic model of stress. In J. C. Quick & L. E. Tetrick (Eds.), *Handbook of occupational health psychology* (2nd ed., pp. 55– 74). Washington, DC: American Psychological Association.

Nemeroff, C. B., & Schatzberg, A. F. (2007). Pharmacologic treatments for unipolar depression. In P. E. Nathan & J. M. Gorman (Eds.), *A guide to treatments that work* (3rd ed., pp. 271–287). New York: Oxford University Press.

Nes, L. S., & Segerstrom, S. C. (2006). Dispositional optimism and coping: A meta-analytic review. *Personality and Social Psychology Review, 10,* 235–251.

Nestoriuc, Y., & Martin, A. (2007). Efficacy of biofeedback for migraine: A meta-analysis. *Pain, 128,* 111–127.

Nestoriuc, Y., Rief, W., & Martin, A. (2008). Meta-analysis of biofeedback for tension-type headache: Efficacy, specificity, and treatment moderators. *Journal of Consulting and Clinical Psychology, 76,* 379–396.

Netz, Y., Wu, M.-J., Becker, B. J., & Tenenbaum, G. (2005). Physical activity and psychological well-being in advanced age: A meta-analysis of intervention studies. *Psychology and Aging, 20,* 272–284.

Newman, E., O'Connor, D. B., & Conner, M. (2007). Daily hassles and eating behavior: The role of cortisol reactivity. *Psychoneuroendocrinology, 32,* 125–132.

Newton, T. (1995). *Managing stress: Emotion and power at work.* London, UK: Sage.

Niaura, R., & Goldstein, M. G. (1992). Psychological factors affecting physical condition: Cardiovascular disease literature review: Part II: Coronary artery disease and sudden death and

hypertension. *Psychosomatics, 33,* 146–155.

Nidich, S., Rainforth, M. V., Haaga, D. A. F., Hagelin, J., Salerno, J. W., Travis, F., . . . Schneider, R. H. (2009). A randomized controlled trial on effects of the Transcendental Meditation program on blood pressure, psychological distress, and coping in young adults. *American Journal of Hypertension, 22,* 1326–1331.

Nieman, D. C. (1995). Upper respiratory tract infections and exercise. *Thorax, 50,* 1229–1231.

Nieman, D. C., Henson, D. A., Austin, M. D., & Brown, V. A. (2005). The immune response to a 30-minute walk. *Medicine and Science in Sports and Exercise, 37,* 57–62.

NIH Consensus Development Panel on Physical Activity and Cardiovascular Health. (1996). Physical activity and cardiovascular health. *Journal of the American Medical Association, 276,* 241–246.

NIH State-of-the-Science Panel. (2006). National Institutes of Health state-of-the-science conference statement: Multivitamin/mineral supplements and chronic disease prevention. *Annals of Internal Medicine, 145,* 364–371.

Nolen-Hoeksema, S. (1991). Responses to depression and their effects on the duration of depressive episodes. *Journal of Abnormal Psychology, 100,* 569–582.

Norris, P. A., Fahrion, S. L., & Oikawa, L. O. (2007). Autogenic biofeedback training in psychophysiological therapy and stress management. In P. M. Lehrer, R. L. Woolfolk, & W. E. Sime (Eds.). *Principles and practice of stress management* (3rd ed., pp. 175–205). New York: The Guilford Press.

Novaco, R. W. (1975). Anger control: The development and evaluation of an experimental treatment. Lexington, MA: D. C. Health.

O'Cleirigh, C., Ironson, G., Weiss, A., & Costa, P. T., Jr. (2007). Conscientiousness predicts disease progression (CD4 number and viral load) in people living with HIV. *Health Psychology, 26,* 473–480.

O'Connor, D. B., Jones, F., Ferguson, E., Conner, M., & McMillan, B. (2008). Effects of daily hassles and

eating style on eating behavior. *Health Psychology, 27,* S20–S31.

O'Connor, P. G., & Spickard, A., Jr. (1997). Physician impairment by substance abuse. *The Medical Clinics of North America, 81,* 1037–1052.

Ogden, C., & Carroll, M. D. (2010). National Health and Nutritional Examination Survey (NHANES). *Prevalence of overweight, obesity, and extreme obesity among adults: United States, trends 1976–1980 through 2007–2008.* Retrieved from http://www.cdc.gov/NCHS/data/hestat/obesity_adult_07_08/obesity_adult_07_08.pdf.

Olatunji, B. O., Cisler, J. M., & Tolin, D. F. (2007). Quality of life in the anxiety disorders: A meta-analytic review. *Clinical Psychology Review, 27,* 572–581.

Oliver, G., Wardle, J., & Gibson, E. L. (2000). Stress and food choice: A laboratory study. *Psychosomatic Medicine, 62,* 853–865.

Ornish, D., Brown, S. E., Scherwitz, L. W., Billings, J. H., Armstrong, W. T., Ports, T. A., . . . Gould, K. L. (1990). Can lifestyle changes reverse coronary heart disease? The Lifestyle Heart Trial. *Lancet, 336,* 129–133.

Ornish, D., Scherwitz, L. W., Billing, J. H., Gould, K. L., Merritt, T. A., Sparler, S., . . . Brand, R. J. (1998). Intensive lifestyle changes for reversal of coronary heart disease. *Journal of the American Medical Association, 280,* 2001–2007.

Ornish, D., Weidner, G., Fair, W. R., Marlin, R., Pettengill, E. B., Raisin, C. J., . . . Carroll, P. R. (2005). Intensive lifestyle changes may affect the progression of prostate cancer. *The Journal of Urology, 174,* 1065–1069; discussion, 1069–1070.

Orth, U., Robins, R. W., & Meier, L. L. (2009). Disentangling the effects of low self-esteem and stressful events on depression: Findings from three longitudinal studies. *Personality Processes and Individual Differences, 97,* 307–321.

Otake, S., Takeda, H., Yasukuni, S., Fukui, T., Wantanabe, S., Ishihama, K., . . . Kawata, S. (2005). Association of visceral fat accumulation and plasma adiponectin with colorectal adenoma: Evidence for participation of insulin resistance. *Clinical Cancer Research, 11,* 3642–3646.

Ouellette, S. C., & DiPlacido, J. (2001). Personality's role in the protection and enhancement of health: Where the research has been, where it is stuck, how it might move. In A. Baum, T. A. Revenson, & J. E. Singer (Eds.), *Handbook of health psychology* (pp. 175–193). Mahwah, NJ: Erlbaum.

Ouimet, A. J., Gawronski, B., & Dozois, D. J. A. (2009). Cognitive vulnerability to anxiety: A review and an integrative model. *Clinical Psychology Review, 29,* 549–570.

Paffenbarger, R. S., Jr., Gima, A. S., Laughlin, M. E., & Black, R. A. (1971). Characteristics of long-shoremen related to fatal coronary heart disease and stroke. *American Journal of Public Health, 61,* 1362–1370.

Paffenbarger, R. S., Jr., Laughlin, M. E., Gima, A. S., & Black, R. A. (1970). Work activity of longshoremen as related to death from coronary heart disease and stroke. *New England Journal of Medicine, 282,* 1109–1114.

Paffenbarger, R. S., Jr., Wing, A. L., & Hyde, R. T. (1978). Physical activity as an index of heart attack risk in college alumni. *American Journal of Epidemiology, 108,* 161–175.

Pagnoni, G., & Cekic, M. (2007). Age effects on gray matter volume and attentional performance in Zen meditation. *Neurobiology of Aging, 28,* 1623–1627.

Paharia, M. I. (2008). Chronic disease prevention. In B. A. Boyer & M. I. Pharia (Eds.), *Comprehensive handbook of clinical health psychology* (pp. 55–80). Hoboken, NJ: John Wiley and Sons.

Paharia, M. I. (2008). Tobacco cessation. In B. A. Boyer & M. I. Paharia (Eds.), *Comprehensive handbook of clinical health psychology* (pp. 105–124). Hoboken, NJ: John Wiley & Sons.

Paharia, M. I., & Kase, L. (2008). Obesity. In B. A. Boyer & M. I. Paharia (Eds.), *Comprehensive handbook of clinical health psychology* (pp. 81–103). Hoboken, NJ: John Wiley & Sons.

Palmer, S. C., & Coyne, J. C. (2004). Examining the evidence that psychotherapy improves the survival of cancer patients. *Biological Psychiatry, 56,* 61–62.

Pargament, K. I. (1999). The psychology of religion and spirituality? Yes and no. The *International Journal for the Psychology of Religion, 9,* 3–16.

Pargament, K. I., Koenig, H. G., & Perez, L. M. (2000). The many methods of religious coping: Development and initial validation of RCOPE. *Journal of Clinical Psychology, 56,* 519–543.

Pargament, K. I., Koenig, H. G., Tarakeshwar, N., & Hahn, J., (2001). Religious struggle as a predictor of mortality among medically ill elderly patients: A 2-year longitudinal study. *Archives of Internal Medicine, 161,* 1881–1885.

Pargament, K. I., Smith, B. W., Koenig, H. G., & Perez, L. (1998). Patterns of positive and negative coping with major life stressors. *Journal for the Scientific Study of Religion, 37,* 710–724.

Park, C. L. (2005). Religion as a meaning-making framework in coping with life stress. *Journal of Social Issues, 61,* 707–729.

Park, C. L. (2008). Testing the meaning making model of coping with loss. *Journal of Social and Clinical Psychology, 27,* 970–994.

Park, C. L., & Folkman, S. (1997). Meaning in the context of stress and coping. *Review of General Psychology, 1,* 115–144.

Parker, J. C., Smarr, K. L., Buckelew, S. P., Stucky-Ropp, R. C., Hewett, J. E., Johnson, J. C., ... Walker, S. E. (1995). Effects of stress management on clinical outcomes in rheumatoid arthritis. *Arthritis & Rheumatism, 38,* 1807–1818.

Pascoe, E. A., & Richman, L. S. (2009). Perceived discrimination and health: A meta-analytic review. *Psychological Bulletin, 135,* 531–554.

Pavot, W., & Diener, E. (1993). Review of the Satisfaction with Life Scale. *Psychological Assessment, 5,* 164–172.

Pavot, W., Diener, E., & Fujita, F. (1990). Extraversion and happiness. *Personality and Individual Differences, 11,* 1299–1306.

Pearce-McCall, D., & Newman, J. P. (1986). Expectation of success following noncontingent punishment in introverts and extraverts. *Journal of Personality and Social Psychology, 50,* 439–446.

Pelletier, K. (1977). *Mind as healer, mind as slayer.* New York: Delacorte Press/Seymour Lawrence.

Pelletier, K., & Herzing, D. (1988). Psychoneuroimmunology: Toward a mind-body model. *Advances, 5,* 27–56.

Pennebaker, J. W., Kiecolt-Glaser, J. K., & Glaser, R. (1988). Disclosures of traumas and immune function: Health implications for psychotherapy. *Journal of Consulting and Clinical Psychology, 56,* 239–245.

Peralta-Ramirez, M. I., Jimenez-Alonzo, J., Goody-Garcia, J. F., & Perez-Garcia, M. (2004). The effects of daily stress and stressful life events on the clinical symptomotology of patients with lupus erythematosus. *Psychosomatic Medicine, 66,* 788–794.

Pereira, D. B., Antoni, M. H., Danielson, A., Simon, T., Efantis-Potter, J., Carver, C., ... O'Sullivan, M. J. (2003). Stress as a predictor of symptomatic genital herpes virus recurrence in women with human immunodeficiency virus. *Journal of Psychosomatic Research, 54,* 237–244.

Pereira, M. A., O'Reilly, E., Augustsson, K., Fraser, G. E., Goldbourt, U., Heitmann, B. L., ... Ascherio, A. (2004). Dietary fiber and risk of coronary heart disease: A pooled analysis of cohort studies. *Archives of Internal Medicine, 164,* 370–376.

Perez, M. I., Linden, W., Perry, T., Jr., Puil, L. J., & Wright, J. M. (2009). Failure of psychological interventions to lower blood pressure: A randomized controlled trial. *Open Medicine, 3,* 92–100.

Perkins, K. A. (2010). Pharmacology and behavior: The case of tobacco dependence. In J. M. Suls, K. W. Davidson, & R. M. Kaplan (Eds.), *Handbook of health psychology and behavioral medicine* (pp. 527–543). New York: The Guilford Press.

Perkins, K. A., Karelitz, J. L., Conklin, C. A., Sayette, M. A., & Giedgowd, G. E. (2010). Acute negative affect relief from smoking depends on the affect measure and situation, but not on nicotine. *Biological Psychiatry, 67,* 707–714.

Perozzo, P., Savi, L., Castelli, L., Valre, W., Lo Giudice, R., Gentile, S., . . . Pinessi, L.(2005). Anger and emotional distress in patients with migraine and tension-type-headache. *Journal of Headache and Pain, 6,* 392–399.

Perry, R. P., Hechter, F. J., Menec, V. H., & Weinberg, L. E. (1993). Enhancing achievement motivation and performance in college students: An attributional retraining perspective. *Research in Higher Education, 34,* 687–723.

Perry, R. P., Stupnisky, R. H., Hall, N. C., Chipperfield, J. G., & Weiner, B. (2010). Bad starts and better finishes: Attributional retraining and initial performance in competitive achievement settings. *Journal of Social and Clinical Psychology, 29,* 668–700.

Peterson, C. (2006). *A primer in positive psychology.* New York: Oxford University Press.

Peterson, C., & Park, N. (2009). Classifying and measuring strengths of character. In S. J. Lopez & C. R. Snyder (Eds.), *Handbook of positive psychology* (2nd ed., pp. 25–33). New York: Oxford University Press.

Peterson, C., & Seligman, M. E. P. (1984). Causal explanations as a risk factor for depression: Theory and evidence. *Psychological Review, 91,* 347–374.

Peterson, C., & Seligman, M. E. P. (2004). *Character strengths and virtues: A handbook and classification.* New York: Oxford University Press.

Peterson, C., Maier, S. F., & Seligman, M. E. P. (1993). *Learned helplessness: A theory for the age of personal control.* New York: Oxford University Press.

Petticrew, M., Fraser, J. M., & Regan, M. F. (1999). Adverse life-events and risk of breast cancer: A meta-analysis. *British Journal of Health Psychology, 4,* 1–17.

Phillips, A. C., Carroll, D., Burns, V. E., Ring, C., Macleod, J., & Drayson, M. (2006). Bereavement and marriage are associated with antibody response to influenza vaccination in the elderly. *Brain, Behavior, and Immunity, 20,* 279–289.

Phillips, A. C., Der, G., & Carroll, D. (2008). Stressful life-events exposure is associated with 17-year

mortality, but it is health-related events that prove predictive. *British Journal of Health Psychology, 13,* 647–657.

Pieterse, A. L., & Carter, R. T. (2007). An examination of the relationship between general life stress, racism-related stress, and psychological health among black men. *Journal of Consulting Psychology, 54,* 101–109.

Pigeon, W. R., & Perlis, M. L. (2008). Cognitive behavioral treatment of insomnia. In W. O'Donohue & J. E. Fisher (Eds.), *Cognitive behavior therapy: Applying empirically supported techniques in your practice* (2nd ed., pp. 283–295). Hoboken, NJ: John Wiley & Sons.

Pinel, J. P. J., Assanand, S., & Lehman, D. R. (2000). Hunger, eating, and ill health. *American Psychologist, 55,* 1105–1116.

Plato. (1999). *Plato: The symposium* (C. Gill, Trans.). New York: Penguin Classics.

Player, M. S., King, D. E., Mainous, A. G., & Geesey, M. E. (2007). Psychosocial factors and progression from prehypertension to hypertension or coronary heart disease. *Annals of Family Medicine, 5,* 403–411.

Pleis, J. R., Lucas, J. W., & Ward, B. W. (2009). Summary health statistics for U.S. adults: National Health Interview Survey, 2008. National Center for Health Statistics. *Vital and Health Statistics* 10(242). Washington, DC: U.S. Government Printing Office.

Post, S. G. (2005). Altruism, happiness, and health: It's good to be good. *International Journal of Behavioral Medicine, 12,* 66–77.

Prasad, A. S. (2009). Impact of the discovery of human zinc deficiency on health. *Journal of the American College of Nutrition, 28,* 257–265.

Preston, S. H., & McDonald, J. (1979). The incidence of divorce within cohorts of American marriages contracted since the Civil War. *Demography, 16,* 1–26.

Prochaska, J. O., & Norcross, J. C. (2010). *Systems of psychotherapy: A transtheoretical analysis* (7th ed.). Belmont, CA: Brooks/Cole.

Public Health Agency of Canada. (2011). *Canada's handbook for physical activity guide to healthy*

active living. Retrieved from http://www.phac-aspc.gc.ca/hp-ps/hl-mvs/pag-gap/pdf/handbook-eng.pdf.

Quadrilatero, J., & Hoffman-Goetz, L. (2003). Physical activity and colon cancer: A systematic review of potential mechanisms. *The Journal of Sports Medicine and Physical Fitness, 43,* 121–138.

Quale, A. J., & Schanke, A-K. (2010). Resilience in the face of coping with a severe physical injury: A study of trajectories of adjustment in a rehabilitation setting. *Rehabilitation Psychology, 55,* 12–22.

Rabin, B. S. (1999). *Stress, immune function, and health: The connection.* New York: Wiley-Liss.

Raes, F. (2010). Rumination and worry as mediators of the relationship between self-compassion and depression and anxiety. *Personality and Individual Differences, 48,* 757–761.

Raglin, J. S. (1997). Anxiolytic effects of physical activity. In W. P. Morgan (Ed.), *Physical activity and mental health* (pp. 107–126). Washington, DC: Taylor & Francis.

Rahe, R. H. (1968). Life-change measurement as a predictor of illness. *Proceedings of the Royal Society of Medicine, 61,* 1124–1126.

Rand, K. L., & Cheavens, J. S. (2009). Hope theory. In S. J. Lopez & C. R. Snyder (Eds.), *Oxford handbook of positive psychology* (2nd ed., pp. 323–333). New York: Oxford University Press.

Ransford, C. P. (1982). A role for amines in the antidepressant effect of exercise: A review. *Medicine and Science in Sports and Exercise, 14,* 1–10.

Rasmussen, B. K., Jensen, R., Schroll, M., & Olesen, J. (1991). Epidemiology of headache in a general population—a prevalence study. *Journal of Clinical Epidemiology, 44,* 1147–1157.

Rasmussen, H. N., Scheier, M. F., & Greenhouse, J. B. (2009). Optimism and physical health: A meta-analytic review. *Annals of Behavioral Medicine, 37,* 239–256.

Rees, K., Bennett, P., West, R., Davey, S. G., & Ebrahim, S. (2004). Psychological interventions for coronary heart disease. *The Cochrane Database of Systematic Reviews* (2).

doi: 10.1002/14651858. CD002902.pub2.

Reid, K. J., Baron, K. G., Lu, B., Naylor, E., Wolfe, L., & Zee, P. C. (2010). Aerobic exercise improves self-reported sleep and quality of life in older adults with insomnia. *Sleep Medicine, 11,* 934–940.

Renaud, S., & de Lorgeril, M. (1992). Wine, alcohol, platelets, and the French paradox for coronary heart disease. *Lancet, 339,* 1523–1526.

Renner, M. J., & Mackin, R. S. (1998). A life stress instrument for classroom use. *Teaching of Psychology, 25,* 46–48.

Rhodewalt, F., & Zone, J. B., (1989). Appraisal of life change, depression, and illness in hardy and nonhardy women. *Journal of Personality and Social Psychology, 56,* 81–88.

Rice, P. L. (1999). *Stress and health* (3rd ed.). Belmont, CA: Wadsworth.

Richman, J. A., Rospenda, K. M., Nawyn, S. J., Flaherty, J. A., Fendrich, M., Drum, M. L., & Johnson, T. P. (1999). Sexual harassment and generalized workplace abuse among university employees: Prevalence and mental health correlates. *American Journal of Public Health, 89,* 358–363.

Richman, L. S., Pek, J., Pascoe, E., & Bauer, D. J. (2010). The effects of perceived discrimination on ambulatory blood pressure and affective responses to interpersonal stress modeled over 24 hours. *Health Psychology, 29,* 403–411.

Ridker, P. M., Rifai, N., Pfeffer, M., Sacks, F., Lepage, S., & Braunwald, E. (2000). Elevation of tumor necrosis factor-alpha and increased risk of recurrent coronary events after myocardial infarction. *Circulation, 101,* 2149–2153.

Rimm, D., & Masters, J. (1974). *Behavior therapy.* New York: Academic Press.

Rimm, E. B., Ascherio, A., Giovannucci, E., Spiegelman, D., Stampfer, M. J., & Willett, W. C. (1996). Vegetable, fruit, and cereal fiber intake and risk of coronary heart disease among men. *Journal of the American Medical Association, 275,* 447–451.

Roberts, B. W., & Mroczek, D. (2008). Personality trait change in adulthood. *Current Directions in Psychological Science, 17,* 31–35.

Robitaille, J., Yoon, P. W., Moore, C. A., Liu, T., Irizarry-Delacruz, M., Looker, A. C., & Khoury, M. J. (2008). Prevalence, family history, and prevention of reported osteoporosis in U.S. women. *American Journal of Preventive Medicine, 35,* 47–54.

Robles, T. F., Glaser, R., & Kiecolt-Glaser, J. K. (2005). Out of balance: A new look at chronic stress, depression, and immunity. *Current Directions in Psychological Science, 14,* 111–115.

Roger, C. J., Colbert, L. H., Greiner, J. W., Perkins, S. N., & Hursting, S. D. (2008). Physical activity and cancer prevention: Pathways and targets for intervention. *Sports Medicine, 38,* 271–296.

Romeo, J., Warnberg, J., Nove, E., Diaz, I., Gomez-Martinez, S., & Marcos, A. (2007). Moderate alcohol consumption and the immune system: A review. *British Journal of Nutrition, 98*(Suppl. 1), S111–S115.

Romero, C., Kalidas, M., Elledge, R., Chang, J., Liscum, K. R., & Friedman, L. C. (2006). Self-forgiveness, spirituality, and psychological adjustment in women with breast cancer. *Journal of Behavioral Medicine, 29,* 29–36.

Rona, R. J., Smeeton, N. C., Amigo, H., & Vargas, C. (2007). Do psychological distress and somatization contribute to misattribution of asthma? A Chilean study. *Journal of Psychosomatic Research, 62,* 23–30.

Rook, K. S. (1990). Parallels in the study of social support and social strain. *Journal of Social and Clinical Psychology, 9,* 118–132.

Rosa-Alcazar, A. I., Sanchez-Meca, J., Gomez-Conesa, A., & Marin-Martinez, F. (2008). Psychological treatment of obsessive-compulsive disorder: A meta-analysis. *Clinical Psychology Review, 28,* 1310–1325.

Rosen, G. M., & Lilienfeld, S. O. (2008). Posttraumatic stress disorder: An empirical evaluation of core assumptions. *Clinical Psychology Review, 28,* 837–868.

Rosengren, A., Hawken, S., Ounpuu, S., Sliwa, K., Zubaid, M., Almahmeed, W. A., . . . Yusuf, S. (2004). Association of psychosocial risk factors with risk of acute myocardial infarction in 11119 cases and 13648 controls from 52 countries (the INTERHEART study): Case-control study. *Lancet, 364,* 953–962.

Rosenman, R. H. (1990). Type A behavior pattern: A personal overview. *Journal of Social Behavior and Personality, 5,* 1–24.

Rosenman, R. H. (1993). Relationships of the Type A behavior pattern with coronary heart disease. In L. Goldberger & S. Breznitz (Eds.), *Handbook of stress: Theoretical and clinical aspects* (pp. 449–476). New York: Free Press.

Rosenman, R. H., Brand, R. J., Jenkins, D., Friedman, M., Straus, R., & Wurm, M. (1975). Coronary heart disease in the Western Collaborative Group Study: Final follow-up experience of 8½ years. *Journal of the American Medical Association, 233,* 872–877.

Rosenman, R. H., Friedman, M., Straus, R., Wurm, M., Kositcheck, R., Hahn, W., & Verthessen, N. T. (1964). A predictive study of coronary heart disease: The Western Collaborative Group Study. *Journal of the American Medical Association, 189,* 15–22.

Rospenda, K. M., & Richman, J. A. (2005). Harassment and discrimination. In J. Barling, E. K. Kelloway, & M. R. Frone (Eds.), *Handbook of work stress* (pp. 149–188). Thousand Oaks, CA: Sage.

Ross, C. E., Mirowsky, J., & Goldsteen, K. (1990). The impact of the family on health: The decade in review. *Journal of Marriage and Family, 52,* 1059–1078.

Roth, T., & Roehrs, T. (2000). Disorders of sleep and wakefulness. In E. R. Kandel, J. H. Schwartz, & T. M. Jessell (Eds.), *Principles of neural science* (4th ed., pp. 948–959). New York: McGraw-Hill.

Rotter, J. B. (1966). Generalized expectancies for internal versus external control of reinforcement. *Psychological Monographs, 80* (1, Whole No. 609).

Rotter, J. B. (1990). Internal versus external control of reinforcement: A case history of a variable. *American Psychologist, 45,* 489–493.

Rouch, I., Wild, P., Ansiau, D., & Marquie, J.-C. (2005). Shiftwork experience, age and cognitive performance. *Ergonomics, 48,* 1282–1293.

Roy, B., Diez-Roux, A. V., Seeman, T., Ranjit, N., Shea, S., & Cushman, M. (2010). Association of optimism and pessimism with inflammation and hemostasis in the Multi-Ethnic Study of Atherosclerosi (MESA). *Psychosomatic Medicine, 72,* 134–140.

Roy-Byrne, P. P., & Cowley, D. S. (2007). Pharmacological treatments for panic disorder, generalized anxiety disorder, specific phobia, and social anxiety disorder. In P. E. Nathan & J. M. Gorman (Eds.), *A guide to treatments that work* (3rd ed., pp. 395–430). New York: Oxford University Press.

Royer, A. (1994). The role of the transcendental meditation technique in promoting smoking cessation: A longitudinal study. *Alcoholism Treatment Quarterly, 11,* 221–239.

Rugh, J. D., & Solberg, W. K. (1975). Electromyographic studies of bruxist behavior before and during treatment. *California Dental Association Journal, 3,* 56–59.

Russell, W. D. (2001). An examination of flow state occurrence in college athletes. *Journal of Sport Behavior, 24,* 83–107.

Rutledge, T., & Hogan, B. E. (2002). A quantitative review of prospective evidence linking psychological factors with hypertension development. *Psychosomatic Medicine, 64,* 758–766.

Rutledge, T., Stucky, E., Dollarhide, A., Shively, M., Jain, S., Wolfson, T., . . . Dresselhaus, T. (2009). A real-time assessment of work stress in physicians and nurses. *Health Psychology, 28,* 194–200.

Ryan, R. M., & Deci, E. L. (2000). Self-determination theory and the facilitation of intrinsic motivation, social development and well-being. *American Psychologist, 55,* 68–78.

Ryff, C. D. (1989). Happiness is everything or is it? Explorations on the meaning of psychological well-being. *Journal of Personality and Social Psychology, 57,* 1069–1081.

Ryff, C. D. (1995). Psychological well-being in adult life. *Current Directions in Psychological Science, 4,* 99–104.

Ryff, C. D., & Singer, B. (1996). Psychological well-being: Meaning, measurement, and implications for psychotherapy research. *Psychotherapy and Psychosomatics, 65,* 14–23.

Ryff, C. D., Love, G. D., Urry, H. L., Muller, D., Rosenkranz, M. A., Friedman, E. M., . . . Singer, B. (2006). Psychological well-being and ill-being: Do they have distinct or mirrored biological correlates? *Psychotherapy and Psychosomatics, 75,* 85–95.

Sacks, F. M. (2011). Ask the expert: Omega-3 fatty acids. *Harvard School of Public Health: The Nutrition Source.* Retrieved from http://www.hsph.harvard.edu/nutritionsource/questions/omega-3/index.html.

Sacks, F. M., Bray, G. A., Carey, V. J., Smith, S. R., Ryan, D. H., Anton, S. D., . . . Williamson, D. A. (2009). Comparison of weight-loss diets with different compositions of fat, protein, and carbohydrates. *The New England Journal of Medicine, 360,* 859–873.

Saleem, T. S. M., & Basha, S. D. (2010). Red wine: A drink to your heart. *Journal of Cardiovascular Disease Research, 1,* 171–176.

Salt, W. B., II, & Neimark, N. F. (2002). *Irritable bowel syndrome and the mind body spirit connection: Seven steps for living a healthy life with a functional bowel disorder, Crohn's disease or colitis.* Columbus, OH: Parkview.

Sanchez-Meca, J., Rosa-Alcazar, A. I., Marin-Martinez, F. M., & Gomez-Conesa, A. (2010). Psychological treatment of panic disorder with or without agoraphobia: A meta-analysis. *Clinical Psychology Review, 30,* 37–50.

Sandvik, E., Diener, E., & Seidlitz, L. (1993). Subjective well-being: The convergence of stability of self-report and non-self-report measures. *Journal of Personality, 61,* 317–342.

Saulsman, L. M., & Page, A. C. (2004). The five-factor model and personality disorder empirical literature: A meta-analytic review. *Clinical Psychology Review, 23,* 1055–1085.

Sauro, K. M., & Becker, W. J. (2009). The stress and migraine interaction. *The Journal of Head and Face Pain, 49,* 1378–1386.

Sausen, K. P., Lovallo, W. R., Pincomb, G. A., & Wilson, M. F. (1992). Cardiovascular responses to occupational stress in male medical students: A paradigm for ambulatory monitoring studies. *Health Psychology, 11,* 55–60.

Schapira, D. V., Clark, R. A., Wolff, P. A., Jarrett, A. R., Kumbar, N. B., & Aziz, N. M. (1994). Visceral obesity and breast cancer risk. *Cancer, 74,* 632–639.

Scheier, M. F., & Carver, C. S. (1985). Optimism, coping, and health: Assessment and implications of generalized outcome expectancies. *Health Psychology, 4,* 219–247.

Scheier, M. F., & Carver, C. S. (1992). Effects of optimism on psychological and physical well-being: Theoretical overview and empirical update. *Cognitive Therapy and Research, 16,* 201–228.

Scheier, M. F., Carver, C. S., & Bridges, M. W. (1994). Distinguishing optimism from neuroticism (and trait anxiety, self-mastery, and self-esteem): A reevaluation of the Life Orientation Test. *Journal of Personality and Social Psychology, 67,* 1063–1078.

Scherg, H., & Blohmke, M. (1988). Associations between selected life events and cancer. *Behavioral Medicine, 14,* 119–124.

Schernhammer, E. S., Laden, F., Speizer, F. E., Willett, W. C., Hunter, D. J., Kawachi, I., . . . Colditz, G. A. (2003). Night-shift work and risk of colorectal cancer in the Nurses' Health Study. *Journal of the National Cancer Institute, 95,* 825–824.

Schernhammer, E. S., Laden, F., Speizer, F. E., Willett, W. C., Hunter, D. J., Kawachi, I., & Colditz, G. A. (2001). Rotating night shifts and risk of breast cancer in women participating in the Nurses' Health Study. *Journal of the National Cancer Institute, 93,* 1563–1568.

Schneider, S. L. (2001). In search of realistic optimism: Meaning, knowledge, and warm fuzziness. *American Psychologist, 56,* 250–263.

Schneiderman, N., Ironson, G., & Siegel, S. D. (2005). Stress and health: Psychological, behavioral, and biological determinant. *Annual Review of Clinical Psychology, 1,* 607–628.

Schousboe, K., Visscher, P. M., Erbas, B., Kyvik, K. O., Hopper, J. L., Henriksen, J. E., . . . Sorensen, T. I. A. (2004). Twin study of genetic and environmental influences on adult body size, shape, and composition. *International Journal of Obesity, 28,* 39–48.

Schroeder, D., & Costa, P. T. (1984). Influence of life event stress on physical illness: Substantive effects or methodological flaws. *Journal of Personality and Social Psychology, 46,* 853–863.

Schuler, J., & Brunner, S. (2009). The rewarding effect of flow experience on performance in a marathon race. *Psychology of Sport and Exercise, 10,* 168–174.

Schulman, P. (1999). Applying learned optimism to increase sales productivity. *Journal of Personal Selling and Sales Management, 19,* 31–37.

Schultz, J. H. (1932). *Das Autogene Training-Konzentrative Selbstentspannung.* Leipzig, Germany: Thieme.

Schumann, N. P., Zeiner, U., & Nebrich, A. (1988). Personality and quantified muscular activity of the masticatory system in patients with temporomandibular joint dysfunction. *Journal of Oral Rehabilitation, 15,* 35–47.

Schwartz, G. E., & Weiss, S. M. (1977). *Yale Conference on Behavioral Medicine.* Washington, DC: Department of Health, Education and Welfare/National Heart, Lung and Blood Institute.

Schwartz, M.S. (2003). Intake decisions and preparation of patients for therapy. In M. S. Schwartz & F. Andrasik (Eds.), *Biofeedback: A practitioner's guide* (3rd ed., pp. 105–127). New York: The Guilford Press.

Schwartz, M. S., & Andrasik, F. (2003). Headache. In M. S. Schwartz & F. Andrasik (Eds.), *Biofeedback: A practitioner's guide* (3rd ed., pp. 275–348). New York: The Guilford Press.

Schwartz, M. S., & Olson, R. P. (2003). A historical perspective on the field of biofeedback and applied psychophysiology. In M. S. Schwartz & F. Andrasik (Eds.), *Biofeedback: A practitioner's guide* (3rd ed., pp. 3–19). New York: The Guilford Press.

Schwartz, M. S., & Sedlacek, K. (2003). Raynaud's disease and Raynaud's phenomenon. In M. S. Schwartz & F. Andrasik (Eds.), *Biofeedback: A practitioner's guide* (3rd ed., pp. 369–381). New York: The Guilford Press.

Schwartz, S. M., Schmitt, E. P., Ketterer, M. W., & Trask, P. C. (1999). Lipid levels and emotional distress among healthy male college students. *Stress Medicine, 15,* 159–165.

Scott, D. S., & Lundeen, T. F. (1980). Myofacial pain involving the masticatory muscles: An experimental model. *Pain, 8,* 207–215.

Scully, J. A., Tosi, H., & Banning, K. (2000). Life event checklists: Revisiting the Social Readjustment Rating Scale after 30 years. *Educational and Psychological Measurement, 60,* 864–876.

Searle, A., & Bennett, P. (2001). Psychological factors and inflammatory bowel disease: A review of a decade of literature. *Psychology, Health, and Medicine, 6,* 121–135.

Segal, Z. V., Williams, J. M., & Teasdale, J. D. (2002). *Mindfulness-based cognitive therapy for depression: A new approach to preventing relapse.* New York: The Guilford Press.

Segerstrom, S. C., & Miller, G. E. (2004). Psychological stress and the human immune system: A meta-analytic study of 30 years of inquiry. *Psychological Bulletin, 130,* 601–630.

Seligman, M. E. P. (1990). *Learned optimism.* New York: Knopf.

Seligman, M. E. P. (2002). *Authentic happiness: Using the new positive psychology to realize your potential for lasting fulfillment.* New York: Free Press.

Seligman, M. E. P. (2011). *Flourish: A visionary new understanding of happiness and well-being.* New York: Simon & Schuster.

Seligman, M. E. P., & Csikszentmihalyi, M. (2000). Positive psychology: An introduction. *American Psychologist, 55,* 5–14.

Seligman, M. E. P., Reivich, K., Jaycox, L., & Gillham, J. (1995). *The optimistic child.* New York: Houghton Mifflin.

Seligman, M. E. P., Steen, T. A., Park, N., & Peterson, C. (2005). Positive psychology progress: Empirical validation of interventions. *American Psychologist, 60,* 410–421.

Seligman, M. E. P., Walker, E. F., & Rosenhan, D. L. (2001). *Abnormal psychology* (4th ed.). New York: Norton.

Selye, H. (1956a). *The stress of life.* New York: McGraw-Hill.

Selye, H. (1956b). What is stress? *Metabolism: Clinical and Experimental, 5,* 525–530.

Shafi, M., Lavely, R. A., & Jaffe, R. D. (1974). Meditation and marijuana. *American Journal of Psychiatry, 131,* 60–63.

Shapiro, F. S. (2002). *Eye movement desensitization and reprocessing* (2nd ed.). New York: The Guilford Press.

Shapiro, S. L., Astin, J., Bishop, S., & Cordova, M. (2005). Mindfulness-based stress reduction for health care professionals: Results from a randomized trial. *International Journal of Stress Management, 12,* 164–176.

Shapiro, S. L., Schwartz, G. E., & Bonner, G. (1998). Effects of mindfulness-based stress reduction on medical and premedical students. *Journal of Behavioral Medicine, 21,* 581–599.

Sheikh, A. I. (2004). Posttraumatic growth in the context of heart disease. *Journal of Clinical Psychology in Medical Settings, 11,* 265–273.

Shekelle, R. B., Gale, M., Ostfeld, A. M., & Oglesby, P. (1983). Hostility, risk of coronary heart disease, and mortality. *Psychosomatic Medicine, 45,* 109–114.

Shekelle, R. B., Hulley, S., Neaton, J., Billings, J., Borhani, N., Gerace, T., . . . the MRFIT Research Group (1985). The MRFIT behavior pattern study II. Type A behavior pattern and incidence of coronary heart disease. *American Journal of Epidemiology, 122,* 559–570.

Shepherd, G. M. (1979). *The synaptic organization of the brain* (2nd ed.). New York: Oxford University Press.

Shipley, B. A., Weiss, A., Der, G., Taylor, M. D., & Deary, I. J. (2007). Neuroticism, extraversion, and mortality in the UK health and lifestyle survey: A 21-year prospective cohort study. *Psychosomatic Medicine, 69,* 923–931.

Shirom, A. (2011). Job-related burnout: A review of major research foci and challenges. In J. C. Quick & L. E. Tetrick (Eds.), *Handbook of occupational health psychology* (2nd ed., pp. 223–241). Washington, DC: American Psychological Association.

Shirom, A., Melamed, S., Rogowski, O., Shapria, I., & Berliner, S. (2009). Workload, control, and social support effects on serum lipids: A longitudinal study among apparently healthy employed adults. *Journal of Occupational Health Psychology, 14,* 349–364.

Shirtcliff, E. A., Coe, C. L., & Pollak, S. D. (2009). Early childhood stress is associated with elevated antibody levels to herpes simplex virus type 1. *Proceedings of the National Academy of Sciences USA, 106,* 2963–2967.

Shraga, O., & Shirom, A. (2009). The construct validity of vigor and its antecedents: A qualitative study. *Human Relations, 62,* 271–291.

Siegel, R. D. (2010). *The mindfulness solution: Everyday practices for everyday problems.* New York: The Guilford Press.

Siegrist, J. (1996). Adverse health effects of high-effort/low-reward conditions. *Journal of Occupational Health Psychology, 1,* 27–41.

Sigal, R. J., Kenny, G. P., Boule, N. G., Wells, G. A., Prud'homme, D., Fortier, M., . . . Jaffey, J. (2007). Effects of aerobic training, resistance training, or both on glycemic control in type 2 diabetes. *Annals of Internal Medicine, 147,* 357–369.

Sigurdson, K., & Ayas, N. T. (2007). The public health and safety consequences of sleep disorders. *Canadian Journal of Physiology and Pharmacology, 85,* 179–183.

Simon, A. E., Palmer, S. C., & Coyne, J. C. (2007). Cancer and depression. In A. Steptoe (Ed.), *Depression and physical illness* (pp. 211–237). New York: Cambridge University Press.

Simopoulos, A. P. (2006). Evolutionary aspects of diet, the omega-6/omega-3 ratio and genetic variation: Nutritional implications of chronic diseases. *Biomedicine & Pharmacotherapy, 60,* 502–507.

Sklar, L. S., & Anisman, H. (1980). Social stress influences tumor growth. *Psychosomatic Medicine, 42,* 347–365.

Small, G., & Vorgan, G. (2008). Meet your ibrain. *Scientific American Mind, 19,* 42–49.

Smith, P. J., Blumenthal, J. A., Hoffman, B. M., Cooper, H., Strauman, T. A., Welsch-Bohmer, K., . . . Sherwood, A. (2010). Aerobic exercise and neurocognitive performance: A meta-analytic review of randomized controlled trials. *Psychosomatic Medicine, 72,* 239–252.

Smith, P. L., & Moss, S. B. (2009). Psychologist impairment: What is it, how can it be prevented, and what can be done to address it? *Clinical Psychology: Science and Practice, 16,* 1–15.

Smith, T. W., & MacKenzie, J. (2006). Personality and risk of physical illness. *Annual Review of Clinical Psychology, 2,* 435–467.

Smyth, J. M, & Pennebaker, J. W. (2008). Exploring the boundary conditions of expressive writing: In search of the right recipe. *British Journal of Health Psychology, 13,* 1–7.

Smyth, J. M., Stone, A., Hurewitz, A., & Kaell, A. (1999). Effects of writing about stressful experiences on symptom reduction in patients with asthma or rheumatoid arthritis: A randomized trial. *Journal of the American Medical Association, 281,* 1304–1309.

Snyder, C. R. (1989). Reality negotiation: From excuses to hope and beyond. *Journal of Social and Clinical Psychology, 8,* 130–157.

Snyder, C. R., Harris, C., Anderson, J. R., Holleran, S. A., Irving, L. M., Sigmon, S. T., . . . Harney, P. (1991). The will and the ways: Development and validation of an individual-differences measure of hope. *Journal of Personality and Social Psychology, 60,* 570–585.

Snyder, C. R., Sympson, S. C., Ybasco, F. C., Borders, T. F., Babyak, M. A., & Higgins, R. L. (1996). Development and validation of the State Hope Scale. *Journal of Personality and Social Psychology, 70,* 321–335.

Solberg Nes, L., & Segerstrom, S. C. (2006). Dispositional optimism and coping: A meta-analytic review. *Personality and Social Psychology Review, 10,* 235–251.

Solomon, G. F., & Moos, R. (1964). Emotions, immunity, and disease. *Archives of General Psychiatry, 11,* 657–674.

Sopori, M. (2002). Effects of cigarette smoke on the immune system. *Nature Reviews Immunology, 2,* 372–377.

Sotile, W. M., & Sotile, M. O. (1996). *The medical marriage: A couple's survival guide.* New York: Carol.

Spiegel, D. (2002). Effects of psychotherapy on cancer survival. *National Review of Cancer, 2,* 383–389.

Spiegel, D., & Giese-Davis, J. (2003). Depression and cancer: Mechanisms and disease progression. *Biological Psychiatry, 54,* 269–282.

Spiegel, D., Bloom, J. R., Kraemer, H. C., & Gottheil, E. (1989). Effect of psychosocial treatment on survival of patients with metastatic breast cancer. *Lancet, 2,* 888–891.

Stallone, D. D., & Stunkard, A. J. (1991). The regulation of body weight: Evidence and clinical implications. *Annals of Behavioral Medicine, 13,* 220–230.

Steel, P., Schmidt, J., & Shultz, J. (2008). Refining the relationship between personality and subjective well-being. *Psychological Bulletin, 134,* 138–161.

Steger, M. F. (2009). Meaning in life. In S. J. Lopez & C. R. Snyder (Eds.), *Handbook of positive psychology* (2nd ed., pp. 679–687). New York: Oxford University Press.

Steptoe, A. (2000). Psychological factors in the development of hypertension. *Annals of Medicine, 32,* 371–375.

Steptoe, A., & Brydon, L. (2007). Psychosocial factors and coronary heart disease: The role of psychoneuroimmunological processes. In R. Ader (Ed.), *Psychoneuroimmunology* II (4th ed., pp. 945–973). Boston: Elsevier Academic Press.

Steptoe, A., Gibson, E. L., Vounonvirta, R., Williams, E. D., Hamer, M., Rycroft, J. A., . . . Wardle, J. (2007). The effects of tea on psychophysiological stress responsivity and post-stress recovery: A randomised double-blind trial. *Psychopharmacology, 190,* 81–89.

Steptoe, A., Hamer, M., & Chida, Y. (2007). The effects of acute psychological stress on circulating inflammatory factors in humans: A review and meta-analysis. *Brain, Behavior, and Immunity, 21,* 901–912.

Sterling, P., & Eyer, J. (1988). Allostasis: A new paradigm to explain arousal pathology. In S. Fisher & J. Reason (Eds.), *Handbook of life stress, cognition, and health* (pp. 629–649). New York: John Wiley.

Sternberg, R. J. (1986). A triangular theory of love. *Psychological Review, 93,* 119–135.

Stetter, F., & Kupper, S. (2002). Autogenic training: A meta-analysis of clinical outcome studies. *Applied Psychophysiology and Biofeedback, 27,* 45–98.

Stone, A. A., Schwartz, J. E., Shiffman, S., Neale, J. M., Marco, C. A., Hickcox, M., . . . Cruise, L. J. (1998). A comparison of coping assessed by ecological momentary assessment and retrospective recall. *Journal of Personality and Social Psychology, 74,* 1670–1680.

Straub, R. H., & Kalden, J. R. (2009). Stress of different types increases the proinflammatory load in rheumatoid arthritis. *Arthritis Research and Therapy, 11,* 114.

Strawbridge, W. J., Deleger, S., Roberts, R. E., & Kaplan, G. A. (2002). Physical activity reduces the risk of subsequent depression for older adults. *American Journal of Epidemiology, 156,* 328–334.

Strike, P. C., & Steptoe, A. (2005). Behavioral and emotional triggers of acute coronary syndromes: A systematic review and critique. *Psychosomatic Medicine, 67,* 179–186.

Stunkard, A. J., Harris, J. R., Pedersen, N. L., & McClean, G. E. (1990). The body-mass index of twins who have been reared apart. *The New England Journal of Medicine, 322,* 1483–1487.

Suarez, E. C., Lewis, J. G., & Kuhn, C. (2002). The relation of aggression, hostility, and anger to lipopolysaccharide-stimulated tumor necrosis factor (TNF)-α by blood monocytes from normal men. *Brain, Behavior, and Immunity, 16,* 675–684.

Suls, J., & Bunde, J. (2005). Anger, anxiety, and depression as risk factors for cardiovascular disease: The problems and implications of overlapping affective dispositions. *Psychological Bulletin, 131,* 260–300.

Suls, J., & Martin, R. (2005). The daily life of the garden-variety neurotic: Reactivity, stressor exposure, mood spillover, and maladaptive coping. *Journal of Personality, 73,* 1–25.

Sulsky, L., & Smith, C. (2005). *Work stress.* Belmont, CA: Thomson-Wadsworth.

Surtees, P. G., Nicholas, W. J., Wainwright, R. L., Khaw, K.-T., & Day, N. E. (2006). Mastery, sense of coherence, and mortality: Evidence of independent associations from the EPIC-Norfolk prospective cohort study. *Health Psychology, 25,* 102–110.

Swickert, R. J., & Gilliland, K. (1998). Relationship between brain-stem auditory evoked response and extraversion, impulsivity, and sociability. *Journal of Research in Personality, 32,* 314–330.

Taktek, K. (2004). The effects of mental imagery on the acquisition of motor skills and performance: A literature review with theoretical implications. *Journal of Mental Imagery, 28,* 79–114.

Talley, N. J., & Spiller, R. (2002). Irritable bowel syndrome: A little understood organic bowel disease. *Lancet, 360,* 555–564.

Tamres, L. K., Janicki, D., & Helgeson, V. S. (2002). Sex differences in coping behavior: A meta-analytic review and an examination of relative coping. *Personality and Social Psychology Review, 6,* 2–30.

Tanasecu, M., Leitzmann, M. F., Rimm, E. B., Willett, W. C., Stampfer, M. J., & Hu, F. B. (2002). Exercise type and intensity in relation to coronary heart disease in men. *Journal of the American Medical Association, 288,* 1994–2000.

Taris, T. W. (2006). Is there a relationship between burnout and objective performance? A critical review of 16 studies. *Work and Stress, 20,* 316–334.

Tatar, M. (2009). Teachers turning for help to school counsellors and colleagues: Toward a mapping of relevant predictors. *British Journal of Guidance & Counselling, 37,* 107–127.

Taylor, S. E. (2006). Biobehavioral bases of affiliation under stress. *Current Directions in Psychological Science, 15,* 273–277.

Taylor, S. E., & Brown, J. (1988). Illusion and well-being: A social psychological perspective on mental health. *Psychological Bulletin, 103,* 193–210.

Taylor, S. E., Klein, L. C., Lewis, B. P., Gruenewald, T. L., Gurung, R. A. R., & Updegraff, J. A. (2000). Biobehavioral responses to stress in females: Tend-and-befriend, not fight-or-flight. *Psychological Review, 107,* 411–429.

Taylor, S. E., Lewis. B. P., Gruenewald, T. L., Gurung, R. A. R., Updegraff, J. A., & Klein, L. C. (2002). Sex differences in biobehavioral responses to threat: Reply to Geary and Flinn (2002). *Psychological Review, 109,* 751–753.

Teasdale, J. D., Segal, Z. V., Williams, J. M. G., Ridgeway, V. A., Soulsby, J. M., & Lau, M. A. (2000). Prevention of relapse/recurrence in major depression by mindfulness-based cognitive therapy. *Journal of Consulting and Clinical Psychology, 68,* 615–623.

Tedeschi, R. G., & Calhoun, L. G. (2004). Posttraumatic growth: Conceptual foundations and empirical evidence. *Psychological Inquiry, 15,* 1–18.

Terry, D. J., & Hynes, G. J. (1998). Adjustment to a low-control situation: Reexamining the role of coping responses. *Journal of Personality and Social Psychology, 74,* 1078–1092.

Tessler, R., & Mechanic, D. (1978). Psychologic distress and perceived health status. *Journal of Health and Social Behavior, 19,* 254–262.

Thompson, D. L. (2007). Nutrition. In E. T. Howley & B. D. Franks (Eds.), *Fitness professional's handbook* (5th ed., pp. 103–117). Champaign, IL: Human Kinetics.

Thompson, L. Y., Snyder, C. R., Hoffman, L., Michael, S. T., Rasmussen, H. N., Billings, L. S., . . . Roberts, D. E. (2005). Dispositional forgiveness of self, others, and situations. *Journal of Personality, 73,* 313–359.

Thompson, M., & Thompson, L. (2007). Neurofeedback for stress management. In P. M. Lehrer, R. L. Woolfolk, & W. E. Sime (Eds.), *Principles and practice of stress management* (3rd ed., pp. 249–287). New York: The Guilford Press.

Tindle, H. A., Chang, Y-F., Kuller, L. H., Manson, J. E., Robinson, J. G., Rosal, M. C., . . . Matthews, K. A. (2009). Optimism, cynical hostility, and incident coronary heart disease and mortality in the Women's Health Initiative. *Circulation, 120,* 656–662.

Toker, S., Shirom, A., Shapira, I., Berliner, S., & Melamed, S. (2005). The association between burnout, depression, anxiety, and inflammation biomarkers: C-reactive protein and fibrinogen in men and women. *Journal of Occupational Health Psychology, 10,* 344–362.

Toneatto, T., & Nguyen, L. (2007). Does mindfulness meditation improve anxiety and mood symptoms? A review of the controlled research. *Canadian Journal of Psychiatry, 52,* 260–266.

Totterdell, P. (2005). Work schedules. In J. Barling, E. K. Kelloway, & M. R. Frone (Eds.), *Handbook of work stress* (pp. 35–62). Thousand Oaks, CA: Sage.

Trakhtenberg, E. C. (2008). The effects of guided imagery on the immune system: A critical review. *International Journal of Neuroscience, 118,* 839–855.

Trapmann, S., Hell, B., Hirn, J.-O. W., & Schuler, H. (2007). Meta-analysis of the relationship between the Big Five and academic success at university. *Zeitschrift für Psychologie/Journal of Psychology, 215,* 132–151.

Trautmann, E., Lackschewitz, H., & Kroner-Herwig, B. (2006). Psychological treatment of recurrent headache in children and adolescents—a meta-analysis. *Cephalagia, 26,* 1411–1426.

Treating depression along with alcohol dependence. (2010). *Harvard Mental Health Letter, 27*(1), 7.

Trost, S. G., Owen, N., Bauman, A. E., Sallis, J. F., & Brown, W. (2002). Correlates of adults? Participation in physical activity: Review and update. *Medicine & Science in Sports & Exercise, 34,* 1996–2001.

Trumbo, P., Schlicker, S., Yates, A. A., & Poos, M. (2002). Dietary reference intakes for energy, carbohydrate, fiber, fat, fatty acids, cholesterol, protein and amino acids. *Journal of the American Dietetic Association, 102,* 1621–1630.

Tryon, W. W. (2005). Possible mechanisms for why systematic desensitization and exposure therapy work. *Clinical Psychology Review, 25,* 67–95.

Tulpule, T. (1971). Yogic exercises in the management of ischemic heart disease. *Indian Heart Journal, 23,* 259–264.

Turner, D. (1989, April 15). Spring's hope—Amazingly, some are unmoved even by this marvelous season. *The Seattle Times,* p. C9.

U.S. Department of Agriculture and U.S. Department of Health and Human Services (USDA & USDHHS). (2010). *Dietary Guidelines for Americans, 2010* (7th ed.). Washington, DC: U.S. Government Printing Office.

U.S. Department of Health and Human Services (USDHHS). (2000). *Healthy People 2010: Understanding and improving health* (2nd ed.). Washington, DC: U.S. Government Printing Office.

U.S. Department of Health & Human Services (2008). *Physical activity guidelines for Americans.* Retrieved from http://www.health.gov/paguidelines.

U.S. Department of Health & Human Services. (2011). *Physical activity guidelines for Americans.* Retrieved from http://www.health.gov/paguidelines/factsheetprof.aspx.

U.S. Merit Systems Protection Board (USMSPB). (1995). *Sexual harassment in the federal workplace: Trends, progress, continuing challenges.* Washington, DC: Author.

Uchino, B. N. (2006). Social support and health: A review of physiological processes potentially underlying links to disease outcomes. *Journal of Behavioral Medicine, 29,* 377–387.

Uchino, B. N., Cacioppo, J. T., & Kiecolt-Glaser, J. K. (1996). The relationship between social support and physiological processes: A review with emphasis on underlying mechanisms and implications for health. *Psychological Bulletin, 119,* 488–531.

Utay, J., & Miller, M. (2006). Guided imagery as an effective therapeutic technique: A brief review of its history and efficacy research. *Journal of Instructional Psychology, 33,* 40–43.

Vainio, H., & Weiderpass, E. (2006). Fruit and vegetables in cancer prevention. *Nutrition and Cancer, 54,* 11–142.

Val, E. B., & Linley, P. A. (2006). Posttraumatic growth, positive changes, and negative changes in Madrid residents following the March 11, 2004, Madrid train bombings. *Journal of Loss and Trauma, 11,* 409–424.

van Dam, R. M., Li, T., Spiegelman, D., Franco, O. H., & Hu, F. B. (2008, September 16). Combined impact of lifestyle factors on mortality: Prospective cohort study in US women. *British Medical Journal, 337*:a1440. Retrieved from http://www.bmj.com/cgi/content/full/337/sep16_2/a1440?eaf.

van der Hal-van Raalte, E. A. M., van IJzendoorn, M. H., & Bakermans-Kranenburg, M. J. (2008). Sense of coherence moderates late effects of early childhood Holocaust exposure. *Journal of Clinical Psychology, 64,* 1352–1367.

Van der Hulst, M. (2003). Long work hours and health. *Scandinavian Journal of Work, Environment and Health, 29,* 171–188.

Van der Kooy, K., Hout, H. V., Marwijk, H., Marten, H., Stehouwer, C., & Beckman, A. (2007). Depression and the risk for cardiovascular diseases: Systematic review and meta-analysis. *International Journal of Geriatric Psychiatry, 22,* 613–626.

van Dierendonck, D., Schaufeli, W. B., & Buunk, B. P. (1998). The evaluation of an individual burnout intervention program: The role of inequity and social support. *Journal of Applied Psychology, 83,* 392–407.

Vealey, R. S., & Geenleaf, C. A. (2006). Seeing is believing: Understanding and using imagery in sport. In J. M. Williams (Ed.), *Applied sport psychology: Personal growth to peak performance* (5th ed., pp. 306–348). New York: McGraw-Hill.

Venable, V. L., Carlson, C. R., & Wilson, J. (2001). The role of anger and depression in recurrent headache. *Headache, 41,* 21–30.

Vener, K. J., Szabo, S., & Moore, J. G. (1989). The effect of shift work on gastrointestinal (GI) function: A review. *Chronobiologica, 16,* 421–439.

Vicennati, V., Pasqui, F., Cavazza, C., Pagotto, U., & Pasquali, R. (2009). Stress-related development of obesity and cortisol in women. *Obesity, 17,* 1678–1683.

Virues-Ortega, J., & Buela-Casal, G. (2006). Psychophysiological effects of human-animal interaction: Theoretical issues and long-term interaction effects. *Journal of Nervous and Mental Disease, 194,* 52–57.

Vitaliano, P. P., Zhang, J., & Scanlon, J. (2003). Is caregiving hazardous to one's health? A meta-analysis. *Psychological Bulletin, 129,* 946–972.

Wacker, J., Chavanon, M-L., & Stemmler, G. (2006). Investigating the dopaminergic basis of extraversion in humans: A multilevel approach. *Journal of Personality and Social Psychology, 91,* 171–187.

Waldie, K. E. (2001). Childhood headache, stress in adolescence, and primary headache in young adulthood: A longitudinal cohort study. *Headache, 41,* 1–10.

Wallace, R. K. (1970). Physiological effects of transcendental meditation. *Science, 167,* 1751–1754.

Wallace, R. K., Benson, H., & Wilson, A. F. (1971). A wakeful hypometabolic state. *American Journal of Physiology, 221,* 795–799.

Wallis, D. J., & Hetherington, M. M. (2004). Stressed eating: The effects of ego-threat and cognitive demand on food intake in restrained and emotional eaters. *Apetite, 43,* 39–46.

Wallston, K. A., & Wallston, B. S. (1981). Health locus of control scales. In H. M. Lefcourt (Ed.), *Research with the locus of control construct: Assessment methods* (Vol. 1, pp. 189–243). New York: Academic Press.

Walsh, R. (2011, January 17). Lifestyle and mental health. *American Psychologist.* Advance online publication. doi: 10.1037/a0021769.

Walters, G. (2009). Anger management training in incarcerated male offenders: Differential impact on proactive and reactive criminal thinking. *The International Journal of Forensic Mental Health, 8,* 214–217.

Wang, H. X., Leineweber, C., Krikeeide, R., Svane, B., Schenck-Gustafsson, K., Theorell, T., & Orth-Gomer, K. (2007). Psychosocial stress and atherosclerosis: Family and work stress accelerate progression of coronary disease in women. The Stockholm Female Coronary Angiography Study. *Journal of Internal Medicine, 261,* 245–254.

Warburton, D. E. R., Charlesworth, S., Ivey, A., Nettlefold, L., & Bredin, S. S. D. (2010). A systematic review of the evidence for Canada's physical activity guidelines for adults. *International Journal of Behavioral Nutrition and Physical Activity, 7,* 1–220.

Ward, M. M., Mefford, I. N., Parker, S. D., Chesney, M. A., Taylor, C. B., Keegen, D. L., & Barchas, J. D. (1983). Epinephrine and norepinephrine responses in continuously collected human plasma to a series of stressors. *Psychosomatic Medicine, 45,* 471–486.

Warr, P. (2005). Work, well-being, and mental health. In J. Barling, E. K. Kelloway, & M. R. Frone (Eds.), *Handbook of work stress* (pp. 547–573). Thousand Oaks, CA: Sage.

Watkins, P. C., Van Gelder, M., & Frias, A. (2009). Furthering the science of gratitude. In S. J. Lopez & C. R. Snyder (Eds.), *Handbook of positive psychology* (2nd ed., pp. 437–445). New York: Oxford University Press.

Watson, D., & Naragon, K. (2009). Positive affectivity: The disposition to experience positive emotional states. In S. J. Lopez & C. R. Snyder (Eds.), *Oxford handbook of positive psychology* (2nd ed., pp. 207–215). New York: Oxford University Press.

Watten, R. G., Syversen, J. F., & Myhrer, T. (1995). Quality of life, intelligence, and mood. *Social Indicators Research, 36,* 287–299.

Weiss, A., & Costa, P. T., Jr. (2005). Domain and facet personality predictors of all-cause mortality among Medicare patients aged 65 to 100. *Psychosomatic Medicine, 67,* 724–733.

Weissman, M. M., & Olfson, M. (1995). Depression in women: Implications for health care research. *Science, 269,* 799–801.

Wenger, M. A., & Bagchi, B. K. (1961). Studies of autonomic functions in practitioners of yoga in India. *Behavioral Science, 6,* 312–323.

Whaley, M. H., Kaminsky, L. A., Dwyer, G. B., Getchell, L. H., & Norton, J. A. (1992). Predictors of over- and under-achievement of age-predicted maximal heart rate. *Medicine & Science in Sports & Exercise, 24,* 1173–1179.

White, C., Kolble, R., Carlson, R., & Lipson, N. (2005). The impact of a health campaign on hand hygiene and upper respiratory illness among college students living in residence halls. *Journal of American College Health, 53,* 175–181.

Wichianson, J. R., Bughi, S. A., Unger, J. B., Spruijt-Metz, D., & Nguyen-Rodriguez, S. T. (2009). Perceived stress, coping and night-eating in college students. *Stress and Health, 25,* 235–240.

Wiener, H. (1977). *Psychobiology and human disease.* New York: Elsevier.

Wilbert-Lampen, U., Leistner, D., Greven, S., Pohl, T., Sper, S., Volker, C., . . . Stenbeck, G. (2008). Cardiovascular events during World Cup soccer. *The New England Journal of Medicine, 358,* 475–485.

Wilde, B. E., Sidman, C. L., & Corbin, C. B. (2001). A 10,000 step count as a physical activity target for sedentary women. *Research Quarterly for Exercise & Sport, 72,* 411–414.

Willenbring, M. L., Levine, A. S., & Morely, J. E. (1986). Stress induced eating and food preference in humans: A pilot study. *International Journal of Eating Disorders, 5,* 855–864.

Willett, W. C. (2007). The role of dietary n-6 fatty acids in the prevention of cardiovascular disease. *Journal of Cardiovascular Medicine, 8,* S42–S45.

Williams, J. E., Nieto, F. J., Sanford, C. P., Couper, D. J., & Tyroler, H. A. (2002). The association between trait anger and incident stroke risk: The Atherosclerosis Risk in Communities (ARIC) Study. *Stroke, 33,* 13–19.

Williams, R. B., Haney, T. L., Kerry, L. L., Kong, Y-H., Blumenthal, J. A., & Whalen, R. E. (1980). Type

A behavior, hostility, and coronary atherosclerosis. *Psychosomatic Medicine, 42,* 539–549.

Wilson, R. S., Krueger, K. R., Gu, L., Bienias, J. L., De Leon, C. F. M., & Evans, D. A. (2005). Neuroticism, extraversion, and mortality in a defined population of older persons. *Psychosomatic Medicine, 67,* 841–845.

Wipfli, B. M., Rethorst, C. D., & Landers, D. M. (2008). The anxiolytic effects of exercise: A meta-analysis of randomized trials and dose-response analysis. *Journal of Sport & Exercise Psychology, 30,* 392–410.

Witter, R. A., Okun, M. A, Stock, W. A., & Haring, M. J. (1984). Education and subjective well-being: A meta-analysis. *Education Evaluation and Policy Analysis, 6,* 165–173.

Witvliet, C. v. O., Ludwig, T. E., & Vander Laan, K. L. (2001). Granting forgiveness or harboring grudges: Implications for emotion, physiology, and health. *Psychological Science, 12,* 117–123.

Wolitzky-Taylor, K. B., Horowitz, J. D., Powers, M. B., & Telch, M. J. (2008). Psychological approaches in the treatment of specific phobias: A meta-analysis. *Clinical Psychology Review, 28,* 1021–1037.

Wolpe, J. (1958). *Psychotherapy by reciprocal inhibition.* Stanford, CA: Stanford University Press.

Wood, A. M., Joseph, S., & Maltby, J. (2008). Gratitude uniquely predicts satisfaction with life: Incremental validity above the domains and facets of the five factor model. *Personality and Individual Differences, 45,* 49–54.

Woods-Giscombe, C, L., & Lobel, M. (2008). Race and gender matter: A multidimensional approach to conceptualizing and measuring stress in African American women. *Cultural Diversity and Ethnic Minority Psychology, 14,* 173–182.

World Health Organization. (2011). *WHO definition of health.* Retrieved from http://www.who.int/about/definition/en/print.html.

Wright, J. D., Hirsch, R., & Wang, C.-Y. (2009). One-third of U.S. adults embraced most heart healthy behaviors in 1999–2002. *NCHS data brief, 17.* Hyattsville, MD: National Center for Health Statistics. Retrieved from http://www.cdc.gov/nchs/data/databriefs/db17.htm.

Yalom, I. D. (1980). *Existential psychotherapy.* New York: Basic Books.

Yates, L. B., Djousse, L., Kurth, T., Buring, J. E., & Gaziano, J. M. (2008). Exceptional longevity in men: Modifiable factors associated with survival and function to age 90 years. *Archives of Internal Medicine, 168,* 284–290.

Yerkes, R. M., & Dodson, J. D. (1908). The relation of strength of stimulus to rapidity of habit formation. *Journal of Comparative and Neurological Psychology, 18,* 459–482.

Young, J. E., Beck, A. T., & Weinberger, A. (1993). Depression. In D. H. Barlow (Ed.), *Clinical handbook of psychological disorders: A step-by-step treatment manual* (2nd ed., pp. 240–277). New York: The Guilford Press.

Yu, X., Bao, Z., Zou, J., & Dong, J. (2011). Coffee consumption and risk of cancers: A meta-analysis of cohort studies. *BMC Cancer, 11,* 96. Retrieved from http://www.biomedcentral.com/1471-2407/11/96.

Yusuf, S., Hawken, S., Ounpuu, S., Bautista, L., Fanzosi, M. G., Commerford, P., . . . Anand, S. S. (2005). Obesity and the risk of myocardial infarction in 27000 participants from 52 countries: A case-control study. *Lancet, 366,* 1640–1649.

Yusuf, S., Hawken, S., Ounpuu, S., Dans, T., Avenzum, A. Lanas, F., . . . Lisheng, L. (2004). Effect of potentially modifiable risk factors associated with myocardial infarction in 52 countries (the INTERHEART study): Case-control study. *Lancet, 364,* 937–952.

Zabora, J., BrintzenhofeSzoc, K., Curbow, B., & Hooker, C. (2001). The prevalence of psychological distress by cancer site. *Psychooncology, 10,* 19–28.

Zautra, A. J., Reich, J. W., & Guarnaccia, C. (1990). Some everyday life consequences of disability and bereavement for older adults. *Journal of Personality and Social Psychology, 59,* 350–361.

Zautra, A. J., Sheets, V. L., & Sandler, I. N. (1996). An examination of the construct validity of coping dispositions for a sample of recently divorced mothers. *Psychological Assessment, 8,* 256–264.

Zohar, J., & Westenberg, H. G. (2000). Anxiety disorders: A review of tricyclic antidepressants and selective serotonin reuptake inhibitors. *Acta Psychiatrica Scandinavica, Supplementum, 403,* 39–49.

Zorrilla, E. P., Luborsky, L., McKay, J. R., Rosenthal, R., Houldin, A., Tax, A., . . . Schmidt, K. (2001). The relationship of depression and stressors to immunological assays: A meta-analytic review. *Brain, Behavior, and Immunity, 15,* 199–226.